Advanced Polymers in Medicine

Francesco Puoci
Editor

Advanced Polymers in Medicine

Springer

Editor
Francesco Puoci
Department of Pharmacy,
Health and Nutritional Sciences
University of Calabria
Rende
Italy

ISBN 978-3-319-12477-3 ISBN 978-3-319-12478-0 (eBook)
DOI 10.1007/978-3-319-12478-0

Library of Congress Control Number: 2014956571

Springer Cham Heidelberg New York Dordrecht London

Printed on acid-free paper

Springer International Publishing AG Switzerland is part of Springer Science+Business Media (www.springer.com)

Preface

Life is a perfect equilibrium between mind and body. It is a whole of different variables that, during our life we have to set up. In this challenge the safe maintenance of the human body represents one of our most important goal. In this sense, science and technology play a key role in the extended life expectancy. In the last century and especially in the last years, the medical area, in order to afford the new challenge in health care, was subject to necessary and deep changes (improvements), thanks also to a cross-fertilization of several disciplines.

Surgery, for example, has developed with a wide range of innovative techniques and new devices (implants and surgical instruments) resulting in a reduction of morbidity and mortality.

The use of drug delivery systems to improve the efficacy of bioactive molecules remains an important strategy for achieving progress against the disease and progress in this field has been remarkable. Over the past 20 years, the number of novel therapeutic approaches has expanded from traditional small chemical medicinals to a wide variety of biomolecules, including peptide/protein- and nucleic acid-based therapeutics. All of these therapies require the administration of stable dosage forms in adequate concentrations and exposure periods with the aim to realize their potential.

At the same time new medical categories are widely expanded: tissue engineering has made great strides in the replacement of worn out organs and tissues due to disease, injury, etc. in order to have real efficiency and efficacy, medical therapy needs efficient and effective biomaterials both for intra and extracorporeal treatments.

Biomaterials and in particular polymeric ones are the focus of this scientific revolution and represent one of the major researches around the world.

One of the reasons for the great popularity in the use of polymers in medicine is that their properties can be tailored to meet specific needs by varying the “atomic composition” of the repeat structure, molecular weight, or performing chemical modifications of natural polymers.

The rationale of this contributed book stems from the premise to have an important instrument that can be a knowledge bridge between teaching experience and scientific research.

This idea represents a true answer to the natural question: What is the novelty in *Advanced Polymers in Medicine*? The first part of the book reviews the relevant background information on polymer chemistry and the physicochemical characterization and represents the scientific support for the following chapters. The second part is devoted to a complete overview of "Medically" oriented polymers and every chapter is dedicated to a medical specialty. In my opinion, this type of approach will provide a better overview of polymers and medical applications and allows an effective use both for teaching that scientific reference book. Therefore, this book is intended for students and researchers who work in the area of biomaterials. I am conscious that a successful book is a product of several integrated expertises; in this contributed volume, many of these were given by contributing authors, all of which are listed in the bibliography. Thank you!

Francesco Puoci

Contents

Chapter 1
Polymer Chemistry and Synthetic Polymers

Ortensia Ilaria Parisi, Manuela Curcio and Francesco Puoci

Abstract Polymers are macromolecules derived by the combination of one or more chemical units (monomers) that repeat themselves along the molecule. The IUPAC Gold Book defines a polymer as "A molecule of high relative molecular mass, the structure of which essentially comprises the multiple repetition of units derived, actually or conceptually, from molecules of low relative molecular mass." Several ways of classification can be adopted depending on: their source (natural and synthetic), their structure (linear, branched and crosslinked), the polymerization mechanism (step-growth and chain polymers) and molecular forces (Elastomers, fibres, thermoplastic and thermosetting polymers). In this chapter, the molecular mechanisms and kinetic of polymer formation reactions were explored and particular attention was devoted to the main polymerization techniques. Finally, an overview of the most employed synthetic materials in biomedical field is performed.

Keywords Step-growth polymerization · Chain polymerization · Homogeneous polymerization · Heterogeneous polymerization · Biomedical applications

---

O.I. Parisi (✉) · M. Curcio · F. Puoci
Department of Pharmacy, Health and Nutritional Sciences,
University of Calabria, 87036 Rende, CS, Italy
e-mail: ortensiailaria.parisi@unical.it

O.I. Parisi
Department of Informatics, Modeling, Electronics and Systems Engineering,
University of Calabria, 87036 Rende, CS, Italy

F. Puoci (ed.), *Advanced Polymers in Medicine*, DOI 10.1007/978-3-319-12478-0_1

Abbreviations

AIBN	Azobisisobutyronitrile
ATRP	Atom transfer radical polymerization
HDI	Hexamethylene diisocyanate
HDPE	High density polyethylene
i-PP	Isotactic polypropylene
LDPE	Low density polyethylene
MDI	4,4′-methylenediphenyl diisocyanate
MDPE	Medium-density polyethylene
PCL	Poly(caprolactone)
PE	Polyethylene
PGA	Polyglycolide
PLA	Polylactide
PLGA	Poly(lactide-co-glycolide)
PPC	Poly(propylene carbonate)
PTMC	Poly(trimethylene carbonate)
PTMO	Poly(tetramethylene oxide)
PVC	Polyvinyl chloride
RAFT	Reversible addition-fragmentation chain transfer polymerization
TDI	Toluene diisocyanate
UHMWPE	Ultra high molecular weight polyethylene

Introduction

Polymers are macromolecules characterized by high relative molecular mass and formed by linking large numbers of small molecules together. They essentially consist of repeating chemical units which are held by covalent bonds and derived, actually or conceptually, from molecules of low relative molecular mass called monomers. Thus, the term *monomer* refers to the small starting molecule from which a polymer is constructed and has not to be confused with the *repeat unit*. This last one represents, indeed, the basic structural unit whose repetition would produce the complete polymeric chain, except for the end-groups.

The length of the polymer chain is specified by the number of repeat units in the main chains and this number is called *degree of polymerization* $\overline{X_n}$.

A monomer must have one or more reactive sites to form bonds with other monomers in order to prepare a polymer and may or may not be equivalent to the repeat unit. The small monomeric units are, indeed, connected to each other through the chemical reactions and the chemical process used for the synthesis of polymers is called the *polymerization*.

The simplest example of polymer is represented by PE which is obtained from its monomer ethylene (Fig. 1.1).

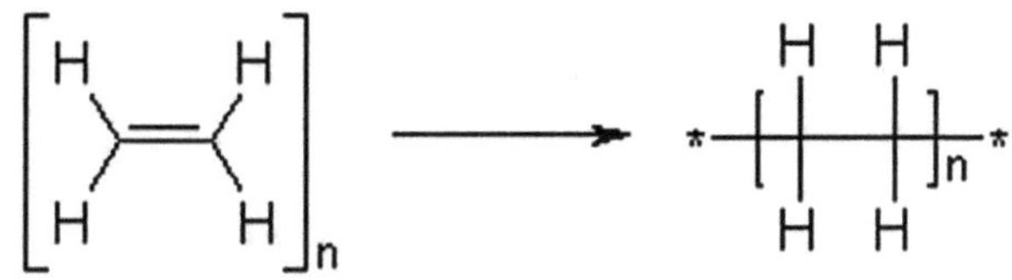

Fig. 1.1 Synthesis of polyethylene starting from ethylene monomer

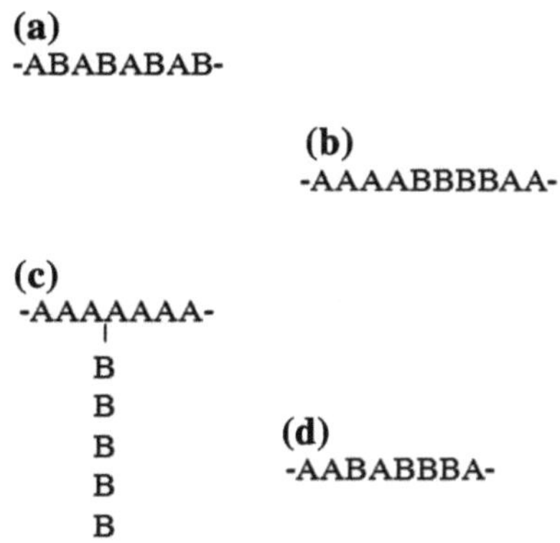

Fig. 1.2 Schematic structures of: **a** alternating copolymers, **b** block copolymers, **c** graft copolymers and **d** random copolymers

The molecular structure of polyethylene chain contains connected tetrahedral sp^3 hybridized C atoms and it can be viewed as an extension of the covalently bound molecule ethane. Thus, in this case, the chemical structure of the repeat unit is different from the structure of ethylene monomer from which the polymer is produced.

Several ways of *classifying polymers* can be adopted depending on different parameters, such as the type of monomer, the source, the structure, the polymerization mechanism, the molecular forces and tacticity (the way pendent groups are arranged on a polymeric backbone).

- *Type of Monomer*
  - *Homopolymers,* polymers formed from only a single type of monomer;
  - *Copolymers,* polymers prepared from more than one type of monomers which can be further divided according to the arrangements of the different repeat units in the chain (Fig. 1.2):

    alternating copolymers: the repeat units of two different monomers are arranged in alternating sequence within the chain;

    block copolymers: in these polymers, two or more long linear sequences of different homopolymers (blocks) are linked together;

    graft copolymers: they are branched block copolymers in which the backbone is one type of block and the other type of blocks are attached to the main chain as pendant groups;

    random copolymers: they consist of two or more different repeat units attached in a random order.

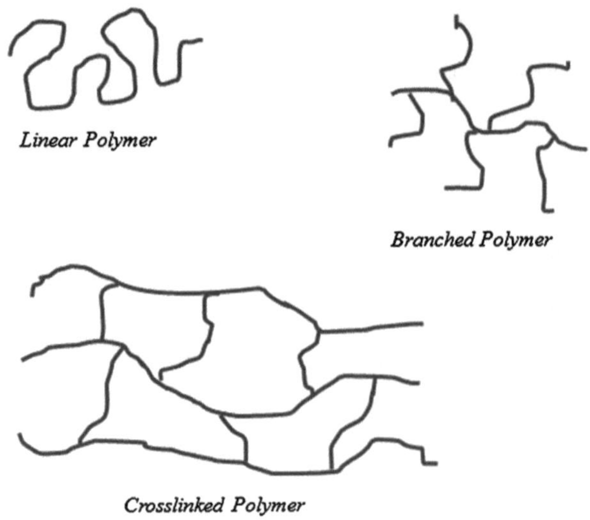

Fig. 1.3 Macromolecule structures

- *The Source*
  - *Natural polymers*: occur in plants and animals, in which play an essential role for life, and include starch, cellulose, silk, chitin, proteins, nucleic acids and natural rubber;
  - *Synthetic polymers*: are artificially synthesized in the laboratory and they can be defined as "man-made polymers". In daily life, this kind of macromolecules finds several applications in a wide range of fields, such as cosmetics, pharmaceutics, medicine, packaging, food processing, textile. Examples include polyethylene, polystyrene, PVC, nylon and polyurethanes;
  - *Semi-synthetic polymers*: these are mostly derived from naturally occurring polymers by chemical modifications. An example is cellulose acetate, a derivative of cellulose which forms due to acetylation of cellulose and used for making threads, films and glasses.
- *The Chain Structure*
  - *Linear polymers*: repeat units are joined together in the form of a single long straight chain (Fig. 1.3). The starting monomers have only two functional groups if the polymer is a step-growth polymer or a single double bond if it is a chain polymer. Examples are polythene, polyvinyl chloride, etc.;
  - *Branched polymers*: linear side chains get branches of different length along the main chain (Fig. 1.3). Branches are caused by the presence of small amounts of trifunctional monomers for step-growth or two unsaturations for chain polymers;
  - *Crosslinked polymers*: three-dimensional networks consisting of long linear chains connected to each other with multifunctional units (Fig. 1.3). The interconnections between chains can be formed during the polymerization process (by choice of a crosslinking agent) or after polymerization (by adding a specific reagent).

- *The Molecular Forces*
  - *Elastomers*: they are amorphous polymers with high degree of elasticity and characterized by weak attraction forces between polymeric chains. An elastomer should be flexible and able to return to its original dimensions;
  - *Fibres*: they have strong intermolecular attraction forces between polymeric chains, high tensile strength, least elasticity, good pliability and are able to hold their shape;
  - *Thermoplastics*: they are characterized by intermediate intermolecular force of attraction between molecules. Linear and slightly branched chains become soft when the temperature is increased, but again gets rigidness after cooling, thus they can be safely processed by melting. These polymeric materials, indeed, can be reshaped with further application of heat and pressure because no changes in the chemical composition and no bond formation occur during heating and cooling processes. Some examples of thermoplastics include polythene, polyvinyl chloride, Teflon, polystyrene;
  - *Thermoset polymers*: unlike thermoplastics, they can not be melted and reshaped with the application of heat due to crosslinking reactions which take place during heating. Therefore, heating must be the last stage of processing due to irreversible changes in the chemical composition. Examples are Bakelite and urea-formaldehyde resin.
- *The Molecular Weight*
  - *Oligomers*: molecules consisting of a few repeat units and characterized by a molecular weight ranged from 500 to 5,000 g mol^{-1}. Dimers, trimers, and tetramers are oligomers composed of two, three and four monomers, respectively;
  - *High polymers*: have a molecular weight in the range of 10^4–10^6 g mol^{-1}.
- *The Polymerization Mechanism*
  - *Step-growth polymers*: polymers that differ from their monomer(s) and are formed when two di- or polyfunctional molecules react and condense producing macromolecules with the elimination of a small molecule, such as water or alcohols (polyamides and polyesters);
  - *Chain polymers*: produced by chain reactions of double-bonded monomers in which the chain carrier can be a radical or an ion.
- *Tacticity*
  - *Atactic polymers*: pendant groups are arranged randomly;
  - *Syndiotactic polymers*: pendant groups are arranged alternately;
  - *Isotactic polymers*: pendant groups are arranged on the same side of the polymer backbone.

On the basis of the reaction mechanisms, polymerizations can be classified into *step-growth* and *chain polymerization*. In the first case, the polymerization mechanism involves a series of chemical condensation reactions between monomers with functional groups leading to the elimination of small molecules (water, alcohol, hydrogen). In chain polymerization, monomeric units incorporating double chemical bond are rapidly added to the reactive sites onto the growing polymeric chain. This reaction mechanism requires an initiator which forms the first active unit.

The present book chapter aims to explore the molecular mechanisms and kinetics of polymer formation reactions with a particular attention devoted to the main polymerization techniques which can be included into two main groups, such as *homogeneous polymerization systems* and *heterogeneous polymerization systems*.

Nowadays, several types of synthetic polymers or copolymers are produced in the laboratories and these macromolecules can find applications in every branch of medicine, thus, the most employed synthetic materials in biomedical field were also reviewed.

Mechanisms of Polymer Synthesis

The mechanisms of polymer synthesis reactions can be classified into two main categories: step-growth and chain polymerization.

Step-growth polymerization occurs when monomers bond together through an extension of normal organic condensation reactions in which side products, characterized by low molar weight such as water or alcohol, are eliminated as the link is formed. These reactions can be achieved through reacting molecules incorporating functional groups including carboxylic acid, carboxyl derivative, alcohol or amine. Therefore, step-growth polymers can be degraded to their starting monomers upon the addition of the eliminated small molecules.

On the other hand, *chain polymerization* involves the linking of unsaturated monomers by the opening of the π double bond. The monomeric units are added to the reactive sites onto the growing polymeric chain consisting of an all-carbon backbone of single σ bonds. This reaction mechanism requires an initiator able to generate the first active unit and start the chain growth. Chain polymerization is involved in the production of a large share of the most employed synthetic polymers including polyethene, polypropylene, polystyrene and PVC.

Step-growth Polymerization

Kinetics of Step-growth Polymerization

Polyesters are formed by typical condensation reactions involving the elimination of water and an example of polyester synthesis from a diol and a diacid is reported as follows:

$$\mathrm{HO{-}R{-}OH + HOOC{-}R'{-}COOH \rightarrow HO{-}R{-}OCO{-}R'{-}COOH + H_2O}$$

The obtained dimer might form a trimer, by reaction with a diol monomer or with a diacid monomer, but it could also react with itself to form a tetramer. Then, the tetramer and trimer proceed to react with themselves, with each other, with the monomer and the dimer [1].

The rate of a step-growth polymerization is the sum of the rates of reactions which take place between molecules of different size, therefore, in this case the kinetics is difficult to analyze. However, the kinetics of step-growth polymerization can be considered identical to those of analogous small molecule reaction and can be expressed as follows:

$$\begin{aligned} &-\mathrm{A} + \mathrm{B}- + \text{catalyst} \rightarrow -\mathrm{AB}- + \text{catalyst} \\ &R = K[A][B]\left[catalyst\right] \end{aligned} \quad (1.1)$$

If the reaction is acid-catalyzed (catalyst = H^+) and if stoichiometry of the groups A and B is assumed, the previous Eq. (1.1) becomes:

$$R = -\frac{d[A]}{dt} = K\left[H^+\right][A]^2 \quad (1.2)$$

Mechanisms of Step-growth Polymerization

In a step-growth polymerization, the monomers polymerize following different reaction mechanisms, such as carbonyl addition-elimination, carbonyl addition-substitution, nucleophilic substitution, double bond addition or free radical coupling [2].

Carbonyl addition-elimination represents the most important reaction employed for the synthesis of polymeric molecules including polyamides, polyacetals, phenol–, urea–, and melamine–formaldehyde polymers. Carbonyl addition-elimination includes:

- the direct reaction of a dibasic acid and a glycol (to form a polyester) or a dibasic acid and a diamine (to form a polyamide);
- interchange (the reaction between a glycol and an ester);
- the reaction of acid chloride or anhydride with a glycol or an amine;
- interfacial condensation (the reaction of an acid halide with a glycol or a diamine proceeds rapidly to high molecular weight polymer if carried out at the interface between two immiscible liquid phases each containing one of the reactants);
- ring versus chain formation (bifunctional monomers react intramolecularly to produce a cyclic product).

The other step-growth mechanisms include [3]:

- *Carbonyl addition-substitution reactions*: the reaction of aldehydes with alcohols involving addition followed by substitution at the carbonyl group leading to the formation of polyacetals;
- *Nucleophilic substitution reactions*: the reaction of an electron pair donor (the nucleophile) with an electron pair acceptor (the electrophile);
- *Free radical coupling*: for the synthesis of polymers containing acetylene units and arylenealkylidene polymers.

Chain Polymerization

In *chain polymerization*, monomeric units incorporating double bond are rapidly added to the reactive sites onto the growing polymeric chain.

Three main categories of chain polymerization mechanisms can be considered:

- free radical polymerization;
- ionic polymerization, which can be further divided into cationic and anionic;
- coordination polymerization.

In general, all these types of polymerization reactions are characterized by three main steps including:

- an *initiation stage*, in which a reactive species is generated and attacks the first monomer molecule;
- a *propagation stage*, in which a large number of monomers are added to the growing polymer chain retaining the active end-group;
- a *termination stage*, in which the reactive end-site is deactivated.

Free Radical Polymerization

In *free radical polymerization* the monomer double bond opens homolytically, the initiator is a radical and the propagating reactive site is a carbon radical.

Free radicals are species containing unpaired electrons that are highly reactive and undergo reactions to extract an electron from another substrate. In this kind of polymerization, each polymer chain grows by addition of monomer to the free radical of the growing chain and, upon addition of the monomer, the radical is transferred to the new chain end.

Free radical polymerization consists of three stages, such as initiation, propagation and termination.

In the initiation stage, free radicals are produced from an initiator molecule and, then, react with the monomer. Initiators can decompose due to the application of heat or electromagnetic radiations (e.g., UV) and can be divided into two main classes, including peroxides and hydroperoxides and azo compounds, in which radicals are generated by the scission of a single bond or by an electron transfer to or from an ion or molecule during a redox reaction. *Peroxides* and *hydroperoxides* are frequently used as initiators because of the instability of the O–O bond. An example of organic peroxide is represented by benzoyl peroxide which decomposes on heating; at 100 °C, indeed, it has a half-life of 30 min. On the contrary, potassium persulphate $K_2S_2O_8$ is an inorganic peroxide and, thus, water-soluble. In the case of *azo compounds*, the process is driven by the release of N_2. The most common employed *azo compound* is AIBN (Fig. 1.4) which decomposes at relatively low temperatures (60 °C) and also at room temperature by irradiating with ultraviolet light (360 nm).

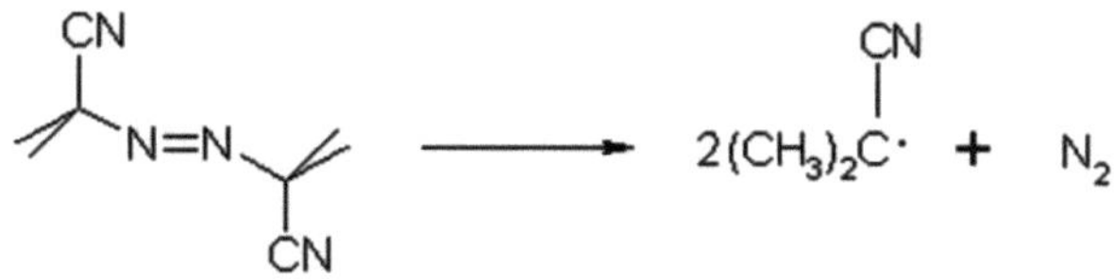

Fig. 1.4 Chemical structure of AIBN and its decomposition

The *initiation step* involves the dissociation of an initiator (I) with the formation of two radicals (R·) with a dissociation rate constant k_d:

$$I \overset{K_d}{\rightarrow} 2R\cdot \tag{1.3}$$

This radical then reacts with the monomer molecule to generate the first activated monomer (RM·):

$$R\cdot + M \overset{K_i}{\rightarrow} RM\cdot \tag{1.4}$$

where k_i is the rate constant of initiation.

During the *propagation step,* the formed activated monomer (RM·) immediately reacts with more monomer molecules leading to growing macroradicals. In the polymerization mechanism, it is assumed that all growing chains have the same propagation constant (k_p) and for most monomers it is in the range of 10^2–10^4 L mol^{-1} s^{-1}:

$$RM_n\cdot + M \overset{K_p}{\rightarrow} RM_{n+1}\cdot \tag{1.5}$$

Termination stage consists of the deactivation of the growth process occurs by combination or disproportionation reactions. Combination is coupling of two radical species to produce a single "dead" polymer molecule:

$$RM_n\cdot + RM_m\cdot \overset{K_{tc}}{\rightarrow} RM_{n+m} \tag{1.6}$$

where k_{tc} is the rate constant for termination by combination.

In disproportionation reaction, a hydrogen atom is abstracted and exchanged between the growing chains leaving behind two terminated chains and producing one deactivated polymer molecule with a saturated end-group and another one with a double bond as end-group:

$$RM_n\cdot + RM_m\cdot \overset{K_{td}}{\rightarrow} RM_n + RM_m \tag{1.7}$$

where k_{td} is the rate constant for termination by disproportionation.

Kinetics of Free Radical Polymerization

In radical polymerization reactions, the initiator decomposition proceeds more slowly than the reaction of the free radical with the monomer molecule. Therefore, this is the rate-determining step.

The *rate of initiation (R_i)* is expressed by the following Eq. (1.8):

$$R_i = -\left(\frac{d[I]}{dt}\right) = \left(\frac{d[R\cdot]}{dt}\right) = 2fK_i[I] \tag{1.8}$$

where f represents the initiator efficiency that indicates the fraction of the radicals successful in initiating chains (0 < f < 1), k_d is the rate constant for initiator dissociation, [I] is the concentration of the initiator and the constant 2 defines that two radicals are formed from one initiator molecule. The initiator efficiency decreases when side reactions terminates the radicals [4].

In the propagation step, the rate of monomer loss can be equated to the *rate of propagation (R_p)* which is represented by the Eq. (1.9):

$$R_p = -\left(\frac{d[M]}{dt}\right) = K_p[R\cdot][M] \tag{1.9}$$

Finally, the *rate of termination (R_t)* is represented as:

$$R_t = -\left(\frac{dRM\cdot}{dt}\right) = 2K_t[RM\cdot]^2 \tag{1.10}$$

where k_t is the overall rate constant for termination and the factor 2 comes from the fact that the two growing chains are terminated by each termination reaction.

At the start of the polymerization, the rate of formation of radicals exceeds the rate of loss of radicals by termination. As the reaction proceeds, the rate of initiation becomes equal to the rate of termination ($R_i = R_t$) leading to the "Steady State":

$$[M\cdot] = \left(\frac{fK_i[I]}{K_t}\right)^{1/2} \tag{1.11}$$

Degree of Polymerization

The *degree of polymerization* ($\overline{X_n}$) is defined as the average number of monomer molecules added to the polymer molecule.

Kinetic chain length ν is defined as the number of monomer molecules used per active center and it is represented as $R_p/R_i = R_p/R_t$ [3]:

$$\nu = \frac{K_p[M]}{2K_t[M\cdot]} \tag{1.12}$$

If the propagating radicals terminate by combination $\overline{X_n} = 2\nu$, while if termination involves a disproportionation $\overline{X_n} = \nu$.

Ionic Polymerization

Chain polymerization of monomers containing double bond can also be achieved with growing centers which can be negatively (anionic) or positively (cationic) charged.

Due to the ionic charge of the active center, these ionic polymerizations are more selective than free radical polymerization in which termination occurs by combination or disproportionation. Initiation stage, indeed, depends on the presence of appropriate substituent groups on the monomer molecule able to stabilize the active center, and on their inductive or resonance characteristics. For cationic active centers, electron-donating substituents (D), including alkoxy, alkyl or phenyl, are needed because they increase the electron density on double bond facilitating the linking to cationic species. On the other hand, electron-withdrawing substituents (W), such as cyano and carbonyl, stabilize the negative charge in anionic polymerization.

Radical species are neutral while in ionic polymerization charged species are involved; therefore, the type of solvent is of significant importance. High dielectric solvents, indeed, allow to completely separate the ions which are less sterically hindered and, thus, able to react and propagate faster than ion pairs.

Since the required activation energy for ionic polymerization is small, these reactions may occur at very low temperatures.

Another difference between radical and ionic polymerizations is that in the last one the termination step does not occur by a reaction between two ionic active centers because they are of similar charge [5].

Cationic Polymerization

In cationic polymerization typical catalysts are represented by strong electron acceptors including Lewis acids, Friedel-Crafts halides, Brönsted acids and stable carbenium-ion salts. However, many of them are not sufficient to initiate the polymerization and, therefore, require small amounts of a co-catalyst, usually a proton donor such as alcohols.

In Fig. 1.5 the mechanism of cationic polymerization is shown.

The propagation stage is usually very fast and, therefore, polymerizations are in solution at low temperature ranged from −80 to −100 °C. The employed solvent is important because it affects the activity of the ion at the end of the growing polymeric chain.

Regarding the termination step, chain transfer to a monomer, polymer, solvent or counterion can terminate the growth of chains. If X^+ is not loss and rejoins the anion to reform the acid catalyst, the termination is called "transfer to counterion"; if X^+ initiates another monomer molecule to start a new chain, termination is defined as "transfer to monomer" [6]. When a distinct termination reaction does not occur, "living" cationic polymers are obtained.

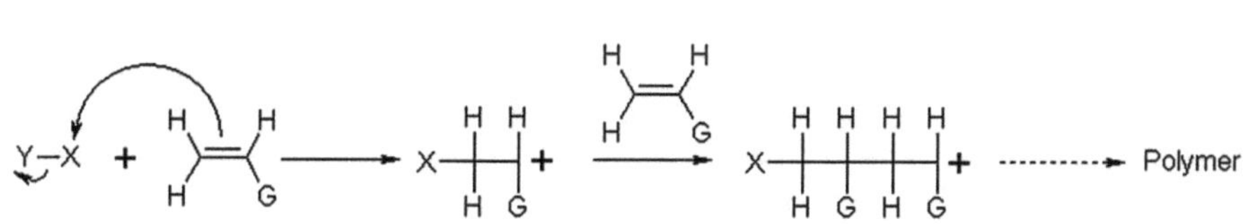

Fig. 1.5 Mechanism of cationic polymerization

Kinetics of Cationic Polymerization

The generation of active species can be described as follows:

$$AX + BH \rightarrow \left[H^{+}\right] + [BAX]^{-}$$

while, the attack of the first monomer molecule is reported as follows:

$$\left[H^{+}\right] + M \rightarrow \left[MH^{+}\right]$$

where AX is the Lewis acid, BH is the Lewis base and M is the monomer.

The propagation step consists of the sequential addition of monomers to the active complex [MH^{+}]:

$$[MH]^{+} + M \rightarrow [M_2H]^{+} \quad \text{or} \quad [M_n]^{+} + M \rightarrow \left[M_{n+1}\right]$$

The kinetics of the propagation stage depends on the strength of the acid and the dielectric constant of the solvent. Indeed, the rate of the process is faster as stronger is the acid and higher is the dielectric constant that means more ions and a larger separation of the ions, respectively.

Kinetics of isobutene initiated by BF_3/H_2O system can be expressed as follows:

$$\textit{Initiation}: \quad R_i = K_i[M][C] \tag{1.13}$$

where C represents the catalyst/co-catalyst system.

$$\textit{Propagation}: \quad R_p = \left[MH^{+}\right][M] \tag{1.14}$$

$$\textit{Termination by rearrangement}: \quad R_t = K_t\left[MH^{+}\right] \tag{1.15}$$

$$\textit{Termination by transfer monomer}: \quad R_{tr} = K_{tr}\left[MH^{+}\right][M] \tag{1.16}$$

Therefore, for both the termination processes, the dependence of rate and molar mass on the initial concentration of initiator and starting monomer are less complex than those of radical polymerization.

Anionic Polymerization

Monomers susceptible to this type of polymerization should be characterized by the presence of an electron-withdrawing group (W) able to stabilize the carbanion (Fig. 1.6).

The reaction is initiated by strong nucleophiles and the most employed anionic initiators include Grignard reagents and other organometallic compounds, such as

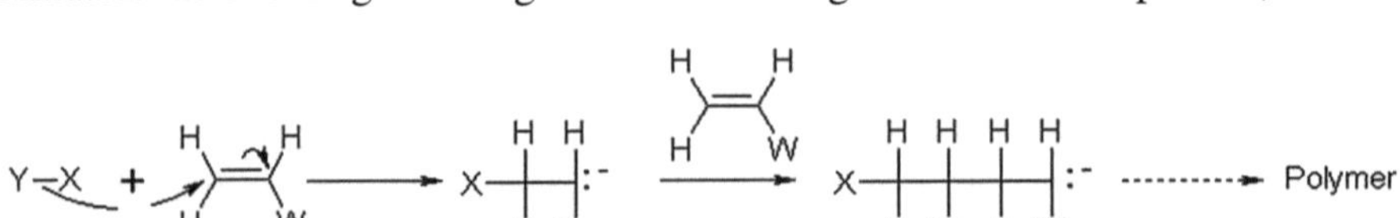

Fig. 1.6 Mechanism of anionic polymerization

organolithium compounds which are air-sensitive, soluble in hydrocarbon solvent and very reactive towards molecules with labile protons.

In particular reaction conditions, characterized by a rigorous exclusion of starting reagents impurities, oxygen and water, the polymeric backbone chain can grow until all the monomer is disappeared, therefore, no termination or chain transfer occur. For this reason, anionic polymerization is sometimes called "living" polymerization and termination takes place only by the deliberate introduction of oxygen, carbon dioxide, methanol or water. The absence of a termination step during a living polymerization leads to a very narrow molecular weight distribution [7].

Kinetics of Anionic Polymerization

The reaction between styrene and potassium amide (KNH_2) represents the first anionic polymerization studied. The kinetics of the three steps, initiation, propagation and termination, can be expressed by the following equations, respectively:

$$\text{Initiation:} \quad R_i = K_i\left[NH_2^-\right][M] \tag{1.17}$$

$$\text{Propagation:} \quad R_p = K_p[M]\left[M^-\right] \tag{1.18}$$

$$\text{Termination:} \quad R_{tr} = K_{tr}\left[M^-\right][NH_3] \tag{1.19}$$

The initiation step is followed by propagation and termination takes place by a transfer process involving the extraction of a proton from the solvent ammonia by the growing anion.

Coordination Polymerization

The use of special catalysts may lead to the formation of very orderly structured polymers characterized by high stereospecificity.

The polymerization processes used in the synthesis of both isotactic polypropylene (i-PP) and high density polyethylene (HDPE) involve the use of transition-metal catalysts called Ziegler-Natta catalysts, which utilize a coordination type mechanism reaction.

Ziegler-Natta catalysts are organometallic complexes prepared by reaction of an alkil of a metal from Groups I to III in the Periodic Table (e.g. $Al(C_2H_5)_3$) with a halide of transition metal from Groups IV to VIII (e.g., $TiCl_4$) which are dissolved in a hydrocarbon solvent, such as toluene or n-heptane, at room temperature. The possible reactions, which take place during the preparation of a coordination complex catalyst from $Al(C_2H_5)_3$ and $TiCl_4$, are reported in Fig. 1.7.

Several mechanisms for coordination polymerization were proposed and an early one was represented by the Natta's bimetallic mechanism, which is reported in Fig. 1.8.

This mechanism was replaced by Cossee's monometallic mechanism (Fig. 1.9): the Ti (III) species has a vacancy in its coordination sphere; the alkene molecule coordinates (in the first time) through the π bond, before reacting with the anionic

$$(C_2H_5)_3Al + TiCl_4 \longrightarrow (C_2H_5)_2AlCl + C_2H_5TiCl_3$$

$$C_2H_5TiCl_3 \longrightarrow {}^{\bullet}C_2H_5 + TiCl_3$$

$$(C_2H_5)_3Al + TiCl_3 \longrightarrow (C_2H_5)_2AlCl + C_2H_5TiCl_2$$

$$C_2H_5TiCl_2 \longrightarrow {}^{\bullet}C_2H_5 + TiCl_2$$

$$(C_2H_5)_3Al + C_2H_5TiCl_3 \longrightarrow (C_2H_5)_2AlCl + (C_2H_5)_2TiCl_2$$

$$(C_2H_5)_2TiCl_2 \longrightarrow {}^{\bullet}C_2H_5 + C_2H_5TiCl_2$$

Fig. 1.7 Preparation of Ziegler-Natta coordination complex

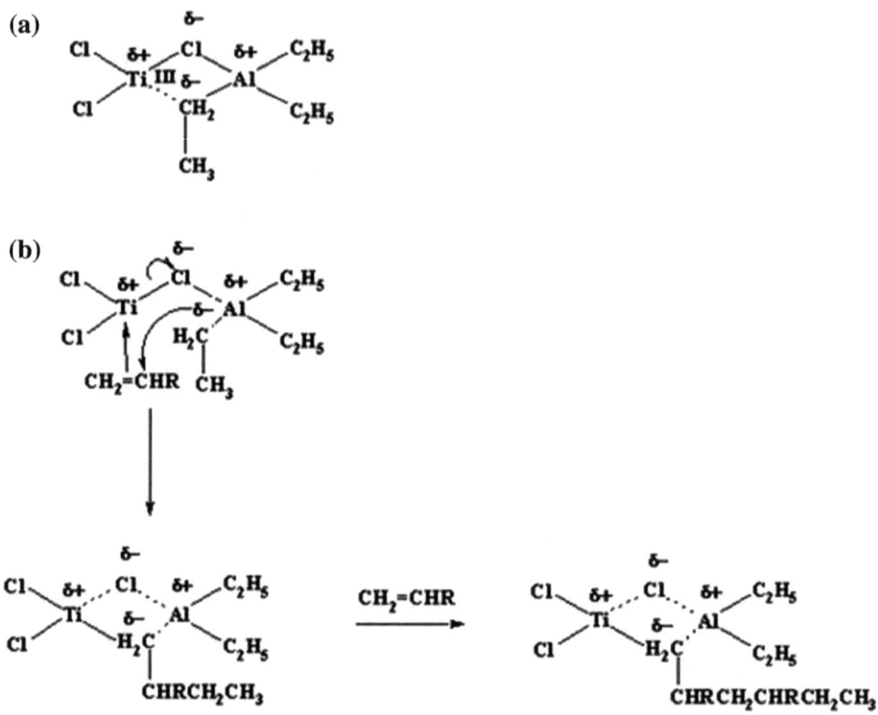

Fig. 1.8 Natta's bimetallic mechanism: **a** catalyst complex after initial exchange reactions before monomer ingress; **b** polymerization reaction mechanism

end of the alkyl unit, in order to get a σ bond with the Ti. The vacancy shifts and as the next monomer approaches for coordination, followed by addition to the chain, the vacancy flips again.

The coordination of the monomer leads to the stereospecificity of the synthesized polymeric material and this kind of polymerizations can be terminated by the introduction of water, hydrogen, aromatic alcohol or metals [7].

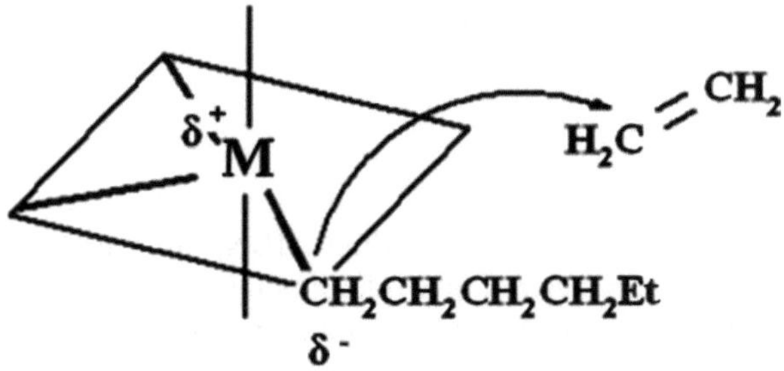

Fig. 1.9 Cossee's monometallic mechanism

Other Polymerization Mechanisms

Atom Transfer Radical Polymerization (ATRP)

Atom transfer radical polymerization is one of the most commonly employed techniques for controlled/living radical polymerization due to its high efficiency in obtaining well-defined polymers characterized by a predetermined molecular weight, narrow molecular weight distribution and high degree of chain end functionality.

Monomer, initiator with a transferable atom (halogen) and catalyst (transition metal with suitable ligands) are the main components of ATRP and, sometimes, an additive such as a metal salt in a higher oxidation state may be employed.

Radical generation and halogen transfer are catalyzed by the metal complex, which makes the halogen transfer much more efficient, according to a reversible redox mechanism.

The propagation stage consists of the repetitive addition of alkenes to the radical species while termination reactions occur by combination or disproportionation, or the active species is reversibly deactivated by the higher oxidation state metal complex.

Examples of ATRP catalysts are represented by transition metal complexes of copper, ruthenium, palladium, nickel and iron [8–10].

Reversible Addition-Fragmentation Chain Transfer Polymerization (RAFT)

Reversible addition-fragmentation chain transfer polymerization is a reversible deactivation radical polymerization and it represents one of the most versatile methods for providing living characteristics to radical polymerization and polymers of predictable chain length and narrow molecular weight distribution.

A RAFT polymerization system consists of an initiator, monomer, solvent and a chain transfer agent, defined as RAFT agent, which mediates the polymerization via a reversible chain transfer process. RAFT agents are thiocarbonylthio compounds, including dithioesters, dithiocarbamates, trithiocarbonates and xanthates, and characterized by the presence of two different functionalities: a Z group, which affects the stability of the C=S bond and controls the effectiveness radicals addition to the growing chain, and a R group, able to initiate new polymeric chains (Fig. 1.10).

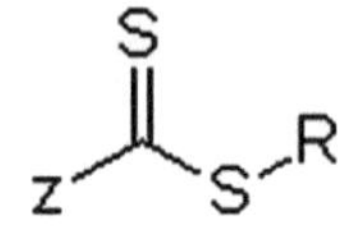

Fig. 1.10 General structure of RAFT agents

Radical initiators, including AIBN, are widely employed as initiators in this kind of polymerization while, among the monomers, methacrylates, methacrylamides, acrylonitrile, styrene and derivatives are commonly used.

The main stages of a RAFT polymerization are initiation, addition-fragmentation, reinitiation and equilibration. In the initiation stage, the reaction is started by the decomposition of a radical initiator, such as AIBN, that generates two fragments which react with a monomer molecule producing the actively polymerizing chain. During addition-fragmentation step, the active chain reacts with the dithioester, which releases the hemolytic leaving group. This stage is reversible because of the presence of an intermediate species capable of losing either the leaving group or the active species. Reinitiation process takes place when the leaving group radical reacts with another monomer species, starting another active polymer chain. In the equilibration step, active polymer chains are in equilibrium between the active and dormant stages. In the dormant one, active polymer chains are bound to the thiocarbonyl compound [11–13] and this limits the possibility of chain termination.

Step-growth Versus Chain Polymerization

These two types of polymerization reactions differ each other by several points including the rate at which the size of polymer molecules increases, the time required for high monomer conversion, the reaction mechanism, the presence of an active center and a termination reaction.

In a *step-growth polymerization*, the average molecular weight of polymeric molecules increases at a slow rate, thus, the chain growth proceeds slowly from monomer to dimer, trimer, tetramer, until the formation of full-sized polymer. In this kind of polymerization, any two molecular species, such as monomer, oligomer or polymer, can be linked involving the same reaction mechanism, the polymeric chain grows from both ends with polymerization times of the order of hours and the presence of an initiator is not required. Monomer disappears early in the reaction and no termination step occurs, therefore, both the chain ends of the polymer molecule remains active to a further polymerization process. Usually, but not always, the repeat units incorporated into the synthesized polymer have fewer atoms than had the starting monomer.

On the other hand, polymeric molecules obtained by *chain polymerization* grow more slowly than time required for high monomer conversion. Indeed, the lifetime of a growing polymeric chain may be in the range of second to microseconds. The molar mass of the polymer backbone increases rapidly at early stage and remains approximately the same throughout the polymerization. A chain polymerization can take place by following different mechanisms operating at different stages of the reaction (i.e. initiation, propagation and termination) and all of them require an active center, including radical species, cations or anions generated by an initiator. Backbone growth occurs only by addition of monomer to the one active chain end and some monomer remains even at long reaction times, therefore, it is present throughout but its concentration decreases gradually. Reaction medium, indeed, generally contains long and dead chains and monomers. The polymeric chain grows extremely rapidly until the termination reaction occurs deactivating the reactive end-group. Usually, but not always, polymer repeat units have the same atoms as had the starting monomer.

The two categories of polymerization mechanisms differ in the relationship between polymer molecular weight and the percent of monomer conversion. In chain polymerization, high molecular weight polymers are present at all percent of monomer conversion, there are no intermediate sized molecules in the reaction mixture, only monomer and high polymer, and just the number of polymer molecules increases with conversion. In step-growth, high molecular weight polymer is obtained at the end of the reaction at 98 % of conversion [1, 14, 15]. Based on these considerations, longer polymerization durations are of relevant importance in obtaining high molecular weight step-growth polymers while, in chain polymerization, long reaction times allows to obtain high yields but do not affect the molecular weight significantly.

The physical properties of polymeric materials depend on the polymerization mechanism involved in the synthetic process due to the difference in molecular masses.

How to Synthesize a Polymer?

From the practical point of view, the synthesis of a polymeric material is performed by adding the monomeric units in reactors o vessels with or without application of heat. On the basis of the phases forming the reaction medium, the polymerization processes can be classified as homogeneous and heterogeneous systems and both category include different polymerization techniques. In general, in a homogeneous polymerization systems all chemicals participating to the reaction, form a single homogeneous mixture in which polymer formation occurs. This technique includes bulk and solution polymerization processes. On the other hand, a heterogeneous polymerization takes place when the reactants form more than one phase, creating heterogeneous media. Suspension, emulsion and polymerizations are typical example of this kind of systems.

Homogeneous Polymerization

Bulk (or Mass) Polymerization

Bulk polymerization is the simplest polymerization technique and it is carried out without using any solvent, dispersant or diluting agent and solubilizing the initiator in one or more monomers in liquid state. As the reaction proceeds, the viscosity of the system increases and, when the process is terminated, the resulting material is passed to another vessel for polymer isolation, unreacted monomer recovery, etc. The resulting polymers, obtained in high yields, are either partially or completely soluble in their starting monomers and are characterized by a broad molecular weight distribution due to the high viscosity and lack of good heat transfer.

This technique is generally used in mildly exothermic reactions when less viscous products are formed and therefore, mixing, heat transfer, and control of the process is easy, e.g. in step-growth polymerization processes. On the other hand, the application of this method offers some disadvantages when the viscosity of the mass reaction increases because heat transfer and mixing become difficult.

Solution Polymerization

In a solution polymerization, monomers are dissolved in a no reactive solvent within an initiator. Although it requires purification and removal of the solvent, this procedure is more versatile than bulk polymerization because it is suitable for chain or step-growth polymerization reactions. Due to the presence of the solvent, the viscosity of the reaction mixture, indeed, is reduced, and the mixing, heat transfer, and control of the process is easier than bulk polymerization. The disadvantages of this procedure are ascribable to the solvent toxicity, flammability and boiling point, which restrict the choice of system, and to the chain transfer to solvent phenomena, affecting the relative molecular mass of the resulted material.

Heterogeneous Polymerization

Suspension Polymerization

In this process, also referred to as bead or pearl polymerization, the monomer, or a mixture of monomers, is dispersed as droplets (size 50–500 mm) by mechanical agitation in a liquid phase (usually water), in which they are insoluble, in the presence of the stabilizers, such as methyl cellulose, gelatine or polyvinyl alcohol (which prevent the monomer droplets from the coalescing) and a free radical initiator. This one is soluble in the monomer phase, and therefore, the mechanism in the droplet is very similar to bulk polymerization. The water: monomer weight ratio varies from 1:1 to 4:1 in most polymerizations while the levels of stabilizers are typically less than 0.1 weight percent (wt %) of the aqueous phase [16].

The resulting product consists of opaque microparticles with irregular surface, and a substantial internal porosity. The beads particles produced in a suspension polymerization are roughly of the same size as the original monomer droplets, with diameters on the order of 10^{-3} to 0.5 cm. Styrene, acrylic and methacrylic esters, vinyl chloride, vinyl acetate, and tetrafluoroethylene are polymerized by the suspension method.

In the vast majority of cases, the suspending medium for suspension polymerization is water, although inverse-suspension polymerizations are also known and used commercially to produce very high molecular weight polymers and copolymers based on the comonomer acrylamide. Here a water-soluble monomer is dispersed in a hydrophobic organic suspending medium, usually in the presence of water in the disperse phase.

Emulsion Polymerization

In this procedure, conceptually similar to suspension polymerization, the polymerization starts in the aqueous phase in presence of a water soluble initiator system, an immiscible monomer forming droplets upon agitation, and a surfactant, to stabilize the droplets in the emulsion.

The initiators can be water-soluble molecules (potassium or ammonium persulfate, hydrogen peroxide, and 2,2′-azobis(2-midinopropane) dihydrochloride), partially water-soluble peroxides (i.e. succinic acid peroxide and t-butyl hydroperoxide) or azo compounds, such as 4,4′-azobis(4-cyanopentanoic acid). As regards the surfactants, anionic species, such as sodium or potassium stearate, laurate, palmitate, or sulfate and sulfonates (sodium lauryl sulfate and sodium dodecylbenzene sulfonate) are the most commonly used in emulsion polymerization [16, 17]. By enhancing the surfactants concentration, the particle size decreases, while the particle number increases.

Emulsion polymerization can also be carried out as an inverse emulsion polymerization [18]. Here, an aqueous solution of a hydrophilic monomer is emulsified in a nonpolar organic solvent such as xylene or paraffin and polymerization initiated with an oil-soluble initiator. The two types of emulsion polymerizations are referred to as oil-in-water (o/w) and water-in-oil (w/o) emulsions, respectively. Inverse emulsion polymerization is used in various commercial polymerizations and copolymerizations of acrylamide as well as other water-soluble monomers.

Finally, miniemulsion and microemulsion polymerization are two subcategories of emulsion polymerization with monomer droplets in water with much smaller droplets than in emulsion polymerization (about 50–1,000 nm in miniemulsion polymerization and 10–100 nm in microemulsion process, compared to 1–100 mm in diameter) [19, 20]. Water-insoluble costabilizers such as hexadecane and cetyl alcohol are present along with the surfactant to stabilize the monomer droplets against diffusional degradation [16].

Precipitation Polymerization

In a precipitation polymerization, the system initially is in a homogeneous phase, because monomer and initiator are completely soluble in the initial reaction medium, but, upon initiation, the formed polymer precipitates as soon as it forms. After precipitation, the polymerization proceeds by absorption of monomer and initiator into the polymer particles. Bulk polymerization of vinyl chloride and solution polymerization of acrylonitrile in water are examples of precipitation polymerization. Precipitation polymerizations are often referred to as powder or granular polymerizations because of the forms in which the final polymer products are obtained.

Table 1.1 Advantages and disadvantages of each polymerization process

Polymerization process	Advantages	Disadvantages
Bulk	Simple Purity of the formed polymer	Exothermic Difficult to control High viscosity Broad molecular weight distribution
Solution	Low viscosity Better heat control May be used directly as solution	Potential toxicity, flammability and environmental pollution of solvents Polymer product contains solvent impurities Yield lower than in bulk polymerization Expensive due to additional solvent costs
Suspension	Heat rapidly dispersed Low viscosity Polymer obtained in granular form	Washing or drying needed Agglomeration Possibility of contamination
Emulsion	High molecular weight polymers made at fast polymerization rates Heat easily dispersed Low viscosity May be used directly as emulsion	Contamination by surfactants or other polymerization adjuvants Washing/drying needed Cannot be used for condensation, ionic or Ziegler-Natta polymerization, although some exceptions are known. Chain transfer agents needed to control the relative molar mass of the products
Precipitation	Heat rapidly dispersed Polymer obtained in granular form	Washing or drying needed Agglomeration Possibility of contamination

In Table 1.1 a resumen of the advantages and disadvantages of each cited polymerization processes is reported.

Polymers in Biomedical Applications

Among others, polymers represent the main and most promising type of biomaterials to be applied in biomedical area. Their widespread use in this field is due to the relative ease and the low cost with which they can be designed and prepared. This great flexibility in chemistry gives rise to materials with a wide variety of structures and appropriate physical, chemical, surface and biomimetic properties. According to their degradation properties, biopolymers can be classified into biodegradable and non-biodegradable. Polymers are applied as medical supplies, as support or replacement of malfunctioning body parts or as a drug reservoir providing a local therapeutic effect. The specifications for the selected material strongly depend on the application.

This section provides a brief overview of the use of polymeric materials in biomedical field, with particular emphasis to non-biodegradable and biodegradable synthetic materials.

Non-biodegradable Polymers in Biomedical Applications

Non degradable synthetic polymers are used in a wide range of medical devices, where long-term structural stability and biocompatibility are needed [21].

The spectrum of applications includes coatings on devices (e.g., to improve blood compatibility), implantable drug delivery systems, artificial heart, implants (e.g., bone pins and screws, articulating surface in artificial joints), catheters and dialysis tubing, vascular graft, membranes for oxygenation and detoxification, injectable drug delivery and imaging systems, membrane and porous scaffolds for tissue regenerative applications.

The most commonly used inert medical polymers include polyethylenes, polyacrylates, polypropylenes, polyamides (nylons), polyurethanes and polysiloxanes (silicone).

Polyethylene

Polyethylene polymers are obtained by chain polymerization processes. Depending on the reaction time, temperature and pressure, polyethylene with different molecular weight, crystallinity and degree of branching can be obtained. They are commonly employed as catheter tubes, facial implants, artificial tendons, or bearing components in total joint replacements. The molecular weight of polyethylene can vary from 30,000 to 6,000,000 g mol^{-1}, density can range from 0.91 to 0.98 g cm^{-3}, and crystallinity can span 30–90 %. The melting temperature is typically in the range of 120–147 °C and the glass transition temperature is on the order of 80 °C. Polyethylene is generally classified in different subcategories based on its density and branching. In particular, LDPE, MDPE, HDPE and UHMWPE are the main classes of polyethylene materials. Among others, UHMWPE possesses the better properties in terms of energetic toughness, low coefficient of friction and wear resistance. It was widely employed as medical polymer in fabrication of orthopedic bearings. UHMWPE remains the gold standard as a bearing material in total joint replacements for hips, knees, shoulders, and elbows.

Polyacrylate

Polyacrylates can be easily polymerized by bulk polymerization in mild conditions. The acrylate and methacylates esters form glassy materials with a broad range of molecular weight (from 200,000 to 700,000 g mol^{-1}), depending on processing conditions this group of polymers is widely used for intraocular lenses, bone cement, dentures and middle ear prostheses. Acrylate polymers are widely

Table 1.2 Biomedical applications of the main classes of non biodegradable polymers

Polymer	Application
Poly(methyl methacrylate) 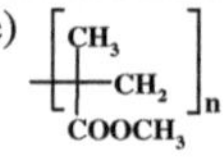	Intraocular lenses, bone cement, orthopedic surgery, middle ear prostheses
Poly(2-hydroxyethyl)methacrylate 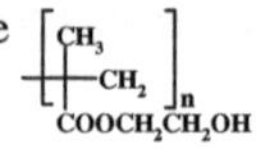	Contact lenses, vehicle in drug delivery, burn treatment
Poly(2-dymethylamino)ethyl methacrylate 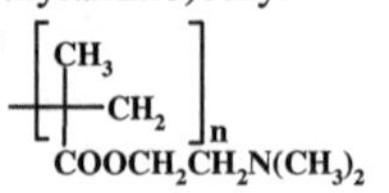	Drug delivery systems, radical scavenger
Poly(methyl metacrylate)-*co*-(methacrylic acid) 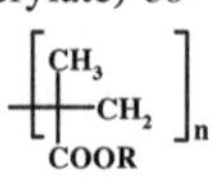 R= H or CH_3	Medical implants, enteric coatings in tablets

used in dentistry and in bone cements. In Table 1.2 the applications of the different kind of polyacrylates are summarized.

Polypropylene

Polypropylene is a thermoplastic polymer also generated through chain polymerization of propylene in presence of suitable catalysts, generally aluminum alkyl and titanium tetrachloride. Polypropylene polymers have a chemical structure similar to polyethylene but have demonstrated certain advantages in improved strength, stiffness and higher temperature capability. Typically, the molecular weight spans 200,000–700,000 $gmol^{-1}$ and the density spans 0.85–0.98 g cm^{-3}. Its melting temperature spans 125–167 °C and its glass transition temperature is on the order of 10 °C. This material has exceptional fatigue life in flexion and is commonly used in finger joint prostheses, grafts, and nondegradable sutures.

Polyamide

Polyamide polymers (Nylons) are obtained by step-growth polymerization. These materials have a broad range of properties, depending on the specific chemistry and processing, and may be amorphous or semicrystalline. The melting temperature is ranged from 190 to 350 °C, and the glass transition temperature is on the order of 45 °C. These polymers are susceptible to swelling in aqueous solutions but are often employed in short-term applications such as catheters and catheter balloons in angioplasty procedures or stent deployment. The most commonly used form of nylon are nylon 6 and nylon 6,6. Nylon is commonly used as the outer layer of balloon angioplasty catheters and also as the balloon used for deployment of a stent or the expansion of an occluded artery. Nylons offer strength and stiffness to balloon angioplasty systems.

Silicone

Silicone polymers, more properly called polysiloxanes, are inorganic-organic polymers with the chemical formula $[R_2SiO]_n$, where R is an organic group such as methyl, ethyl, or phenyl. By varying the -Si-O- chain lengths, side groups, and crosslinking, silicones can be synthesized with a wide variety of properties and compositions. They can be classified as fluids, elastomers, and resins. Polymers of moderate molecular weight are fluids, while high molecular weight, slightly cross-linked polymers are elastomeric.

Silicones have a number of medical applications because of their biocompatibility and chemical inertness. The FDA has approved many medical silicone-based medical devices such as catheters, tubing, gastric bags, drains, and endoscopic windows. The gel form is used in bandages and dressings, breast implants, testicle implants, pectoral implants, contact lenses, and a variety of other medical uses.

Polyurethane

Polyurethanes represent a major class of synthetic elastomers and are constituted of chains of organic units joined by carbamate links. They are generated through a step-growth polymerization reaction of three basic components: a diisocyanate, a sort chain diol and a long-chain diol. The structure of the linear polymeric chain of polyurethane is characterized by an alternation of hard segments, formed by the reaction of the diisocyanate and the short-chain diol, and soft segments, formed by the reaction of the diisocyanate and the long-chain diol.

Depending from the processing mode, the ratio between the hard and soft segments is modified and the resulting polyurethanes can span a full range of structural properties, ranging from elastomeric (rubber-like) to glassy. Although they require sophisticated and quite expensive manufacturing processes, the employment of polyurethanes in biomedical applications is dramatically growing, because they can be used in applications where other materials do not work. They are tough, biocompatible, and hemocompatible and have been evaluated for a variety of medical implants, particularly for long-term implants [22].

They are used in the fabrication of medical implants such as cardiac pace makers and vascular grafts. Recent developments in siloxane-based polyurethanes, which have greater in vivo stability than conventional polyetherurethanes (e.g., PTMO-based) have provided opportunities for development of a range of medical implants for chronic applications [23].

Biodegradable Polymers in Biomedical Applications

Biodegradable synthetic polymers find their biomedical applications mostly in tissue engineering, to provide temporary structure support, regenerative medicine, or in controlled gene and drug delivery [24].

Biodegradation takes place through the action of enzymes and/or chemical deterioration associated with living organisms. This event occurs in two steps. The first one is the fragmentation of the polymers into lower molecular mass species by means of either abiotic reactions, i.e. oxidation, photodegradation or hydrolysis, or biotic reactions, i.e. degradations by microorganisms. This is followed by bioassimilation of the polymer fragments by microorganisms and their mineralization [25].

Biodegradable synthetic polymers offer a number of advantages over other materials because of the possibility to tailor mechanical properties and degradation kinetics, and because they can be fabricated into various shapes with desired pore morphologic features conducive to tissue in-growth.

Biodegradable synthetic polymers such as poly(glycolic acid), poly(lactic acid) and their copolymers, and copolymers of trimethylene carbonate and glycolide have been used in a number of clinical applications [26–30]. The major applications include resorbable sutures, drug delivery systems and orthopaedic fixation devices such as pins, rods and screws [31, 32].

Polyglycolide

PGA belongs to the family of polyesters. The polyesters have been attractive for applications in tissue engineering and drug delivery because of their ease of degradation by hydrolysis of ester linkage, degradation products being resorbed through the metabolic pathways in some cases and the potential to tailor the structure to alter degradation rates. Polyesters have also been considered for development of tissue engineering applications [33–36], particularly for bone tissue engineering [37, 38].

PGA is the simplest linear aliphatic polyester. It is prepared by ring opening polymerization of a cyclic lactone, glycolide. It is highly crystalline, with a crystallinity of 45–55 % and thus is not soluble in most organic solvents. It has a high melting point (220–225 °C) and a glass transition temperature of 35–40 °C.

The attractiveness of PGA as a biodegradable polymer in medical application is that its degradation product glycolic acid is a natural metabolite. A major application of PGA is in resorbable sutures (Dexon, American Cyanamide Co). Numerous studies [39–41] have established a simple degradation mechanism via homogeneous erosion. The degradation process occurs in two stages, the first involves the diffusion of water into the chain scission of the ester groups. The second stage of degradation involves largely the crystalline areas of the polymer, which becomes predominant when the majority of the amorphous regions have been eroded.

Polylactide

PLA is obtained from polycondensation of D- or L-lactic acid or from ring opening polymerization of lactide, a cyclic dimer of lactic acid.

Poly(lactic acid) is present in three isomeric forms D(−), L(+) and racemic (D,L). and the polymers are usually abbreviated to indicate the chirality. Poly(L)LA and poly(D)LA are semi-crystalline solids, with similar rates of hydrolytic degradation as

PGA. Due to the presence of $-CH_3$ side groups, PLA is more hydrophobic than PGA, and is more resistant to hydrolytic attack than PGA. For most applications the (L) isomer of lactic acid is chosen because it is preferentially metabolized in the body. The main disadvantage of PLA is its brittleness and poor thermal stability.

Poly(lactide-co-glycolide)

L-lactide and DL-lactide have been used for copolymerization with glycolic acid monomers. Varying the ratio between these two components, PLGA materials have been commercially developed, obtaining materials with different mechanical properties.

PLGA is the most investigated degradable polymer for biomedical applications and has been used in sutures, drug delivery devices and tissue engineering scaffolds [42].

PLGA demonstrates great cell adhesion and proliferation properties making it an excellent candidate for application in tissue engineering. PLGA has been fabricated into scaffolds by a number of different techniques including gas foaming [43, 44], microsphere sintering [45], porogen leaching [46, 47], electrospinning [48–50], polymer printing [51] or a combination of these techniques [52, 53] in order to create unique nano- and microstructured materials that can facilitate tissue development.

Polycaprolactones

PCL is a semicrystalline polymer prepared by the ring-opening polymerization of ε-caprolactone. It is characterized by a glass transition temperature of about −60 °C and a low melting temperature (59–64 °C). PCL degrades at a much lower rate that PLA and is a useful base polymer for developing long term, implantable drug delivery systems. Capronor® is a commercial contraceptive PCL product that is able to deliver levonorgestrel in vivo for over a year and has been on the market for over 25 years [54].

PCL has found numerous application in tissue engineering. PCL has low tensile strength (~23 MPa), but very high elongation at breakage (4,700 %) making it a very good elastic biomaterial. 41 PCL's processability allows for the formation of scaffolds composed of adhered microspheres [55, 56], electrospun networks created by porogen leaching [57–59]. PCL and PCL composites have been used as tissue engineering scaffolds for regeneration of bone [60, 61] ligament [62, 63] cartilage [64], skin [65], nerve [66, 67], and vascular tissues [68, 69].

Polyurethanes

The biodegradation of polyurethanes depends on the chemical nature of the soft and hard segments.

If the polyol is a polyester, indeed, the polyurethanes are readily biodegradable [70]. Biodegradable polyesters used are PCL, PLA and PGA [71, 72].

Polyurethanes can also be designed to have chemical linkages that are degradable in the biological environment [73]. However, a major problem has been the toxicity of degradation products, particularly those derived from the diisocyanate component. For example, degradation products of polyurethanes based on diisocyanates such as MDI and TDI are toxic [74]. Accordingly, in designing degradable polyurethanes diiscoyanates such as lysine diisocyanate [75] and other aliphatic diisocyanates like HDI [76] and 1,4-butanediisocyanate have been used.

Polycarbonate

Polycarbonates are linear polymers that have two geminal ether bonds and a carbonyl bond susceptible of enzymatic degradation in vivo [76]. PTMC a widely studied elastomeric aliphatic polymer with great flexibility and a slow degradation profile, but poor mechanical strength. Its degradation into biocompatible, non-acidic 1,3-propanediol and carbonic acid make it an ideal candidate for drug delivery applications. PTMC has been fabricated into microparticles [77], discs [78] and gels [79, 80] for the delivery of angiogenic agents and antibiotics. To enhance the delivery potential of PTMC, it is often copolymerized with PLA [81], PCL [81], polyether [82], or poly(L-glutamic acid) [83, 84], to allow for the fabrication of sutures, micelles, and polymersomes with superior mechanical and degradation properties. Other polycarbonate possessing good properties such as compatibility and impact resistance is PPC, synthesized via copolymerization of propylene oxide and carbon dioxide.

Tyrosine-based polycarbonates have been reported as promising degradable polymers for use as tissue engineering scaffolds in orthopaedic applications [85]. These polymers possess three potentially hydrolysable bonds: amide, carbonate and ester. Studies have shown [85] that the carbonate group hydrolyzes at a faster rate than the ester group, and the amide bond is not labile in vitro.

Polyanhydrides

Polyanhydrides are a widely studied class of biodegradable materials interesting biodegradable materials with demonstrated biocompatibility and excellent controlled release characteristics. They have two hydrolysable sites in the repeating unit. Polyanhydrides degrades by surface erosion [86] and the degradation rate depends on the polymer backbone. Aromatic polyanhydrides will degrade slowly over a long period, while aliphatic polyanhydrides can degrade in a few days. The main applications of these materials are in controlled drug delivery [87]. Polyanhydrides have limited mechanical properties that restrict their use in load–bearing applications such as in orthopaedics. For this reason they are often combined with other materials. For example, to combine good mechanical properties of polyimides with surface-eroding characteristics of polanhydrides, poly(anhydrides-co-imides) have been developed [88], particularly for orthopaedic applications. Examples include poly-[trimellitylimidoglycine-co-bis(carboxyphenoxy) hexane], and poly [pyromellitylimidoalanine-co-1,6-bis(carboph-enoxy)-hexane].

Another approach is the incorporation of acrylic functional groups in the monomeric unit. This leads to photocrosslinkable polyanhydrides. The mechanical strength and degradation rate of these crosslinked polyanhydrides depend on the nature of the monomeric species.

Conclusions

Polymers are macromolecular systems constituted by a large number of structural units joined by the same type of linkage. Synthetic polymers are an extraordinarily versatile class of materials and their enormous heterogeneity in consistence, shape and chemical-physical properties is due to the great number of polymerization mechanisms, monomers and initiators which can be used as well as polymerization processes. The biomedical area is widely exploiting the enormous potential of these materials in many applications such as tissue engineering and drug delivery. This chapter is concerned with the basis of polymer chemistry, with particular emphasis on the polymerization mechanisms and the different synthetic processes. Moreover, in the last section the applications of the main class of non-biodegradable and biodegradable polymers in medical area are discussed.

References

1. Odian, G. (ed.): Principles of Polymerization, 4th edn. Wiley, New York (2004)
2. Billmeyer, F.W. (ed.): Textbook of Polymer Science. Wiley, New York (1984)
3. Hasirci, V., Yilgor, P., Endogan, T., Eke, G., Hasirci, N.: Polymer fundamentals: polymer synthesis. In: Ducheyne, P., Healy, K.E., Hutmacher, D.W., Grainger, D.W., Kirkpatrick, C.J. (eds.) Comprehensive Biomaterials, 1st edn, pp. 350–371. Elsevier Ltd, Oxford (2011)
4. Hiemenz, P.C., Lodge, T.P. (eds.): Polymer Chemistry, 2nd edn. CRC Press, Boca Raton (2007)
5. Young, R.J., Lovell, P.A. (eds.): Introduction to Polymers, 2nd edn. Chapman and Hall, London (1995)
6. Walton, D.J., Lorimer, J.P.: Polymers. Oxford University Press, Oxford (2001)
7. Fried, J.R. (ed.): Polymer Science and Technology. Prentice Hall, Englewood Cliffs (1995)
8. Fischer, H.: The persistent radical effect in "living" radical polymerization. Macromolecules **30**, 5666–5762 (1997)
9. Matyjaszewski, K., Xia, J.: Atom transfer radical polymerization. Chem. Rev. **101**, 2921–2990 (2001)
10. Matyjaszewski, K., Davis, T.P. (eds.): Handbook of Radical Polymerization. Wiley, Hoboken (2002)
11. Lubnin, A., O'Malley, K., Hanshumaker, D., Lai, J.: Waterborne RAFT polymers. Eur. Polym. J. **46**, 1563–1575 (2010)
12. Moad, G., Rizzardo, E., Thang, S.H.: Radical addition-fragmentation chemistry in polymer synthesis. Polymer **49**, 1079–1131 (2008)

13. Mya, K.Y., Lin, E.M.J., Gudipati, C.S., Gose, H.B.A.S., He, C.: Self-assembly of block copolymer micelles: synthesis via reversible addition-fragmentation chain transfer polymerization and aqueous solution properties. J. Phys. Chem. B **114**, 9128–9134 (2010)
14. Braun, D., Cherdron, H., Rehahn, M., Ritter, H., Voit, B. (eds.): Polymer Synthesis: Theory and Practice, Fundamentals, Methods, Experiments, 4th edn. Springer, New York (2005)
15. Moad, G., Solomon, D.H. (eds.): The Chemistry of Radical Polymerization, 2nd edn. Elsevier, Oxford (2006)
16. Odian, G. (ed.): Principles of Polymerization, 4th edn. Wiley Interscience, New York (2004)
17. Blackley, D.C. (ed.): Emulsion Polymerization. Applied Science, London (1975)
18. Poehlein, G.W.: Emulsion polymerization. In: Mark, H.F., Bikales, N.M., Overberger, C.G., Menges, G. (eds.) Encyclopedia of Polymer Science and Engineering, vol. 6, pp. 1–51. Wiley-Interscience, New York (1986)
19. Antonietti, M., Landfester, K.: Polyreactions in miniemulsions. Prog. Polym. Sci. **27**, 689–757 (2002)
20. Asua, J.M.: Miniemulsion polymerization. Prog. Polym. Sci. **27**, 1283–1346 (2002)
21. Pruitt, L.A.: Structural biomedical polymers (Nondegradable). In: Ducheyne, P., Healy, K.E., Hutmacher, D.W., Grainger, D.W., Kirkpatrick, C.J. (eds.) Comprehensive Biomaterials, 1st edn, pp. 373–379. Elsevier Ltd, Oxford (2011)
22. Pinchuk, L.: A review of the biostability and carcinogenicity of polyurethanes in medicine and the new generation of 'biostable' polyurethanes. J. Biomater. Sci. Polym. Ed. **3**, 225–267 (1994)
23. Gunatillake, P.A., Meijs, G.F., McCarthy, S.J.: Developments in design and synthesis of biostable polyurethanes. In: Vermette, P., Griesser, H.J., Laroche, G., Guidoin, R. (eds.) Biomedical Applications of Polyurethanes, pp. 160–170. Landes Bioscience, Georgetown (2001)
24. Gunatillake, Pathiraja A., Adhikari, R.: Biodegradable synthetic polymers for tissue engineering. Eur. Cells Mater. **5**, 1–16 (2003)
25. Vroman, I., Tighzert, L.: Biodegradable Polymers. Materials **2**, 307–344 (2009)
26. Shalaby, S.W.: Bioabsorbable polymers. In: Swarbrick, J., Boylan, J.C. (eds.) Encyclopedia of Pharmceutical Technology, pp. 465–476 (1988)
27. Holland, S.J., Tighe, B.J.: Biodegradable polymers. Advances in Pharmaceutical Science, pp. 101–164. Academic Press, London (1992)
28. Kohn, J., Langer, R.: Bioresorbable and bioerodible materials. In: Ratner, B.D., Hoffman, A.S., Schoen, F.J., Lemon, J.E. (eds.) An Introduction to Materials in Medicine, pp. 65–73. Academic Press, San Diego (1997)
29. Ashammakhi, N., Rokkanen, P.: Absorbable polyglycolide devices in trauma and bone surgery. Biomaterials **18**, 3–9 (1997)
30. Kohn, J., Langer, R.: Bioresorbable and bioerodible materials. In: Ratner, B.D., Hoffman, A.S., Schoen, F.J., Lemon, J.E. (eds.) An Introduction to Materials in Medicine, pp. 65–73. Academic Press, San Diego (1997)
31. Behravesh, E., Yasko, A.W., Engle, P.S., Mikos, A.G.: Synthetic biodegradable polymers for orthopaedic applications. Clin. Orthop. **367S**, 118–185 (1999)
32. Middleton, J.C., Tipton, A.J.: Synthetic biodegradable polymers as orthopaedic devices. Biomaterials **21**, 2335–2346 (2000)
33. Hubbell, J.: Biomaterials in tissue engineering. Biotechnology **13**, 565–576 (1995)
34. Thomson, R.C., Wake, M.C., Yaszemski, M.J., Mikos, A.G.: Biodegradable polymer scaffolds to regenerate organs. Adv. Polym. Sci. **122**, 245–274 (1995)
35. Yazemski, M.J., Yasko, A.W., Engel, P.S., Mikos, A.G.: *In vitro* degradation of a poly(propylene fumarate)/ßtricalcium phosphate composition orthopaedic scaffold. Tissue Eng. **3**, 207–215 (1997)
36. Wong, W.H., Mooney, D.J.: Synthesis and properties of biodegradable polymers used as synthetic matrices for tissue engineering. In: Atala, A., Mooney, D. (eds.) Synthetic Biodegradable Polymer Scaffolds, pp. 51–84. Burkhäuser, Boston (1997)
37. Kohn, J., Langer, R.: Bioresorbable and bioerodible materials. In: Ratner, B.D., Hoffman, A.S., Schoen, F.J., Lemon, J.E. (eds.) An Introduction to Materials in Medicine, pp. 65–73. Academic Press, San Diego (1997)

38. Burg, K.J.L., Porter, S., Kellam, J.F.: Biomaterials development for bone tissue engineering. Biomaterials **21**, 2347–2359 (2000)
39. Chu, C.C.: An in-vitro study of the effect of buffer on the degradation of poly(glycolic acid) sutures. J. Biomed. Mater. Res. **15**, 19–27 (1981)
40. Chu, C.C.: The *in-vitro* degradation of poly(glycolic acid) sutures-effect of pH. J. Biomed. Mater. Res. **15**, 795–804 (1981)
41. Chu, C.C.: Hydrolytic degradation of polyglycolic acid: tensile strength and crystallinity study. J. Appl. Polym. Sci. **26**, 1727–1734 (1981)
42. Ulery, B.D., Nair, L.S., Laurencin, C.T.: Biomedical applications of biodegradable polymers. J. Polym. Sci. B Polym. Phys. **12**, 832–864 (2011)
43. Chung, H.J., Kim, I.K., Kim, T.G., Park, T.G.: Highly open porous biodegradable microcarriers: *In Vitro* cultivation of chondrocytes for injectable delivery. Tissue Eng. Part A **14**, 607–615 (2008)
44. Zhu, X.H., Lee, L.Y., Jackson, J.S.H., Tong, Y.W., Wang, C.H.: Characterization of porous poly(d, l-lactic-co-glycolic acid) sponges fabricated by supercritical CO_2 gas-foaming method as a scaffold for three-dimensional growth of Hep3B cells. Biotechnol. Bioeng. **100**, 998–1009 (2008)
45. Simpson, R.L., Wiria, F.E., Amis, A.A., Chua, C.K., Leong, K.F., Hansen, U.N., Chandrasekaran, M., Lee, M.W.: Development of a 95/5 poly(l-lactide-co-glycolide)/hydroxylapatite and β-tricalcium phosphate scaffold as bone replacement material via selective laser sintering. J. Biomed. Mater. Res. Part B Appl. Biomater. 84B, 17–25 (2008)
46. Arnold, M.M., Gorman, E.M., Schieber, L.J., Munson, E.J., Berkland, C.: NanoCipro encapsulation in monodisperse large porous PLGA microparticles. J. Control Release **121**, 100–109 (2007)
47. Narayan, D., Venkatraman, S.S.: Effect of pore size and interpore distance on endothelial cell growth on polymers. J. Biomed. Mater. Res. Part A **87A**, 710–718 (2008)
48. Bashur, C.A., Dahlgren, L.A., Goldstein, A.S.: Effect of fiber diameter and orientation on fibroblast morphology and proliferation on electrospun poly(d, l-lactic-co-glycolic acid) meshes. Biomaterials **27**, 5681–5688 (2006)
49. Moffat, K.L., Kwei, A.S.-P., Spalazzi, J.P., Doty, S.B., Levine, W.N., Lu, H.H.: Novel nanofiber-based scaffold for rotator cuff repair and augmentation. Tissue Eng. Part A **15**, 115–126 (2009)
50. Aviss, K.J., Gough, J.E., Downes, S.: Aligned electrospun polymer fibres for skeletal muscle regeneration. Eur Cell Mater **19**, 193–204 (2010)
51. Ge, Z., Wang, L., Heng, B.C., Tian, X.-F., Lu, K., Fan, V.T.W., Yeo, J.F., Cao, T., Tan, E.: Proliferation and differentiation of human osteoblasts within 3D printed poly-lactic-co-glycolic acid scaffolds. J. Biomater. Appl. **23**, 533–547 (2009)
52. Yoon, J.J., Chung, H.J., Lee, H.J., Park, T.G.: Heparin-immobilized biodegradable scaffolds for local and sustained release of angiogenic growth factor. J. Biomed. Mater. Res., Part A **79A**, 934–942 (2006)
53. Perron, J.K., Naguib, H.E., Daka, J., Chawla, A., Wilkins, R.J.: A study on the effect of degradation media on the physical and mechanical properties of porous PLGA 85/15 scaffolds. Biomed. Mater. Res. Part B **91B**, 876–886 (2009)
54. Nair, L.S., Laurencin, C.T.: Biodegradable polymers as biomaterials. Prog. Polym. Sci. **32**, 762–798 (2007)
55. Garkhal, K., Verma, S., Tikoo, K., Kumar, N.: Surface modified poly(L-lactide-*co*-ε-caprolactone) microspheres as scaffold for tissue engineering. J. Biomed. Mater. Res., Part A **82A**, 747–756 (2007)
56. Danhier, F., Vroman, B., Lecouturier, N., Crokart, N., Pourcelle, V., Freichels, H., Jerome, C., Marchand-Brynaert, J., Feron, O., Preat, V.J.: Targeting of tumor endothelium by RGD-grafted PLGA-nanoparticles loaded with Paclitaxel. J. Control Release **140**, 166–173 (2009)
57. Pankajakshan, D., Philipose, L.P., Palakkal, M., Krishnan, K., Krishnan, L.K.J.: Development of a fibrin composite-coated poly(ε-caprolactone) scaffold for potential vascular tissue engineering applications. J. Biomed. Mater. Res., Part B **87B**, 570–579 (2008)

58. Chen, H., Huang, J., Yu, J., Liu, S., Ge, P.: Electrospun chitosan-*graft*-poly (ε-caprolactone)/ poly (ε-caprolactone) cationic nanofibrous mats as potential scaffolds for skin tissue engineering. Int. J. Biol. Macromol. **48**, 13–19 (2011)
59. Guarino, V., Ambrosio, L.: The synergic effect of polylactide fiber and calcium phosphate particle reinforcement in poly ε-caprolactone-based composite scaffolds. Acta Biomater. **4**, 1778–1787 (2008)
60. Plikk, P., Malberg, S., Albertsson, A.-C.: Design of resorbable porous tubular copolyester scaffolds for use in nerve regeneration. Biomacromolecules **10**, 1259–1264 (2009)
61. Zuo, Y., Yang, F., Wolke, J.G.C., Li, Y., Jansen, J.A.: Incorporation of biodegradable electrospun fibers into calcium phosphate cement for bone regeneration. Acta Biomater. **6**, 1238–1247 (2010)
62. Mountziaris, P.M., Tzouanas, S.N., Mikos, A.G.: Dose effect of tumor necrosis factor-α on in vitro osteogenic differentiation of mesenchymal stem cells on biodegradable polymeric microfiber scaffolds. Biomaterials **31**, 1666–1675 (2010)
63. Hayami, J.W.S., Surrao, D.C., Waldman, S.D., Amsden, B.G.: Design and characterization of a biodegradable composite scaffold for ligament tissue engineering. J. Biomed. Mater. Res., Part A **92A**, 1407–1420 (2010)
64. Vaquette, C., Kahn, C., Frochot, C., Nouvel, C., Six, J.-L., Isla, N.D., Luo, L.-H., Cooper-White, J., Rahouadj, R., Wang, X.J.: Aligned poly(l-lactic-*co*-e-caprolactone) electrospun microfibers and knitted structure: A novel composite scaffold for ligament tissue engineering. Biomed. Mater. Res. Part A **94A**, 1270–1282 (2010)
65. Li, W.-J., Chiang, H., Kuo, T.-F., Lee, H.-S., Jiang, C.-C., Tuan, R.S.: Evaluation of articular cartilage repair using biodegradable nanofibrous scaffolds in a swine model: a pilot. J. Tissue Eng. Regen Med. **3**, 1–10 (2009)
66. Jeong, S.I., Lee, A.-Y., Lee, Y.M., Shin, H.: Electrospun gelatin/poly(l-lactide-co-ε-caprolactone) nanofibers for mechanically functional tissue-engineering scaffolds. J. Biomater. Sci. Polym. Ed. **19**, 339–357 (2008)
67. Nisbet, D.R., Rodda, A.E., Horne, M.K., Forsythe, J.S., Finkelstein, D.I.: Neurite infiltration and cellular response to electrospun polycaprolactone scaffolds implanted into the brain. Biomaterials **30**, 4573–4580 (2009)
68. Liu, J.J., Wang, C.Y., Wang, J.G., Ruan, H.J., Fan, C.Y.: Peripheral nerve regeneration using composite poly(lactic acid-caprolactone)/nerve growth factor conduits prepared by coaxial electrospinning. J. Biomed. Mater. Res. A 96a, 13–20 (2011)
69. Heydarkhan-Hagvall, S., Schenke-Layland, K., Dhanasopon, A.P., Rofail, F., Smith, H., Wu, B.M., Shemin, R., Beygui, R.E., MacLellan, W.R.: Three-dimensional electrospun ECM-based hybrid scaffolds for cardiovascular tissue engineering. Biomaterials **29**, 2907–2914 (2008)
70. Nakajima-Kambe, T., Shigeno-Akutsu, Y., Nomura, N., Onuma, F., Nakarahara, T.: Microbial degradation of polyurethane, polester polyurethanes and polyether polyurethanes. Appl. Microbiol. Biotechnol. **51**, 134–140 (1999)
71. Guelcher, S.A., Gallagher, K.M., Didier, J.E., Klinedinst, D.B., Doctor, J.S., Goldstein, A.S.: Synthesis of biocompatible segmented polyurethanes from aliphatic diisocyanates and diurea diol chain extenders. Acta Biomater. **1**, 471–484 (2005)
72. Hassan, M.K., Mauritz, K.A., Storey, R.F., Wiggins, J.S.: Biodegradable aliphatic thermoplastic polyurethane based on poly(ε-caprolactone) and l-lysine diisocyanate. J. Polym. Sci. A-Polym Chem. **44**, 2990–3000 (2006)
73. McGill, D.B., Motto, J.D.: An industrial outbreak of toxic hepatitis due to methylenedianiline. New Engl. J. Med. **291**, 278–282 (1974)
74. Gogolewski, S., Pennings, A.J.: Biodegradable materials of polylactides, 4. Porous biomedical materials based on mixtures of polylactides and polyurethanes. Makromol. Chem., Rapid Commun. **3**, 839–845 (1982)
75. Storey, R.F., Taylor, A.E.: Effect of stannous octoate on the composition, molecular weight, and molecular weight distribution of ethyleneglycol-initiated poly(ecaprolactone). J. Macromol. Sci. Pure Appl. Chem. **A35**, 723–750 (1998)

76. Ekholm, M., Helander, P., Hietanen, J., Lindqvist, C., Salo, A., Kellomaki, M., Suuronen, R.: A histological and immunohistochemical study of tissue reactions to solid poly(ortho ester) in rabbits. Int. J. Oral Maxillofac. Surg. **35**, 631–635 (2006)
77. Zhang, Z., Foks, M.A., Grijpma, D.W., Feijen, J.: PTMC and MPEG-PTMC microparticles for hydrophilic drug delivery. J. Control Release **101**, 392–394 (2005)
78. Kluin, O.S., Mei, H.C.vd., Busscher, H.J., Neut, D.: A surface-eroding antibiotic delivery system based on poly-(trimethylene carbonate). Biomaterials **30**, 4738–4742 (2009)
79. Timbart, L., Tse, M.Y., Pang, S.C., Babasola, O., Amsden, B.G.: Low viscosity poly(trimethylene carbonate) for localized drug delivery: rheological properties and in vivo degradation. Macromol. Biosci. **9**, 786–794 (2009)
80. Amsden, B.G., Timbart, L., Marecak, D., Chapanian, R., Tse, M.Y., Pang, S.C.: VEGF-induced angiogenesis following localized delivery via injectable, low viscosity poly(trimethylene carbonate) J. Controlled Release **145**, 109–115 (2010)
81. Zurita, R., Puiggali, J., Rodriguez-Galan, A.: Loading and release of ibuprofen in multi- and monofilament surgical sutures. Macromol. Biosci. **6**, 767–775 (2006)
82. Chen, W., Meng, F., Li, F., Ji, S.-J., Zhong, Z.: pH-responsive biodegradable micelles based on acid-labile polycarbonate hydrophobe: synthesis and triggered drug release. Biomacromolecules **10**, 1727–1735 (2009)
83. Sanson, C., Schatz, C., Meins, J.-F.L., Brulet, A., Soum, A., Lecommandoux, S.: Biocompatible and biodegradable poly(trimethylene carbonate)-*b*-poly(L-glutamic acid) polymersomes: size control and stability. Langmuir **26**, 2751–2760 (2010)
84. Sanson, C., Schatz, C., Meins, J.-F.L., Soum, A., Thevenot, J., Garanger, E., Lecommandoux, S.: A simple method to achieve high doxorubicin loading in biodegradable polymersomes. J. Control Release **147**, 428–435 (2010)
85. Muggli, D.S., Burkoth, A.K., Keyser, S.A., Lee, H.R., Anseth, K.S.: Reaction behavior of biodegradable, photo cross-linkable polyanhydrides. Macromolecules **31**, 4120–4125 (1998)
86. Kohn, J., Langer, R.: Bioresorbable and bioerodible materials. In: Ratner, B.D., Hoffman, A.S., Schoen, F.J., Lemon, J.E. (eds.) An Introduction to Materials in Medicine, pp. 65–73. Academic Press, San Diego (1997)
87. Brem, H., Piantadosi, S., Burger, P.C., Walker, M., Selker, R., Vick, N.A., Black, K., Sisti, M., Brem, G., Mohr, G., Muller, P., Morawetz, R., Schold, S.C.: Interventions affect aortic wall stiffness. Lancet **345**, 1008 (1995)
88. Attawia, M.A., Uhrich, K.E., Botchwey, E., Fan, M., Langer, R., Laurencin, C.T.: Cytotoxocity testing of poly(anhydride) for orthopaedic applications. J. Biomed. Mater. Res. **29**, 1233–1240 (1995)

Chapter 2
Biodegradable Natural Polymers

Sindhu Doppalapudi, Sameer Katiyar, Abraham J. Domb and Wahid Khan

Abstract Natural polymers have proved to be useful in versatile applications, including controlled drug delivery, gene delivery, regenerative medicine, and other biomedical applications. These polymers are obtained primarily from plants, animals, and microbial sources which are again classified based on their chemistry into polysaccharide, protein, polyester, polyamide-based polymers. The in-depth surveys of these polymers reveals their malleable nature to be modified for various applications. Also, their responsive chemical linkages provide ease of biodegradability, which in turn makes them biocompatible. Their desirable features of ample abundance, biocompatibility, and biodegradability make them potential material for various uses. The eco-friendly profile of these polymers makes researchers inclined towards alluring natural polymers. This chapter describes natural polymers obtained from different sources and provides insights on the origin, chemistry, key features, applications, and marketed products of natural polymers that are being explored as adaptable materials in multifaceted areas.

Keywords Natural polymers · Polysaccharide · Protein · Polyester · Polyamide · Biodegradability · Biocomaptibility

List of Abbreviations

CDs	Cyclodextrin
HPMC	Hydroxy propyl methyl cellulose
MCC	Micro crystalline cellulose

S. Doppalapudi · S. Katiyar · W. Khan (✉)
Department of Pharmaceutics, National Institute of Pharmaceutical Education and Research (NIPER), Hyderabad 500037, India
e-mail: wahid@niperhyd.ac.in

A.J. Domb · W. Khan
School of Pharmacy-Faculty of Medicine, The Hebrew University of Jerusalem, Jerusalem 91120, Israel

F. Puoci (ed.), *Advanced Polymers in Medicine*, DOI 10.1007/978-3-319-12478-0_2

GFR	Glomerular filtration rate
DE	Degree of esterification
SPIONs	Super paramagnetic iron oxide nanoparticles
CaPG	Calcium pectinate gel
KGM	Konjac glucomannan
BSA	Bovine serum albumin
AG	Arabinogalactan
AGP	Arabinogalactan protein
GAG	Glycosaminoglycan
HA	Hyaluronic acid
CS	Chondroitin sulphate
ECM	Extracellular matrix
HAS	Hyaluronan synthases
IdoA	L-iduronic acid
TC	Tropocollagen
FACITs	Fibril associated collagens with interrupted triple helices
MACITs	Membrane associated collagens with interrupted triple helices
MULTIPLEXINS	Multiple triple helix domains and interruptions
HSA	Human serum albumin
EPR	Enhanced permeability and retention effect
BMMNCs	Bone marrow mono-nuclear cells
ADSCs	Adipose derived stem cells
bFGF	Basic fibroblast growth factor
FH	Fibrin-H-chain
FL	Fibrin-L-chain
RSF	Regenerated silk fibroin
SFCS	Silk fibroin chitosan scaffold
GalCS	Galactosylated chitosan scaffold
PHA	Poly hydroxy alkanoate
PHB	Poly hydroxy butyrate
PHBV	Poly (hydroxybutyrate-co-hydroxyvalerate)
PHBH	Poly (hydroxybutyrate-co-hydroxyhexanoate)
PHBO	Poly (hydroxybutyrate-co-hydroxyoctanoate)
sCL	Short chain length
mCL	Medium chain length

Introduction

Natural polymers have been used in diverse applications due to their desirable characteristics, such as abundant availability, biodegradability, and renewability. These polymers are known to produce fewer toxic effects when compared with synthetic polymers. Research into these polymers has been conducted to improve existing applications by the fine tuning of properties and by improving the stability of the polymers. These polymers have left their own mark in various fields, from acting as food additives to applications in tissue engineering, regenerative medicine, controlled drug delivery, gene delivery, cell delivery, etc. Thus, the potential of these materials in versatile areas makes them attractive for research and development to make them suitable for various food and pharmaceutical applications.

Classification

Biodegradable natural polymers classification is represented in Fig. 2.1 and chemical structures of natural polymers represented in Fig. 2.2.

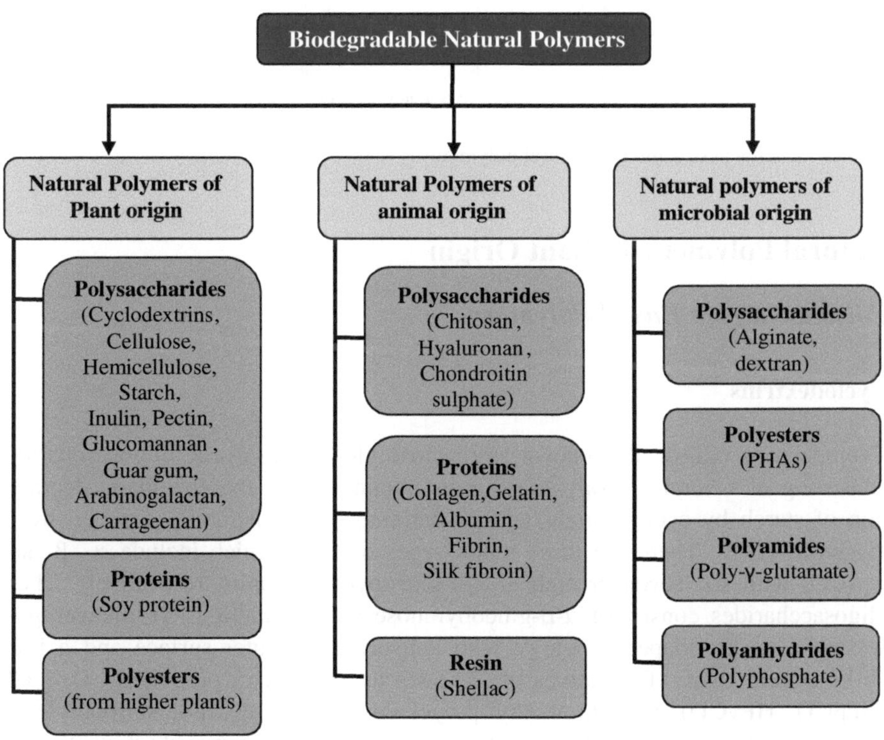

Fig. 2.1 Classification of biodegradable natural polymers

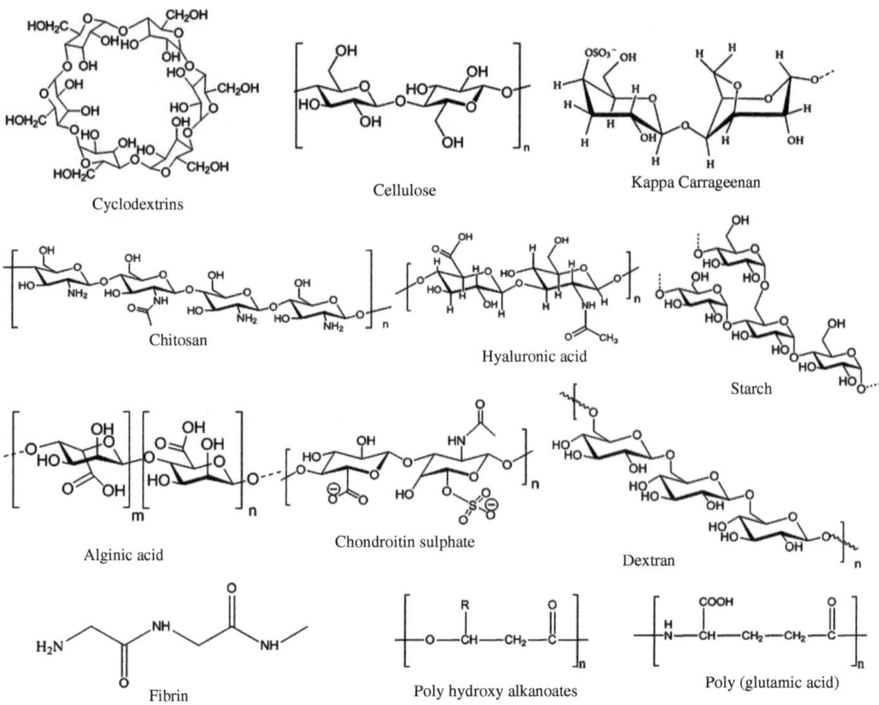

Fig. 2.2 Chemical structures of natural polymers

Natural Polymers of Plant Origin

Polysaccharide Based Polymers

Cyclodextrins

Cyclodextrins (CDs), also known as (cycloamyloses) are cyclic oligosaccharides consisting of several glucopyranose units obtained from the enzymatic degradation of starch by cyclomaltodextrin glucanotransferase, naturally secreted by *B. macerans* [1–3]. There are three major types of CDs, which include α-, β- and γ- (CD) with six, seven or eight *d*-(+)-glucopyranose units, respectively. These oligosaccharides consist of α-D-glucopyranose units with (α-1, 4)-linkages possessing a basket-shaped topology with a hydrophilic outer surface and a lipophilic central cavity. Derivatives of CD such as (2-hydroxy propyl) β-CD, γ-CD (HPβCD, HPγCD), random methyl-β-cyclodextrin (RM-β-CD), sulfobutylether CD (SBEβCD) and many other hydrophilic, hydrophobic, ionizable derivatives of CD are being explored. CDs are chemically stable in neutral and basic conditions, whereas they undergo non-enzymatic hydrolysis in acid conditions to yield glucose, maltose, and non-cyclic oligosaccharides [4, 5].

CDs exhibit multiple applications in versatile areas [6–8]. CD inclusion complexes containing guest molecules improve physicochemical properties, which in turn increase the bioavailability of drugs. The release of drugs is mediated by action of heat/enzymes/pH changes. The dimethyl derivatives of CDs are extremely water soluble, which enhances the bioavailability of lipophilic drugs. They also act as absorption and solubilization enhancers in nasal drug delivery [5, 9, 10]. The use of random methyl CD avoids in vivo crystallization due to its amorphous nature. These polymers were also being investigated for application in intestinal gene transfer. The use of CDs as non-viral vectors for gene delivery results in increased transfection efficiency with high levels of reporter gene expression and low toxicity [11–13]. CDs also serve as promising carriers for anti-cancer drug delivery in tumour therapy [14]. They also have proven suitability as an additive in ophthalmic preparations, and rectal and dermal delivery systems. They are responsible for improving the stability and solubility of various ophthalmic preparations. The problem, however, of decreased bioavailability associated with the use of CDs can be overcome by using viscosity enhancers in the final formulation [15, 16]. They also serve as carriers for peptides, oligonucleotides and proteins because of their cellular interactions. Due to their ability to recognize the surface properties of lipoprotein particles, they have also been explored as diagnostic tools for cholesterol measurement. Recent research has shown greater control of drug release by incorporation of CDs into polymeric drug delivery systems [17].

Cellulose and Hemicellulose

Cellulose is an organic polysaccharide with the formula $(C_6H_{10}O_5)_n$, consisting of a linear chain of several hundred to over ten thousand β (1 → 4) linked D-glucose units [18, 19]. Cellulose is the most abundant organic polymer and is the essential structural component of cell wall in plant cells. The parallel aligned cellulose molecule forms crystalline microfibril that provides mechanical strength and resistance to enzymatic attack. Cellulose is insoluble in water and indigestible by the human body [19, 20]. Cellulose obtained from fibrous materials such as wood and cotton can be mechanically disintegrated to produce powdered cellulose, which has been used in the pharmaceutical industry as filler in tablets. Many cellulose derivatives have been prepared by the hydroxyl moieties on the D-glucopyranose unit of cellulose. Microcrystalline cellulose, cellulose esters, cellulose ethers, and cross linked or graft copolymers are widely used in the pharmaceutical industry.

Microcrystalline cellulose (*MCC*) is mainly used in the pharmaceutical industry as a diluent/binder in tablets for both granulation and direct compression processes. Treating high quality cellulose with hydrochloric acid to the desired level yields purified microcrystalline cellulose which is a partially depolymerized cellulose [21]. Membrane controlled systems or monolithic matrix drug delivery systems obtained from cellulose derivatives provide controlled release of drugs. Film coating techniques are employed for the manufacture of membrane controlled release systems, which include enteric coated dosage forms and semi-permeable membranes in osmotic pump delivery systems.

Hydroxypropylmethylcellulose (*HPMC*) is a partly O-methylated and O-(2-hydroxypropylated) cellulose ether derivative. It is a widely used cellulose derivative, used as excipient in controlled release drug delivery systems owing to its gel forming properties. *Carboxymethylcellulose* has been employed for controlling the release of soluble drugs; the polymer can sustain release over an extended period of time enabling a zero order release profile [22]. Hydroxypropylmethylcellulose monolithic matrix systems show similar dissolution profiles as a commercial osmotic pump system for glipizide, a drug with low solubility. In addition it provides superior in vivo performance in terms of matrix resistance to the destructive forces within the gastrointestinal tract [23].

Hemicellulose is a heteropolymer consisting of a matrix of polysaccharides, such as arabinoxylans, present along with cellulose in almost all plant cell walls. Unlike cellulose, hemicellulose has a random, amorphous structure with little mechanical strength. Hemicelluloses include xyloglycans, xylans, mannans and glucomannans, and β-(1 → 3, 1 → 4)-glucans [24]. Their extraction from the plant cell wall is carried out with the aid of strong alkali. Hemicellulose consists of shorter chains and 500–3,000 sugar units. It is branched, unlike cellulose which is unbranched. Hemicelluloses have β-(1 → 4)-linked backbones with an equatorial configuration. Although xyloglycans have a similar backbone as cellulose, they contain xylose branches in 3 of every 4 glucose monomers, while the β-1, 4-linked D-xylan backbone of arabinoxylan contains arabinose branches [25].

Starch

Starch is a common polysaccharide that is found mainly in plants. Starch acts as a storage material in plants. Chemically, it is composed of recurring units of glucopyranose in an alpha D-(1,4) linkage. It is comprised of two polymers, namely *amylose* (a non-branching helical polymer consisting of α-1, 4 linked D-glucose monomers) and *amylopectin* (a highly branched polymer consisting of both α-1, 4 and α-1, 6 linked D-glucose monomers), on hydrolysis it yields the monosaccharide, glucose [26].

> Usually, a plasticizer is added to starch to overcome brittleness and to make it easily processed. The amount of plasticizer added determines final physical properties of starch. Generally water is the common plasticizer used. Other plasticizers like low molecular weight alcohols are added to produce thermoplastic starches.

This abundantly available polymer has been investigated for various biomedical applications such as scaffolds for bone tissue engineering applications, bone cements, and as drug delivery systems. Starch based microparticles and fiber mesh scaffolds are used as carriers for osteoblasts, bone marrow stromal cells and endothelial cells facilitating bone tissue engineering and vascularization [26]. Moreover, starch is blended with other natural or synthetic polymers to improve properties and make it suitable for various applications. For instance, starch–alginate beads were developed to obtain a detained release of model peptide drug phenylalanine. The release of drugs can be altered by the number of alginate coatings outside the bead. Similarly, blends of starch with other polymers like poly lactic acid, polycaprolactone, polyethylene have been researched for various specific indications. These modified derivatives of starch exhibit altered properties related to degradation profile and physical properties of the polymer [27–29].

Inulin

Inulins are a group of naturally occurring polysaccharides produced by many types of plants including onion, garlic, chicory, and artichoke. Chicory acts as a major source for industrial production. They belong to a group of carbohydrates known as fructans. Structurally, inulins consist of 2 to more than 60 fructose molecules linked by β-2, 1-bonds and a glucosyl unit at the reducing end. Due to its ability to maintain inertness in upper GIT, it is applicable in developing colon specific drug delivery systems. It is degraded by colonic microflora (more specifically, *bifidobacteria*). The rate of degradation of inulin derivatives depend on the degree of substitution. Highly substituted inulin has higher mechanical strength, which in turn slows the degradation process [30].

For colon specific delivery, polysaccharides like inulin, pectin, dextran, etc., remain intact in GIT and show specific digestion and degradation at the colon by microflora in that region. The β-2,1 osidic bonds are not significantly hydrolyzed by enzymes from the endogenous secretion of the human digestive tract. For this purpose, biodegradable colon-specific films were developed in combination with Eudragit® RS. Apart from this, methylated inulin derivatives and inulin-azo hydrogels were investigated for colon specific delivery. Research to enhance the dissolution rate and to control the rate of drug release for poorly water soluble drug *Irbesartan* has proven successful. Inulin and its analog sinistrin are used to help measure kidney function by determining the glomerular filtration rate. Inulin-based glycopolymers have great potentials as cell-targeted drug carriers. Also, inulin is a superior lyoprotectant of PEGylated lipoplexes compared with dextran [30–33].

Pectin

Pectin is a complex heteropolysaccharide, found both in the cell walls of plants and between the cell walls. It is produced commercially as a white to light brown powder, mainly extracted from citrus fruits. Pectins are anionic polysaccharides composed of a backbone of poly-(1-4)-α-D-galacturonic acid [34].

Pectins are commercially available as low methoxy (LM) pectin (degree of esterification (DE) <50 %) and high methoxy (HM) pectin (DE > 50 %). LM pectins form a gel in the presence of divalent ions such as Ca^{2+}, and can gel in the absence of Ca^{2+} when the pH is below about 3.3.

Pectin remains intact in the upper GIT and is degraded by colonic microflora, which makes it suitable for designing colon specific drug delivery systems administered via oral route [35, 36]. Amidated pectins in which some of the carboxylic acid groups are amidated are more tolerant to pH variations. They are used to develop a multiparticulate system (hydrogel beads) for site specific delivery to the colon [37]. The properties of this system can be altered using chitosan, which controls the release rate of the drug [38]. The potential of in situ gelling xyloglucan/pectin mixture has been explored for the oral administration of paracetamol. The reported gelation characteristics of this mixture are a result of a combination of both thermal and ion responsiveness due to a synergistic interaction between these two polymers [39]. There have also been efforts to develop nanocarrier based anti-cancer drug delivery systems. Fabricated pectin nanocarriers loaded with oxaliplatin have been investigated as a potential targeted anticancer-drug therapy by incorporating super paramagnetic iron oxide nanoparticles (SPIONs) [40]. Pectin has also been explored as a carrier to develop an intra gastric floating drug delivery system using calcium pectinate gel (CaPG) beads containing carbonate salts. All the types of pectin (LM, HM, and AM) protect the liposomes against aggregation during storage. Pectin coated liposomes have been investigated as potential drug delivery systems [41]. Other possibilities include pectin–chitin/nano $CaCO_3$ composite scaffolds in tissue engineering and freeze-dried chitosan/pectin nasal inserts for antipsychotic drug delivery [42, 43]. It is used in food industry as a gelling agent particularly in jams and jellies. It is also used in fillings, medicines, sweets, as a stabilizer in fruit juices and milk drinks, and as a source of dietary fiber.

Glucomannan

Konjac glucomannan (KGM) is a straight chained hydrocolloidal polysaccharide of the mannan family. Glucomannan consists of β-1,4 linked D-mannose and D-glucose with an acetyl side chain on some backbone units (8 % branching of glucosyl linkage). The mannose: glucose ratio may differ depending on the source [44]. The presence of *acetyl group* contributes to its swelling capacity and solubility, thus making it a soluble natural polymer with high viscosity and water retaining capacity. *Konjac glucomannan* is the most commonly used glucomannan, which is obtained through the extraction of tubers from the plant *Amorphophallus konjac* belonging to the ulmaceae family.

KGM has been investigated as an excipient for a controlled release drug delivery system with or without combination with other polymers. Modification of the chemical structure is another approach for increasing its effectiveness as an excipient for controlled release delivery devices. The combination of KGM and xanthan gum in matrix tablets has been shown to effectively retard drug release by stabilization of the gel phase of the tablets by a network of intermolecular hydrogen bonds between the two polymers [45]. KGM gels also control the release of theophylline and diltiazem for 8 h, but they are region dependent, since the degree of acetylation changes in KGM [46]. KGM is used to form hydrophilic cylinders and particles for the controlled release of DNA [47]. Cross linked KGM with disodium trimetaphosphate forms cross linking density and enzymatic degradation dependent upon the hydrogel system with sustained release of hydrocortisone [45]. The use of a drug binding effector like graphene oxide to functionalize hydrogel based on KGM/sodium alginate has been found to effectively control the release rate of 5-Fluorouracil. Gels based on copolymers of KGM with acrylic acid have been investigated for colon specific drug delivery. A pulsatile capsule based on KGM/HPMC/lactose has also been designed to deliver 5-ASA specifically to the colon.

Guar Gum

Guar gum, also called *guaran*, is a galactomannan and a non-ionic polysaccharide obtained from the seeds of *Cyamopsis tetragonolobus* and is composed of mannose and galactose sugars. It consists of a linear backbone with (1, 4) mannose residues to which 1, 6-linked galactose residues are linked to every second mannose, thereby forming short side branches on the backbone [48]. DAVANAT®, a modified version of guar-gum, is being developed by Pro-pharmaceuticals, Inc. It is not affected by ionic strength but is sensitive to changes in pH and temperature extremes. The pH of 1 % w/v aqueous dispersion varies from 5 to 7. Strong acids and strong alkaline conditions tend to reduce viscosity due to acid/base catalytic reactions. It is dispersed in hot and cold water, and forms a highly viscous thixotropic gel. It is insoluble in organic solvents [49].

Guar-gum exhibits potential applications in various industries such as pharmaceutical formulations, cosmetic, food, textile industries, etc. This hydro colloidal agent is used as a binder and disintegrant in solid dosage forms, and as a suspending, thickening and stabilizing agent in liquid formulations [48]. It is a non-toxic, biodegradable polysaccharide applicable for colon targeting drug delivery, controlled matrix for intestinal delivery of peptides, potential hydrophilic carrier for oral controlled release for drugs with variable solubility, site specific targeting interpenetrating network hydrogels formed from cross-linked guar gum derivatives, and as a compression coat [50, 51]. Synthetic derivatives of hydrogels like guar acetate, guar phthalate, and guar acetate phthalate have been investigated for various pharmaceutical applications. Low-swelling index derivatives of guar-gum are used to retard premature drug release. Such derivatives are obtained by cross-linking gum with glutaraldehyde/trisodiumtrimetaphosphate. These derivatives have been explored for colon specific targeting. The properties of swelling (to retard the drug release in gastric environment) and ability to release the drug at colon (by enzymatic degradation of polymer by colonic microflora) make it a potential material for colon specific delivery [51, 52]. There are potential applications of this polysaccharide: hydrogel based on acryloyl guar gum as a carrier for the slow release of L-DOPA and L-tyrosine, hydrophilic carrier for metoprolol tartarate, trimetazidine hydrochloride etc., pH sensitive hydrogels based on guar-gum/poly (acrylic acid), poly (N-Iso propyl acrylamide), glutaraldehyde cross-linked derivatives, alginate-guar gum based controlled matrix delivery system for delivery of bovine serum albumin (BSA), and colon targeted system of 5-Fluorouracil [50, 51, 53–57]. Other applications include use as a thickener in toothpaste, conditioner in shampoos, and retardation of ice crystal growth.

Arabinogalactan

Arabinogalactan (AG) is a highly branched natural polysaccharide comprised of arabinose and galactose monosaccharides present in furanose configuration. This biopolymer is obtained from both plant (*Larix occidentalis*) and microbial origin. The arabinan portion of the polymer is a complex branched structure possessing α-(1–3), α-(1–5), and β-(1–2) glycosidic linkages, usually capped with mycolic acids. The microbial AG is a major structural component of the mycobacterial cell wall. It is often found attached to proteins. The resulting arabinogalactan protein (AGP) functions as an intercellular signaling molecule. AGPs belong to a class of glycoproteins with a hydroxyproline-rich core protein along with arabinose and galactose-rich polysaccharide units [58–60].

The high water solubility, biocompatibility, biodegradability, and the ease of chemical modification in aqueous media make it a potential material for development of scaffolds applicable in tissue engineering. The oxidized polymer is cross linked with polyamines like chitosan, spermine, and spermidine to form three dimensional scaffolds. The degree of oxidation alters the pore size and degradation rate of these scaffolds. *AG-chitosan sponges* were found to exhibit high swelling behavior in aqueous media; they have suitable pore size for cell growth. This polysaccharide has been explored for hepatic drug delivery [61]. AG has properties that make it suitable as a carrier for delivering diagnostic or therapeutic agents to hepatocytes via the asialoglycoprotein receptor. This polymer also plays a role as a carrier for drug formulations [62]. For instance amphotericin-B (AM-B), a standard antifungal agent, is conjugated to both AG and AGP and investigated in two different studies. These conjugates show increased stability and solubility of AM-B in aqueous media and also reduced toxicity with a high degree of biocompatibility [62–65]. Apart from pharmaceutical applications, it possesses some other industrial uses. It is a major component of many gums, including gum arabic and gum ghatti. Gum arabic finds its application as a valuable additive in the food and candy industries. The extent to which the AGPs in gum arabic are responsible for remarkable properties has yet to be investigated.

Carrageenan

Carrageenans belong to a family of natural linear sulfated carbohydrates extracted from red edible seaweeds. Carrageenans are formed by alternate units of D-galactose and 3, 6-anhydro-galactose (3, 6-AG) joined by α-1, 3 and β-1, 4-glycosidic linkage. There are different types of carrageenans, which are classified according to their differences in solubility, ester sulphate content and amount of 3, 6-AG. Among λ, κ, ι, ε, μ, types kappa, iota, lambda types are major kinds [66–68].

- **Kappa** forms strong, rigid gels in the presence of potassium ions. It has an ester sulfate content of about 25–30 % and a 3, 6-AG content of about 28–35 %. κ is soluble in hot solution.
- **Iota** forms soft gels in the presence of calcium ions. It has an ester sulfate content of about 28–30 % and a 3, 6-AG content of about 25–30 %.
- **Lambda** does not gel and is used to thicken dairy products. It has an ester sulfate content of about 32–39 % and *no content of 3, 6-AG*. λ-type is readily soluble in cold or hot aqueous solution. λ-carrageenan exhibits the highest antioxidant and free radical scavenging activity.

Commercially, it is available as salts of sodium, potassium, calcium or a mixture of these, which in turn determines the physical properties of carrageenan. These salts are generally water soluble and form highly viscous solutions. Viscosity depends on the type of carrageenan, molecular weight, concentration, temperature, and the presence of other solutes. It is depolymerised at low pH (especially pH $\leq$3.0) by hydrolysis of glycosidic linkages at high temperature [69].

They are widely used in the food industry for their gelling, thickening, and stabilizing properties. Their main application is in dairy and meat products due to their strong binding to food proteins. λ and κ combine easily with milk proteins to improve solubility and texture. Carrageenan-induced rat paw edema is a widely used animal model to determine anti-inflammatory activity for evaluation of pain [69]. They have been investigated for use in delivery systems for controlled release of drugs [70]. Gelatin–carageenan hydrogel loaded with Quercetin, cross linked carageenan beads for controlled drug release, temperature responsive κ-carageenan angels, buckle drug delivery by lyophilized wafers comprising carageenan and pluronics acid, trans-sclera delivery of macromolecules by carageenan/methylcellulose polymeric systems, carboxy-methylated kappa-carageenan for intestinal-targeted delivery of bioactive macromolecules, microparticles based on lection-functionalized carboxy-methylated kappa-carageenan for oral insulin delivery, and carageenan–gelatin mucoadhesive systems for ion-exchange based ophthalmic delivery all prove the potential of this sulfated Polyglactin in versatile areas [66, 67, 70–75].

Protein Based Polymers

Soy Bean

The soy or soya bean is rich in protein (40–50 %), carbohydrates (26–30 %), and lipids (20–30 %). It is obtained from an annual plant, *Glycine max*, a species of legume native. Soy flour, soy concentrate and soy isolate are different soy bean products with different protein content among which isolated soy protein has the highest protein proportion (90 %) on dry weight basis. The major soy proteins in the isolate are *glycine* or 11S and *β-conglycinin* or 7S; it also contains isoflavones like *genistein* and *daidzein* [76]. There are many desirable characteristics associated with this protein, which makes it an excellent material of investigation for making drug delivery devices and tissue engineering applications. Soy bean exhibits excellent thermal stability, hydrolytic stability, melt processability, storage stability, biodegradability, and abundant availability, all of which make it an adaptable material for various purposes [77]. Soy bean also exhibits tailoring flexibility where the degree of cross linking can be modified to make it suitable for a particular purpose. Highly versatile properties of soy protein based thermoplastics make them suitable for many biomedical applications [78]. Soy protein based double layered control delivery devices have also been investigated [77].

Transgenic Plant Based Collagen

Collagen is a group of naturally occurring proteins present in the form of fibrils and forms a major part of the connective tissue. This is generally derived from animal sources, but collagen derived from these sources exhibits immunogenicity. Type I human collagen obtained from transgenic tobacco is a breakthrough technology invented by *Collplant Ltd.* of NesTziyona, Israel. There are several challenges to be met, for example development of transgenic tobacco plants that are able to develop human collagen, and extraction methods successfully overcome by *Collplant* from this new source. This development requires high-level genetic engineering combined with general plant genetics [79]. Plant engineering based pharmaceuticals are feasible alternatives to conventional fermentation based expression models. Vergenix™ wound dressing, a tobacco-derived collagen sponge, is used for chronic wounds and skin ulcers (pressure sores and diabetic wounds). Collagen plays a major role from medical devices to tissue repair [80]. A detailed review of collagen types and their applications is given in later sections.

Polyesters from Higher Plants

Polyesters, namely cutin and suberin, respectively present in epidermal cell walls and the inner periderm layer in the higher plants protect them from physical, chemical, and biological factors in the environment. These are glycerolipid polymers associated with cell walls in higher plants. Cutin, an insoluble cuticular polymer, is composed of hydroxy and hydroxy epoxy fatty acids, whereas suberin is composed of aromatic and aliphatic domains. These polyesters are degraded by enzymatic degradation/alkaline hydrolysis of ester linkages. These polyesters allow the tailoring of specific properties, making them suitable for drug delivery applications. Abundant availability, sustainability, renewability and biodegradability are some of the desirable characteristics of these biopolymers [81].

Natural Polymers of Animal Origin

Polysaccharide Based Polymers

Chitosan

Chitosan is a linear polysaccharide composed of randomly distributed β-linked D-glucosamine and N-acetyl-D-glucosamine. It is a naturally occurring cationic polysaccharide derived by partial N-deacetylation of chitin from shrimp and crustacean shells. The pKa value of chitosan is about 6.2–7; it is insoluble in neutral and alkaline pH solutions. The degradation rate mainly depends on the degree of deacetylation that occurs by hydrolysis of glycosidic links of acetylated residues in the presence of lysozyme. Chitosan adopts a more extended and coiled conformation at a high or low degrees of deacetylation respectively. Chemical modifications due to the presence of amino group at C-2 and primary and secondary hydroxyl groups at C-6 and C-3 improve mechanical properties and impart new biological activities in chitosan. The chief constituent in chitosan is glucosamine, a natural material present in the body and used to produce glycosaminoglycans. Chitosan and its derivatives are the most extensively investigated materials for pharmaceutical and biomedical applications. The cationic property of chitosan imparts key bioactive properties like biodegradability, biocompatibility, and a microbicidal and mucoadhesive nature. Amenability of chitosan to different chemical modifications makes it suitable for a broad range of therapeutic applications. Each modification imparts a different biomedical or pharmaceutical application. For example, sulfated chitosan exhibits antioxidant activity [6, 7, 82, 83].

Chitin consists mostly of N-acetyl-D-glucosamine-unit. Most units are deacetylated to D-glucosamine-units during the preparations of chitosan. Chitosan is a linear polymer of β-D glucopyranose units characterized by a degree of deacetylation. It is structurally similar to cellulose, but it has –$NHCOCH_3$ (acetamide groups) at C-2 position [84].

Key features of chitosan: The amino and hydroxyl groups of chitosan that are chemically modifiable make it a highly versatile molecule for various applications (Table 2.1). The metabolism of chitosan by lysozyme makes it biodegradable. Chitosan exhibits a pH-sensitive behavior as a weak poly-base because of the large quantities of amino groups on its chain. At low pH conditions, the amino groups of chitosan are protonated and exhibit pH-sensitive swelling.

Table 2.1 Applications of chitosan [82, 86, 87]

Application	Role of chitosan
Biological properties	Wound healing, osteogenesis, biodegradation
Vaccine and drug delivery by chitosan particles:	Mucoadhesive property of chitosan improves the bioavailability of peptide in GIT
1. Peptide drug delivery	Antigen encapsulated chitosan microparticles and nanoparticles
2. Ophthalmic drug delivery	
3. Targeted drug delivery	Promising carriers for nasal and mucosal vaccine delivery
	Cyclosporine A loaded chitosan nanoparticles
	Colon targeting by corticosteroid loaded chitosan microspheres
Gene delivery vehicle	Topical application of plasmid-DNA based chitosan nanoparticles
Regenerative medicine	Chitosan-gelatin wound dressings
	Regeneration of various tissues like skin, bone, liver, cartilage and nerve
Hydrogels	Chitosan/β-glycerophosphate hydrogel loaded with anti cancer agents against breast cancer/cervical cancer

Chitosan dissolves easily at low pH, while it is insoluble at higher pH ranges. Dialdehydecrosslinkers like glyoxal are used to cross link chitosan molecules to modify the properties of the molecules. Glutaraldehyde reduces the antigenicity of the material. Natural crosslinkers like genipin are gaining wide acceptance for crosslinking chitosan. Chitosan is found to be biologically renewable, bioadhesive, biocompatible, biofunctional, nonantigenic, and nontoxic. Chitosan, which is structurally similar to glycosaminoglycan (GAG) found in extracellular matrices (ECM) available in native articular cartilage, plays a key role in modulating chondrocytes morphology, differentiation and function, and has application in cartilage engineering. It also exhibits biosensor and antihyperlipidemic actions [82, 83, 85].

Hyaluronan

Hyaluronic acid (HA), also called hyaluronan, is a high molecular weight (10^5–10^7 Da) naturally occurring biodegradable polymer. This name is derived from “hyalos” (Greek for glass + uric acid). HA is an unbranched non-sulfated glycosaminoglycan (GAG) composed of repeating disaccharides (β-1, 4-D-glucuronic acid (known as uronic acid) and β-1, 3-N-acetyl-D-glucosamide). HA is a polyanion that can self-associate and that can also bind water molecules when not bound to other molecules. HA, one of the major elements in the ECM of vertebrate tissues is also found in almost all body fluids and tissues, such as the synovial fluid, the vitreous humor of the eye, and hyaline cartilage. HA is involved in several important biological functions, such as regulation of cell adhesion and cell motility, manipulation of cell differentiation and proliferation, and providing biomechanical properties of tissues. HA interacts with several cell surface receptors such as CD44, RHAMM, and ICAM-1, and it controls cellular processes including morphogenesis, wound repair, inflammation, and metastasis. HA is responsible for maintenance of viscoelasticity of biofluids (synovial fluid and vitreous humor of the eye) and controlling tissue hydration and water transport [88].

D-glucuronic acid and DN-acetyl glucosamine, in the HA disaccharide structure are connected together through alternative beta-1, 4 and beta-1, 3 glycosidic bonds. The number of repeat disaccharides in a completed hyaluronan molecule can reach 10,000 or more, a molecular mass of ~4 million daltons (each disaccharide is ~400 Da). The average length of a disaccharide is ~1 nm. The structure of the disaccharide is energetically very stable in light of its beta configuration [88].

Key features of hyaluronic acid: HA is naturally synthesized by a class of integral membrane proteins called hyaluronan synthases, of which vertebrates have three types: HAS1, HAS2, and HA. The rheological property (concentration and molecular weight dependent) of HA solutions has made HA ideal for lubrication in biomedical applications. For example, a 1 % solution of high molecular weight HA (Mw $\gtrsim$1,000 kDa) can behave like jelly, but when shear stress is applied it easily shears thin and can be administered via a thin needle. Viscoelasticity is another characteristic of HA, resulting from entanglement and self-association of HA random coils. This property, due to molecular interactions, depends in turn on concentration and molecular weight. Three types of enzymes like hyaluronidase (hyase), β-d-glucuronidase, and β-N-acetyl-hexosaminidase catalyze the enzymatic degradation of HA. Hyase cleaves high molecular weight HA into smaller oligosaccharides, while β-D-glucuronidase and β-N-acetyl hexosaminidase further degrade the oligosaccharide fragments by removing nonreducing terminal sugars. The degradation products of hyaluronan, oligosaccharides and very low molecular weight hyaluronan, exhibit pro-angiogenic properties. By catalyzing the hydrolysis of HA, a major constituent of the interstitial barrier, hyaluronidase lowers the viscosity of HA, thereby increasing tissue permeability. It is, therefore, used in medicine in conjunction with other drugs to speed dispersion and delivery [88]. Applications of HA are represented in Table 2.2.

Chondroitin Sulphate

Chondroitin sulphate (CS), a GAG of the same class as glucosamine, is a disaccharide composed of alternate sequences of differently sulfated residues of D-glucuronic acid (GlcA) and N-acetyl-D-galactosamine (GalNAc) linked by β bonds. Sequences of these disaccharides are formed into polysaccharide chains. Some GlcA residues are epimerized into L-iduronic acid (IdoA); the resulting disaccharide is then referred to as dermatan sulfate. CS found extensively in the extracellular matrix of articular cartilage is obtained by extraction from

Table 2.2 Applications of hyaluronic acid [88, 89]

Application	Role of Hyaluronic Acid
Dermal filler	Recover soft-tissue volume of the skin and remove skin wrinkles
Chondroprotective effects	Effect of a HA injection may be mediated via CD44 interactions
	Potential agent of therapeutic intervention in osteoarthrosis (OA)
Orthopaedic applications	Development of cartilage, the maintenance of the synovial fluid and the regeneration of tendons
	Lubricant and shock absorber
	Viscosupplementation (osteoarthritis treatment)
Antiadhesion applications	Prevent bacterial adhesion to dental implants, intraocular lenses, and catheters
Ophthalmology	HA solutions also serve as a viscosity-enhancing component of eye drops and as an adjuvant to eye tissue repair
Cardiovascular applications	HA increases the blood compatibilities of cardiovascular implants such as vascular grafts and stents. For example, biomaterial surfaces treated with cross-linked HA have been associated with reduced platelet adhesion and thrombus formation

tissues of several animals (bovine, porcine, avian, cartilagenous fishes, etc.). Glycosaminoglycans gather on the core protein and mass attach to HA via a link protein, which makes proteoglycans that are hydrated and resist compression stress. CS chains are linked to hydroxyl groups on serine residues of certain proteins [90].

Key features of chondroitin sulphate: Due to its GAG nature, CS is an attractive natural-origin polymer applied essentially in cartilage tissue engineering. It is non-immunogenic and biodegradable to non-toxic oligosaccharides. These characteristics, together with their defined physical and chemical characteristics, make CS very interesting for tissue engineering. CS can bind with core protein to produce highly absorbent aggregan, which is a major structure inside cartilage and acts as a shock absorber; or, it can produce sydecan, a cell receptor that can interact with adhesion proteins, cells and the extracellular matrix (ECM). CS in negatively charged interaction with positively charged molecules, such as polymers or growth factors, is anticipated to become a key element to facilitate the design of delivery systems. For instance, this characteristic is used to produce chondroitin sulfate–chitosan sponges as delivery systems for platelet-derived growth factor-BB (PDGF-BB) for bone regeneration [90].

Applications of chondroitin sulphate [91].

1. *Chondroprotective effects*: CS exhibit chondroprotective effects through three main mechanisms-stimulation of ECM production by chondrocytes, suppression of inflammatory mediators, and inhibiting cartilage degeneration. Thus, CS plays a key role in the treatment of osteoarthritis. It also exhibits bone regeneration effects.
2. *Anti-inflammatory effects*: CS acts as an anti-inflammatory agent by inhibition of nuclear translocation of nuclear factor-kappaB (NF-kappaB) which is associated with pro-inflammatory activity.

Protein Based Polymers

Collagen

The role of collagen is essential. It is one of the most abundant mammalian proteins accounting for about 20–30 % of total body proteins available in extracellular matrix and tissues of primarily mechanical function. Its mode of interaction in the body and biological features such as excellent biocompatibility, weak antigenicity, formation of fibres through self-aggregation and cross-linking distinguish it from other available synthetic and natural polymers. These two amino acids allow for differentiation between collagen and other protein hydrolysates. Although collagen is the most preferred biomaterial, some disadvantages of collagen-based systems stem from the difficulty of assuring adequate supplies, poor mechanical strength, and ineffectiveness in the management of infected sites [92, 93].

Types of collagen and their occurrence: Collagen can be obtained from porcine, bovine, equine, human or other sources. It offers many biomedical applications. Collagen is synthesized by fibroblasts, which usually originate from pluripotential adventitial or reticulum cells. The spectrum of amino acids resulting from the hydrolysis of collagen differs greatly from that of other proteins by its high content of glycine and proline and low content of histidine, tryptophan and cystine. Collagen also contains two amino acids not found in other proteins, hydroxyproline and hydroxylysine. The properties of collagen that make it suitable for various indications are dependent upon characteristics of amino acid composition and sequence [92, 94].

This fibrous, structural protein comprises a right-handed bundle of three parallel, left-handed polyproline II-type helices. In animals, individual collagen triple helices, known as tropocollagen (TC), assemble in a complex, hierarchical manner that ultimately leads to the macroscopic fibers and networks observed in tissue, bone, and basement membranes. Although the three polypeptide chains in the triple helix of each collagen type can be identical, heterotrimeric triple helices are more prevalent than homotrimeric triple helices. The categories of collagen include classic fibrillar and network-forming collagens, FACITs (fibril-associated collagens with interrupted triple helices), MACITs (membrane associated collagens with interrupted triple helices), and MULTIPLEXINs (multiple triple-helix domains and interruptions). Twenty-nine different types of collagen composed of at least 46 distinct polypeptide chains have been identified in vertebrates. Many other proteins contain collagenous domains [94, 95]. Table 2.3 represents types of collagen.

Degradation of collagen: Collagen is particularly resistant to attack by neutral proteases, probably due to its function as the primary structural protein in the body. At neutral pH only specific collagenases (i.e., zinc containing metalloproteinases) cleave the native helix at a position about three quarters of the way from the N-terminus. Fibrils as aggregates of collagen molecules are degraded starting from the exterior. Collagenase binds tightly to triple-helices at or near the surface, whereas molecules in the interior become accessible to enzymes in the course of progressive degradation from the outside. After the triple-helix is cracked, further degradation of collagen molecules is facilitated by enzymes such as gelatinases and non-specific proteinases, which cleave the primary fragments into small peptides and amino acids [97].

Table 2.3 Types of collagen [96]

Category	Types of collagen
Fibril-forming collagens	Type I, II, III, V, XI
Basement membrane collagen	Type IV
Microfibrillar collagen	Type VI
Anchoring fibrils	Type VII
Hexagonal network forming collagen	Type VIII, X
FACIT collagens	Type IX, XII, XIV, XIX, XX, XXI
Transmembrane collagens	Type XIII, XVII
Multiplexins	Type XV, XVI, XVIII

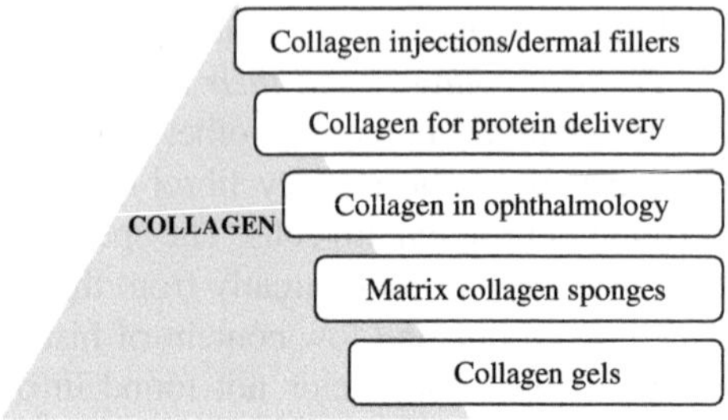

Fig. 2.3 Applications of collagen

Applications of collagen [95, 98, 99]

Collagen is the main structural protein in vertebrates. It plays an essential role by acting as a scaffold for cellular support; it is thereby responsible for maintaining cell attachment, migration, proliferation, differentiation, and survival. As such, it also plays an important role in numerous approaches to the engineering of human tissues for medical applications related to tissue, bone, skin repair, and reconstruction (Fig. 2.3).

Gelatin

Gelatin is defined as a product obtained by the partial hydrolysis of collagen derived from the skin, white connective tissue, and bones of animals. Gelatin is also defined as the product obtained from the acid, alkaline, or enzymatic hydrolysis of collagen, the chief protein component of the skin, bones, and connective tissue of animals, including fish and poultry. Gelatin derived from an acid-treated precursor is known as Type A and gelatin derived from an alkali-treated process is known as Type B. It does not occur free in nature, and it cannot be recovered from horns, hoofs and other noncollagen-containing parts of vertebrate animals. There are no plant sources of gelatin, and there is no chemical relationship between gelatin and other materials referred to as vegetable gelatin, such as seaweed extracts. Gelatin is an important material with application in the food, pharmaceutical and photographic industries as well as diverse technical uses [100].

There are two main gelatin types, referred to as A-(or acid) type and B-(or limed/alkaline) type. This categorization essentially goes back to the pre-treatment of the raw material which will affect the characteristics of the gelatin extracted. Typical differences are the Iso-electrical point (as explained below), as well as viscosity in solution. Type A gelatin has a broad isoelectric range between pH 7 and 9. Type B has a narrower isoelectric range between pH 4.7 and 5.4. It consists of a distribution of polypeptide fragments of different sizes. Gel strength is expressed in (gram) Bloom. Commercial gelatins may vary from low Bloom (<150) and medium Bloom (150–220) to high Bloom (>220) types.

Physicochemical properties of gelatin vary depending on method of extraction, amount of thermal denaturation employed, and electrolyte content of the resulting material. The viscosity of a gelatin solution depends on the type of gelatin, the bloom value, concentration, and temperature of gelatin in solution. Gelatin is sensitive to degradation as long as no gel has been formed. The possible degree of degradation depends on several parameters such as pH, temperature, time, and concentration [91, 100]. Gel strength, which is expressed in gram Bloom, ranges from 80 to 280 Bloom for commercial gelatins:

(A) 80–150 Bloom: low Bloom range
(B) 150–220 Bloom: medium Bloom range
(C) 250–280 Bloom: high Bloom range

Gelatin gels have a thermo-reversible character with a setting point always roughly 5 °C lower than the melting point. For alkaline gelatins, the iso-electric point is almost constant and thus independent of the Bloom value: the IEP is between pH 4.8 and 5.2. The IEP of acid type gelatins is linked to the Bloom value and ranges from about 7 (low Bloom) to about 9 (high Bloom), which means that an acid type gelatin always has a positive charge in a food system [91, 100].

Applications of gelatin [91, 100]: Gelatin has shown to be useful in a great number of fields:

1. Gelatin possesses hemostatic application which produces hemostasis by accelerating the clotting process of blood.
    - Gelfoam (Pharmacia & Upjohn)
    - Surgifoam (Ethicon)
    - Floseal matrix (Baxter healthcare)
2. Capsular material
3. Food industry (gel former, thickening agent, protective colloid)
4. Photographic industry
5. Other technical uses (microencapsulation)

Albumin

Albumins are a family of globular proteins, the most common of which is serum albumin. The albumin family consists of all proteins that are water-soluble, are moderately soluble in concentrated salt solutions, and experience heat denaturation. Albumins are commonly found in blood plasma; they are unique from other blood proteins in that they are not glycosylated. Substances containing albumins, such as egg white, are called albuminoids. Commercially, albumins are obtained insignificant quantities from egg white (ovalbumin), bovine serum (bovine serum albumin, BSA), and human serum (human serum albumin, HSA). They are also available from soybeans, milk, and grains [101–103].

(a) *Ovalbumin*: It has a molecular weight of 47,000 Da and isoelectric point (pI) of 4.8. Due to its pH- and temperature-sensitive properties, it has a high potential for use as a carrier for controlled drug release.
(b) *Bovine serum albumin* (*BSA*) has a molecular weight of 69,323 Da and an isoelectric point (pI) of 4.7 in water. It is widely chosen for drug delivery because of its medical importance, abundance, low cost, and ease of purification.
(c) *Human serum albumin* (*HSA*): This is the most abundant globular monomeric protein with an average half-life of 19 days and molecular weight of 66,500 Da. When HSA is broken down, the amino acids provide nutrition to peripheral tissues. It acts as a substitute to BSA in case of immunogenic responses [101, 102].

Recombinant human serum albumin (Recombumin), an alternative to blood derived albumin, has been developed. A genetically engineered protein expressed in yeast cells has been found, and it shows comparable safety, tolerability, pharmacokinetics, and pharmacaodynamics to native HSA. Albumin is an acidic, very soluble protein that is extremely robust. It is stable in the pH range of 4–9, soluble in 40 % ethanol, and can be heated at 60 °C for up to 10 h without significant effects. These properties as well as its preferential uptake in tumor and inflamed tissue, its ready availability, its biodegradability, and its lack of toxicity and immunogenicity make it an ideal candidate for drug delivery. Serum albumins are important in regulating blood volume by maintaining oncotic pressure (also known as colloid osmotic pressure) of the blood compartment. Recombumin also serves as a carrier for molecules of low water solubility, thus isolating their hydrophobic nature, including lipid soluble hormones, bile salts, unconjugated bilirubin, free fatty acids (apoprotein), calcium, ions (transferrin), and some drugs. Albumin molecules with the presence of different drug binding sites can entrap a significant amount of drug into the particle matrix. Albumin, being non-toxic, non-immunogenic, and with other favorable properties like greater stability and ease of preparation, makes it an excellent candidate for nanoparticulate delivery systems [101, 104].

Applications of albumin [99, 101, 102, 104–107].

1. Albumin as a drug carrier: This macromolecule finds its potential in providing various formulation strategies like drug conjugates, albumin binding drug derivatives, nanoparticles and drug adducts. Being a macromolecule, it shows

an EPR (enhanced permeability and retention) effect in the case of tumors. As the pore size of tumor micro vessels varies from 100 to 1,200 nm in diameter, macromolecules (e.g., serum albumin have an effective diameter of 7.2 nm) employed as carriers for the development of macromolecular prodrugs, allows extravasation into tumor tissue but not into normal tissue. Albumin exhibits various key roles by:

(a) Improving the pharmacokinetic profile of a peptide molecule with the help of three advanced albumin based technologies: albumin fusion, drug affinity complex, and preformed conjugate drug affinity complex.
(b) Development of fatty acid derivative of peptide (myristic acid derivative of insulin) and conjugating it to albumin due to the presence of fatty acid binding sites on it also improves the stability profile of peptide.

2. It acts as a vehicle for the transport of metals, fatty acids, cholesterol, bile pigments, and drugs. It is a key element in the regulation of osmotic pressure and distribution of fluid between different compartments.
3. 99mTc macroaggregated albumin has been used diagnostically for various indications including lymphoscintigraphy sentinel node detection in breast cancer and other solid tumors, as well as rheumatoid arthritis.
4. Nab technology (albumin based nanotechnology) is ideal for encapsulating lipophilic drugs into nanoparticles. An example is Nab-Paclitaxel (Abraxane) an FDA approved formulation for the treatment of breast cancer.
5. Albumin, the most abundant circulating protein in the plasma, exerts important antioxidant activities due to its free radical binding capacity.

The different uses of albumin as a drug carrier that have emerged so far are fascinating and range from extending the half-life of therapeutically active proteins and peptides (e.g., Albuferon Levemir) and drug targeting (e.g., MTX-HSA, Abraxane). The development and market approval of the paclitaxel albumin nanoparticle, Abraxane, can be viewed as a landmark for Nab-technology. Albumin offers many other interesting perspectives such as photodynamic therapy, artificial blood substitute, and ultrasound mediated drug release etc., which are yet to be explored.

Fibrin

Fibrin is a non-globular protein obtained from fibrinogen by the action of thrombin. It is also known as *Factor Ia* which plays a crucial role in blood clotting mechanism. Commercially, fibrinogen and thrombin are available from different sources including human. These preparations are used to produce required fibrin. Homologous fibrin sealant systems are also readily available which are used to produce autologous fibrin components from blood plasma. Tisseel VH® (*Baxter, Deerfield, Illinois, USA*), Cryoseal® (*Thermo Genesis, Rancho Cordova, California, USA*), Vivostat® (*Vivolution, Alleroed, Denmark*) are examples of commercially available fibrin sealant systems [76]. Even autologous thrombin obtained from a single donor can be utilized in producing fibrin components without any immunological and infectious effects [108]. The desirable characteristics of high adhesive and tensile strengths, biocompatibility and resorption make them applicable as sealants, hemostatic systems, bioadhesive, and matrix delivery systems [109]. The concentrations of fibrinogen and thrombin, local pH, and ionic strength influence various characteristics of fibrin clot like adhesive strength, strand strength, permeability, and stability of fibrin components. Varying the above parameters makes specific fibrin components fit for a particular application. Low concentration of thrombin produces loosely woven fibrin strands, whereas higher concentration of thrombin produces tightly woven strands of fibrin [76].

These fibrin components find their application in tissue engineering and controlled matrix systems for cell delivery. Due to their ability to improve cellular interactions, fibrin gels, beads, and scaffolds have been used for vascularization, peripheral nerve regeneration, and bone and cartilage engineering purposes. Rapid degradation of these fibrin matrices, however, presents a problem with shape-specific scaffolds, which can be overcome by optimization of fibrin composition [76]. Its physical and biomimetic characteristics allow fibrin gel to be used as a carrier in cell delivery. The bioavailability and controlled release of bone morphogenetic proteins (BMPs) can be achieved by using heparin loaded fibrin-fibronectin matrix in which heparin acts as reservoir for BMPs released by the gel degradation mechanism [110]. The approach of grafting fibrin matrix with the help of 2-Hydroxy ethyl methacrylate has been explored for wound healing in burn victims; and it has shown to have better healing efficiency than non-grafted matrices [111]. The ease of injectability and ability to avoid immunogenic reactions by autologous fibrin component makes it successful in demonstrating neovascularization, and myocardial regeneration in infracted myocardium using bone marrow mononuclear cell (BMMNCs) in incorporated fibrin implantation matrix [112]. The investigation of freeze dried tetracycline loaded fibrin disc as a biodegradable matrix for local antibiotic therapy demonstrates its suitability as a drug delivery implant [113]. Adipose derived stem cell (ADSCs) therapy is under investigation for future regenerative medicines, where the fibrin gel matrices are used as carriers for ADSCs [114]. The above instances explain the potential applications of this fibrous, non-globular protein.

Silk Fibroin

Silk fibroin is a fibrous protein obtained by the larvae of *Bombyx mori*, other moth genera such as *Antheraea, Cricula,* and many other insects. The silk protein obtained from spiders and silk worms produces the toughest and strongest fibres [115]. Silkworms produce silk whose main components are fibroin and sericin amongst which fibroin constitutes the core of silk, and sericin is glue like protein surrounding the core. Fibroin is composed of various components like fibroin H-chain (FH), fibroin L-chain (FL), and fibro hexamerin. Even transgenic silk worms are developed to produce the modified versions of fibroin, i.e., gene encoding fibroin L-chain fused with basic fibroblast growth factor (bFGF). This is used to produce fibroin layers which are composed of natural fibroin protein and recombinant bFGF. These scaffolds have been investigated for seeding endothelial cells; the results suggest the use of this scaffold in tissue engineering [76]. The source of silk and the processing conditions influence certain properties of silk fibroin like conformation of protein, molecular weight, and amino-acid composition. These properties in turn have an impact on mechanical and biological properties such as the pore size of scaffold, cell adhesion, and inflammatory mediator production.

The properties of biocompatibility, slow biodegradability, mechanical strength, and elasticity make them suitable as surgical sutures, carriers in tissue engineering, drug delivery, artificial tendons, and coatings for metallic medicinal implants [116]. Electrospun nano fibres made from chitin and fibroin are applicable as tissue engineering scaffolds [115]. Novel nanocomposites of biocompatible hydroxyapatite-silk fibroin have been investigated as coatings on metallic (titanium) orthopaedic implants which showed improved physicochemical and biological properties [116]. Poly (D,L-lactic acid) modified with silk fibroin and silk fibroin modified with peptide sequences enhance cell adhesion ability. 3-D porous silk fibroin matrix scaffolds have been investigated in cartilage tissue engineering [117]. One of the interesting subjects in the field of tissue reconstruction is the use of adipose-derived stem cells incorporated silk fibroin–chitosan (SFCS) scaffold [118]. Regenerated silk fibroin (RSF) and galactosylated chitosan (GalCS) scaffolds have been explored for *hepatic* tissue engineering applications; they demonstrated superiority in hepatocyte growth, viability, and metabolic activity [119]. Regenerated silk fibroin has also been investigated for immobilization of enzymes like *peroxidase* [120].

Polymeric Resin

Shellac

Shellac is a natural bioadhesive resin secreted by lac insects (*Lacciferlacca*). It consists mainly of esters of aleuritic acid, butolic acid, jalaric acid, and shellolic acid. Due to its desirable film forming and protective properties, shellac has been used in food and pharmaceutical products. It has been reported as an excipient in the development of matrix tablets for oral controlled release. It is also used in sugar-coating and enteric coating applications. High dissolution pH of shellac makes it suitable for colon delivery applications, whereas when used for enteric coating, additives that enhance drug release must accompany shellac [121, 122]. Lower stability of shellac makes it less attractive; however methods to enhance stability to make it suitable for various applications have been developed. For instance, formation of composite film with gelatin inhibits the polymerization of shellac and thereby enhances the stability of the resin [123].

Natural Polymers of Microbial Origin

Polysaccharides

Alginate

Alginates are linear, anionic, water soluble heteropolysaccharides that form the cell wall constituents of brown algae like *Laminaria sp.*, *Macrocystis sp.*, *Lessonia sp.*, belonging to the family Phaeophyceae. Alginates can be used to develop delivery systems for cationic polyelectrolytes and proteoglycans through simple electrostatic interactions due to its pH dependent anionic nature. It contains blocks of (1–4)-linked β-D-mannuronic acid (M) and α ± -L-guluronic acid (G) monomers, generally composed of three different forms of polymer segments: consecutive G residues, consecutive M residues, and alternating MG residues [124].

The relative composition of guluronic to mannuronic acid residues within an alginate sample determines the strength of the complex which in turn influences the properties of designed delivery systems. Alginates forms more rigid and porous gels with a high guluronic acid content and randomly packed and less porous gels with low guluronic acid content.

The design of an alginate based delivery system is based on the sol-gel transition behavior of alginate in the presence of divalent cations like calcium, strontium, and barium. After this reaction, the water solubility of monovalent alginate is decreased and is converted to water insoluble salt. Alginic acid, its sodium, potassium, ammonium and calcium salts, and propylene glycol alginate have been given INS numbers of 400–405 (E400–E405 in the EU). These salts have many applications in the food, textile, and pharmaceutical industries. For example, sodium alginate is being widely used as an emulsifier, stabilizer, and as an additive in dairy product preparation competing with carrageenan. On the other hand, calcium alginate being water insoluble has been widely employed in the textile industry, production of bandages for wound healing, and preparation of beads to encapsulate certain chemicals in the presence of sodium alginate and calcium chloride solution. The glycosidic linkages of alginates are susceptible to both acid (acid hydrolysis) and alkali (alkaline β-elimination). No alginate degrading enzymes exist in humans, whereas alginate lyases that catalyze the beta-elimination of alginates are found in bacteria. Degradation of alginate chains applied as biomaterials in vivo takes place only by spontaneous beta-elimination.

Moreover, the degradation rate and mechanical properties of alginate-based biomaterials is influenced by the molecular weight (MW) of alginate. Basically, higher MW polymers exhibit a slower degradation rate due to the reduced number of reactive positions susceptible for hydrolysis.

Alginates form a distinct family of polysaccharides that allows tailoring of a variety of biomaterials suitable for tissue engineering. They have been investigated to develop different delivery vehicles like hydrogels, microspheres, microcapsules, sponges, foams, and fibers applicable in regeneration medicine, nutrition supplements, semi permeable separation, and repair and regeneration of various tissues and organs such as skin, cartilage and bone. The pH sensitivity of alginate based hydrogel is applied in the design of oral delivery of peptide or protein drugs. So far, alginates have been investigated for the entrapment of several proteins like IgG, fibrinogen, insulin, melatonin, heparin, hemoglobin, vaccines, etc. This polymer was blended with another natural polysaccharide like guar gum to overcome the rapid dissolution of alginate at high pH, a major limitation during delivery of peptide drugs. Use of alginate based delivery systems for the delivery of cell induction ligands, bioactive signaling molecules, functional DNAs or siRNAs proves the significance of this polyanionic polysaccharide [53, 72, 124].

Dextran

Dextrans are hydrophilic polysaccharides characterized by their moderate to high molecular weight, good water solubility, low toxicity, and immunogenicity. Dextran is synthesized from sucrose by enzymatic conversion with help of *dextransucrase* present in certain lactic-acid bacteria, the best-known being Leuconostoc *mesenteroides* and Streptococcus *mutans*. Dextran obtained from Leuconostoc *mesenteroides* consists of α (1–6)-linked glucan comprising of side chains linked to the 3-positions of the backbone glucose units which is being commercially developed. Generally it is a complex, branched glucan (polysaccharide made of many glucose molecules) composed of chains of varying lengths in which the straight chain consists of α -1,6 glycosidic linkages between glucose molecules, while branches begin from α -1,3 linkages. Due to their uncommon poly-(α-D-1, 6-glucose) linkages, they are resistant to cleavage by most endogenous cellular glycosidases. The physical and chemical properties of dextrans vary depending upon the source from which it is obtained and the type of production method [125, 126].

Dextrans are classified into three classes based on the structural features:

- **Class 1 dextrans** contain the α (1 → 6)-linked D-glucopyranosyl backbone modified with small side chains of D-glucose branches with α (1 → 2), α (1 → 3), and α (1 → 4)-linkage.
- **Class 2 dextrans** (alternans) contain a backbone structure of alternating α (1 → 3) and α (1 → 6)-linked D-glucopyranosyl units with α (1 → 3)-linked branches.
- **Class 3 dextrans** (mutans) have a backbone structure of consecutive α (1 → 3)-linked D-glucopyranosyl units with α (1 → 6)-linked branches.

Dextran is used as an antithrombotic (anti-platelet) to reduce blood viscosity and as a volume expander in anemia. The antithrombotic effect of dextran is due to its capacity to bind with erythrocytes, platelets, and vascular endothelium, thus reducing aggregation of erythrocytes and adhesiveness of platelets. Dextran is used as a blood substitute in case of emergency and as a lubricant in eye drops. It is used to treat hypovolemia that can result from severe blood loss after surgery, injury, or other causes of bleeding. Other uses include immobilization in biosensors, fluorescent labeled dextran for endosomal identification under fluorescent microscope, and anterograde and retrograde tracers in neurons. Dextran also finds application in the design of colloidal drug delivery systems. Nanoparticles prepared from dextran sulfate and quaternized chitosan are being investigated for the delivery of protein drugs to protect the protein molecule from the harsh environment of the stomach [127]. On the other hand, dextran is being explored as an excellent material for colon-specific drug delivery. Glutaraldehydes cross linked dextran and colon degradable dextran fatty acid esters have been employed for this purpose. In another approach, this is utilized to develop prodrugs which release drugs after degradation by colonic bacteria. Examples are Naproxen-dextran, Ketoprofen-dextran, and Ibuprofen-dextran. Biodegradable dextran hydrogels have also been developed using diisocyanate as a crosslinking agent [125, 128–130].

The property of dextran being degraded by *colonic dextranases* present in anaerobic gram-negative intestinal bacteria is being used to design dextran based colon specific drug delivery systems.

Others

Other bacterial polysaccharides like xanthan, gellan and curdlan are worth mentioning. These are used mainly as food additives, i.e., thickeners and gelling agents. Xanthan obtained from *Xanthomonas species* is comprised of β-(1, 4)-linked heteropolymer with pentasaccharide units. Curdlan obtained from *Agrobacterium, Rhizobium and Cellulomonas species* is a β-(1, 3)-linked homopolymer. Gellan obtained from *Sphingomonas species* is a β-(1, 3)-linked heteropolymer containing tetrasaccharide units [131].

Polyesters

Polyhydroxyalkanoates

These belong to a class of intracellular biopolymers synthesized by many bacteria and act as carbon and energy storage granules. They are composed of β-hydroxy fatty acids, where the R group changes from methyl to tridecyl. The main biopolymer of the PHA family is the poly hydroxybutyrate (PHB), but many copolymers have been synthesized based on PHB [poly (hydroxybutyrate-co-hydroxyvalerate) (PHBV), poly (hydroxybutyrate-co-hydroxyhexanoate) (PHBH), poly (hydroxybutyrate-co-hydroxyoctanoate) (PHBO) [132]. PHB is a highly crystalline polyester (above 50 %) with a high melting point, $T_m = 173–180$ °C, compared with other biodegradable polyesters and with T_g around 5 °C. PHAs are generally classified into short-chain-length (4 or 5 carbons)-PHA (sCL-PHA) and medium-chain-length (6 or more carbons)-PHA (mCL-PHA). Biocompatibility and biodegradability by simple hydrolysis of ester bonds in aerobic conditions as well as piezoelectric properties make them suitable for drug delivery, tissue engineering, and orthopaedic applications [133, 134].

Polyamides

Poly-γ-Glutamate

This is a water-soluble, anionic, biodegradable homo-polyamide produced by microbial fermentation. This is actually a copolymer composed of D- and L-glutamic acid in various proportions. Apart from α-amide linkages between α-amino and γ-carboxylic acid groups, they exhibit other types of amide linkages that involve β- and γ-carboxylic groups as well as ε-amino groups. It has been investigated so far as a drug delivery vehicle (delivery of taxol using covalent immobilization technique), scaffolds for tissue engineering application, and as a thermosensitive polymer. A surgical adhesive and haemostatic agent based on gelatin and poly (glutamic acid) has been developed [133, 135, 136].

Others

Other important polyamides include Cyanophycin from *Cyanobacteria* and ε-poly-L-lysine from Streptomyces *albulus*. The former is a repeating heteropolymer comprised of dipeptide units of aspartate and arginine, whereas the latter is a homopolymer with lysine as the main component. Cyanophycin is used as a water softener and dispersant, whereas ε-poly-L-lysine is used as a food [133] preservative as well as an adsorbent [131].

Polyanhydrides

Polyphosphate

This is a linear, unbranched polymer of orthophosphate residues linked by phosphoanhydride bonds. Polyphosphate can be isolated from many species of bacteria, yeast, and plant and animal cells. This polymer accumulates in cells in response to environmental stress and nutritional status. It acts as a substitute for

ATP in many kinase reactions, plays a role in cellular regulation, and also participates in heavy metal detoxification based on metal chelating property [131].

Conclusions

Natural Polymers prove their immense potential in multifaceted applications. Also, they open up many interesting avenues for further development of new strategies and improvement of existing applications. Some drawbacks associated with stability and immunogenicity aspects need to be overcome to make them prime materials of investigation in various biomedical applications. Blends of natural polymers with other synthetic polymers to achieve suitable characteristics are also practised, which is another wide area of research with these attractive materials.

References

1. Laza-Knoerr, A., Gref, R., Couvreur, P.: Cyclodextrins for drug delivery. J. Drug Target. **18**(9), 645–656 (2010)
2. Challa, R., Ahuja, A., Ali, J., Khar, R.: Cyclodextrins in drug delivery: an updated review. Aaps Pharmscitech **6**(2), E329–E357 (2005)
3. Muntimadugu, E., Ickowicz, D.E., Domb, A.J., Khan, W.: Polysaccharide biomaterials. Isr. J. Chem. **53**(9–10), 787–794 (2013)
4. Vyas, A., Saraf, S., Saraf, S.: Cyclodextrin based novel drug delivery systems. J. Incl. Phenom. Macrocycl. Chem. **62**(1–2), 23–42 (2008)
5. Loftsson, T., Jarho, P., Masson, M., Järvinen, T.: Cyclodextrins in drug delivery. Expert Opin. Drug Deliv. **2**(2), 335–351 (2005)
6. Khan, W., Muthupandian, S., Domb, A.J.: Cationic polymers for the delivery of therapeutic nucleotides. Nanotechnology for the Delivery of Therapeutic Nucleic Acids. Pan Stanford Publishing, Singapore (2013)
7. Swami, R., Singh, I., Khan, W., Ramakrishna, S.: Diseases originate and terminate by genes: unraveling nonviral gene delivery. Drug Deliv. Transl. Res. **3**(6), 593–610 (2013)
8. Khan, W., Hosseinkhani, H., Ickowicz, D., Hong, P.D., Yu, D.S., Domb, A.J.: Polysaccharide gene transfection agents. Acta Biomater. **8**(12), 4224–4232 (2012). S1742-7061(12)00459-X[pii]/j.actbio.2012.09.022
9. Merkus, F., Verhoef, J., Marttin, E., Romeijn, S., Van der Kuy, P., Hermens, W., Schipper, N.: Cyclodextrins in nasal drug delivery. Adv. Drug Deliv. Rev. **36**(1), 41–57 (1999)
10. Loftsson, T., Brewster, M.E., Másson, M.: Role of cyclodextrins in improving oral drug delivery. Am. J. Drug Deliv. **2**(4), 261–275 (2004)
11. Redenti, E., Pietra, C., Gerloczy, A., Szente, L.: Cyclodextrins in oligonucleotide delivery. Adv. Drug Deliv. Rev. **53**(2), 235–244 (2001)
12. Neill, M.J., Mahony, A.M., Byrne, C., Darcy, R., Driscoll, C.M.: Gastrointestinal gene delivery by Cyclodextrins—In vitro quantification of extracellular barriers. Int. J. Pharm. **456**(2), 390–399 (2013)
13. Lai, W.-F.: Cyclodextrins in non-viral gene delivery. Biomaterials **35**(1), 401–411 (2014)
14. Tan, H., Qin, F., Chen, D., Han, S., Lu, W., Yao, X.: Study of glycol chitosan-carboxymethyl β-cyclodextrins as anticancer drugs carrier. Carbohydr. Polym. **93**(2), 679–685 (2013)
15. Matsuda, H., Arima, H.: Cyclodextrins in transdermal and rectal delivery. Adv. Drug Deliv. Rev. **36**(1), 81–99 (1999)

16. Loftssona, T., Jarvinen, T.: Cyclodextrins in ophthalmic drug delivery. Adv. Drug Deliv. Rev. **36**(1), 59–79 (1999)
17. Bibby, D.C., Davies, N.M., Tucker, I.G.: Mechanisms by which cyclodextrins modify drug release from polymeric drug delivery systems. Int. J. Pharm. **197**(1), 1–11 (2000)
18. Nishiyama, Y., Langan, P., Chanzy, H.: Crystal structure and hydrogen-bonding system in cellulose Iβ from synchrotron X-ray and neutron fiber diffraction. J. Am. Chem. Soc. **124**(31), 9074–9082 (2002)
19. Aguilera J.M., Stanley D.W.: Microstructural principles of food processing and engineering, pp. 166–168. Springer, New York (1999)
20. Cosgrove, D.J.: Growth of the plant cell wall. Nat. Rev. Mol. Cell Biol. **6**(11), 850–861 (2005)
21. Hon, D.N.S.: Cellulose and its derivatives: structures, reactions, and medical uses. In: Severian D. (ed.) Polysaccharides in Medicinal Applications, pp. 87–105. Marcel Dekker, New York (1996)
22. Conti, S., Maggi, L., Segale, L., Ochoa Machiste, E., Conte, U., Grenier, P., Vergnault, G.: Matrices containing NaCMC and HPMC: 1. Dissolution performance characterization. Int. J. Pharm. **333**(1), 136–142 (2007)
23. Jamzad, S., Fassihi, R.: Development of a controlled release low dose class II drug-Glipizide. Int. J. Pharm. **312**(1), 24–32 (2006)
24. Scheller, H.V., Ulvskov, P.: Hemicelluloses. Plant Biol. **61**(1), 263–289 (2010)
25. Lerouxel, O., Cavalier, D.M., Liepman, A.H., Keegstra, K.: Biosynthesis of plant cell wall polysaccharides—a complex process. Curr. Opin. Plant Biol. **9**(6), 621–630 (2006)
26. Elvira, C., Mano, J., San Roman, J., Reis, R.: Starch-based biodegradable hydrogels with potential biomedical applications as drug delivery systems. Biomaterials **23**(9), 1955–1966 (2002)
27. Malafaya, P., Elvira, C., Gallardo, A., San Roman, J., Reis, R.: Porous starch-based drug delivery systems processed by a microwave route. J. Biomater. Sci. Polym. Ed. **12**(11), 1227–1241 (2001)
28. Santander-Ortega, M., Stauner, T., Loretz, B., Ortega-Vinuesa, J., Bastos-González, D., Wenz, G., Schaefer, U., Lehr, C.: Nanoparticles made from novel starch derivatives for transdermal drug delivery. J. Controlled Release **141**(1), 85–92 (2010)
29. Vilivalam, V.D., Illum, L., Iqbal, K.: Starch capsules: an alternative system for oral drug delivery. Pharm. Sci. Technol. Today **3**(2), 64–69 (2000)
30. Izawa, K., Akiyama, K., Abe, H., Togashi, Y., Hasegawa, T.: Inulin-based glycopolymer: its preparation, lectin-affinity and gellation property. Bioorg. Med. Chem. **21**(11), 2895–2902 (2013)
31. Akhgari, A., Farahmand, F., Afrasiabi Garekani, H., Sadeghi, F., Vandamme, T.F.: Permeability and swelling studies on free films containing inulin in combination with different polymethacrylates aimed for colonic drug delivery. Eur. J. Pharm. Sci. **28**(4), 307–314 (2006)
32. Maris, B., Verheyden, L., Van Reeth, K., Samyn, C., Augustijns, P., Kinget, R., Van den Mooter, G.: Synthesis and characterisation of inulin-azo hydrogels designed for colon targeting. Int. J. Pharm. **213**(1), 143–152 (2001)
33. Pitarresi, G., Giacomazza, D., Triolo, D., Giammona, G., San Biagio, P.L.: Rheological characterization and release properties of inulin-based hydrogels. Carbohydr. Polym. **88**(3), 1033–1040 (2012)
34. Mohnen, D.: Pectin structure and biosynthesis. Curr. Opin. Plant Biol. **11**(3), 266–277 (2008)
35. Liu, L., Fishman, M.L., Kost, J., Hicks, K.B.: Pectin-based systems for colon-specific drug delivery via oral route. Biomaterials **24**(19), 3333–3343 (2003)
36. Jung, J., Arnold, R.D., Wicker, L.: Pectin and charge modified pectin hydrogel beads as a colon-targeted drug delivery carrier. Colloids Surf. B Biointerfaces **104**, 116–121 (2013)
37. Munjeri, O., Collett, J., Fell, J.: Hydrogel beads based on amidated pectins for colon-specific drug delivery: the role of chitosan in modifying drug release. J. Controlled Release **46**(3), 273–278 (1997)

38. Fernandez-Hervas, M., Fell, J.: Pectin/chitosan mixtures as coatings for colon-specific drug delivery: an in vitro evaluation. Int. J. Pharm. **169**(1), 115–119 (1998)
39. Itoh, K., Yahaba, M., Takahashi, A., Tsuruya, R., Miyazaki, S., Dairaku, M., Togashi, M., Mikami, R., Attwood, D.: In situ gelling xyloglucan/pectin formulations for oral sustained drug delivery. Int. J. Pharm. **356**(1), 95–101 (2008)
40. Dutta, R.K., Sahu, S.: Development of oxaliplatin encapsulated in magnetic nanocarriers of pectin as a potential targeted drug delivery for cancer therapy. Results Pharma Sci. **2**, 38–45 (2012)
41. Smistad, G., Boyum, S., Alund, S.J., Samuelsen, A.B.C., Hiorth, M.: The potential of pectin as a stabilizer for liposomal drug delivery systems. Carbohydr. Polym. **90**(3), 1337–1344 (2012)
42. Kumar, P., Ramya, C., Jayakumar, R., Lakshmanan, V.-K.: Drug delivery and tissue engineering applications of biocompatible pectin-chitin/nano $CaCO_3$ composite scaffolds. Colloids Surf. B Biointerfaces **106**, 109–116 (2013)
43. Luppi, B., Bigucci, F., Abruzzo, A., Corace, G., Cerchiara, T., Zecchi, V.: Freeze-dried chitosan/pectin nasal inserts for antipsychotic drug delivery. Eur. J. Pharm. Biopharm. **75**(3), 381–387 (2010)
44. Katsuraya, K., Okuyama, K., Hatanaka, K., Oshima, R., Sato, T., Matsuzaki, K.: Constitution of konjac glucomannan: chemical analysis and 13C NMR spectroscopy. Carbohydr. Polym. **53**(2), 183–189 (2003)
45. Fan, J., Wang, K., Liu, M., He, Z.: In vitro evaluations of konjac glucomannan and xanthan gum mixture as the sustained release material of matrix tablet. Carbohydr. Polym. **73**(2), 241–247 (2008)
46. Alvarez-Mancenido, F., Landin, M., Lacik, I., Martinez-Pacheco, R.: Konjac glucomannan and konjac glucomannan/xanthan gum mixtures as excipients for controlled drug delivery systems. Diffusion of small drugs. Int. J. Pharm. **349**(1), 11–18 (2008)
47. Wen, X., Wang, T., Wang, Z., Li, L., Zhao, C.: Preparation of konjac glucomannan hydrogels as DNA-controlled release matrix. Int. J. Biol. Macromol. **42**(3), 256–263 (2008)
48. Prabaharan, M.: Prospective of guar gum and its derivatives as controlled drug delivery systems. Int. J. Biol. Macromol. **49**(2), 117–124 (2011)
49. Shukla, R.K., Tiwari, A.: Carbohydrate polymers: Applications and recent advances in delivering drugs to the colon. Carbohydr. Polym. **88**(2), 399–416 (2012)
50. Krishnaiah, Y., Satyanarayana, S., Rama Prasad, Y., Narasimha Rao, S.: Evaluation of guar gum as a compression coat for drug targeting to colon. Int. J. Pharm. **171**(2), 137–146 (1998)
51. Prasad, Y., Krishnaiah, Y., Satyanarayana, S.: In vitro evaluation of guar gum as a carrier for colon-specific drug delivery. J. Controlled Release **51**(2), 281–287 (1998)
52. Li, X., Wu, W., Wang, J., Duan, Y.: The swelling behavior and network parameters of guar gum/poly (acrylic acid) semi-interpenetrating polymer network hydrogels. Carbohydr. Polym. **66**(4), 473–479 (2006)
53. George, M., Abraham, T.: pH sensitive alginate-guar gum hydrogel for the controlled delivery of protein drugs. Int. J. Pharm. **335**(1), 123–129 (2007)
54. Krishnaiah, Y., Karthikeyan, R., Gouri Sankar, V., Satyanarayana, V.: Three-layer guar gum matrix tablet formulations for oral controlled delivery of highly soluble trimetazidine dihydrochloride. J. Controlled Release **81**(1), 45–56 (2002)
55. Krishnaiah, Y., Karthikeyan, R., Satyanarayana, V.: A three-layer guar gum matrix tablet for oral controlled delivery of highly soluble metoprolol tartrate. Int. J. Pharm. **241**(2), 353–366 (2002)
56. Li, X., Wu, W., Liu, W.: Synthesis and properties of thermo-responsive guar gum/poly (N-isopropylacrylamide) interpenetrating polymer network hydrogels. Carbohydr. Polym. **71**(3), 394–402 (2008)
57. Thakur, S., Chauhan, G.S., Ahn, J.-H.: Synthesis of acryloyl guar gum and its hydrogel materials for use in the slow release of l-DOPA and l-tyrosine. Carbohydr. Polym. **76**(4), 513–520 (2009)
58. Ponder, G.R.: Arabinogalactan from Western larch. Part IV. Polymeric products of partial acid hydrolysis. Carbohydr. Polym. **36**(1), 1–14 (1998)

59. Showalter, A.: Arabinogalactan-proteins: structure, expression and function. Cell. Mol. Life Sci. **58**(10), 1399–1417 (2001)
60. Parveen, S., Gupta, A.D., Prasad, R.: Arabinogalactan protein from Arachis hypogaea: Role as carrier in drug-formulations. Int. J. Pharm. **333**(1), 79–86 (2007)
61. Prescott, J.H., Enriquez, P., Jung, C., Menz, E., Groman, E.V.: Larch arabinogalactan for hepatic drug delivery: isolation and characterization of a 9 kDa arabinogalactan fragment. Carbohydr. Res. **278**(1), 113–128 (1995)
62. Avramoff, A., Khan, W., Mizrahi, B., Domb, A.J.: Preparation and characterization of a novel once-daily formulation of diltiazem using arabinogalactan as a channeling agent. J. Appl. Polym. Sci. **126**(S1), E197–E203 (2012)
63. Ehrenfreund-Kleinman, T., Azzam, T., Falk, R., Polacheck, I., Golenser, J., Domb, A.: Synthesis and characterization of novel water soluble amphotericin B-arabinogalactan conjugates. Biomaterials **23**(5), 1327–1335 (2002)
64. Ehrenfreund-Kleinman, T., Gazit, Z., Gazit, D., Azzam, T., Golenser, J., Domb, A.: Synthesis and biodegradation of arabinogalactan sponges prepared by reductive amination. Biomaterials **23**(23), 4621–4631 (2002)
65. Ehrenfreund-Kleinman, T., Golenser, J., Domb, A.J.: Conjugation of amino-containing drugs to polysaccharides by tosylation: amphotericin B-arabinogalactan conjugates. Biomaterials **25**(15), 3049–3057 (2004)
66. Daniel-da-Silva, A.L., Ferreira, L., Gil, A.M., Trindade, T.: Synthesis and swelling behavior of temperature responsive κ-carrageenan nanogels. J. Colloid Interface Sci. **355**(2), 512–517 (2011)
67. Keppeler, S., Ellis, A., Jacquier, J.: Cross-linked carrageenan beads for controlled release delivery systems. Carbohydr. Polym. **78**(4), 973–977 (2009)
68. Sukhlaaied, W., Riyajan, S.-A.: Synthesis and properties of carrageenan grafted copolymer with poly (vinyl alcohol). Carbohydr. Polym. **98**(1), 677–685 (2013)
69. Necas, J., Bartosikova, L.: Carrageenan: a review. Vet. Med. **58**(4), 187–205 (2013)
70. Hezaveh, H., Muhamad, I.I.: Controlled drug release via minimization of burst release in pH-response kappa-carrageenan/polyvinyl alcohol hydrogels. Chem. Eng. Res. Des. **91**(3), 508–519 (2013)
71. Kianfar, F., Antonijevic, M., Chowdhry, B., Boateng, J.S.: Lyophilized wafers comprising carrageenan and pluronic acid for buccal drug delivery using model soluble and insoluble drugs. Colloids Surf. B Biointerfaces **103**, 99–106 (2013)
72. Kulkarni, R.V., Boppana, R., Krishna Mohan, G., Mutalik, S., Kalyane, N.V.: pH-responsive interpenetrating network hydrogel beads of poly (acrylamide)-carrageenan and sodium alginate for intestinal targeted drug delivery: synthesis, in vitro and in vivo evaluation. J. Colloid Interface Sci. **367**(1), 509–517 (2012)
73. Leong, K.H., Chung, L.Y., Noordin, M.I., Mohamad, K., Nishikawa, M., Onuki, Y., Morishita, M., Takayama, K.: Carboxymethylation of kappa-carrageenan for intestinal-targeted delivery of bioactive macromolecules. Carbohydr. Polym. **83**(4), 1507–1515 (2011)
74. Makino, K., Idenuma, R., Murakami, T., Ohshima, H.: Design of a rate-and time-programming drug release device using a hydrogel: pulsatile drug release from κ-carrageenan hydrogel device by surface erosion of the hydrogel. Colloids Surf. B Biointerfaces **20**(4), 355–359 (2001)
75. Leong, K.H., Chung, L.Y., Noordin, M.I., Onuki, Y., Morishita, M., Takayama, K.: Lectin-functionalized carboxymethylated kappa-carrageenan microparticles for oral insulin delivery. Carbohydr. Polym. **86**(2), 555–565 (2011)
76. Malafaya, P.B., Silva, G.A., Reis, R.L.: Natural-origin polymers as carriers and scaffolds for biomolecules and cell delivery in tissue engineering applications. Adv. Drug Deliv. Rev. **59**(4), 207–233 (2007)
77. Vaz, C.M., Van Doeveren, P., Reis, R., Cunha, A.: Development and design of double-layer co-injection moulded soy protein based drug delivery devices. Polymer **44**(19), 5983–5992 (2003)
78. Vaz, C., Fossen, M., Van Tuil, R., De Graaf, L., Reis, R., Cunha, A.: Casein and soybean protein-based thermoplastics and composites as alternative biodegradable polymers for biomedical applications. J. Biomed. Mater. Res. Part A **65**(1), 60–70 (2003)

79. Ruggiero, F., Exposito, J.-Y., Bournat, P., Gruber, V., Perret, S., Comte, J., Olagnier, B., Garrone, R., Theisen, M.: Triple helix assembly and processing of human collagen produced in transgenic tobacco plants. FEBS Lett. **469**(1), 132–136 (2000)
80. Shoseyov O., Amitai H., Posen Y., Yaari A., Shilo S., Roth S., Dgany O., Tal T., Lapidot N.: Large-scale molecular farming of recombinant human collagen in transgenic tobacco (2010)
81. Kolattukudy P.E.: Polyesters in higher plants. In: Biopolyesters, pp. 1–49. Springer, New York (2001)
82. Dutta, P.K., Dutta, J., Tripathi, V.: Chitin and chitosan: chemistry, properties and applications. J. Sci. Ind. Res. **63**(1), 20–31 (2004)
83. Rinaudo, M.: Chitin and chitosan: properties and applications. Prog. Polym. Sci. **31**(7), 603–632 (2006)
84. de Alvarenga E.S.: Characterization and properties of chitosan. In: Biotechnology of Biopolymers, p. 91. (2011)
85. Bansal P., Verma S., Khan W., Kumar N.: Global patent and technological status of biodegradable polymers in drug delivery and tissue engineering. In: Biodegradable Polymers in Clinical Use and Clinical Development, pp. 665–725. Wiley, New York. doi:10.1002/9781118015810.ch18
86. Di Martino, A., Sittinger, M., Risbud, M.V.: Chitosan: a versatile biopolymer for orthopaedic tissue-engineering. Biomaterials **26**(30), 5983–5990 (2005)
87. Malafaya, P., Pedro, A., Peterbauer, A., Gabriel, C., Redl, H., Reis, R.: Chitosan particles agglomerated scaffolds for cartilage and osteochondral tissue engineering approaches with adipose tissue derived stem cells. J. Mater. Sci. Mater. Med. **16**(12), 1077–1085 (2005)
88. Necas, J., Bartosikova, L., Brauner, P., Kolar, J.: Hyaluronic acid (hyaluronan): a review. Vet. Med. **53**(8), 397–411 (2008)
89. Burdick, J.A., Prestwich, G.D.: Hyaluronic acid hydrogels for biomedical applications. Adv. Mater. **23**(12), H41–H56 (2011)
90. Sintov, A., Di-Capua, N., Rubinstein, A.: Cross-linked chondroitin sulphate: characterization for drug delivery purposes. Biomaterials **16**(6), 473–478 (1995)
91. Chang, C.H., Liu, H.C., Lin, C.C., Chou, C.H., Lin, F.H.: Gelatin-chondroitin-hyaluronan tri-copolymer scaffold for cartilage tissue engineering. Biomaterials **24**(26), 4853–4858 (2003)
92. Lee, C.H., Singla, A., Lee, Y.: Biomedical applications of collagen. Int. J. Pharm. **221**(1), 1–22 (2001)
93. Khan W., Yadav D., Domb A.J., Kumar N.: Collagen. Biodegradable polymers in clinical use and clinical development: 59–89 (2011)
94. Gelse, K., Pöschl, E., Aigner, T.: Collagens—structure, function, and biosynthesis. Adv. Drug Deliv. Rev. **55**(12), 1531–1546 (2003)
95. Neel, E.A.A., Bozec, L., Knowles, J.C., Syed, O., Mudera, V., Day, R., Hyun, J.K.: Collagen—emerging collagen based therapies hit the patient. Adv. Drug Deliv. Rev. **65**(4), 429–456 (2013)
96. Brown, J., Timpl, R.: The collagen superfamily. Int. Arch. Allergy Immunol. **107**(4), 484–490 (1995)
97. Friess, W.: Collagen–biomaterial for drug delivery. Eur. J. Pharm. Biopharm. **45**(2), 113–136 (1998)
98. von der Mark, K.: Structure, biosynthesis and gene regulation of collagens in cartilage and bone, pp. 3–26. Academic Press, Orlando (1999)
99. Das, S., Khan, W., Mohsin, S., Kumar, N.: Miltefosine loaded albumin microparticles for treatment of visceral leishmaniasis: formulation development and in vitro evaluation. Polym. Adv. Technol. **22**(1), 172–179 (2010). doi:10.1002/pat.1710
100. Ledward D., Phillips G., Williams P.: Gelatin. In: Handbook of Hydrocolloids, pp. 67–86. (2000)
101. Kratz, F.: Albumin as a drug carrier: design of prodrugs, drug conjugates and nanoparticles. J. Controlled Release **132**(3), 171–183 (2008)

102. Elzoghby, A.O., Samy, W.M., Elgindy, N.A.: Albumin-based nanoparticles as potential controlled release drug delivery systems. J. Controlled Release **157**(2), 168–182 (2012)
103. Domb A.J., Khan W.: Biodegradable polymers as drug carrier systems. In: Dumitriu S., Popa C. (eds) Polymeric Biomaterials, pp. 135–176. CRC Press, Boca Raton (2013)
104. Fasano, M., Curry, S., Terreno, E., Galliano, M., Fanali, G., Narciso, P., Notari, S., Ascenzi, P.: The extraordinary ligand binding properties of human serum albumin. IUBMB Life **57**(12), 787–796 (2005)
105. Hu, Y.J., Liu, Y., Sun, T.Q., Bai, A.M., Lü, J.Q., Pi, Z.B.: Binding of anti-inflammatory drug cromolyn sodium to bovine serum albumin. Int. J. Biol. Macromol. **39**(4), 280–285 (2006)
106. Roche, M., Rondeau, P., Singh, N.R., Tarnus, E., Bourdon, E.: The antioxidant properties of serum albumin. FEBS Lett. **582**(13), 1783–1787 (2008)
107. Khan, W., Kumar, N.: Drug targeting to macrophages using paromomycin-loaded albumin microspheres for treatment of visceral leishmaniasis: an in vitro evaluation. J. Drug Target. **19**(4), 239–250 (2011). doi:10.3109/1061186X.2010.492524
108. Haisch, A., Loch, A., David, J., Pruss, A., Hansen, R., Sittinger, M.: Preparation of a pure autologous biodegradable fibrin matrix for tissue engineering. Med. Biol. Eng. Comput. **38**(6), 686–689 (2000)
109. Furst, W., Banerjee, A., Redl, H.: Comparison of structure, strength and cytocompatibility of a fibrin matrix supplemented either with tranexamic acid or aprotinin. J. Biomed. Mater. Res. B Appl. Biomater. **82**(1), 109–114 (2007)
110. Han, D., Liu, W., Ao, Q., Wang, G.: Optimal delivery systems for bone morphogenetic proteins in orthopedic applications should model initial tissue repair structures by using a heparin-incorporated fibrin-fibronectin matrix. Med. Hypotheses **71**(3), 374–378 (2008)
111. Sathian, J., Sastry, T., Suguna, L., Lakshminarayana, Y., Radhakrishnan, G.: Fibrin as a matrix for grafting 2-hydroxyethyl methacrylate: Preparation and characterization of the graft and its in vivo evaluation for wound healing. J. Biomed. Mater. Res., Part A **65**(4), 435–440 (2003)
112. Ryu, J.H., Kim, I.-K., Cho, S.-W., Cho, M.-C., Hwang, K.-K., Piao, H., Piao, S., Lim, S.H., Hong, Y.S., Choi, C.Y.: Implantation of bone marrow mononuclear cells using injectable fibrin matrix enhances neovascularization in infarcted myocardium. Biomaterials **26**(3), 319–326 (2005)
113. Kumar, T., Vasantha Bai, M., Krishnan, L.K.: A freeze-dried fibrin disc as a biodegradable drug release matrix. Biologicals **32**(1), 49–55 (2004)
114. Shim, G., Im, S., Lee, S., Park, J.Y., Kim, J., Jin, H., Lee, S., Im, I., Kim, D.-D., Kim, S.W.: Enhanced survival of transplanted human adipose-derived stem cells by co-delivery with liposomal apoptosome inhibitor in fibrin gel matrix. Eur. J. Pharm. Biopharm. **85**(3), 673–681 (2013)
115. Jin, J., Hassanzadeh, P., Perotto, G., Sun, W., Brenckle, M.A., Kaplan, D., Omenetto, F.G., Rolandi, M.: A biomimetic composite from solution self-assembly of chitin nanofibers in a silk fibroin matrix. Adv. Mater. **25**(32), 4482–4487 (2013)
116. Miroiu, F., Socol, G., Visan, A., Stefan, N., Craciun, D., Craciun, V., Dorcioman, G., Mihailescu, I., Sima, L., Petrescu, S.: Composite biocompatible hydroxyapatite–silk fibroin coatings for medical implants obtained by matrix assisted pulsed laser evaporation. Mater. Sci. Eng. **B169**(1), 151–158 (2010)
117. Wang, Y., Bella, E., Lee, C.S., Migliaresi, C., Pelcastre, L., Schwartz, Z., Boyan, B.D., Motta, A.: The synergistic effects of 3-D porous silk fibroin matrix scaffold properties and hydrodynamic environment in cartilage tissue regeneration. Biomaterials **31**(17), 4672–4681 (2010)
118. Altman, A.M., Gupta, V., Ríos, C.N., Alt, E.U., Mathur, A.B.: Adhesion, migration and mechanics of human adipose-tissue-derived stem cells on silk fibroin-chitosan matrix. Acta Biomater. **6**(4), 1388–1397 (2010)
119. Kasoju, N., Bora, U.: Silk fibroin based biomimetic artificial extracellular matrix for hepatic tissue engineering applications. Biomed. Mater. **7**(4), 045004 (2012)

120. Liu, Y., Liu, H., Qian, J., Deng, J., Yu, T.: Regenerated silk fibroin membrane as immobilization matrix for peroxidase and fabrication of a sensor for hydrogen peroxide utilizing methylene blue as electron shuttle. Anal. Chim. Acta **316**(1), 65–72 (1995)
121. Farag, Y., Leopold, C.S.: Development of shellac-coated sustained release pellet formulations. Eur. J. Pharm. Sci. **42**(4), 400–405 (2011)
122. Limmatvapirat, S., Limmatvapirat, C., Puttipipatkhachorn, S., Nunthanid, J., Luangtana-anan, M., Sriamornsak, P.: Modulation of drug release kinetics of shellac-based matrix tablets by in-situ polymerization through annealing process. Eur. J. Pharm. Biopharm. **69**(3), 1004–1013 (2008)
123. Soradech, S., Limatvapirat, S., Luangtana-anan, M.: Stability enhancement of shellac by formation of composite film: effect of gelatin and plasticizers. J. Food Eng. **116**(2), 572–580 (2013)
124. Yu, C.-Y., Yin, B.-C., Zhang, W., Cheng, S.-X., Zhang, X.-Z., Zhuo, R.-X.: Composite microparticle drug delivery systems based on chitosan, alginate and pectin with improved pH-sensitive drug release property. Colloids Surf. B Biointerfaces **68**(2), 245–249 (2009)
125. Hornig, S., Bunjes, H., Heinze, T.: Preparation and characterization of nanoparticles based on dextran–drug conjugates. J. Colloid Interface Sci. **338**(1), 56–62 (2009)
126. Saboktakin, M.R., Tabatabaie, R., Maharramov, A., Ramazanov, M.A.: Synthesis and characterization of superparamagnetic chitosan–dextran sulfate hydrogels as nano carriers for colon-specific drug delivery. Carbohydr. Polym. **81**(2), 372–376 (2010)
127. Shu, S., Zhang, X., Wu, Z., Wang, Z., Li, C.: Delivery of protein drugs using nanoparticles self-assembled from dextran sulfate and quaternized chitosan. J. Controlled Release **152**, e170–e172 (2011)
128. Brondsted, H., Andersen, C., Hovgaard, L.: Crosslinked dextran—a new capsule material for colon targeting of drugs. J. Controlled Release **53**(1), 7–13 (1998)
129. Cortesi, R., Esposito, E., Osti, M., Menegatti, E., Squarzoni, G., Spencer Davis, S., Nastruzzi, C.: Dextran cross-linked gelatin microspheres as a drug delivery system. Eur. J. Pharm. Biopharm. **47**(2), 153–160 (1999)
130. Hovgaard, L., Brondsted, H.: Dextran hydrogels for colon-specific drug delivery. J. Controlled Release **36**(1), 159–166 (1995)
131. Rehm, B.H.: Bacterial polymers: biosynthesis, modifications and applications. Nat. Rev. Microbiol. **8**(8), 578–592 (2010)
132. Averous L., Pollet E.: Biodegradable polymers. In: Environmental Silicate Nano-Biocomposites, pp. 13–39. Springer, New York
133. Nair L.S., Laurencin C.T.: Polymers as biomaterials for tissue engineering and controlled drug delivery. In: Tissue Engineering I, pp. 47–90. Springer, New York (2006)
134. Ueda, H., Tabata, Y.: Polyhydroxyalkanonate derivatives in current clinical applications and trials. Adv. Drug Deliv. Rev. **55**(4), 501–518 (2003)
135. Nair, L.S., Laurencin, C.T.: Biodegradable polymers as biomaterials. Prog. Polym. Sci. **32**(8), 762–798 (2007)
136. Ashiuchi M., Misono H.: Poly γ glutamic Acid. Biopolymers Online (2002)

Chapter 3
Chemical and Physical Properties of Polymers for Biomedical Use

Vincenzo Guarino, Marica Marrese and Luigi Ambrosio

Abstract Polymers have been widely used to develop innovative and high-throughput solutions for biomedical applications. As a function of specific bio-functionalities, they have been successfully employed to fabricate biocompatible devices (i.e., prostheses components, porous/nonporous scaffolds) with structural properties able to resist to external stimuli under physiological conditions (i.e., degradation from body fluids). This wide application field depends upon the peculiar polymer chemistry and physical properties (i.e., thermal, mechanical, etc.), which significantly concur to define the ultimate properties of the polymer for a specific biomedical use. In this chapter, we aim at introducing the fundamental concepts regarding chemical and physical properties of polymers to provide the basic knowledge and better predict the structure occurring in manufacturing processes involving biomaterials. For this reason, we discuss the main correlations occurring between physical and chemical structure to establish structure-property-function relationships. Meanwhile, we describe the methods for the estimation and prediction of properties of polymers (i.e., thermal, mechanical) at different physical state, which are essential to set process conditions to properly design polymers in biomedical applications.

Keywords Intermolecular forces · Intramolecular forces · Biopolymers

Abbreviations

$+\delta$	Partial positive charge
ACL	Anterior cruciate ligament
D	Dispersity

V. Guarino (✉) · M. Marrese · L. Ambrosio
Institute for Polymers, Composites and Biomaterials, National Research Council of Italy, Mostra D'Oltremare, Pad.20, V.Le Kennedy 54, 80125 Naples, Italy
e-mail: vguarino@unina.it; vincenzo.guarino@cnr.it

L. Ambrosio
e-mail: ambrosio@unina.it

F. Puoci (ed.), *Advanced Polymers in Medicine*, DOI 10.1007/978-3-319-12478-0_3

E	Elastic modulus
E	Energy
E_o	Minimum energy
F	Force
F_a	Attractive force
F_r	Repulsive force
HA	Hyaluronic acid
IPN	Interpenetrating networks
M_e	Average molecular weight of the polymer segments between two entanglements in solution
M_i	Molecular weight of $species_i$
M_K	A series of average molecular weights
M_N	Average molecular weight
M_n	Polymer number average molecular weight
M_v	Viscosity average molecular weight
M_W	Weight average molecular weight
$n_{e,sol}$	M_n/M_e ratio
N_i	Number of moles of $species_i$
PAA	Polyacrylic acid
PAAm	Polyacrylamide
PCL	Polycaprolactone
PEG	Polyetheleneglycol
PEO	Poly(ethylene) oxide
PHA	Polyhydroxy acid
PLA	Polylactic acid
PMMA	Polymethylmetacrilate
PTFE	Polytetrafluoroethylene
PVA	Polyvinyl alcohol
PVP	Polyvinylpyrrolidone
r_o	Equilibrium spacing
T_g	Glass transition temperature
TIPS	Thermally induced phase separation
T_m	Melting temperature
ε	Strain
η	Viscosity
σ	Standard deviation
σ	Stress
ϕ	Volume fraction

Introduction

Polymers are one of the major functional components in a number of biomedical devices for applications ranging from clinical diagnosis, extracorporeal procedures up to in vivo applications such as tissue engineering, biosensors and drug delivery.

Their application in medical surgery fall into three broad categories: (a) extracorporeal uses (catheters, tubing, and fluid lines; dialysis membranes/artificial kidney; ocular devices; wound dressings and artificial skin) [1, 2], (b) permanently implanted devices (sensory devices; cardiovascular devices; orthopedic and dental devices) [3, 4], and (c) temporary implants (degradable sutures; implantable drug delivery systems; polymeric scaffolds for cell or tissue transplants; temporary vascular grafts and arterial stents; temporary small bone fixation devices, transdermal drug delivery) [5–7]. This incites chemists and materials scientists to increasingly investigate biopolymers with new functionalities to explore their properties under different biological conditions in order to satisfy the enormous demand in the area of medical science. Recently, a large number of biopolymers have been variously used in biomedical field, including natural polymers such as polysaccharides (starch, cellulose, chitin, alginate, hyaluronate, etc.) or proteins (collagens, gelatins, caseins, albumins) and/or synthetic and biodegradable polymers (Polyvinyl alcohol (PVA), Polyvinylpyrrolidone (PVP), Polyetheleneglycol (PEG), Polylactic acid (PLA), Polyhydroxy acid (PHA) etc.). However, despite the apparent proliferation of biopolymers in clinical surgery, the modern science and technology of biopolymers is still in its early stages of development due to the large heterogeneity of chemical properties of polymers which makes difficult to completely understand dynamic structure-processing condition-property relationship required for the design of medical devices.

For instance, different approaches have been investigated to design novel devices which may be in turn able to directly or indirectly interact with the host tissues and to replace the functional tissue through the mimicry of morphological characteristics of natural systems [8]. Starting from the basic principle of "*learning from nature*", polymers have been chemically designed to reproduce the native chemical/physical behavior of soft/hard tissues under the specific biomechanical and physiological conditions at the interface with the surrounding tissues. In particular, tailor-made polymers with different fluid transport and degradation properties have been synthesized to bio-molecularly interact with cells: they may finely control basic cell functions, guiding the spatially and temporally complex multicellular processes of tissue formation and regeneration or facilitating the restoration of structure and function of damaged or dysfunctional tissues [9, 10].

Still, several drawbacks of current synthesized polymers have been recognized in terms of durability of mechanical response over time [11] so making their use in load bearing applications often unsatisfactory. This may be referred to a not efficient control of the material properties mediated by specific molecular interactions, i.e., side reactions coupled with the presence of un-reacted pendant groups and physical bonds—which unclearly affect degradation mechanisms thus compromising the biomechanical performance after implantation, with potential effects on the required response of materials to the external stimuli [12]. In this context, it is mandatory to identify and adequately investigate all the interactions which occur between macromolecules and macromolecular assemblies in order to properly address the properties to the specific application need.

As a general rule, it is possible to recognize two types of molecular interactions generated by intramolecular and intermolecular forces respectively.

In detail, the macroscopic properties of polymer for biomedical use, are determined to a great extent by the physical/chemical characteristics of individual polymer chains, related to the presence of specific chemical moieties able to influence the elasticity or the mechanical stability of covalent bonds as well as of molecular conformations [13]. Meanwhile, intermolecular forces between adjacent polymer chains in the bulk also contribute to the properties of the chains assembly, and influence the local interactions between specific groups along the backbone, thus negatively influencing and sometimes compromise the materials biocompatibility for specific use. The intramolecular forces influence the properties of single polymer molecules, which result from the entropic and enthalpic elasticity of the polymers, as well as from specific structural changes along the stretched polymer chain, so, governing the elastic response of single polymer chains. Otherwise, intermolecular forces involve all processes in which the interaction is transmitted through the surrounding medium such as unbinding mechanisms of intermolecular aggregates based on non-covalent interactions (i.e., in ligand-receptor pairs, coordination complexes, hydrogen bonded systems, ion pairs or hydrophobically assembled structures). So, they govern the stability of intermolecular aggregates such as polymeric micelles or hydrophobic domains, folding of proteins or polymer crystals packing. In order to better understand the macroscopic properties of polymeric biomaterials and their potential use in biomedical applications, it is therefore necessary to properly frame the microscopic interactions occurring inter and intra molecular chains, so identifying the peculiar contribution of intramolecular and intermolecular forces which may optimize the ultimate properties of the biomedical device. In this chapter, it is proposed an accurate description of chemical and physical properties of biopolymers elucidating their origin from inter- or intra-molecular interactions (Fig. 3.1).

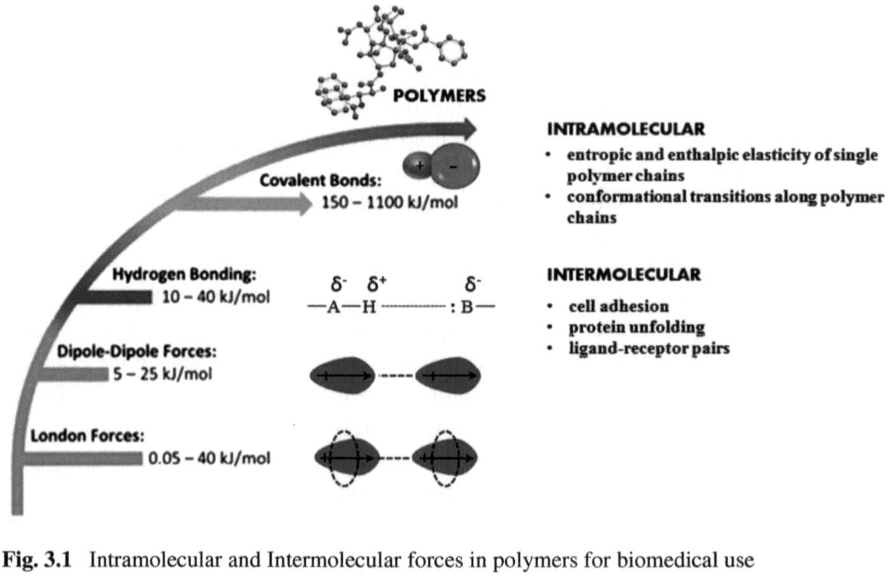

Fig. 3.1 Intramolecular and Intermolecular forces in polymers for biomedical use

Intra and Inter Polymer Molecular Interactions

A correct understanding of many physical and chemical properties of polymeric materials is linked to the knowledge of the intra and inter molecular interactions. All matter is held together by force and its property results from the properties of individual molecules and from how they act collectively. Preeminently, it is necessary to distinguish the types of forces acting within and between molecules: including *intramolecular* interactions that occur between macromolecular groups itself that are responsible for the complex chemical properties and the *intermolecular* interactions, responsible for the physical properties. At atomic level, considering the interaction between two isolated atoms as they are brought into close proximity from an infinite separation. At large distances interactions are negligible but as the atoms approach, each exerts forces on the other. These forces are of two types attractive force (F_a) and repulsive force (F_r) and the magnitude of each is a function of interatomic distance. The origin of attractive part depends on the particular type of bonding. The repulsion between atoms is related to the Pauli principle: when the electronic clouds surrounding the atoms, they start to overlap and the energy of the system increases suddenly. The sum of attractive and repulsive components is the net force F, and then when F_a and F_r become equal there is no net force and a state of equilibrium exists. Sometimes it is more convenient to work with potential energies between two atoms instead of forces considering that energy and force for atomic systems are mathematically related:

$$E = \int F dr \tag{3.1}$$

At equilibrium spacing r_0, the force F is zero and net energy corresponds to minimum energy E_0 [14]. The binding energy require to separate two atoms from their equilibrium spacing to an infinite distance apart is the minimum energy E_0. A large of material properties depend on E_0, curve shape and bonding type [15].

As already said, the potential curve is the result of two terms: the contribution of attractive force at long ranges (Van der Waals force) and the repulsive term at short ranges. The curves indicate the strength of the bond based on the depth of the potential well: more deep is the well more stable is the molecule [15].

By *chemical bonding* is meant the effect that causes the energy of two atoms close to each other to be significantly lower than when they are apart. The effect arises from the sharing of the outer (valence) electrons of these atoms which, in the presence of two or more positively charged nuclei, rearrange themselves into spatial distributions (orbitals) where the electrons are, on the average, closer to the nuclei. The strength and length of a chemical bond are related to potential distance curve in which the minimum value of energy, the *bond energy,* is defined as the amount of energy required to increase the separation of the atoms forming the bond to infinity. However, what is lacking from the curves is the fact that chemical bonds, due to the redistributed electron clouds, have distinct directionality. The most widely used model for chemical bonding is the *covalent bond* or *shared electron* model. Different elements have different tendencies to draw electrons toward their nuclei. This ability is called *electronegativity*. Thus, in general the shared electron cloud is not evenly distributed in the space between the bonding nuclei. The difference in the electronegativities of the bonding atoms quantifies the extent how evenly or unevenly the bond electrons are shared. A purely covalent bond (i.e., completely evenly shared electrons) can only be obtained when the bonding atoms are of the same element. The atom with a smaller electronegativity, can be viewed as having a partial positive charge $+\delta$, as the positive charge of its nuclei is not fully screened anymore by the valence electrons. The formation of one or more chemical bonds allows atoms to form energetically stable *molecules* which are characterized by their structure and composition. Since chemical bonds result in increased localized electron densities, it can be assumed that the spatial regions associated with different chemical bonds repel each other electrostatically. As became apparent from the discussion on chemical bonds above, many molecules contain polar chemical bonds that can be associated with electric dipoles, comprising of atomic partial charges. The molecules, in turn, as collections of these partial charges, can be associated with electric dipoles, quadrupoles, and higher multipoles. Many chemical groups in molecules may also be charged, and then the electrostatic effects are important in a wide range of molecular systems. It turns out that relating the intricate intermolecular forces to simple electrostatic interactions between charges, dipoles, and higher multipoles works surprisingly well in understanding the structure and dynamics of condensed matter systems. The long chains are held together either by secondary bonding forces such as van der Waals and hydrogen bonds or primary covalent bonding forces through cross links between chains. In general, the intermolecular interactions could be or a dipole-dipole interaction or dispersion (London) interaction. Dipole-dipole forces are referred to an electrostatic interaction acting between two permanent dipoles, averaged over different orientations due to the thermal motion of the molecules. These interactions tend to align the molecules in order to increase the attraction reducing potential energy. London dispersion interactions, instead, are of purely quantum-mechanical origin. They are caused by correlated movements of the electrons in interacting molecules. Finally, hydrogen bond occurs between molecules that have a permanent net dipole resulting from hydrogen being covalently bonded to relatively electronegative atoms (fluorine, oxygen or nitrogen). Hydrogen bonds are a stronger intermolecular force than either dispersion forces or dipole-dipole interactions. Inter and intramolecular interactions are generally present in several polymers largely used for biomedical applications, which have very long chain molecules, formed by covalent bonding along the backbone chain. In addition, each chain can have side groups, branches, and copolymeric chains or blocks which can also interfere with the long-range ordering of chains. In the case of branched polymers in which side chains are attached to the main backbone chain, chain packing is limited by the steric hindrance of side chains resulting in a not ordered structure.

Molecular Weight Polidispersivity and Effects on Polymer Viscosity

Because polymers are long-chain molecules, their properties tend to be more complex than their short-chain counterparts. Thus, in order to choose a polymer type for a particular application, microscopic properties of polymers must be understood [16]. Among them, polymer molecular weight is important because it determines many physical properties. Some examples include the transitions temperatures from liquids to rubbers, solids and mechanical properties such as stiffness, strength, viscoelasticity, toughness, and viscosity. If molecular weight is too low, the transition temperatures and the mechanical properties will generally not be adequate for the use in commercial applications in terms of transition temperatures or mechanical properties for load bearing application. Unlike small molecules, however, the molecular weight of a polymer is not one unique value. Rather, a given polymer will have a distribution of molecular weights that will depend on the way the polymer is produced. For polymers we should not speak of a molecular weight, but rather of the distribution of molecular weight or of the average molecular weight. There are many ways, however, to calculate an average molecular weight. The question therefore is how ones can define the average molecular weight for a given distribution of molecular weights.

The answer is that the type of property being studied will determine the desired type of average molecular weight. For example, strength properties may be influenced more by high molecular weight molecules than by low molecular weight molecules and thus the average molecular weight for strength properties should be weighted to emphasize the presence of high molecular weight polymer. The molecular weight of polymer is described by two statistically useful definitions: the number average and weight average molecular weights. The number average molecular weight is correlated to the number of molecules present in the mixture. This average molecular weight follows the conventional definition for the mean value of any statistical quantity. In polymer science is called the number average molecular weight (M_N) that therefore is an average over the number of molecules.

$$M_N = \frac{\sum N_i M_i}{\sum N_i} \tag{3.2}$$

where N_i is the number of moles of species, and M_i is the molecular weight of species$_i$. By considering the polymer property which depends on the size or weight of each polymer molecule, it is possible to define the weight average molecular weight (M_W). It represents an average over the weight of each polymer chain.

$$M_w = \frac{\sum N_i M_i^2}{\sum N_i M_i} \tag{3.3}$$

where N_i is the number of moles of species$_i$, and M_i, is the molecular weight of species$_i$ [17]. In general, a series of average molecular weights can be defined by the equation:

$$M_k = \frac{\sum N_i M_i^{k+1}}{\sum N_i M_i^k} \tag{3.4}$$

where

$k = 0$ gives M_N
$k = 1$ gives M_W
$k = 2$ gives M_z
$k = 3$ gives M_{z+1}

One average molecular weight which does not fit into the general expression of M_k is the viscosity average molecular weight, M_v that is given by the Mark-Houwink and defined as:

$$M_v = \left(\frac{\sum N_i M_i^{a+1}}{\sum N_i M_i^a} \right)^{\frac{1}{a}} \tag{3.5}$$

Here a represents a constant that depends on the polymer/solvent pair used in the viscosity experiments.

For all synthetic polydisperse polymers, the various average molecular weights always rank in the follow order:

$$M_N < M_v < M_W < M_k < M_{k+1} \tag{3.6}$$

For monodisperse polymers all molecules have the same molecular weight, then all molecular weight averages are equal [18]. To measure an average molecular weight, it is possible to use a colligative property which yields M_N or light scattering which yields M_W. A molecular weight distribution for a typical polymer is shown in Fig. 3.2; it seems like a probability distribution curve.

Standard deviation of molecular weight is used in order to characterize the spread of the distribution function.

$$\sigma = M_N \sqrt{\frac{M_W}{M_N} - 1} \tag{3.7}$$

A key term in the standard deviation is the ratio of M_W to M_N. This term is known as the **polydispersivity index** and it is used as a measure of the breadness of the molecular weight distribution. The polydispersity index or dispersity D is commonly used to measure the distribution of molecular mass in a given polymer sample:

$$D = \frac{M_W}{M_N} \tag{3.8}$$

So, the dispersity calculated is the weight average molecular weight (M_W) divided by the number average molecular weight (M_N) indicating in this way the distribution of individual molecular masses in a batch of polymers [19].

Linear polymers used for biomedical applications generally have M_N in the range of 25,000–100,000 and M_N from 50,000 to 30,000. Higher or lower molecular weights may be necessary, depending on the ability of the polymer chains to exhibit secondary interactions such as hydrogen bonding which may concur to additional strength. In general, increase molecular weight corresponds to an increase of physical properties [16] such as viscosity. Equally the intrinsic viscosity can be related to the molecular weight of the solute and gives an idea of molecular weight. For solutions of polymers with $M_N > 10{,}000$ Dalton, it is possible to consider the Mark-Houwink relation:

$$[\eta] = KM^a \tag{3.9}$$

where K and a are constants characteristic of the particular system investigated. K is referred to the particular solvent-solute pair and "a" is particularly related to the shape of the solute molecule.

Values of these parameters have been determined for a large number of polymer-solvent pairs in the range of molecular weights normally of interest for characterization purposes [20]. For instance molecular weight of the polymer also has an important effect on morphologies of electrospun scaffold. Here, the electric field forces permit to modify the size scale of fibres from micro to nano-meter in order to obtain micro or nanostructured scaffolds. In these applications, molecular weight is correlated with the solution viscosity, then considering the same concentration of the same polymer increasing molecular weight is possible to switch from microspheres to fibres. Interestingly, during the electrospinning and electrospraying process, the morphology from beads to fibres changes as the solution viscosity: droplet shape in the case of lower viscosity until smooth fibres when the sufficient viscosity is achieved [21], as shown in Fig. 3.2. In the case of intermediate values of viscosities, Zong et al. [22] have demonstrated the formation of droplets (i.e., beads) along the fibres, also underlining the possibility to control the spacing between the beads as the viscosity changes. In particular, it has been observed that by properly choosing polymer molecular weight and concentration, it is possible to discriminate between the formation of fibres or particles. In addition, chain entanglements may strongly affect size and morphology of the obtained particles, thus offering tunable release kinetics suitable for different drug delivery systems [23, 24]. It is well-known that particle morphology obtained by electrospraying is mainly determined by the competition between chain entanglement and Coulomb fission within a single droplet. More in detail, as the solvent evaporates from the droplet, two competing factors occur: the increase of polymer concentration and, consequently, of entanglements which stabilize the droplet from further subdivision thus preserving its spherical shape—and, secondly the increase of surface charge which can overcome the surface tension thus leading to droplet fission and the formation of "*offspring droplets*". Considering that polymer chain entanglements oppose the Coulomb fission during the electrospraying

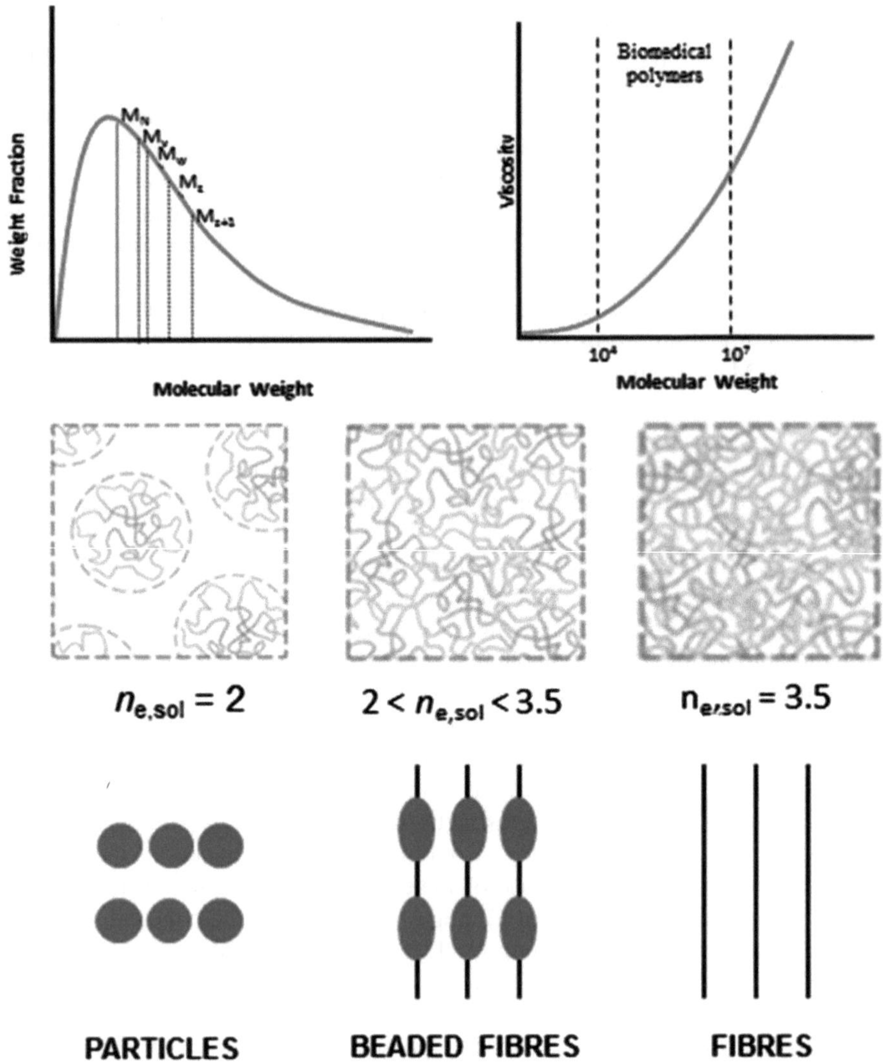

Fig. 3.2 Typical molecular weight distribution and viscosity dependence for biomedical polymers. Effect of entanglement molecular weight and viscosity on the morphology of electrospinning/spraying products

process, some researchers [25] have identified a not dimensional parameter to describe the transition between fibre and bead formation and, consequently, between electrospraying and electrospinning process—as a function of the entanglements forming among chains in solution. This parameter $n_{e,sol}$ is defined as the ratio between polymer number average molecular weight (M_n) and M_e, which is the average molecular weight of the polymer segments between two entanglements in solution. So, it is possible to distinguish three different regimes in the electrospinning/spraying process of polymer solutions: $n_{e,sol} < 2$, in this case, particle formation occurs; $n_{e,sol} > 3.5$, regular electrospinning with fibre formation appears. In the intermediate case, $2 < n_{e,sol} < 3.5$, a mixed regime yielding beads and fibres takes place [26] (Fig. 3.2).

Furthermore, molecular weight and viscosity are extremely important parameters for the processing of melt polymers at different temperatures. In scaffold design for tissue engineering, polymer blends have been largely investigated to obtain porous substrates with high control of pores interconnections and anisotropy. The mixing and extrusion of immiscible blends composed of polymers with different molecular weight, i.e., polycaprolactone (PCL) and poly (ethylene oxide) (PEO) is an interesting example where the sage balance of viscosity and relative composition play a crucial role on the final morphology of the scaffold. In this case, to reach a co-continuous phase organization—i.e., fully percolation of polymer phases,—it is possible to study ab initio the viscosity ratio, depending upon the relative volume fraction of components in the binary polymer blend as follows.

$$\frac{\eta_1(\gamma)}{\eta_2(\gamma)} = \frac{\phi_1}{\phi_2} \tag{3.10}$$

In agreement with basic rules of co-continuous blends, a viscosity ratio equal to 1 should lead to a phase inversion at a 50:50 composition. However, when two components have different viscosities, the less viscous component (i.e., lower molecular weight) usually tends to encapsulate the more viscous one (i.e., higher molecular weight), thus pushing the phase inversion point toward a blend that is richer in the most viscous component [27]. In the case the viscosity gap between the blend components is relatively modest, a phase inversion point close to 50/50 (% vol) may be expected. According to this idea [28], through the complex viscosity curve, it is possible to reach the isoviscosity condition that represents the essential requirement to obtain an optimal mixing of the polymer blend.

Thermal Properties: Effect of Crystalline and Amorphous Phases

Molecular shape arrangements are important factors in determining the physical properties of polymers. The molecular structure, conformation and orientation of the polymers have a relevant effect on the organization of molecules on the micro and macroscopic scale as they aggregate into more ordered structures. In order to explain this phenomena, crystalline and amorphous phase are generally recognized. In particular, polymer whose molecular structure lacks a definite repeating form, shape or structure is called amorphous polymer and has no definite shape while the polymer in which a unit structure repeats itself is called crystalline and has a definite shape, form and structure. There are some polymers that are completely amorphous, but most are a combination with the tangled and disordered regions surrounding the crystalline areas, called semicrystalline polymers. The presence of crystallites in the polymer usually leads to enhanced mechanical properties, unique thermal behavior, and increased fatigue strength. These properties make semicrystalline polymers desirable materials for biomedical applications.

As a function of the peculiar chain organization is possible to identify three important physical transitions: glass transition, melting point and crystallization. These phenomena are important with respect to the design and processing of polymeric materials and maybe controlled by thermal conditions. Crystallization is the process by which, upon cooling, an ordered solid phase is produced from liquid melt having a highly random molecular structure. The melting transformation is the reverse process that occurs when a polymer is heated and the glass transition occurs with amorphous or non crystallizable polymers. Of course, during the physical steps of crystallization, melting and glass transition it is possible to observe changes in physical and mechanical properties of polymers. In the case of semi-crystalline polymers, the non-crystalline regions undergo the phenomenon of the glass transition, while the crystalline regions are affected by the melt phenomenon. The understanding of the mechanism and dynamics of crystallization in polymers is important since the degree of crystallinity affects the thermal and mechanical properties of these materials. Crystallization from a melt is the most fundamental of all phase transformations in materials that occurs through the nucleation and growth processes. Furthermore, the crystallization is a process associated with partial alignment of polymer molecular chains. These chains fold together and form ordered regions called lamellae, which compose larger spheroidal structures named spherulites. The crystallization proceeds with the formation of isolated spherulites, which then grow until their mutual impingement with further slow crystallization. In a sample of crystalline polymer there are billions of spherulities. There is an initial induction time required for the formation of spherulitic nuclei, followed by a period of accelerated crystallization in which spherulites grow in radius. When the spherulites begin to touch each other, crystallization rates slow down again. Complete crystallinity is almost never achieved, and the final degree of crystallinity is molecular-weight-dependent. Crystallization at low temperature nucleates a great number of spherulites which grow slowly while at high temperature crystallization results in rapid growth of relatively few spherulites, influencing in this manner the morphology of polymers.

Other two important parameters for polymers characterization are the glass transition temperature T_g and the melting point T_m. The term melting point, when applied to polymers suggests the transition from a crystalline phase or semi crystalline phase to a solid amorphous phase. The process of melting occurs in a specific range of temperature and not at a fixed temperature. Furthermore the melting behavior depends on the previous history of the polymers and, in particular, on the temperature at which crystallization occurs. Moreover, since the thickness of chain-folded lamellae depends on crystallization temperature; greater is the thickness of the lamellar structure much greater is also the melting temperature. Then, the polymeric materials react to thermal treatments with modifications of their structure and their properties. In addition, it is possible to get an increase in the lamellae thickness annealing the piece just below the melting temperature. The process of annealing, consecutively, increases the melting temperature of the polymer.

The phenomenon of the glass transition, instead, occurs in amorphous and semicrystalline polymers. It is due to a reduction in motion of large segments of molecular chains as the temperature decreases. Upon cooling, the glass transition corresponds to the gradual transformation from a liquid into a rubbery material, and then into a rigid solid; the last step corresponds to the glass transition. In particular, the temperature at which the polymer undergoes the transformation from a rubbery into a rigid state is called the glass transition temperature T_g. It is important to note that the glass transition does not occur suddenly, but usually takes place over a temperature range. The value of T_g depends on the mobility of the polymer chain, the more immobile the chain, the higher the value of T_g. Both melting temperature and glass transition temperature are very important parameters for the industrial applications of polymeric materials. They define, respectively, the upper and lower temperature limits for many applications, especially for semicrystalline polymers. The glass transition temperature, moreover, defines the upper limit temperature for glassy amorphous materials. In addition, T_m and T_g also influence the fabrication and processing of polymers and polymer matrix composites. The temperatures at which the phenomena occur for polymer are determined by a plot where the specific volume (the reciprocal of the density) is a function of temperature (Fig. 3.3).

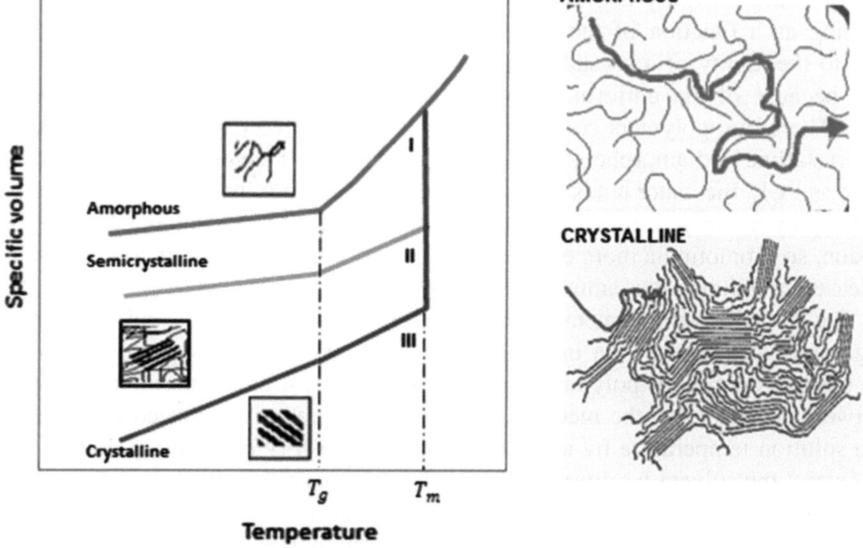

Fig. 3.3 Specific volume of polymers as a function of temperature for totally amorphous (**a**), semicrystalline (**b**), and crystalline (**c**) polymers and schematic representation of diffusion mechanisms of small molecules amorphous and crystalline domains

For crystalline polymers, there is a discontinuous change in specific volume at the melting temperature. The curve for the totally amorphous material is continuous but with a slight decrease in slope at the glass transition temperature. In the case of a semicrystalline polymer, there is the coexistence of crystalline and amorphous phases. The exact temperatures at which the polymer chains undergo these transitions depend on the structure of the polymer, which means that molecular chemistry and structure are factors able to influence melting and glass transition temperatures.

Both the melting and the glass transition temperatures are influenced from the molecular structure and the inter chain bonds of polymers. During the melting process, in fact, there is a rearrangement of the molecules in the transformation from ordered to disordered molecular states. Molecular chemistry and structure influence the ability of polymer chain molecules to make these rearrangements affecting the melting temperature. Chain stiffness also has a pronounced effect on melting temperature because of double bonds in the polymer backbone, in fact, rigid chains have higher T_m. Moreover, the melting temperature and glass transition temperature also depend on molecular weight. At low molecular weights T_m decrease, since low polymer molecular weight have shorter chain length comparing to higher polymer molecular weight. Less significantly, even an increase of molecular weight generally is coupled to the increase of T_g.

The control of amorphous and crystalline domains by thermal process conditions into a polymer system is extremely important to properly design the final properties of devices for biomedical use. For instance, polymer based carriers for drug delivery applications are generally designed by using different polymers in terms of degradability and crystallinity, which allows different drug and growth loading as a function of the relative crystalline/amorphous phase ratio. This is due to the ability of a crystalline polymer to degrade slowly than an amorphous one because of the uniform arrangement of its chains within the lattice structure. Therefore, polymers commonly used in drug delivery are usually a mixture of crystalline and amorphous forms [29]. Indeed, into a semi-crystalline polymer such as PCL, the water tends to easily penetrate only into the amorphous domains of the polymer matrix, thus facilitating the release of the water soluble drug by diffusion, so promoting a more efficient encapsulation of drug as well as a controlled release through polymer amorphous regions.

The peculiar arrangement of polymer chains in crystalline and amorphous regions is also relevant on influencing mechanisms of phase separation induced by thermal cooling of polymer solutions to design scaffolds with multiscale pore network. In this case, the mechanism of phase separation is induced by lowering the solution temperature by a controlled thermal history or adding a non-solvent to extract the solvent by different thermodynamic affinity of components. Indeed, thermally induced phase separation (TIPS) of polymer solution is a complex process, depending on the interplay between thermodynamic and kinetic evolution of the polymer solution cooling process. In particular, a liquid–liquid phase separation occurs when the applied temperature is higher than the solvent crystallization temperature or higher than the freezing point, while a solid–liquid phase separation takes place when the solvent crystallization temperature exceeds the coolant temperature. The strict control of physical transition of polymer component by applying appropriate thermal histories can significantly influence the final aspect of the scaffold in terms of morphological and mechanical properties. For example, the cooling kinetics can affect the degree of crystallinity of the polymer matrix, promoting the formation of scaffolds with high mechanical properties in comparison with products obtained by conventional techniques. During liquid–liquid phase separation, the presence of semi-crystalline polymers in solution (e.g., polylactide and polycaprolactone) may frequently initiate a gelation process. This leads to the formation of small crystallites, which act as physical crosslinks; these can stabilize the 3D polymer network and may also enhance the mechanical properties. The study of the behavior of binary systems becomes more complex in the presence of a solid–liquid separation mechanism. This is because of the formation of microcellular domains, which grow preferentially during cooling of the polymer solution until the solvent crystallization temperature is reached. Moreover, solvent removal by freeze drying promotes the formation of macropores as consequence of the solvent sublimation, preserving the crystal shape previously formed.

Mechanical Properties of Polymers

Basic Aspects: Toughness and Viscoelasticity

The mechanical response of polymers is the result of several force contributions: the properties of single polymer chains mediated by intramolecular forces and the properties of polymer chains assembly in the bulk system governed by intermolecular forces. However, it is really complex to identify separately the contribution of different forces which often mutually concur to the final mechanical response offering a multiplicity of different behavior as a function to the specific force activity. From macroscopic point of view, the mechanical behavior of polymers is generally classified into three categories: brittle, ductile, and rubbery (Fig. 3.4). Brittle polymers show a high modulus and high ultimate tensile strength but low ductility and toughness and are generally characterized by a glass transition T_g that is much higher than room temperature, (i.e., Polymethylmetacrilate, PMMA). Ductile polymers are semicrystalline polymers such as polyethylene or polytetrafluoroethylene (PTFE) that have a T_g below room temperature for the amorphous polymer content. The intrinsic crystalline regions confer the strength to the polymer while the amorphous regions determine the capability of energy adsorption before failure (toughness). These polymers have generally lower strength and modulus but greater toughness than brittle polymers. Finally, rubbery polymers show low moduli since they have a T_g well below room temperature, but they can return to their original shape following high extensions since cross-links prevent significant polymer chain translations.

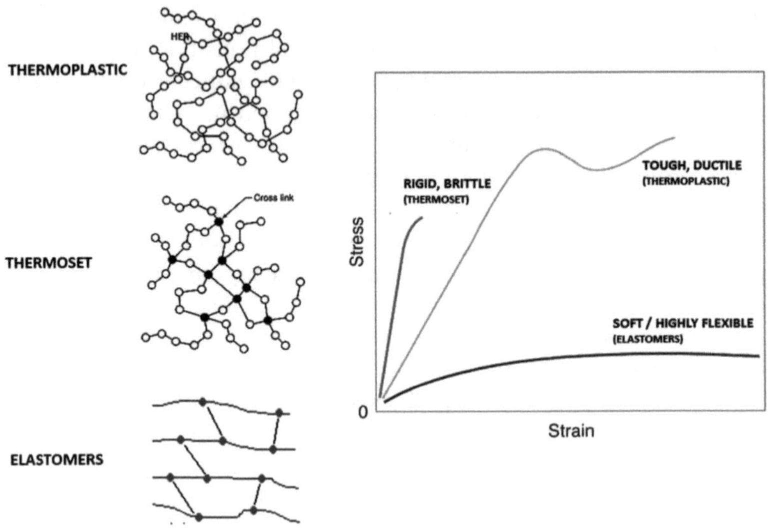

Fig. 3.4 Stress versus strain curves of three different polymer classes characterized by different molecular interactions

According to this classification, it is possible to recognize three different groups of polymers namely thermoplastic, thermoset and elastomers, respectively (Fig. 3.4) which may be classified as a function of peculiar intra and inter molecular interactions. Thermoplastic polymers are made of individual polymer chains that are held together by relatively weak van der Waals and dipole-dipole forces. They are generally processed into products by melt processing such as injection molding and extrusion, but may be also dissolved in solvents to form films and other devices by casting technique. Thermosetting polymers contain cross-links between polymer chains. Cross-links are covalent bonds between chains and can be formed using monomers with at least two free-functionalities during synthesis (i.e., polyurethanes, silicones). Depending on the cross-link density, thermosets can swell in certain solvents, whereas may degrade prior to reach the theoretical melting point. Sometimes, cross-links may be created after the polymer is formed (i.e., Vulcanization) with the support of cross-linking agent (i.e., sulfurs) but in this case they are named rubbers or elastomers. Their mechanical properties are strongly influenced by the peculiar organization/conformation of chains and their interactions at atomic, microscopic, and macroscopic scales, thus allowing to variously resist against stretching (i.e., tensile strength), compression (i.e., compressive strength), bending (i.e., flexural strength), sudden stress (i.e., impact strength), and dynamic loading (fatigue). As function of molecular weight and the level of intramolecular forces, polymers may display different mechanical properties under an applied stress. For instance, flexible polymers work better under stretching rather than a rigid polymer working better under compression. In the case of thermoset polymers, as cross-link density increases, the slope of the stress/strain line become steeper, corresponding to higher elastic moduli, and ultimately, to higher polymer strength or stiffness. In the case of thermoplastic polymers as melt or viscous solutions may be handled with more difficulty as their molecular weight increases due to the occurrence of topological interactions called entanglement, which limit the sliding of adjacent polymer chains.

The most part of polymers shows mechanical properties which are also highly strain rate and temperature dependent. In this case, polymers are no purely elastic but are viscoelastic materials and stiffness increases with increasing strain rate and decreasing temperature. For an elastic solid, stress σ is a linear function of the applied strain, and there is no strain-rate dependence. Elastic modulus E is the slope of the stress versus strain curve. For viscous materials, instead, stress is proportional to strain rate and unrelated to strain and viscosity η is the slope of the stress versus strain rate curve. Polymers generally exhibit both viscous and solid mechanical behavior simultaneously, namely viscoelasticity, and the degree of viscous behavior depends on temperature and strain rate. Below the T_g, polymers will behave more or less as elastic solids with very little viscous behavior. Above T_g, polymers exhibit viscoelastic behavior until they reach their melting temperature, behaving as liquids. This is relevant on the design of polymer gels which are liquid embedded network with liquid appearance but have to transform into relatively rigid network structures by a change in temperature or by addition of ionic cross-linking agents. They are largely used for cell interaction studies due to their excellent biocompatibility but mainly to fabricate injectable systems able to release molecular species in vivo.

Moreover, many polymers may deform differently with time when they are under a continuous load (creep mechanism). Ideal elastic solids do not show any creep since strain is proportional to stress, and there is no time dependence. Viscous materials (liquids) deform at a constant rate with a constant applied stress. Viscoelastic polymers may show both mechanisms so variously behave in terms of modulus, ductility, and strength as a function of the strain rate. This is the basic working mechanisms of hydrogels such as hyaluronic acid which are largely used as dumping systems in the place of damaged articular cartilage, for nucleus substitution in spine surgery or ocular therapies. For example, the physical properties of hyaluronic acid (HA) and its derivate compounds, including viscosity, elasticity and highly negative charge, make it useful in various therapeutic uses including tissue engineering and viscosupplementation for osteoarthritis treatment. HA's structural characteristics hinge on this random coiled structure in solution. At very low concentrations, chains entangle each other, leading to a mild viscosity which is strictly dependent upon the molecular weight of polymer. On the other hand, HA solutions at higher concentrations are very highly viscous due to greater HA chain entanglement which confer to the polymer a shear-dependent mechanical behavior. Indeed, the most distinctive property of HA is its peculiar viscoelasticity in the hydrated state as a function of shear rate stimulation. For example, the viscosity of a 1 % solution of HA, having a molar mass of 3–4 $\times$ 10^6 Da, is about 500,000 times that of water at low shear rate, but can drop 1,000-fold when forced through a fine needle. As a consequence, high shear rates promote a reduction of

HA viscosity, which is reflected in the force required to overcome internal friction. This also increases the elasticity, namely stored energy, thus permitting the polymer chain recovery after deformation. In consideration of these peculiar viscosity and elasticity properties, HA have been largely used in various surgical or medical preparations to replace the vitreous body after surgery, to manipulate the retina in retinal detachment surgery or protect the corneal endothelium in corneal transplantation (viscoprotection) [30, 31]. Indeed, HA solutions may be intraocularly implanted by different surgical practices as a function of viscoelastic properties; high viscosity at low shear rate allows to maintain space and manipulate tissues; moderate viscosity at medium shear rates allows easily for the manipulation of surgical instruments and intraocular lenses within the polymer solution. Very low viscosity at high shear rates allows to minimize the pressure needed to expel the solution through a thin cannula. Meanwhile, high degree of elasticity is fundamental to protect adjacent intraocular tissues, especially the endothelial cells of the cornea, from contact with surgical instruments. For example, highly visco-elastic HA solutions (i.e., Healon®) are commercially available for therapeutic use in alleviating discomfort in "dry eye syndrome". Although HA is not present in tears, in many aspects sodium hyaluronate is similar to mucin, a major component of tears. Mucin with a mean molar mass of about 2 MDa shows, similarly to HA, typical visco-elastic and shear-thinning behavior. This glycoprotein plays an important role in the lubricating, cleansing, and water-retaining properties of tears. In this case, the usefulness of an HA solution as a tear substitute resides in its water-entrapment capacity (hydration) and its function as a visco-elastic barrier between the corneal and conjunctival epithelia. Indeed, the HA eye drops are elastically deformed during eye blinking, but not removed from the surface of the eye with blinking movements.

HAs have been also successfully used to support the normal activity of pathological articular cartilage when the synovial fluid in osteoarthritis joints lacks sufficient shock absorption and lubrication properties mostly due to the not adequate viscosity of fluid at the interface (i.e., viscosupplementation) [30]. In particular, a large series of HA injectable preparations are commercially available to modify the local properties of the joint fluid with different viscoelasticity in order to stimulate the production of endogenous HA, to inhibit the effects of inflammatory mediators, and to decrease cartilage degradation also promoting cartilage matrix synthesis.

Referring to structural applications, viscoelastic properties of polymers are historically used to reproduce the mechanical properties of natural ligament into a synthetic prosthesis which have to develop the knee function after injury. Indeed, natural ligaments exhibit significant time and history dependent viscoelastic properties with different strain-rate sensitivity as a function of the proximity to the bone tissue joint, which is crucial to preserve it from uncontrolled failure under different loading conditions [32]. The composite structure of native tissue also contributes to mediate the viscoelastic properties of natural ligaments, which regulate important biomechanical functions of the knee during dynamic loading [33]. In particular, the viscous dissipation evident at low strain and/or low loading frequency is presumably due to the mechanical interaction (friction) between collagen fibres and the hydrated matrix of proteoglycans and glycoproteins [34] as suggested by the dependence of the loss modulus upon the static stress [35]. Current devices for ligament augmentation characterized by fibrous in woven non woven tissues made of monolithic polymers are suitable to replace many of its biomechanical functions due to the intrinsic viscoelastic properties of constituent materials [36, 37]. However, its simplified architecture does not reproduce completely the mechanical features of the natural tissue. Hence recently enabled to develop soft composite materials fabricated by reinforcing hydrogel-like matrixes with rigid polymeric fibres have been proposed alternatively [38]. In this case, the mechanical response is strictly controlled by the structural arrangement of the reinforcing fibres and by the properties of the components so that the static and dynamic mechanical behavior of natural ligaments can be reproduced [39]. Noteworthy, the viscoelastic response of device is also affected by intermolecular forces which concur to the macroscopic mechanical response including fibre hydration, fibre–matrix interaction, and fibre–fibre interaction, which influence the mechanical parameters (i.e., static, storage, loss moduli) of the composite materials and preserve the same constitutive dependency upon the kinematics variables (i.e., strain, frequency) as natural tissues. More recently degradable polymers typically used for tissue engineering approaches [40] allow to design ligament devices where the viscoelastic response progressively changes as the polymer begin to degrade in vivo, opening new advantages in terms of biocompatibility for in vivo ACL reconstruction.

Mechanical Properties Mediated by Intermolecular Forces

Mechanical properties are among the most fundamental properties of polymeric materials [41] in biomedical applications. In traditional applications, polymers firstly have to meet the basic mechanical criteria such as strength (modulus), energy-dissipating capacity (toughness) and elasticity. With the tremendous progress made in polymer science in the last century, a wide range of synthetic polymers with excellent mechanical properties have been developed for various applications including plastic, fibre, and elastomers [42, 43]. Whereas synthetic polymers can be prepared to meet particular mechanical parameter one at a time, it is still challenging to design advanced polymeric materials that show peculiar mechanical properties as a function of the specific application.

In this context, the approach based on the learning for nature allows to design synthetic polymers mimicking the natural biopolymers on natural tissues that combine important mechanical properties including strength, toughness, and elasticity. For example, cell adhesion proteins and connective proteins existing in both soft and hard tissues such as muscle [44], and bone [45] exhibit a remarkable combination of high strength, toughness, and sometimes elasticity as well—three properties that are rarely found in one synthetic polymer. Starting from this approach, recent advanced structural analysis and single-molecule nanomechanical studies revealed that the combination of these mechanical properties in natural materials originates from their unique molecular and nanoscopic structures [46]. These mechanistic understandings at molecular level provide inspiration to materials scientists for designing biomimetic polymers that have a balance of advanced mechanical properties.

One important strategy nature adopted to enhance mechanical properties is the use of non-covalent weak forces in addition to covalent bonds. By programming weak forces, such as hydrogen bonds, hydrophobic interactions, and ionic interactions, etc., biopolymers can achieve combined mechanical performances that synthetic polymers still cannot rival. Among the weak forces, inter-molecular interactions among biopolymers chains are particularly interesting to enhance mechanical properties. For instance, the exceptional mechanical properties of silk produced by spiders have recently attracted much attention from scientists in various disciplines to investigate the molecular origin of its mechanical properties mainly ascribable to intermolecular forces. For example, natural silk produced by spiders shows an exceptional strength (tensile strength of 1.5 GPa) and toughness (150 MJ/m), which makes it stronger than steel compared on a weight basis and has a tensile strength similar to Kevlar. Moreover, it is also characterized by high elasticity and exceptionally high toughness values never attained in synthetic high-performance fibres which are directly ascribable to the peculiar polymer chain organization. Indeed, spider silk is a semicrystalline material made of amorphous segments reinforced by strong and stiff crystalline domains. Molecular studies [47] indicate that the crystalline domains are made of hydrophobic poly (alanine) and poly (alanine-glycine) repeat motifs whereas the amorphous segments are composed of glycine-rich peptides formed both inter- and intramolecularly (Fig. 3.5). This peculiar microscopic organization explain the species-specific silk mechanical response well represented by a characteristic nonlinear stress–strain (σ–ε) curve which show four distinct regimes characteristic of silk: (a) stiff initial response governed by homogeneous stretching; (b) entropic unfolding of semi-amorphous protein domains; (c), stiffening regime as molecules align and

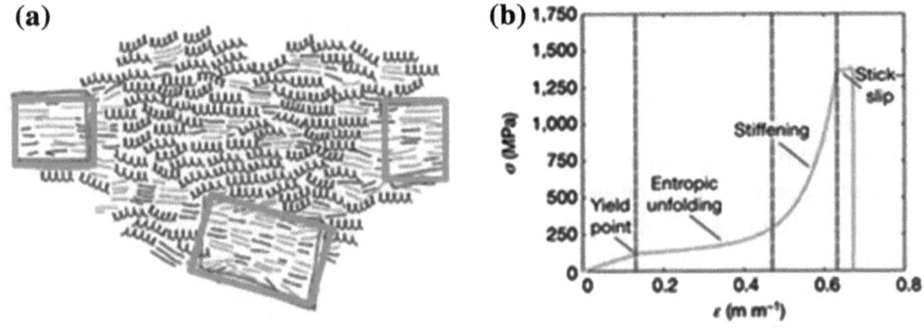

Fig. 3.5 **a** Spider silk microscopic model to reproduce chain arrangement of spider silk. **b** Stress–strain curve to describe the mechanical behavior of spider silk (adapted from [48])

load is transferred to the β-sheet crystals; and (d) stick–slip deformation of β-sheet crystals until failure [48].

Based on X-ray evidence, spider silk is characterized by a large number of nanocrystallites separated by amorphous regions made of flexible chains. This allows to underline the important role of crystallites, which act as multifunctional crosslinks playing an analogous role of carbon black in carbon-reinforced elastomers, creating inside the amorphous regions a thin layer with modulus higher than in the bulk. This is an excellent example of using a combination of inter and intramolecular weak forces (hydrogen bonds) to assemble polymers into more ordered structures for enhanced mechanical properties and have inspired many researchers to design biomimetic fibres that hopefully can mimic both its structure and mechanical properties. Sogah and coworkers [43] have proposed a synthesis of peptide and synthetic modules to imitate the crystalline and amorphous silk structures based on the assembly of phenoxathiin-templated parallel β-sheet peptide building blocks which are linked into polymers through polymerization. However, the design of a synthetic polymer that imitate both the structure and mechanical properties of spider dragline silk is still far due to the difficulty to effectively balance of various molecular parameters that control polymer secondary structures to achieve optimal mechanical properties.

In this direction, stimuli responsive polymers are emerging as a versatile solution to adapt the properties of materials to the biological context, by properly imparting external stimuli [49, 50]. Their recent success rises from the low costs of materials combined with the ease to tailor, better than tradition materials classes specific functionalities, by the responsive behavior to pH, temperature, ionic strength, electric or magnetic field, light and/or other chemical or biological stimuli. Indeed, this offers the opportunity to design highly customizable materials with a large variety of properties to be fruitfully used in biomedical applications from drug delivery to tissue engineering [51, 52].

Among them, crosslinked hydrogels based on interpenetrating networks (IPN) are extremely interesting for their peculiar mechanical properties. They consist of two covalently linked polymer networks which are bound together by physical entanglement as opposed to covalent bonds. This is possible by the polymerization of both networks simultaneously and results in two intermixed networks that can only be separated by breaking bonds. As a consequence, this confers to the polymer the ability to improve the intrinsic mechanical properties by controlling two networks interactions or maintain two different properties when acting independently. This approach is also particularly interesting in drug delivery application where the drug release may be controlled by thermosensitive properties of IPN gel [53]. Specifically, an interpenetrating network of polyacrylic acid (PAA) and polyacrylamide (PAAm) above the transition temperature break the hydrogen bonding among chains which assure the water retention at lower temperature, inducing the networks to swell thus giving the possibility of increasing drug release with increased temperature. Recent work on the same IPN with grafted β-cyclodextrin showed a faster response for lower transition temperature (35 °C) promoting a more efficient swelling at body temperature [54].

Concluding Remarks

The basic mechanisms at molecular level used in nature to design natural materials are increasingly inspiring chemists and materials scientists to design biomimetic polymers to imitate both the structures and properties of their natural counterparts. Due to the complexity and subtlety of biopolymer structures, it remains a major challenge but the rapid improvement of advanced analytical techniques open new insights to develop truly effective synthetic polymers that can rival the biomimetic performance of their natural analogs. Despite many techniques are available to synthesize and process polymers for biomedical applications, there is still a need to either develop novel methodologies or expand their employment to more polymers, in the light of knowledge of chemical and physical interactions and recent discovery of effects of micro environmental stimuli, thus giving the opportunity to design a greater variety of modified polymers that can be used as innovative systems in pharmaceutics and medicine.

Acknowledgments This study was financially supported by BEYOND-NANO (PON A3_00363), POLIFARMA (PON02_3203241) and NEWTON (FIRB-RBAP11BYNP).

References

1. Handa, H., Major, T.C., Brisbois, E.J., Amoako, K.A., Meyerhoff, M.E., Bartlett, R.H.: Hemocompatibility comparison of biomedical grade polymers using rabbit thrombogenicity model for preparing nonthrombogenic nitric oxide releasing surfaces. J. Mater. Chem. B. Mater. Biol. Med. **2**, 1059–1067 (2014)
2. Fujiwara, T., Nagaoka, E., Watanabe, T., Miyagi, N., Kitao, T., Sakota, D., Mamiya, T., Shinshi, T., Arai, H., Takatani, S.: New generation extracorporeal membrane oxygenation with MedTech Mag-Lev, a single-use, magnetically levitated, centrifugal blood pump: preclinical evaluation in calves. Artif. Organs. **37**, 447 (2013)
3. Pandis, N., Fleming, P.S., Kloukos, D., Polychronopoulou, A., Katsaros, C., Eliades, T.: Survival of bonded lingual retainers with chemical or photo polymerization over a 2-year period: a single-center, randomized controlled clinical trial. Am. J. Orthod. Dentofacial. Orthop. **144**, 169 (2013)
4. Goyal, A., Hurkadle, J., Magegowda, S., Bhatia, P.: Use of light-curing units in orthodontics. J. Investig. Clin. Dent. **4**, 137 (2013)
5. Wan Abdul Khodir, W.K., Guarino, V., Alvarez-Perez, M.A., Cafiero, C., Ambrosio, L.: Trapping of tetracycline loaded nanoparticles into PCL fibre networks in periodontal regeneration therapy. J. Bioact. Compat. Polym. **28**, 258 (2013)
6. Pires, L.R., Guarino, V., Oliveira, M.J., Ribeiro, C.C., Barbosa, M.A., Ambrosio, L., Pego, A.P.: Loading poly(trimethylene carbonate-co-ε-caprolactone) fibers with ibuprofen towards nerve regeneration. J. Tissue Eng. Reg. Med. (2013). doi:10.1002/term.1792
7. Guarino, V., Alvarez-Perez, M.A., Borriello, A., Napolitano, T., Ambrosio, L.: Conductive PEGDA/pani macroporous hydrogels for nerve regeneration. Adv. Healthc. Mater. **2**, 218 (2013)
8. Lutolf, M.P., Hubbell, J.A.: Synthetic biomaterials as instructive extracellular microenvironments for morphogenesis in tissue engineering. Nat. Biotechnol. **23**, 47 (2005)
9. Zustiak, S.P., Leach, J.B.: Hydrolytically degradable poly(ethylene glycol) hydrogel scaffolds with tunable degradation and mechanical properties. Biomacromolecules **11**, 1348 (2010)

10. Nie, T., Baldwin, A., Yamaguchi, N.: Production of heparin-functionalized hydrogels for the development of responsive and controlled growth factor delivery systems. J. Control. Release **122**, 287 (2007)
11. Kopecek, J., Yang, J.: Hydrogels as smart materials. Polym. Int. **56**, 1078 (2007)
12. Matthew, H.W., Salley, S.O., Peterson, W.D.: Complex coacervate microcapsules for mammalian cell culture and artificial organ development. Biotechnol. Prog. **9**, 510 (1993)
13. Hugel, T., Seitz, M.: The study of molecular interactions by AFM force spectroscopy. Macromol. Rapid Commun. **22**, 989 (2001)
14. Callister, W.D.: Material Science and Engineering: An Introduction, 7th edn. Wiley, Hoboken (2008)
15. Padmavathi, D.A.: Energy curves and material properties. Mater. Sci. Appl. **2**, 97 (2011)
16. Ratner, B.D., Hoffman, A.S., Schoen, F.J., Lemons, J.E.: Biomaterials science: an introduction to materials in medicine. Biomaterials Sci. Academic press, New York (1996)
17. Ambrosio, J.: Polymer molecular weight. Chap. 3 online version, p. 43 (2011)
18. Agilent Technologies: Polymer molecular weight distribution and definitions of MW averages. Technical Overview (2011)
19. Gilbert, R.G., Hess, M., Jenkins, A.D., Jones, R.G., Kratochvil, P., Stepto, R.F.T.: Dispersity in polymer science. IUPAC recommendations 2009. Pure Appl. Chem. **81**, 351 (2009)
20. Zhang, Z., Yang, G.: A new method for estimation of weight average molecular weight of polymer from the intrinsic viscosity and chromatogram. Chin. J. Polym. Sci. **2**, 142 (1986)
21. Zander, N.E.: Hierarchically structured electrospun fibers. Polymers **5**(1), 19 (2013)
22. Zong, X.H., Kim, K., Fang, D.F., Ran, S., Hsiao, B.S., Chu, B.: Structure and process relationship of electrospun bioabsorbable nano membranes. Polymers **43**, 4403 (2002)
23. Guarino, V., Cirillo, V., Taddei, P.: Tuning size scale and crystallinity of PCL electrospunfibres via solvent permittivity to address hMSC response. Macromol. Biosci. **11**, 1694 (2011)
24. Wu, Y., Clark, R.L.: Electrohydrodynamic atomization: a versatile process for preparing materials for biomedical applications. J. Biomater. Sci. Polym. **19**, 573 (2008)
25. Shenoy, S.L., Bates, W.D., Frisch, H.L., Wneak, G.E.: Role of chain entanglements on fiber formation during electrospinning of polymer solutions: good solvent, non-specific polymer–polymer interaction limit. Polymers **46**, 3372 (2005)
26. Mayol, L., Borzacchiello, A., Guarino, V.: Design of electrospayed non-spherical poly (L-lactide-co-glicolide) microdevices for sustained drug delivery. J. Mater. Sci. Mater. Med. (2013). doi:10.1007/s10856-013-5080-5
27. Doi, M., Ohta, T.: Dynamics and rheology of complex interfaces. J. Chem. Phys. **95**, 1242 (1991)
28. Guarino, V., Guaccio, A., Ambrosio, L.: Anipulating co-continuous polymer blends to create PCL scaffolds with fully interconnected and anisotropic pore architecture. J. Appl. Biomater. Biomech. **9**(1), 34 (2011)
29. Coccoli, V., Luciani, A., Orsi, S.: Engineering of poly(*e*-caprolactone) microcarriers to modulate protein encapsulation capability and release kinetic. J. Mater. Sci. Mater. Med. **19**, 1703 (2008)
30. Volpi, N., Schiller, J., Stern, R., Soltes, L.: Role, metabolism, chemical modifications and applications of hyaluronan. Curr. Med. Chem. **16**(14), 1718 (2009)
31. Shen, B., Wei, A., Bhargav, D., Kishen, T., Diwan, A.D.: Hyaluronan: its potential application in intervertebral disc regeneration. Orthop. Res. Rev. **10**, 217 (2010)
32. Kwan, M.K., Lin, T.H.C., Woo, S.L.Y.: On the viscoelastic properties of the anteromedial bundle of the anterior cruciate ligament. J. Biomech. **26**, 447 (1993)
33. Woo, S.H.: Mechanical properties of tendons and ligaments: quasi-static and nonlinear viscoelastic properties. Biorheology **19**, 385 (1982)
34. Haut, R.C.: The mechanical and viscoelastic properties of the anterior cruciate ligament and of ACL fascicles. In: Jackson, D.W. (ed.) The Anterior Cruciate Ligament, p. 63. Raven Press, New York (1993)
35. Netti, P., D'Amore, A., Ronca, D., Ambrosio, L., Nicolais, L.: Structure–mechanical properties relationship of natural tendons and ligaments. J. Mater. Sci. Mater. Med. **7**, 525 (1996)

36. Cooper, J.A., Lu, H.H., Ko, F.K., Freeman, J.W., Laurencin, C.T.: Fiber-based tissue-engineered scaffold for ligament replacement: design considerations and in vitro evaluation. Biomaterials **26**(13), 1523 (2005)
37. Freeman, J.W., Kwansa, A.L.: Recent advancements in ligament tissue engineering: the use of various techniques and materials for ACL repair. Recent Pat. Biomed. Eng. **1**, 18 (2008)
38. Guarino,V., Causa, F., Ambrosio, L.: Bioactive scaffolds for bone and ligament tissue. Expert Rev. Med. Devices **4**(3), 405 (2007). http://informahealthcare.com/doi/abs/10.1586/17434440.4.3.405
39. Ambrosio, L., De Santis, R., Iannace, S.: Viscoelastic behavior of composite ligament prostheses. J. Biomed. Mater. Res. **42**, 6 (1998)
40. Vunjak-Novakovic, G., Altman, G., Horan, R.: Tissue engineering of ligaments. Ann. Rev. Biomed. Eng. **6**, 131 (2004)
41. Hearle, J.W.S.: Polymers and Their Properties, Vol 1: Fundamentals of Structure and Mechanics. Halstead Press, New York (1982)
42. Krejchi, M.T., Atkins, E.D.T., Waddon, A.J., Fournier, M.J., Mason, T.L., Tirrell, D.A.: Chemical sequence control of beta-sheet assembly in macromolecular crystals of periodic proteins. Science **265**, 1427 (1994)
43. Rathore, O., Sogah, D.Y.J.: Self-assembly of beta-sheets into nanostructures by poly(alanine) segments incorporated in multiblock copolymers inspired by spider silk. Am. Chem. Soc. **123**, 5231 (2001)
44. Rief, M., Gautel, M., Oesterhelt, F., Fernandez, J.M., Gaub, H.E.: Reversible unfolding of individual titin immunoglobulin domains by AFM. Science **276**, 1109 (1997)
45. Thompson, J.B., Kindt, J.H., Drake, B., Hansma, H.G., Morse, D.E., Hansma, P.K.: Bone indentation recovery time correlates with bond reforming time. Nature **414**, 773 (2001)
46. Marszalek, P.E., Lu, H., Li, H., Carrion-Vazquez, M., Oberhauser, A.F., Schulten, K., Fernandez, J.M.: Mechanical unfolding intermediates in titin modules. Nature **402**, 100 (1999)
47. Van Beek, J.D., Hess, S., Vollrath, F., Meier, B.H.: The molecular structure of spider dragline silk: folding and orientation of the protein backbone Proc. Natl. Acad. Sci. U.S.A **99**(16):10266 (2002)
48. Keten, S., Xu, Z.P., Ihle, B., Buehler, M.J.: Nanoconfinement controls stiffness, strength and mechanical toughness of beta-sheet crystals in silk. Nat. Mater. **9**(4), 359 (2010)
49. Stile, R.A., Healy, K.E.: Thermo-responsive peptide-modified hydrogels for tissue regeneration. Biomacromolecules **2**(1), 185 (2001)
50. Twaites, B.R., Alarcon, C.D.H., Lavigne, M., Saulnier, A., Pennadam, S.S., Cunliffe, D., Gorecki, D.C., Alexander, C.: Thermoresponsive polymers as gene delivery vectors: cell viability DNA transport and transfection studies. J. Control. Release **108**, 472 (2005)
51. Liu, F., Urban, M.W.: Recent advances and challenges in designing stimuli-responsive polymers. Prog. Polym. Sci. **35**, 3 (2010)
52. Klouda, L., Mikos, A.G.: Thermoresponsive hydrogels in biomedical applications. Eur. J. Pharm. Biopharm. **68**, 34 (2008)
53. Shin, H.S., Kim, S.Y., Lee, Y.M.: Indomethacin release behaviors from pH and thermoresponsive poly(vinyl alcohol) and poly(acrylic acid) IPN hydrogels for site-specific drug delivery. J. Appl. Polym. Sci. **65**(4), 685 (1997)
54. Wang, Q.F., Li, S.M., Wang, Z.Y., Liu, H., Li, C.: Preparation and characterization of a positive thermoresponsive hydrogel for drug loading and release. J. Appl. Polym. Sci. **111**(4), 1417 (2009)

Chapter 4
Overview on Cell-Biomaterial Interactions

Sara Gonçalves, Fernando Dourado and Lígia R. Rodrigues

Abstract Biomaterials, a name given to express materials used as medical implants, indwelling devices, extracorporeal ones and other categories in several medical fields, have increasingly played a significant role when aiming at improving the quality of life in humans. The behavior of a biomaterial with the surrounding physiologic environment is of major relevance for determining the in vivo performance and host acceptance of any device. Indeed, the biocompatibility and bio-functionality of implantable devices remains a serious challenge in establishing the device's function and lifetime. Several research efforts have been conducted to further understand and control the interactions between biomaterials and cell-mediated processes, aiming at the definition of the main guidelines that regulate materials biocompatibility. Several criteria should be met when considering a biomaterial for a specific application. On the materials' perspective, its composition, mechanical, physicochemical, thermal, electrical properties must be well understood. In parallel, knowledge on the cell-biomaterial interaction mechanisms (including specific adhesion proteins and cell receptors, signal transduction, cell differentiation, tissue development, host immune response mechanisms, to name a few processes) must be attained, to better characterize, follow up and control cell-biomaterial interactions. This review attempts to define the basic phenomenon that take place when a biomaterial comes into contact with host living tissues. Numerous strategies have been investigated to overcome body reactions induced by the implantation of devices. These strategies, their advantages and limitations, along with the fundamentals underlying biomaterials-tissue interactions and current research on biomaterial surface modification are discussed. Besides, the use of polymeric biomaterials for use in age-related macular degeneration will be presented as a case study.

S. Gonçalves · F. Dourado · L.R. Rodrigues (✉)
CEB-Centre of Biological Engineering, University of Minho, 4710-057 Braga, Portugal
e-mail: lrmr@deb.uminho.pt

F. Puoci (ed.), *Advanced Polymers in Medicine*, DOI 10.1007/978-3-319-12478-0_4

Keywords Biomaterials · Cell-biomaterial interactions · Extracellular matrix · Integrins · Adhesion · Immune response · Biocompatibility · Biomaterial surface modifications · Topography · Morphology · Porosity · Hydrophobicity · Age-related macular degeneration · Retinal pigmented epithelial cells · Retina · Bruch's membrane

Abbreviations

AFM	Atomic force microscopy
AMD	Age-related macular degeneration
ATRP	Atom transfer radical polymerization
BM	Bruch's membrane
CCMS	4-(N-cinnamoylcarbamide)methylstyrene
DNA	Deoxyribonucleic acid
ECM	Extracellular matrix
EGF	Epithelial cell growth factor
FBGCs	Foreign body giant cells
FGF	Fibroblast growth factor
Fn	Fibrinogen
GAGs	Glycosaminoglycans
GOD	Glucose oxidase
HLC	Human lens capsule
ICAMs	Intracellular adhesion molecules
IPAAm	N-isopropylacrylamide
IPE	Iris pigment epithelium
IPNs	Interpenetrating polymer networks
LB	Langmuir-Blodgett
MAdCAM	Mucosal addressin cell adhesion molecule
OSs	Photoreceptor outer segments
PDMS	Polydimethylsiloxane
PGS	Poly(glycerol sebacate)
PHBV8	Poly(hydroxybutyrate-co-hydroxyvalerate)
PLC	Porcine lens capsule
PLGA	Poly(lactic-co-glycolic) acid
PLLA	Poly(L-lactide)
PMMA	Poly(methyl methacrylate)
PMN	Polymorphonuclear leukocytes
RFGD	Radio frequency gas discharge
RGD	Tripeptide Arg-Gly-Asp
RPCs	Retinal progenitor cells
RPE	Retinal pigment-epithelium
SAMs	Self-assembly monolayers
SIP	Surface-initiated polymerization

STM	Scanning tunnelling microscopy
UV	Ultra-violet
VCAM	Vascular cell adhesion molecule
VEGF	Vascular endothelial cell growth factor
θ	Contact angle

Biomaterials

Biomaterials are materials foreign to the human body that are used in medicine to replace, support and restore body function [1]. A great amount of materials with distinct features have been used for different biomedical purposes ranging from tissue engineering to drug delivery systems. These however, are still far from being "ideal" materials [1, 2]. Indeed, great demands are posed to materials that are ought to be used as biomedical implants or prostheses. Whereas the desired bulk properties in terms of strength or elasticity can often be achieved, tailoring the biomaterials surfaces for a perfect interaction with the human body is a complex task. The behaviour of a biomaterial with the surrounding environment is crucial for the performance and host acceptance of any device. Biocompatibility and bio-functionality of implantable devices remains a serious challenge in establishing the device's function and lifetime.

Since biomaterials are intended to contact directly with living tissues and body fluids, they are targets of the protective mechanisms within the body, including protein adsorption, hemostasis, inflammation and foreign body response [3]. In the past decade, it has been accepted that, independently of their nature, all implantable biomaterials invoke similar inflammatory and foreign body responses [4]. Therefore, it is crucial to understand and predict the interactions between biomaterials and tissues or body fluids.

Cell adhesion to a biomaterial surface is a critical step for the integration of implants since it precedes other events, such as cell spreading, cell migration, and often cell differentiation [5]. Most mammalian cells are anchorage-dependent, meaning that they must adhere to a surface in order to survive [6]. On one hand, this adhesion is mediated by serum proteins adsorbed onto the material surface, such as immunoglobulins, vitronectin, fibrinogen and fibronectin [7–9]. On the other hand, the conditioning of the biomaterial's surface with serum proteins is greatly influenced by the physicochemical characteristics of the material and will determine the subsequent biological reactions [2, 10, 11].

Cell-biomaterial interactions involve cell adhesion and spreading (Fig. 4.1), and these are the consequence of a series of molecular events occurring in and around the cells that are regulated by trans-membrane receptors present in the extracellular matrix (ECM) [6, 12–14].

The biological molecules involved in cell adhesion and spreading, including ECM, cell membrane and cytoskeleton proteins, interact to induce signal transduction, promote transcription factors and regulate gene expression [16, 17]. Controlling the interaction between these proteins and biomaterials surfaces is an important factor for the design of biocompatible surfaces [7, 14, 18].

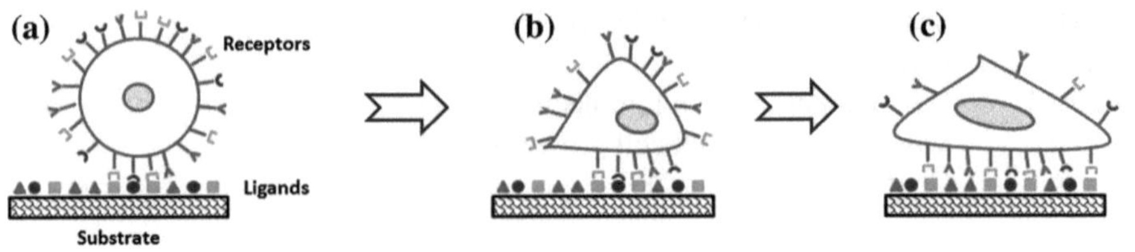

Fig. 4.1 Mammalian cell adhesion onto a biomaterial. **a** Initial contact between the cell and the biomaterial conditioned with serum proteins. **b** Bonding between cell surface receptors and protein adhesion ligands. **c** Cell cytoskeletal reorganization with progressive cell spreading onto the biomaterial surface. (Adapted from Ratner et al. [15])

Cells Involved in the Immune Response

In order to understand and predict cell-biomaterial interactions it is important to know which cells circulating in the blood are actively responding to biomaterials. Red blood cells carry hemoglobin that contains iron and is responsible for oxygen transport. White blood cells, known as leukocytes, are the ones involved in the body's immune response. Generally, the occurrence of an infection is characterized by an increased number of leukocytes. These are grouped into granulocytes, monocytes and lymphocytes. Table 4.1 summarizes these groups of leukocytes, their abundance within the leucocytes' population, function and relevance.

Among the granulocytes, which are the most representative group of white blood cells, the neutrophils are predominant. These cells provide a protective mechanism, as their function is to engulf and destroy foreign material.

Monocytes are also phagocytic cells capable of engulfing and destroying foreign substances. These cells change their morphology and differentiate into macrophages when going into the tissues. When the macrophage fails to phagocytize a given material, it coalesces with other cells and forms a multinucleated giant cell. Among the several types of giant cells, the Foreign Body Giant Cells (FBGCs, a collection of fused macrophages) is of major concern to biomaterials.

Table 4.1 Cells involved in the body's immune response (Adapted from Onuki et al. [3])

Leukocyte	Abundance*(%)	Function	Relevance
Granulocytes			
Neutrophil	65–70	Phagocytosis	Body defense against bacteria and other foreign substances
Eosinophil	3		Allergic response
Basophil	<1		Not well understood
Monocytes	10	Phagocytosis Differentiation into macrophages	Formation of foreign body giant cells
Lymphocytes	20	Production and secretion of immune proteins	Immune system

*Abundance within the leucocytes' population

The presence of FBGCs indicates that the phagocytic system is incapable of eliminating the foreign matter from the body. Tissue destruction often occurs and results in loss of normal tissue, loss of function of the organ, or significant bone resorption, depending on the site of inflammation [3, 19].

The lymphocytes are responsible for our immune system that protects us from disease. These cells are active protein factories and have a large nucleus that almost completely fills the cell. The small amount of cytoplasm contains the factory components for making and secreting immune proteins.

Scattered throughout the blood cells are fragments called platelets that are important in the clotting mechanisms, forming a plug to prevent excessive bleeding when the tissue is injured.

Extracellular Matrix

Normal cells respond to various environmental signals within the ECM. The interaction between cells and ECM is bidirectional and dynamic, meaning that cells are constantly accepting signals from the environment through the ECM, which in turn is often reshaped by the cells. At least three roles have been assigned to the ECM in the control of cell behavior, namely it (a) the provision of adhesion signals; (b) binding sites for growth factors; and (c) local protein breakdown for the occurrence of enzyme activity during cell migration [7, 16].

The ECM secreted by cells that populate a tissue or an organ, consists in a polymeric network of chemical and physical connections between several types of macromolecules. Its composition will be determined by factors like mechanical forces, oxygen requirements and gene expression patterns. Indeed, it is a complex mixture of structural and functional proteins (collagen and fibronectin), glycosaminoglycans (GAGs), glycoproteins and small molecules (Fig. 4.2) arranged in a unique, tissue-specific three-dimensional architecture [7, 16, 20].

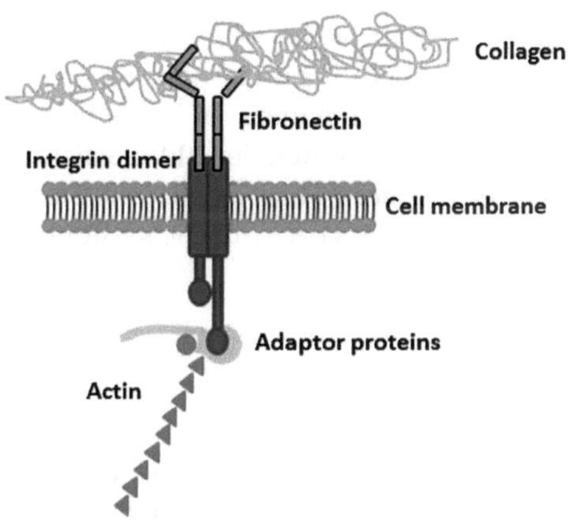

Fig. 4.2 Schematic representation of the extracellular matrix

Efforts have been conducted to mimic the ECM, i.e. by knowing its composition and how the components fit together, and how these will contribute to the advance of the biomaterials field. The rational division of the ECM into structural and functional components is not an easy task since many of these molecules present both structural and functional roles [16]. The most important ECM proteins are briefly described below.

Collagen

Collagen is the most abundant protein within the mammalian ECM, representing over 90 % of the ECM dry weight in most of the tissues and organs. More than 20 different types of collagen have been identified, each with a unique biological function [13–15]. Type I collagen is the main structural protein present in tissues. It is abundant in tendinous and ligamentous structures, and provides the necessary strength to accommodate the mechanical loading to which these tissues are commonly subjected. Furthermore, these tissues provide a convenient source of collagen for many biomedical applications. Other types of collagens can be found in the ECM in much lower amounts than Type I collagen, although providing different mechanical and physical properties to the ECM. One example is the Type IV collagen, which is present within the basement membrane of most vascular structures and tissues with an epithelial cell component [21].

Fibronectin

Fibronectin is the second most abundant protein in the ECM. It is a large dimeric glycoprotein that exists either in the soluble state or as a tissue isoform. The ECM of sub-mucosal structures, basement membranes and interstitial tissues contains great amounts of fibronectin. This protein possesses ligands for the adhesion of several cell types. Fibronectin is rich in the Arg-Gly-Asp (RGD) subunit, the most common adhesion motif, which is recognized by the cell surface receptors (integrins), thus being extremely important for cell adhesion [21]. When bound via integrins, this protein triggers a number of signal transduction pathways that activates events like cell spreading, proliferation, differentiation and migration [13]. The cell friendly features of fibronectin have made it an attractive substrate for in vitro cell culture, but also for its use to coat synthetic scaffold materials to promote biocompatibility [22].

Laminin

Laminin is an adhesion protein that is present in the ECM in numerous forms depending on the specific combination of its peptide chains. This protein is one of the most critical ECM factors in the cell and tissue differentiation [13].

Glycosaminoglycans

Depending on the tissue location, age of the host and microenvironment, several combinations of glycosaminoglycans (GAGs) can be found in the ECM. These macromolecules have various functions such as binding to growth factors and cytokines, promoting water retention and contributing to the gel properties of the matrix. Heparin and hyaluronic acid are examples of two GAGs that are present in the ECM [13].

Growth Factors

Although in small amounts, growth factors and cytokines are also present in the ECM and they act as potent cell behavior modulators. There is an extensive list of growth factors present in the ECM, including the vascular endothelial cell growth factor (VEGF), the fibroblast growth factor (FGF) family, and the epithelial cell growth factor (EGF), among others [23].

Cell Membrane Proteins—Integrins and Adhesion Proteins

The adhesion proteins are comprised of four main classes—selectins, immunoglobulin super family, adhesins and integrins—and are capable of interacting with specific ligands located at the membrane of neighbor cells or on the ECM [24]. Among the adhesion proteins, the integrins are the main cell surface receptors for proteins within the ECM [24, 25].

Integrins are transmembranar proteins that can act as a bridge between surface adsorbed ECM proteins and interacting cells. The cellular recognition of biomaterials and the progression of subsequent cellular events are essentially based on integrin-mediated interactions.

Integrins are composed of two non-covalently associated glycoprotein subunits, namely α- and β- subunits [25]. Different types of α- and β- subunits and different combinations exist, thus a large variety of integrins with the ability to bind to different types of ligands are available (Table 4.2) [26]. Many integrins are also capable of binding to more than one protein, whereas many proteins can act as ligands for more than one integrin [27, 28]. In the integrin structure, each subunit has a large extracellular domain, a transmembrane domain and a short cytoplasmic domain [25].

Integrins bind specifically to ECM proteins binding sites, such as the RGD sequence that is present in most of them (e.g. fibronectin). The fact that many integrins recognize this sequence is probably the explanation for their overlapping specificity [27, 29]. Besides, integrins can interact with components of the cytoskeleton and signaling molecules through their intracellular domain. Indeed, after binding to the ligand, the integrins also bind to several intracellular anchorage proteins including talin, α-actinin and filamin. Those anchorage proteins can

Table 4.2 Integrin types and respective ligands

Subunits		Ligands
β1	α1	Collagens, laminins
	α2	Collagens, laminins
	α3	Laminins, fibronectin, thrombospondin
	α4	Fibronectin, vascular cell adhesion molecule (VCAM)
	α5	Fibronectin
	α6	Laminins
	α7	Laminins
	α8	Fibronectin, tenascin
	α9	Tenascin
	α10	Collagens
	α11	Collagens
	αv	Fibronectin, vitronectin
β2	αL	Intracellular adhesion molecules (ICAMs)
	αM	Fibrinogen, ICAMs
	αX	Fibrinogen
	αD	VCAM, ICAMs
β3	αlib	Collagens, fibronectin, vitronectin, fibrinogen, thrombospondin
	αv	Fibronectin, vitronectin, fibrinogen, thrombospondin, osteopontin, tenascin
β4	α6	Laminins
β5	αv	Vitronectin
β6	αv	Fibronectin, tenascin
β7	α4	Fibronectin, VCAM, Mucosal addressin cell adhesion molecule (MAdCAM)
	αE	E-cadherin
β8	αv	Collagens, laminins, fibronectin

bind directly to actin or to other proteins like vinculin, thereby linking the integrin to actin filaments in the cell cortex. If the proper environmental conditions are in place, this linkage leads to a clustering of integrins and the focal adhesion between the cell and the ECM. The cytoskeletal attachment aids the formation of the integrins cluster providing a stronger aggregate bond [30].

This interaction between integrins and ECM proteins will affect the signal transduction which can induce adhesion, spreading and migration, as well as the expression of transcription factors and specific genes [31]. Besides the recruitment of signaling molecules, integrin activation also leads to changes in the cytoskeleton organization, subsequently affecting cell adhesion and mobility. Signals from different ECM ligands can result in different signaling pathways.

Integrins are promising targets for manipulating cellular and host responses to biomaterials. For instance, controlled integrin binding at the biomaterial interface, in terms of specific integrin receptors may activate specific signaling pathways and adhesive activities that elicit desired cellular and host responses [32]. Therefore, regarding the interaction with a biomaterial, adhesive extracellular ligands for integrins can be adsorbed in the surface from the surrounding environment (e.g. protein adsorption from blood, plasma or serum), deposited by cells on the biomaterial (e.g. fibronectin and collagen deposition), or engineered at the interface [29, 31].

Protein-Biomaterial Interactions

After a biomaterial is implanted in the body, it takes seconds to minutes for proteins to adsorb and cover its surface, forming the so-called conditioning film [11]. Therefore, instead of the original surface of the implanted material, the cells will recognize and interact with this protein layer. It is fair to assume that the adhesion proteins are responsible for converting the biomaterials into biologically recognizable materials. The adsorption of these adhesion proteins is the basis for all the reactions that may further occur in the body [33].

The surface properties of the biomaterials will determine the type, amount and conformation of the adsorbed proteins [2]. The composition of this protein layer can be different, depending on the fluid composition and adsorption time [25]. Besides the composition of the protein layer, the conformation and the orientation of the protein can also change with time [8]. This conditioning protein layer will increase the cell adhesiveness, since the cells have receptors in their membranes that specifically bind to the adhesion proteins. Moreover, the protein layer also increases the cell spreading at the biomaterial surface [6, 10].

Cell-Biomaterial Interactions

Nowadays it is generally accepted that there are no inert biomaterials. Any foreign material that is implanted in the body triggers tissue responses during the healing process that will naturally depend on the nature of the biomaterial and the implant site [3, 34]. Indeed, the host-biomaterial interaction, that controls the biological performance of the implanted device, is a very complex process. Upon device implantation in the body, a wound is formed and the healing process is initiated. The way the implant is more or less accepted by the host, and how well it heals, depends largely on the wound healing process. A cascade of events, common to the body's reaction mechanism to an implanted material is summarized in Fig. 4.3a.

Blood-biomaterial interactions, provisional matrix formation, acute and chronic inflammation, granulation tissue development, foreign body reaction, and fibrosis/fibrous capsule development comprise the series of host reactions occurring after device implantation (Fig. 4.3b) [3].

Inflammation

Inflammation is the first response of any vascularized tissue to tissue damage (surgery trauma or presence of a foreign body). Injury and vascular damage triggers the two branches of the blood coagulation system. The first involves activation of

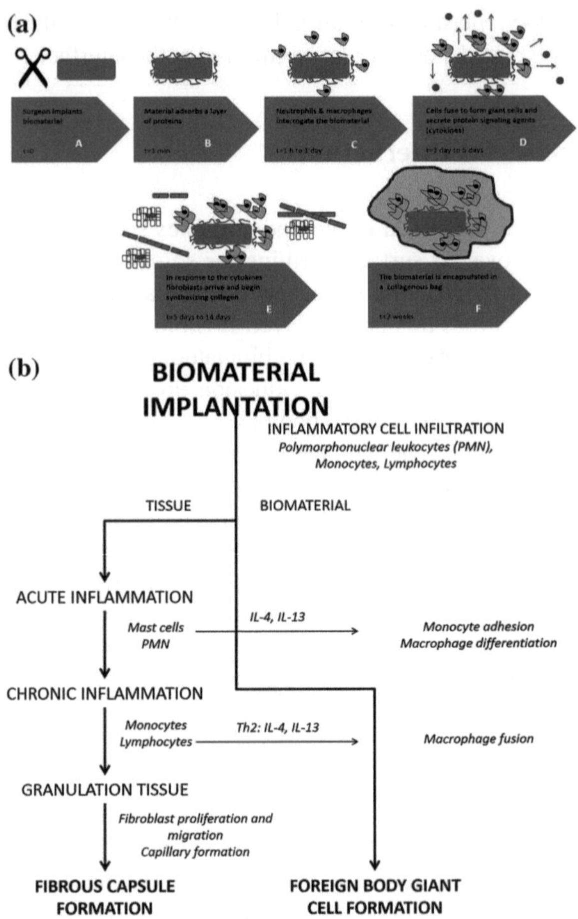

Fig. 4.3 **a** Host reaction to an implanted biomaterial. (*A*) The biomaterial is implanted in the body. (*B*) A layer of serum proteins quickly adsorbs to the implant surface. (*C*) The neutrophils and macrophages approach and attack the biomaterial that is too large to be ingested. (*D*) Macrophages cannot digest the implant and fuse into giant cells to engulf it. The giant cells send out cytokines to attract other cells. (*E*) The fibroblasts arrive and start synthesizing collagen. (*F*) The implant is entrapped in a collagen bag. (Adapted from Castner and Ratner [8]). **b** Schematic summary of the sequence of events involved in inflammatory and wound healing responses leading to Foreign Body Giant cell formation. (Adapted from Anderson et al. [19])

platelets, which stick to exposed surfaces or foreign objects and form a plug. The other involves a series of proteolytic reactions, starting with the activation of proteins circulating in the blood by the exposure to a foreign object. This sequence results in the final pathway of conversion of fibrinogen to fibrin and the formation of a clot [8].

Several cellular and non-cellular responses will occur in the first 24 h after the implantation of a device. The first event corresponds to a non-cellular response; it consists in the vasodilatation of the local vessels, which culminates with the increased permeability of the vascular endothelium and the edema formation. RBCs and fluid are present at this stage and can continue to appear with a maximum response in about 3–5 days after injury, which is characteristic of an acute inflammation). If the source of the injury is removed, then the response stops, and the tissue returns to a normal appearance. If the source of injury is not removed and the response continues, then inflammation progresses through various stages to chronic inflammation [4, 19].

Afterwards, a cellular response is observed corresponding to the recruitment of inflammatory cells through molecular signals that act as chemoattractants at the implant site. The first cells migrating to the injury site are the neutrophils, which are responsible for the phagocytosis, engulfing and degradation of the foreign body. Once the neutrophils initiate their function, the monocytes circulating in the blood enter the tissue and differentiate into macrophages, which are also responsible for the phagocytosis and the release of several biochemical factors that can activate other cells. The activated macrophages adhere to the biomaterial and spread on its surface, trying to phagocyte it. When they cannot do the job, they coalesce into very large, multinucleated giant cells, so called foreign body giant cells. This represents chronic inflammation and is usually associated with a large mass of tissue debris that can be harmful to the tissue. In some circumstances, the response is organized into a mass with a characteristic cellular response, including multinucleated giant cells, and is called a granuloma. These can be very painful, harmful, and a cause for concern [3].

It is important to keep these fundamental biological events in mind when evaluating materials for use in or on the body [35, 36]. Acute inflammation is a necessary response for tissue repair; however, a chronic response is harmful. If a material is not tolerated by the host or is toxic, then chronic inflammation will occur. Any biomaterial implanted into the body must be sterile; otherwise, an infection will occur. Sterilization methods may destroy or alter the material's properties. This is a major issue in developing or adapting materials for use in the biological environment. Infection in the presence of an implanted material is of special concern because often to cure the infection it is necessary to remove the implant [1, 19, 37].

Wound Healing

Whenever there is an injury with destruction of tissue, there must be repair. The first step in the repair process is acute inflammation. Changes occur in the vascular system, and the polymorphonuclear leukocytes (PMN) go into the tissue to clean up the damaged tissue and the foreign material. The platelets get activated and form clots to prevent further leakage of blood into the site. The remaining debris is then phagocytized by the leukocytes. Finally, actual tissue repair begins. In order for the tissue to function, there must be a blood supply to the small vessels starting to grow into the wound. Tissue cells, called fibroblasts, come in and start to synthesize collagen. This forms a structural network called granulation tissue [38].

Healing in the Presence of a Biomaterial

Upon insertion of a biomaterial into the body, all the features above described are involved. First, there is damage to the tissue during the insertion, and then an acute inflammatory response occurs. This is followed by the wound healing response that can proceed normally if the biomaterial is there for a short period of time, otherwise the response is distinct. The normal tissue repair cannot take place since there is a foreign body in the way. The first reaction of the body is to try to eliminate it. At this stage, the phagocytes come in and the acute inflammatory response may progress to chronic response. If it is not a degradable material or prone to phagocytosis, then the reaction will follow one of the two paths. The usual response consists in the formation of a fibrous capsule around the biomaterial by the fibroblasts in an attempt to eliminate it from the body. It is generally accepted that the thickness of the fibrous capsule is an indication of the material's biocompatibility, i.e. a thinner capsule corresponds to a more biocompatible material [38]. There are two types of factors that can influence the wound healing process, the intrinsic factors and the extrinsic factors. The bulk nature of the biomaterial, its porosity, roughness and changes in the surface chemistry are intrinsic factors of the implant [39]. The extrinsic factors are, for example, the surgical procedure, the condition of the patient (diabetic, immunocompromised) and the anatomical location of the implant [4]. The less common response is for the inflammatory process to continue as a chronic inflammatory response and to progress to giant cells and granulomas. This occurs when the material is not biocompatible, and the host reaction is still trying to neutralize it.

At this stage some problems can occur associated with the host reaction to the biomaterial ultimately leading to infection. The formation of the fibrous capsule is an indication that the material is biocompatible and will occur as an early step in healing. Fibrous capsule formation needs to be considered when predicting device function [19]. For instance, if the device is to serve as a drug delivery system, the formation of the fibrous capsule may alter the permeability of the device and the diffusion of the drug so that the function of the device will not be anticipated from laboratory studies. Formation of a fibrous capsule generally does not occur with porous or textured materials [15]. If the interstices are large enough, local vascularized tissue will grow into the pores rather than form the capsule. Long-term percutaneous catheters have been coated with velour to facilitate ingrowth and anchorage. Vascular prostheses made of fabric demonstrate ingrowth of vascular-like tissue [37]. Joint replacement prostheses are sometimes coated with metal beads or wire mesh to facilitate ingrowth of bone and biological anchorage [37]. It is important to notice that acute inflammation and wound healing are necessary steps in the implantation of biomaterials and devices that enter the body, hence the effect of these responses on the function of the device must be considered.

Infection

Whenever there is damage to the skin or mucous membranes and bacteria can enter, there is the risk of infection [40]. The occurrence of infection will prevent the resolution of inflammation, and a chronic inflammatory response will arise. If there is a chronic inflammatory response, the wound healing response will not be completed. The combination of the injury and the presence of the foreign material will initiate the inflammatory response. It is well known that the presence of a foreign body greatly increases the infection risk and markedly decreases the number of bacteria required to cause an infection from 10^6 to 10^2. Not only is there an increased risk of infection but also the infection will be difficult to cure, most often only through the removal of the device [3]. The consequences of this depend on the need for the device. Removal of sutures may cause little impairment to healing, whereas removal of the total artificial heart would result in death [15].

The issues related with implant site infection remain an active area of research in many different fields including microbiology, infectious diseases, material science, device design, among others [37, 41].

Immune Response

The immune system is an important and complex protective system that reacts specifically and with memory [42]. As previously mentioned, the lymphocytes are the key element in the immune system. Although the immune system is an important defence mechanism, sometimes it can cause harm to the host. These reactions are called allergy or autoimmunity [19].

Allergic responses occur to foreign substances through a variety of mechanisms. One type of allergy is called atopic or type I. An inflammatory response occurs, and the nature of the reaction depends on the site. This type of reaction must be avoided by minimizing use of materials with substances that stimulate the reaction [3]. The current concern in this area is with latex materials, such as surgical gloves, which contain a protein that may cause this type of allergy [4]. A second type of reaction is called contact dermatitis (type IV). It is important in evaluating biomaterials to determine that stimulation of allergic responses similar to this does not occur, and it is generally the degradation products from the materials that are of concern [1]. Care is taken to avoid the use of chemicals that are known to cause allergy or to minimize their release into the body. Some of the metals, such as nickel and chromium, are common causes of allergy when contacted as metal salts [1]. Allergic reactions to metallic devices are a concern, but unless there is corrosion and release of metal ions, there will not be allergic responses.

The issue of autoimmunity is also important in the selection of biomaterials and evaluation of responses. In autoimmune reactions, there is an immune reaction that causes damage to the host tissue. This occurs because the material altered the host tissue in some manner or the immune response to the biomaterial also reacted with the host tissue [19, 42].

Biocompatibility Determined by Cell-Material Interactions

Currently, a biocompatible material is defined as a material that is able to perform an appropriate host response in a specific application [1]. Nevertheless, for many years the term "biocompatibility" was associated to the biological "inertness" of the material. The main goal behind the design of such biological inert materials was to reduce or virtually eliminate any unfavorable immune response to the foreign body or biomaterial. However, for some applications it is required that cells interact with such biomaterials, for example to promote cell adhesion and proliferation [4], and to promote cells and tissue ingrowth. In these cases, the strategy adopted to improve the material's biocompatibility is to incorporate specific bioactive molecules on the polymer surfaces in order to promote or support of a favorable cell-material interaction [5, 10]. Therefore, for searching biomaterials able to provide the best performance in each application it is crucial to understand the cell-material interactions, namely the chemical, biochemical, physiological, physical or other mechanisms involved in such interactions, as well as their consequences [2, 37, 41].

Effect of the Materials Properties on Cell Behaviour

Today, there are already several (bio)materials available for use in tissue engineering applications and as medical implants [43–45], these include dental fillings, coating for tablets or capsules, contact lenses, kidney dialyzers, vascular grafts, cardiac pacemakers, maxillofacial prosthesis, to name a few examples. A wide variety of biodegradable polymers (natural or synthetic), bioactive ceramics, wear-resistant metal alloys have become available for use in a variety of human conditions [46–50]. From the previous sections it is reasonable to assume that all materials to be used as biomaterials, medical devices, or prostheses inevitably undergo a host tissue response, following implantation. This occurs as a consequence of the interaction of cells and tissues with the outermost surface layers of the materials. One of the first phenomena observed in tissue culture assays was the response of cells to the topography of the substratum to which they were attached [51, 52], these surfaces exhibited a topography measured on the micro scale. Subsequent research has shown that, along with topography, the surface chemistry, microstructure, porosity, surface area, thermal, mechanical and electrical properties of the biomaterial play a significant role on cell behaviour [43, 44, 47, 50, 53–60].

Morphological Properties

Surface Topography

Surface roughness (Fig. 4.4a) can essentially be divided into nano-roughness (<100 nm), micro-roughness (100 nm–100 μm) and macro-roughness (from 100 μm to several millimetres) [61]. The cells response to roughness will vary with the cell type and roughness scale (i.e. size, shape and distribution on the materials' surface). Hence, surface roughness regulates the biological response of cells and tissues that are in contact with the implanted material. It provides cues to promote cell adhesion, orientation, migration and production of ECM. For instance, cells grown on micro-rough surfaces spread more and differentiate better than on smooth ones, as shown by their gene expression [62–64]. Also, on grooved materials, cells can orient themselves in the direction of grooves and proliferate faster than on a smooth surface [43, 65–70].

Nanotopography may provide superior biomimetic cell-modulating cues, as it may further resemble the natural ECM environment in which cells reside and interact. It has been shown that nanopatterned surfaces can improve protein adsorption and cellular response, since as on rougher surfaces, the focal adhesion points are located at cell edges, where the contact with the materials' surface takes place [61, 71–77].

Porosity

Porous structures (Fig. 4.4b) typically consist of irregularly shaped voids with interconnecting channels (voids). The pore size, porosity (the fraction of void

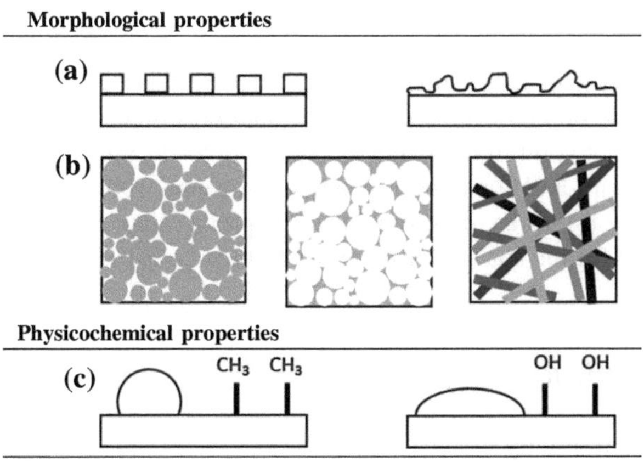

Fig. 4.4 Relevant properties of biomaterials. Morphological properties: **a** surface topography (etched surfaces can be obtained with either specific patterns (*left*) or irregular (*right*); **b** porosity (the *white* regions inside the squares represent the porous (void) fraction of the scaffolds); **c** surface charge and hydrophobicity: a water droplet on a hydrophobic surface (Table 4.4) will have a higher contact angle (*left*) than on a hydrophilic surface (*right*)

Table 4.3 Optimal pore size for cell infiltration and host tissue ingrowth (adapted from Chang and Wang [93])

Cell/tissue type	Optimal pore size (μm)	Scaffold material[a]	Reference
Human skin fibroblasts	<160	PLLA/PLGA[a]	Yang et al. [94]
Bone	450	PMMA[a]	Ashman and Moss [95]
Fibrocartilaginous tissue	150–300	Polyurethane	de Groot et al. [96]
Adult mammalian skin cells	20–125	Collagen-glycocaminoglycan	Yannas et al. [97]
Osteogenic cells	100–150	Collagen-GAG[a]	O'Brien et al. [56]
Smooth muscle cells	60–150	PLLA	Zeltinger et al. [98]
Endothelial cells	<80	Silicon nitride	Salem et al. [99]

[a]*PLLA* Poly(L-lactide); *PLGA* Poly(lactic-co-glycolic) Acid; *PMMA* Poly(methyl methacrylate); *GAG* Glycosaminoglycan

volume) and surface area (also presented as a surface-to-volume ratio parameter when characterizing a biomaterial), pore shape, wall morphology (tortuosity) and pore interconnectivity are important requisites for a scaffold in tissue engineering applications. The tailoring of these properties allows for rapid cell attachment and proliferation, improve nutrient and cell transfer to the scaffolds' center (cell and tissue ingrowth), as well as metabolite dispersal and new tissue formation [78–84]. The open pore structure and interconnected porosity have also been found to disrupt fibrous tissue deposition, minimize the formation of foreign-body capsules, improve tissue healing, and increase vascularization of the tissue surrounding the implant [85–90]. Pore size (microporosity: pore size <10 μm; macroporosity: pore size >50 μm) can be tailored to meet specific applications (Table 4.3); for instance the optimum size for neovascularization is around 5 μm; whereas for fibroblast ingrowth is in the range of 5–15 μm; for hepatocytes ingrowth close to 20 μm; for the regeneration of adult mammalian skin around 20–125 μm; for osteoid ingrowth around 40–100 μm and for bone regeneration around 100–350 μm. On the other hand, fibrovascular tissues require pores sizes greater than 500 μm for a rapid vascularization and for the survival of the transplanted cells [91, 92].

Physico-Chemical Properties

Surface Hydrophobicity

One of the most common techniques used to measure the surface energy of a material is the determination of contact angles, whereby the angle made by a drop of liquid deposited on a surface correlates with its hydrophobicity (Fig. 4.4c). The size and shape of the liquid droplet can be explained as a balance between the force with which the molecules of the liquid drop are being attracted to each other (designated by cohesive force) and, on the other hand, the attraction of the liquid molecules for the surface (adhesive force). The balance between these two opposing forces is expressed by the contact angle value (θ), which in turn translates the hydrophobicity of a given surface. Consequently, relatively more water wettable surfaces (i.e. exhibiting lower θ) are termed hydrophilic (high surface energy); conversely less wettable surfaces (with higher θ) are termed hydrophobic (low surface energy). To establish a borderline between these two terms, it is generally agreed that the criterion of a $\theta = 65°$ separates between the two regimes [100–105].

In the previous sections it was already explained that many proteins adsorb onto an implant surface immediately upon contact with it. This event modulates subsequent cell adhesion and/or foreign-host response (protein adsorption is the first step in the integration of an implanted device with its surrounding tissues). The dominant response will depend largely on the hydrophobicity (also referred to as surface energy or wettability) of the scaffold. The materials hydrophobicity thus affects protein adsorption, platelet adhesion/activation, blood coagulation and cell and bacterial adhesion. For instance, the adsorption of serum proteins (fibrinogen, fibronectin or vitronectin) later affect the adhesion of leukocytes, macrophages or platelets by preventing ECM proteins adsorption, ultimately leading to fibrous encapsulation; thus delaying or even preventing proper cell adhesion. Also, surface wettability (hydrophobicity) was found to regulate cytoskeletal organization and cell morphology. As a general rule, the more hydrophilic a surface is, the more cells adhere to it. Conversely, hydrophobic surfaces are more prone to protein-adsorption. This occurs due to the strong hydrophobic interactions between the material's surface and the protein's hydrophobic groups [6, 93, 106–113]. With respect to contact angle values, literature shows that polymer surfaces exhibiting moderate wettability (i.e. θ in the range 40–70°) enhance cell adhesion [106, 114, 115].

In the biomedical field, protein-surface interactions play key roles for the assembly of interfacial protein constructs, such as biosensors, activators and other functional components at the biological/electronic interface. In analytical sciences, non-specific protein adsorption on sensor surfaces, protein chips, or assay platforms represents a serious problem as adsorbed proteins are responsible for the degradation and thus decrease of the device performance. For example, in biosensors for in situ monitoring of cell culture or blood glucose levels in diabetic patients, specificity and sensitivity levels, and durability depend greatly on the protein adsorption onto the sensor surface. Likewise, in polymeric drug matrix delivery systems the accumulation of adsorbed proteins may impair the diffusion of the drug. In the design of biocompatible materials for surgical implants, adsorption of fibrinogen in particular should be suppressed, to avoid blood agglutination [116–118].

Surface Charge

Surface chemistry is very important for the physiological interactions with biomaterials and it is closely related to surface energy (hydrophobicity); the surface free energy of a material originates from its surface functional groups and electrical charges. The material's surface chemistry mediates cell response given that surface

Table 4.4 The effect of material surface functional groups on proteins, cells and tissue interactions (adapted from Barbosa et al. [127], Faucheux et al. [128], Kamath et al. [129] Keselowsky et al. [120, 130], Kidoaki and Matsuda [131], Lan et al. [132], Lorenz et al. [133], Schmidt et al. [122], Tang et al. [134], Thevenot et al. [2], Verena et al. [135])

Functional group	Effect on proteins, cells and tissues
Neutral charge	
Hydrophobic	
$-CH_3$	Promotes increased leukocyte adhesion and phagocyte migration
	Promotes fibronectin adsorption and exposure of cell-adhesive domains, allowing cell growth
	Promotes nanoparticle uptake
	Reduces inflammatory response and fibrotic capsule formation
	Enhances differentiation and increases osteoblasts mineralization
Hydrophilic	
–OH	Increases osteoblast differentiation
–COOH	Increase osteoblast attachment
	Promotes fibronectin adsorption and exposure of cell-adhesive domains, allowing cell growth
	Increases nanoparticle uptake
	Reduces inflammatory responses and fibrotic capsule formation
	Enhances differentiation and increases osteoblast mineralization
	Leads to thickened fibrotic capsule with high levels of cell infiltration in vivo
$-CH_2NH_2$	Enhance CHO attachment of Chinese hamster ovary cells
Positive charge	
Hydrophilic	
$-NH_2$	Promotes myoblast and endothelial proliferation and osteoblast differentiation
	Enhances fibronectin adsorption leading to increased endothelial cell growth, differentiation and osteoblast mineralization, and myoblast proliferation
	Promotes focal adhesion formation, cell spreading, and matrix formation with fibroblasts
	Increases particle uptake
	Triggers acute inflammatory responses, thick fibrotic capsule formation, and cell infiltration in vivo

chemistry directly impacts on protein adsorption and interaction (i.e. surface chemistry affects the amount and conformation of the adsorbed proteins). All these factors play crucial roles in the later cell interactions and functions [119–122]. Table 4.4 lists some of the material's most common surface groups and describes how they affect proteins, cells and tissue interactions.

So far, no general principles allow the full prediction of the effect of surface chemistry on protein and cell behavior. However, some guidelines could be drawn from extensive research. Methyl ($-CH_3$), nonpolar, hydrophobic groups allow strong binding of fibrinogen and IgG, which causes alterations in the conformations and denaturation of the protein structures, possibly leading to unfavorable cellular interactions. In vivo, methyl groups were also found to induce the recruitment of inflammatory cells to the material's surface. Contrarily, hydroxyl groups reduce the affinity for plasma proteins and induce conformational changes in fibronectin, allowing the exposure of adhesive domains for cell focal adhesion. While polar (hence hydrophilic), amine groups also induce an acute inflammatory response, despite promoting myoblast and endothelial proliferation and osteoblast differentiation. Carboxyl groups (negatively charged in blood serum) interact preferentially with fibronectin and albumin [2, 5, 93, 122–126].

Surface Treatments for Improved Biocompatibility

The surface of a material is of prime importance in determining the in vivo acceptance and performance of an implant, once in contact with blood and tissue. Several of the above-described categorical surface properties interplay, at the molecular, microscopic and macroscopic scale, during the in vitro and in vivo interaction of the materials with the surrounding environment. These surface properties can be further modified to a range of scales, to improve the material's biocompatibility. The following sections will cover the gathered understanding on surface-modification methods to improve the materials biocompatibility. In essence, methods are divided into physical, chemical, mechanical, biological and radiation modifications, although in some cases more than one category applies, due to the use of combined methods for the surface modification of the materials. Table 4.5 summarizes some of the above categorical methods; however this is not an exhaustive description of the currently available techniques.

In general, thin surface modifications (in the range of 3–10 Å of the outermost molecular layers) are preferable. Modified surface layers that are too thick may change the mechanical and functional properties of the material in the bulk. Also, thick coatings are prone to delamination due to mismatch with the substrate in physical properties. However, thicker films are actually prepared to ensure that the original surface is uniformly covered when coatings and treatments are molecularly thin. Also, extremely thin layers are more prone to mechanical erosion and to surface reversal (or rearrangement, whereby surface atoms can diffuse or translate into the bulk of the material, as a response to the external environment). However, there are cases where coatings intrinsically have a specific thickness. For example, the thickness of Langmuir-Blodgett (LB) films depends on the length of the surfactant molecules, and these usually comprise 15–40 Å.

Adsorption is the physical process of the adhesion of atoms, ions, biomolecules, or molecules of a gas, vapour or liquid onto the surface of a solid substrate. Adsorption has been used to modify the surface of polymeric biomaterials by immobilizing a bioactive compound via electrostatic interactions or ligand–receptor pairing. Hydrophilic coatings (with natural or synthetic macromolecules and proteins) promote the formation of a hydration layer through hydrogen bonding between the surface and the solvent, thus acting as anti-biofouling agents.

Table 4.5 Methods for polymer surface modification (adapted from Goddard and Hotchkiss [107], Guney et al. [136], Hoffman [137] and Ratner [138])

I. Physico-chemical methods
(A) Treatment with active gases and vapours, or radiation
Deposition of polymers from active gases and vapours (e.g., RFGD[a], chemical vapour, flame spray)
Active gas or accelerated ion treatments (e.g., etching, ablation or oxidation using RFGD, corona discharge or ion beam; ion implantation, surface micro- and nanopatterning)
Crosslinking of surface molecules (e.g., RFGD, ionizing radiation, UV)
(B) Solution treatments or bulk phase desorption
Solution deposition of polymers and amphiphiles (e.g. polymer coatings such as Langmuir–Blodgett film deposition, IPNs, surfactants, SAMs)
Desorption of surface active compounds from bulk (e.g. desorption of surfactants from bulk to surface)
Chemical treatments to modify surface groups (e.g. oxidation, sulfonation, chlorination, acetylation, quaternization)
Chemical conjugation of molecules to surface groups (e.g. silanating agents, PEG, ATRP)
(C) Combinations of (A) and (B)
Grafting or IPN polymerization (e.g., initiation by ionizing radiation, UV, 0 3, or RFGD, followed by polymerizations)
Patterning or domains of the above(e.g. microlithographic techniques)
II. Mechanical methods
Roughening(e.g., from micro-rough to porous surfaces)
Micromanipulation (e.g. using STM, AFM probes)
III. Biological methods
Physical adsorption of biomolecules (e.g. proteins, peptides, ligands, receptors, drugs, lipids)
Physical adsorption and self-crosslinking of biomolecules (e.g. same biomolecules as above, where feasible)
Chemical conjugation of biomolecules to surface groups (e.g. same biomolecules as above)
Cell seeding and growth to confluence

[a]*RFGD* Radio Frequency Gas Discharge; *UV* ultra-violet; *IPNs* Interpenetrating Polymer Networks; *SAMs* Self-Assembly Monolayers; *AFM* Atomic Force Microscopy; *STM* Scanning Tunnelling Microscopy; *ATRP* Atom Transfer Radical Polymerization

This layer of tightly bounded water molecules will not only act as a physical barrier, but also as an energetic barrier that the proteins have to overcome before adsorbing onto the device surface [107, 136, 137, 139–143].

A major challenge in surface modification is the precise control over functional groups. Many surface modification schemes produce a spectrum of functional groups such as hydroxyl, ether, carbonyl, carboxyl, and carbonate, in contrast to one functional group that was perhaps intended for the surface. Glow-discharge plasmas, corona or chemical oxidation are examples of methods often yielding non-specific reactions. In other surface modifications, post-oxidation and reaction may occur at the material's surface. Glow discharge (plasma) deposition is a technique where thin films can be deposited on most solid substrates through microwave, radio-frequency and acoustic activation. These surface modification techniques can be used to modify surfaces for better cell growth, fractionate

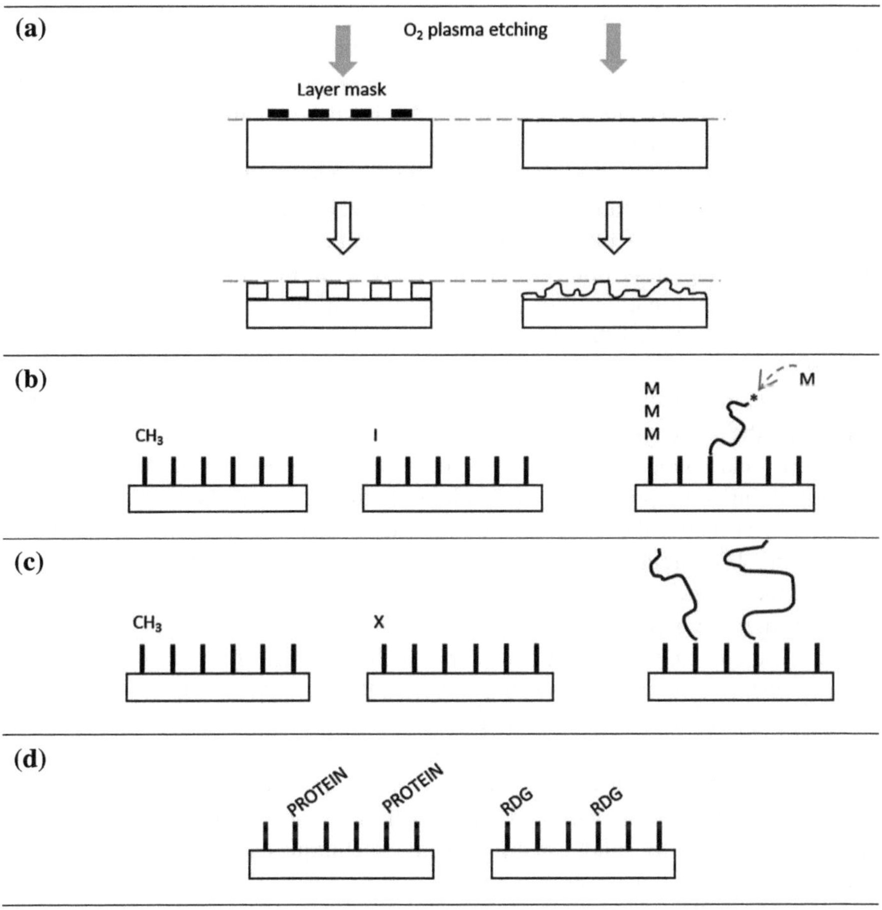

Fig. 4.5 Summary of the examples of surface treatments to improve the biomaterial's biocompatibility. **a** O_2 plasma etching, with (*left*) or without (*right*) the placement of a template for specific surface design (*grey dashed line* aims to show the decrease in the scaffolds thickness due to etching); **b** surface-ATRP ("grafting from approach"); **c** "Grafting to" surface modification; polymers can also be bound to the scaffold's surface by physisorption; **d** Bio-coating: specific proteins such as peptides or peptide sequences (RGD) and other biological molecules can be bound onto surfaces

specific proteins, minimize both blood platelet activation and accumulation of proteinaceous and cellular films.

Plasma (Fig. 4.5a) allows to modifying only the top nanometer depth of a polymer surface, without the need for solvents or generating chemical waste, without degrading or roughening the material's surface. The targeted functionalization can be defined by the selection of the plasma gas (Ar, N_2, O_2, H_2O, CO_2, NH_3) and operating parameters (such as pressure, power, time, gas flow rate). Plasma spraying (like thermal spraying) uses a high temperature plasma jet that projects particles onto the surface of an implant; these particles condense and fuse together thus coating the surface. This technique allows for the structuring of implant surfaces in the range of micron-scale level. In the case of biomedical applications, bio-inert ceramics, such as titania, zirconia or alumina, can be deposited mostly onto titanium based alloys by plasma spraying. This leads to an increase of the surface roughness and also enables changing the surface chemistry. The choice of alumina and zirconia coatings for clinical applications is related with their high wear resistance. However, these coatings cannot bind directly to bone tissues since they are bio-inert. In the case of plasma spraying of titania, coated implant surfaces may show average roughness values of 20 μm. In general, plasma sprayed surfaces are often used in combination with other modification methods such as blasting or etching [107, 136, 137, 139–143].

Another approach to create anti-fouling surfaces is by reducing the diffusive transport region in the protein adsorption process (i.e. by reducing protein adsorption), thus minimizing the amount of proteins arriving at the surface. This can be achieved by surface micro- and nanopatterning, for instance through lithography techniques, micro-contact printing or by printing biomolecules onto the surface of the biomaterial. These techniques can change the topography of a surface in an ordered or random manner.

By using UV radiation, it is also possible to generate reactive sites on polymeric surfaces; once the surface becomes activated, the functional groups created can be further exposed to gas or used to initiate UV-induced graft polymerization. Contrarily to ionized gas treatments, this technique has the ability to tailor the depth of surface reactivity by varying wavelength and exposure time.

Controlled surface modification is as a very interesting approach to modulate the chemical and physical properties of a substrate biocompatibility, wettability and mechanical properties (such as wear and corrosion resistance). The surface functionalization with polymer brushes can be achieved by two strategies: the "grafting to" and "grafting from" techniques (Fig. 4.5b, c). Surface-functionalization using a "grafting from" approach consists of grafted polymer chains (previously prepared) tethered from one of their extremities to a surface by a covalent bond. The "grafting to" approach, also called Surface-Initiated Polymerization" (SIP) takes better control of the nature and amount of monomer, the grafting density, the chain length (i.e. de molecular weight of the final polymer), which in principle, allows the tailoring of a surface to any specific desired functionality. This control can be achieved by a living/controlled radical polymerization process. From the several possible approaches available, surface-initiated ATRP (Atom Transfer Radical Polymerization) is based on the reversible activation/deactivation between alkyl halides (R-X) by means of a metal catalyst complexed with ligands (Mtn/2L). This dynamic equilibrium results in the formation of growing radicals (R*) that propagate by the addition of the monomer (M). Control is achieved by fast initiation relative to slower polymerization rates. In addition, the terminal monomer of the polymerized chain is "dormant", i.e. it has the potential to allow further polymerizations (yielding co-copolymers with region-specific properties such as pH sensitivity, temperature sensitivity, hydrophobicity/hydrophilicity ratio) or even further covalently bind specific bioactive molecules.

Biochemical surface functionalization methods have also been widely investigated in order to immobilize biologic molecules (such as specific proteins, peptides (e.g. RGD-peptides), antibodies, enzymes (such as glucose oxidase (GOD), glutamate oxidase, lactate oxidase), polysaccharides (e.g. chitosan, heparin), DNA) onto surfaces, and regulate specific cell and tissue responses (Fig. 4.5d). Methods for the immobilization of biomolecules onto implant surfaces can be categorized by physical adsorption (via non-specific interaction forces (van der Waals forces or electrostatically), physical entrapment for the controlled release of bioactive substances and covalent immobilization using cross-linker molecules. Typical molecules that can self-organize on surfaces consist of a polar head group (–SH, $-NH_2$, –COOH) that may bind to charged surfaces (previously activated for instance by UV treatment or plasma) as described above, or at least interact by van der Waals forces. Physical adsorption lacks the ability to properly control the bioactive release kinetics and thus its delivery; retention and proper orientation of the adsorbed molecules are hampered, which in case of proper exposure of focal adhesion points, limits a proper cell attachment. These drawbacks coupled with external parameters such as micro-movements of the implant, pH and temperature changes in the host tissue, lead to a reduction of the implants effective purpose. Alternatively, covalent binding of biomolecules onto surfaces, while requiring a more complex surface chemistry, allows higher loading capabilities and, since the bioactive agents are covalently attached onto the surface, show relatively low-loss rates. For the successful covalent surface immobilization of biomolecules, the surface of the materials must first be modified to provide reactive groups (such as –OH, $-NH_2$, –COOH) for the subsequent immobilization steps to occur. Today, there are various methods for the covalent immobilization of biomolecules onto biomedical material surfaces. Common denominators of successful methods (regarding binding and functionality of the modified surface) include the need for a linker molecule that binds covalently both onto the surface and onto the biomolecules (bi-functional cross-linkers), a pre-conditioning (activation or functionalization) of the substratum and finally, the preservation of the biological activity of the bioactive molecules [107, 136, 137, 139–143].

Biomaterials for Treatment of Age-Related Macular Degeneration (AMD)

As a follow up of the previous sections, the following sections will cover a specific scenario, concerning the use of biomaterials for the treatment of AMD. Background information regarding this disease will be provided, followed by an overview on the use of biomaterial scaffolds as supports for retinal pigment epithelium (RPE).

Worldwide, visual impairment is one of the leading causes of human disability. A total of 285 million people are visually impaired, 13.7 % of which are blind and the remaining 86.3 % have low vision (these include severe or moderate visual impairment). A total of 65 % of the visually impaired and 82 % of the blind people are over 50 years of age (this age group representing 20 % of the World population). Roughly 90 % of the World's visually impaired people live in developing countries. Uncorrected refractive errors were identified as the main cause of visual impairment, whereas cataracts represented the leading cause of blindness [144]. Age-Related Macular Degeneration (AMD) comprises a heterogeneous group of disorders that affects central area of vision (macula) and can lead to blurred vision, visual distortions and the appearance of dark spots in the central vision field, ultimately leading to blindness. This disorder affects mostly the macula of elderly individuals. The major sites of AMD pathology are the retinal neurons, including photoreceptors. It is considered a complex disease, in which multiple genes, as well as environmental factors are considered to play key roles in its pathogenesis [145–149].

Anatomy of the Human Retina

In the animal kingdom, perception of the physical World is achieved through the visual system, a set of two functional organs, the eye and the brain, linked by connecting pathways through to the visual cortex. The three major components/of the eye include the external layer (sclera and cornea), a middle layer (a vascular layer divided into choroid, ciliary body and iris) and a inner layer of nerve tissue (the retina). The retina (Fig. 4.6a), a 0.4 mm thick tissue, is responsible for the capture and conversion of light energy into neural signs that are transmitted to the brain via the optic nerve (phototransduction). At the center of the retina, in the optical axis of the eye, it is located the macula lutea, also known as the yellow spot. The macula is responsible for the central vision and contains the fovea, the region of highest visual acuity and high cone cell density. The neuronal layers (Fig. 4.6a) are involved in signal transduction [150–153].

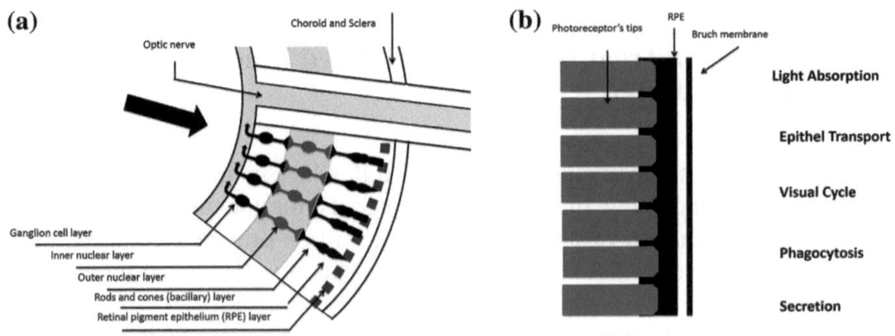

Fig. 4.6 **a** Schematic representation of the human retina (the large *black arrow* indicates the direction of the light path); **b** major functions of the RPE. (Adapted from Edward [151])

Retinal Pigment-Epithelium (RPE)

The retinal pigment epithelium (Fig. 4.6b) consists of a monolayer of hexagonally cuboidal cells located at the outermost layer of the retina, between the neural retina and the choroid. RPE cells are differentiated into apical and basal configurations. The apical side faces the photoreceptor outer segments, whereas its basolateral surface faces the Bruch's membrane, a pentalaminar, 1–4 μm thick structure adjacent to the choroidal capillaries (or choriocapilaries; a capillary bed) of the eye. The RPE's apical side contains long microvilli enveloping the outer segments of the photoreceptors. In turn, the basal membrane has numerous convoluted infolds to increase the surface area for the absorption and secretion of material. RPE is strongly involved in the maintenance of the visual function by closely interacting with photoreceptors cells. This layer regulates the transport of fluid, ions, and metabolites between the neurosensory retina and the retinal vasculature, phagocytose the rods and cones outer segments as they are renewed. RPE can phagocytose roughly 10 % of the photoreceptor outer segments on a daily basis, to maintain optimum function of the photoreceptors. The by-products of this process consist of toxic radicals, photo-damaged proteins and lipids, including lipofuscin and melanin. Both RPE cells and photoreceptors form the functional unit crucial to vision; their layered organization and correct orientation is critical for normal function and survival [154–161].

Bruch's Membrane (BM)

The human BM (Fig. 4.6b) is a thin (2–4 μm thick), acellular, extracellular ECM pentalaminar membrane located between the retina and the choroid. It separates the RPE from the underlying choriocapillaries. BM provides physical support for RPE cell adhesion, migration and differentiation. It also acts as a natural molecular sieve regulating the exchange of biomolecules, nutrient, oxygen and metabolic wastes between the retina and choriocapillaries [162–165].

Age-Related Macular Degeneration (AMD)

It is believed that dysfunction of the RPE interrupts the normal health and function of the neurosensory retina, leading to the appearance of several diseases such as AMD (and others), and to reduced visual function. For instance, with aging, melanin, which is packed in melanosomes in the apical part of the RPE cells, becomes oxidized, allowing the increase (accumulation) of granules (melanolysosomes) containing melanolipofuscin. This phenomenon is accelerated because, the number of RPE cells decreases with age, thus increasing the metabolic burden of the live ones.

While its full composition is still unknown, lipofuscin is a heterogeneous material consisting of a mixture of lipids, proteins and several fluorescent compounds. Along with other by-products from the phagocytic process, lipofuscin generates free radicals, such as the superoxide anion, singlet oxygen and hydrogen peroxide, which damage the DNA of RPE cells leading to their apoptosis [166–171].

As previously mentioned, AMD is considered to be the leading cause of blindness among adults. Its causes are still the focus of intensive research; however, based on both animal and human model studies, development of AMD is a multifactorial disease process, resulting from a combination of intrinsic (i.e. genetic origin) and extrinsic factors (photooxidative damage). The decrease in RPE cell number, the build-up of partially metabolized by-products and drusen (lipid-rich extracellular deposits) lead to the progression of AMD. In parallel, choroidal neovascularization, originating from choroidal blood vessels and progressing through Bruch's membrane into the sub-retinal RPE space, leads to the accumulation of blood and serum beneath the RPE. This causes the detachment of the RPE layer.

Two major forms of AMD exist, namely the "dry" (non-exudative) and the "wet" (exudative). The dry type affects the majority of the patients and is briefly characterized by the occurrence of drusen and atrophy of certain regions of the RPE layer. Over time, dry AMD can progress to the exudative form, where patients lose all central vision caused by the gradual thinning of the macula's photoreceptors and choroidal neovascularization, leading to atrophy and tissue death [147, 154, 166, 172–174]. A recent and extensive review on the ultrastructure of the human retina in aging and various pathological states can be found in Nag and Wadhwa [175].

To date, no curative treatment exists for AMD. Several therapeutic strategies have been proposed based on the possibility of neuroprotection, prevention of oxidative damage and suppression of inflammation. As prophylactic measures against early AMD and the conversion from nonexudative to exudative AMD, possible treatments include supplementation of vitamins and antioxidants (vitamin C, vitamin E, beta-carotene, zinc oxide and cupric oxide) and laser photocoagulation and photodynamic therapy. Intravitreal injections of vascular endothelial growth factor inhibiting pharmacotherapeutics (or anti-VEGF therapies) have recently allowed patients a significant visual improvement and stability (i.e. not only stop disease progression but to reverse its pathologic effects) [172, 176, 177].

Scaffolds for RPE Replacement

A fundamental strategy to improve cell-based RPE therapies consists of using a carrier scaffold on which RPE cells can be cultured and then transported to the implantation site (the sub-retinal space). The scaffold can add the proper structural support, allowing the development of a monolayered organization of RPE cells and with the correct orientation, a critical step for their long-term survival (RPE cells are anchorage-dependent and must quickly re/attach to a support following transplantation) [178, 179]. A key goal is thus to mimic the architecture of the

Table 4.6 Scaffolds for RPE transplantation (adapted from Hynes and Lavik [183])

Polymer	In vitro/in vivo (animal model)	Cell type	Transplanted result
Collagen	In vivo (New Zealand albino rabbit)	Human RPE	Collagen supported RPE integrated with host RPE
	In vitro	Porcine RPE and IPE	RPE cells formed a monolayer with appropriate phenotype
		Adult human RPE (ARPE-19)	RPE cells formed a monolayer with appropriate phenotype and could phagocytose OSs
			RPEs cells formed a monolayer; collagen demonstrated upregulation of angiogenic molecules
PLGA	In vitro	Fetal human RPE	RPE cells formed a monolayer with appropriate phenotype
PLGA/PLLA	In vitro	Fetal human RPE	RPE cells formed a monolayer with appropriate phenotype on PLGA, PLLA scaffolds demonstrated decreased attachment
		Adult human RPE (D407)	RPE cells formed a monolayer with appropriate phenotype
			RPE adhesion and cell morphology is influenced by micropatterned scaffolds
		Adult human RPE; porcine RPE rabbit corneal epithelium	RPE cells formed a monolayer with appropriate phenotype
RPE-ECM	In vitro	Human RPE; Bovine corneal endothelial cells	RPE ECM promotes RPE attachment and inhibits apoptosis
RPE-ECM and adult human BM	In vitro	Adult human RPE	Aged BM demonstrated decreased RPE attachment
Descemet's membrane	In vitro	Porcine RPE; IPE bovine RPE and IPE	RPE and IPE cells formed a monolayer with appropriate phenotype

(continued)

Table 4.6 (continued)

Polymer	In vitro/in vivo (animal model)	Cell type	Transplanted result
CCMS/IPAAm	In vitro	RPE	RPE cells formed a monolayer with appropriate phenotype
Adult HLC; PLC	In vitro	Porcine RPE; IPE	RPE IPE cells formed monolayer with appropriate phenotype. Collagen support was required for RPE but not IPE cell proliferation
Fn	In vitro/in vivo (albino and pigmented rabbits)	Fetal human RPE	RPE adhered to fibrinogen and survived in subretinal space for up to 1 month; retinal degeneration was noted in areas of particles
PDMS		Adult human RPE (ARPE 19)	Scaffolds with microfabricated architectures demonstrated less cell contracts; substrate topography influences RPEs
Gelatin	In vivo	Porcine RPEs	RPEs survived with no inflammation for 3 months. Scaffold did not transplant uniformly, overlapping areas of RPE death
BM	In vivo	Human fetal & Adult human RPE (ARPE-19)	Cleaning and coating of aged BM improves adherence of fetal RPEs, but not adult RPEs

BM—Bruch's membrane; CCMS/IPAAm—4-(N-cinnamoylcarbamide)methylstyrene (CCMS) and N-isopropylacrylamide (IPAAm); Fn—Fibrinogen; IPE—iris pigment epithelium; HLC—human lens capsule; RPE-ECM—retinal pigment epithelial (RPE) cells to provisional extracellular matrices (ECM); OSs—photoreceptor Outer Segments; PDMS—Polydimethylsiloxane; PLC—porcine lens capsule; PLGA—poly(lactic-co-glycolic) acid; PLLA—poly(L-lactide)

human BM (by developing a BM substitute, as this structure is responsible for maintaining the healthy homeostasis of the retina). Among the bulk and surface properties that are necessary for a scaffold to ensure the attachment and survival of RPE cells, it is important that it is extremely thin (5–90 μm) in order to reflect the size of the subretinal space. This further requires proper mechanical properties, not only to hold the monolayer of RPE cells, but also to withstand the surgical manipulation during transplantation. In addition, the ideal scaffold should allow for fluid transport, thus possessing a porosity comparable to the native BM (as a reference, molecules of up to 350 kDa should be able to pass through the scaffold). As with many biomaterials, the scaffold should also be biodegradable or biointegrated over time. The identification of natural or artificial matrices for the attachment and delivery of RPE cells is a topic under intense research (Table 4.6) [179–182].

Gelatin has a long history of use in cell transplantation to the eye and has been shown potential in improving the delivery of retinal tissue, without significant adverse cell reactions. Collagen, being a major component of the BM, was one of the first scaffolds ever tested for RPE transplantation. The successful culture of RPE cells on thin cross-linked collagen films was recorded by the formation of a monolayer of RPE cells, having also the appropriate cell morphology (hexagonal, cobblestone like and closely packed). However, collagen was found to promote an upregulation of angiogenic factors in in vitro RPE cultures. This effect could cause a neovascular response, thus ending in subretinal haemorrhaging and detachment of either the RPE or retina. Descemet membrane, lens capsule, aged BM, amniotic membrane, PMMA, PLLA, PDMS, PLGA, collagen, are also among the many different types of scaffolds prepared for RPE transplantation assays [178, 183–188]. While natural scaffolds are biocompatible, allow obviating host immune response and can better mimic the mechanical properties of native tissues, their availability is limited and have the risk of possible transmission of disease (as is the case with collagen); also their absorption profile cannot be tailored. Contrarily, synthetic matrices are a much more appealing approach given the greater control over the scaffold's properties. Porous PLLA/PLGA films have been shown to be a potential matrix with proper mechanical properties for RPE monolayer formation. However, they are too rigid for proper manipulation during surgical insertion into the subretinal space. Ultra-thin, micro-machined scaffolds of PMMA were used with murine retinal progenitor cells (RPCs). These cells were shown to grow and differentiate well on these scaffolds both in vitro and in wild-type C57BL/6 mice. Porous, ultrathin and elastic scaffolds of poly(ε-caprolactone) and Poly(glycerol sebacate), successfully enabled the growth of murine RPCs, both in vitro and wild-type and degenerative mouse models. Thin (6–100 μm), porous (11–50 μm diameter) and grooved (20–40 μm wide) scaffolds have been fabricated from poly(methyl methacrylate) (PMMA), blends of PLGA and poly(hydroxybutyrate-co-hydroxyvalerate) (PHBV8), and poly(glycerol sebacate) (PGS). The porous scaffolds (PMMA and PGS) showed better cell retention by protecting attached cells during surgical implantation [178, 183–188].

Concluding Remarks

This chapter provided a broad conceptual background on the key principles underlying cell-biomaterial interactions, both from the cellular and from the material's perspective. The chronological chain of events that mediate a biologic response occurring when cells (in vitro and in vivo) come in contact with a foreign body (scaffold); as well as the material's properties that most impact biocompatibility and major strategies to improve the bio-functionality of the (bio)materials were discussed.

Although important achievements have been reported in the biomaterials field, there are still many unsolved issues. In the case of macular regeneration via tissue engineering approaches, the design of a scaffold, thin but mechanically strong, with adequate porosity that not only supports the growth of a well aligned and oriented RPE cell layer, but withstands surgical manipulation and further contributes to maintaining the healthy homeostasis of the retina, remains a challenge. This chapter reviewed the ground breaking approaches used in the design of such materials, as well as the major results obtained so far.

References

1. Williams, D.: On the nature of biomaterials. Biomaterials **30**(5897), 5909 (2009)
2. Thevenot, P., Hu, W., Tang, L.: Surface chemistry influence implant biocompatibility. Curr. Top. Med. Chem. **8**(4), 270–280 (2008)
3. Onuki, Y., Bhardwaj, U., Papadimitrakopoulos, F., Burgess, D.J.: A review of biocompatibility of implantable devices: Current challenges to overcome foreign body response. J. Diab. Sci. Technol. **2**(6), 1003–1015 (2008)
4. Williams, D.: On the mechanisms of biocompatibility. Biomaterials **29**, 2941–2953 (2008)
5. Saltzman, W.M., Kyriakides, T.R.: Cell interactions with polymers. In: Lanza, R., Langer, R., Vacanti, J.P. (eds.) Principles of Tissue Engineering, pp. 221–235. Elsevier Academic Press, New York (2007)
6. Webb, K., Hlady, V., Tresco, P.A.: Relationships among cell attachment, spreading, cytoskeletal organisation and migration rate for anchorage-dependent cells on model surfaces. J. Biomed. Mater. Res. **49**(3), 362–368 (2000)
7. Anselme, K.: Osteoblast adhesion on biomaterials. Biomaterials **21**(7), 667–681 (2000)
8. Castner, D.G., Ratner, B.D.: Biomedical surface science: Foundations to frontiers. Surf. Sci. **500**(1–3), 28–60 (2002)
9. Kooten, T., Spijker, H., Busscher, H.: Plasma-treated polystyrene surfaces: model surfaces for studying cell-biomaterial interactions. Biomaterials **25**(10), 1735–1747 (2004)
10. Chen, H., Yuan, L., Song, W., Wu, Z., Li, D.: Biocompatible polymer materials: role of the protein—surface interactions. Prog. Polym. Sci. **33**(11), 1059–1087 (2008)
11. Rodrigues, L.R.: Inhibition of bacterial adhesion on medical devices. In: Linke, D., Goldman, A. (eds.) Bacterial Adhesion: Biology, Chemistry, and Physics, Series: Advances in Experimental Medicine and Biology, vol. 715, pp. 351–367. Springer, Germany (2011)
12. Badylak, S.F.: Xenogeneic extracellular matrix as a scaffold for tissue reconstruction. Transpl. Immunol. **12**(3–4), 367–377 (2004)
13. Badylak, S.F.: The extracellular matrix as a biologic scaffold material. Biomaterials **28**(25), 3587–3593 (2007)
14. Badylak, S.F., Freytes, D.O., Gilbert, T.W.: Extracellular matrix as a biological scaffold material: structure and function. Acta Biomater. **5**(1), 1–13 (2009)
15. Ratner, B.D., Hoffman, A.S., Schoen, F.J., Lemons, J.E. (eds.): Biomaterials Science: An Introduction to Materials in Medicine. Elsevier Academic Press, New York (2004)
16. Bosman, F.T., Stamenkovic, I.: Functional structure and composition of the extracellular matrix. J. Pathol. **200**, 423–428 (2003)
17. Brown, A.E.X., Discher, D.E.: Conformational changes and signaling in cell and matrix physics. Curr. Biol. **19**, R781–R789 (2009)

18. Janik, M.E., Litynska, A., Vereecken, P.: Cell migration—the role of integrin glycosylation. Biochim. Biophys. Acta **1800**, 545–555 (2010)
19. Anderson, J.M., Rodriguez, A., Chang, D.T.: Foreign body reaction to biomaterials. Semin. Immunol. **20**(2), 86–100 (2008)
20. Lanza, R., Langer, R., Vacanti, J.P. (eds.): Principles of Tissue Engineering, pp. 53–66. Elsevier Academic Press, New York (2007)
21. Brown, B.N., Barnes, C.A., Kasick, R.T., Michel, R., Gilbert, T.W., Beer-Stolz, D., Castner, D.G., Ratner, B.D., Badylak, S.F.: Surface characterization of extracellular matrix scaffolds. Biomaterials **31**(3), 428–437 (2010)
22. Dexter, S.J., Pearson, R.G., Davies, M.C., Cámara, M., Shakesheff, K.M.: A comparison of the adhesion of mammalian cells and Staphylococcus epidermidis on fibronectin-modified polymer surfaces. J. Biomed. Mater. Res. **56**(2), 222–227 (2001)
23. Schultz, G.S., Wysocki, A.: Interactions between extracellular matrix and growth factors in wound healing. Wound Rep. Reg. **17**, 153–162 (2009)
24. Larsen, M., Artym, V.V., Green, J.A., Yamada, K.M.: The matrix reorganized: extracellular matrix remodeling and integrin signaling. Curr. Opin. Cell Biol. **18**, 463–471 (2006)
25. Garcia, A.: Get a grip: integrins in cell-biomaterial interactions. Biomaterials **26**(36), 7525–7529 (2005)
26. Siebers, M., Brugge, P., Walboomers, X., Jansen, J.: Integrins as linker proteins between osteoblasts and bone replacing materials. A Crit. Rev. Biomater. **26**(2), 137–146 (2005)
27. Delon, I., Brown, N.: Integrins and the actin cytoskeleton. Curr. Opin. Cell Biol. **19**(1), 43–50 (2007)
28. Gahmberg, C., Fagerholm, S., Nurmi, S., Chavakis, T., Marchesan, S., Gronholm, M.: Regulation of integrin activity and signaling. Biochemica et Biophysica Acta **1790**(6), 431–444 (2009)
29. Ginsberg, M.H., Partridge, A., Shattil, S.S.: Integrin regulation. Curr. Opin. Cell Biol. **17**(5), 509–516 (2005)
30. Yim, E., Darling, E., Kulangara, K., Guilak, F., Leong, K.: Nanotopography—induced changes in focal adhesions, cytoskeletal organization, and mechanical properties of human mesenchymal stem cells. Biomaterials **31**, 1299–1306 (2010)
31. Sanborn, S., Murugesan, G., Marchant, R.E., Kottke-Marchant, K.: Endothelial cell formation of focal adhesions on hydrophilic plasma polymers. Biomaterials **23**, 1–8 (2002)
32. Vadgama, P.: Surface biocompatibility. Annu. Rep. Prog. Chem. Sect. C **101**, 14–52 (2005)
33. Cole, M.A., Voelcker, N.H., Thissen, H., Griesser, H.J.: Stimuli-responsive interfaces and systems for the control of protein–surface and cell–surface interactions. Biomaterials **30**, 1827–1850 (2009)
34. Werkmeister, J.A., Tebb, T.A., White, J.F., Ramshaw, J.A.M.: Collagenous tissue formation in association with medical implants. Curr. Opin. Solid State Mater. Sci. **5**(2–3), 185–191 (2001)
35. Franz, S., Rammelt, S., Scharnweber, D., Simon, J.C.: Immune responses to implants—a review of the implications for the design of immunomodulatory biomaterials. Biomaterials **32**, 6692–6709 (2011)
36. Morais, J.M., Papadimitrakopoulos, F., Burgess, D.J.: Biomaterials/tissue interactions: possible solutions to overcome foreign body response. AAPS J **12**(2), 188–196 (2010)
37. Webster, J.G. (ed.): Encyclopedia of Medical Devices and Instrumentation. Wiley, New York (2006)
38. Buckley, C.D., Pilling, D., Lord, J.M., Toellner, D.S., Salmon, M.: Fibroblasts regulate the swith from acute to persistent inflammation. Trends Immunol. **22**(4), 199–204 (2001)
39. Bacakova, L., Filova, E., Parizek, M., Ruml, T., Svorcik, V.: Modulation of cell adhesion, proliferation and differentiation on materials designed for body implants. Biotechnol. Adv. **29**(6), 739–767 (2011)
40. Proctor, R.A.: Toward an understanding of biomaterial infections: a complex interplay between the host and bacteria. J. Lab. Clin. Med. **135**, 14–15 (2000)
41. Chan, G., Mooney, D.J.: New materials for tissue engineering: towards greater control over the biological response. Trends Biotechnol. **26**(7), 382–392 (2008)

42. Badylak, S.F., Gilbert, T.W.: Immune response to biologic scaffold materials. Semin. Immunol. **20**, 109–116 (2008)
43. Eisenbarth, E., Meyle, J., Nachtigall, W., Breme, J.: Influence of the surface structure of titanium materials on the adhesion of fibroblasts. Biomaterials **17**, 1399–1403 (1996)
44. Hoerstrup, S.P., Sodian, R., Daebritz, S., Wang, J., Bacha, E.A., Martin, D.P., Moran, A.M., Guleserian, K.J., Sperling, J.S., Kaushal, S., Vacanti, J.P., Schoen, F.J., Mayer Jr, J.E.: Functional living trileaflet heart valves grown in vitro. Circulation **102**, 44–49 (2000)
45. Mendelson, K., Aikawa, E., Mettler, B.A., Sales, V., Martin, D., Mayer, J.E., Schoen, F.J.: Healing and remodeling of bioengineered pulmonary artery patches implanted in sheep. Cardiovasc. Pathol. **16**, 277–282 (2007)
46. Langer, R.: Biomaterials: status, challenges, and perspectives. AIChE J. **46**, 1286–1289 (2000)
47. Patel, N.R., Gohil, P.P.: A review on biomaterials: scope, applications and human anatomy significance. Int. J. Emerg. Technol. Adv. Eng. **2**, 91–101 (2012)
48. Ratner, B.D., Hoffman, A.S., Schoen, F.J., Lemons, J.E.: Introduction—biomaterials science: an evolving, multidisciplinary endeavor. In: Ratner, B.D., Hoffman, A.S., Schoen, F.J., Lemons, J.E. (eds.) Biomaterials Science: An Introduction to Materials in Medicine, 3rd edn. Elsevier Science, Academic Press (2013)
49. Seal, B.L., Otero, T.C., Panitch, A.: Polymeric biomaterials for tissue and organ regeneration. Mater. Sci. Eng. R **34**, 147–230 (2001)
50. Tathe, A., Ghodke, N., Nikalje, A.P.: A brief review: biomaterials and their applications. Int. J. Pharm. & Pharm. Sci. **2**, 19–23 (2010)
51. Harrison, R.G.: On the stereotropism of embryonic cells. Science **34**, 279–281 (1911)
52. Harrison, R.G.: The reaction of embryonic cells to solid structures. J. Exp. Zool. **17**, 521–544 (1914)
53. Chou, L., Firth, J.D., Uitto, V.-J., Brunette, D.M.: Substratum surface topography alters cell shape and regulates fibronectin, mRNA level, mRNA stability, secretion and assembly in human fibroblasts. J. Cell Sci. **108**, 1563–1573 (1995)
54. Engler, A.J., Sen, S., Sweeney, H.L., Discher, D.E.: Matrix elasticity directs stem cell lineage specification. Cell **126**, 677–689 (2006)
55. Fan, Y.W., Cui, F.Z., Hou, S.P., Xu, Q.Y., Chen, L.N., Lee, I.S.: Culture of neural cells on silicon wafers with nano-scale surface topography. J. Neurosci. Methods **120**, 17–23 (2002)
56. O'Brien, F.J., Harley, B.A., Yannas, I.V., Gibson, L.J.: The effect of pore size on cell adhesion in collagen-GAG scaffolds. Biomaterials **26**, 433–441 (2005)
57. Peyton, S.R., Putnam, A.J.: Extracellular matrix rigidity governs smooth muscle cell motility in a biphasic fashion. J. Cell. Physiol. **204**, 198–209 (2005)
58. Ventre, M., Causa, F., Netti, P.A.: Determinants of cell-material crosstalk at the interface: towards engineering of cell instructive materials. J. Roy. Soc. Interface **9**, 2017–2032 (2012)
59. Vilches, J., Vilches-Perez, J.I., Salido, M.: Cell-surface interaction in biomedical implants assessed by simultaneous fluorescence and reflection confocal microscopy. Mod. Res. Educ. Top. Microsc. **1**, 60–67 (2007)
60. Yang, C.Y., Huang, L.Y., Shen, T.L., Yeh, J.A.: Cell adhesion, morphology and biochemistry on nano-topographic oxidized silicon surfaces. Eur. Cells Mater. **20**, 415–430 (2010)
61. Sabrina, M., Antonella, P.: Cell-material Interactions. Biomaterials for Stem Cell Therapy. CRC Press, Boca Raton (2013)
62. Anselme, K., Ponche, A., Bigerekke, M.: Relative influence of surface topography and surface chemistry on cell response to bone implant materials. Part 2: biological aspects. Proc. Inst. Mech. Eng H: J. Eng. Med. **224**, 1487–1507 (2010)
63. Hatano, K., Inoue, H., Kojo, T., Matsunaga, T., Tsujisawa, T., Uchiyama, C., Uchida, Y.: Effect of surface roughness on proliferation and alkaline phosphatase expression of rat calvarial cells cultured on polystyrene. Bone **25**, 439–445 (1999)
64. Lim, J.Y., Hansen, J.C., Siedlecki, C.A., Runt, J., Donahue, H.J.: Human foetal osteoblastic cell response to polymer-demixed nanotopographic interfaces. J. R. Soc. Interface **2**, 97–108 (2005)

65. Brunette, D.M.: Fibroblasts on micromachined substrata orient hierarchically to grooves of different dimensions. Exp. Cell Res. **164**, 11–26 (1986)
66. Dalton, B.A., Walboomers, X.F., Dziegielewski, M., Evans, M.D., Taylor, S., Jansen, J.A., Steele, J.G.: Modulation of epithelial tissue and cell migration by microgrooves. J. Biomed. Mater. Res. **56**, 195–207 (2001)
67. Den Braber, E.T., De Ruijter, J.E., Ginsel, L.A., Von Recum, A.F., Jansen, J.A.: Quantitative analysis of fibroblast morphology on microgrooved surfaces with various groove and ridge dimensions. Biomaterials **17**, 2037–2044 (1996)
68. Rickert, D., Franke, R.P., Lendlein, A., Kelch, S., Moses, M.A.: Influence of the surface structure of a multiblock copolymer on the cellular behavior of primary cell cultures of the upper aerodigestive tract in vitro. J. Biomed. Mater. Res. A **83**, 558–569 (2007)
69. Tamada, Y., Ikada, Y.: Fibroblast growth on polymer surfaces and biosynthesis of collagen. J. Biomed. Mater. Res. **28**, 783–789 (1994)
70. Walboomers, X.F., Croes, H.J., Ginsel, L.A., Jansen, J.A.: Growth behavior of fibroblasts on microgrooved polystyrene. Biomaterials **19**, 1861–1868 (1998)
71. Curtis, A., Wilkinson, C.: Nanotechniques and approaches in biotechnology. Trends Biotechnol. **19**(3), 97–101 (2001)
72. Dalby, M.J., Yarwood, S.J., Riehele, M.O., Johnstone, H.J.H., Affrossman, S., Curtis, A.S.G.: Increasing fibroblast response to materials using nanotopography: morphological and genetic measurements of cell response to 13-nm-high polymer demixed islands. Exp. Cell Res. **276**, 1–9 (2002)
73. Dalby, M.J., Childs, S., Riehle, M.O., Johnstone, H.J.H., Affrossman, S., Curtis, A.S.G.: Fibroblast reaction to island topography: changes in cytoskeleton and morphology with time. Biomaterials **24**, 927–935 (2003)
74. Dalby, M.J., Giannaras, D., Riehele, M.O., Gadegaard, N., Affrossman, S., Curtis, A.S.G.: Rapid fibroblast adhesion to 27 nm high polymer demixed nano-topography. Biomaterials **25**, 77–83 (2004)
75. Flemming, R.G., Murphy, C.J., Abrams, G.A., Goodman, S.L., Nealy, P.F.: Effects of synthetic micro- and nano-structured surfaces on cell behavior. Biomaterials **20**, 573–588 (1999)
76. Lord, M.S., Foss, M., Besenbacher, F.: Influence of nanoscale surface topography on protein adsorption and cellular response. Nano Today **5**, 66–78 (2010)
77. Rechendorff, K., Hovgaard, M.B., Foss, M., Zhdanov, V.P., Besenbacher, F.: Enhancement of protein adsorption induced by surface roughness. Langmuir **22**, 10885–10888 (2006)
78. Levenberg, S., Langer, R.: Advances in Tissue Engineering. Current Topics in Developmental Biology. Academic Press, New York (2004)
79. Ma, P.X., Choi, J.W.: Biodegradable polymer scaffolds with well-defined interconnected spherical pore network. Tissue Eng. **7**, 23–33 (2001)
80. Karageorgiou, V., Kaplan, D.: Porosity of 3D biomaterial scaffolds and osteogenesis. Biomaterials **26**, 5474–5491 (2005)
81. Kim, T.G., Shin, H., Lim, D.W.: Biomimetic scaffolds for tissue engineering. Adv. Funct. Mater. **22**, 2446–2468 (2012)
82. Ranucci, C.S., Kumar, A., Batra, S.P., Moghe, P.V.: Control of hepatocyte function on collagen foams: sizing matrix pores toward selective induction of 2-D and 3-D cellular morphogenesis. Biomaterials **21**, 783–793 (2000)
83. Yang, Y.L., Motte, S., Kaufman, L.J.: Pore size variable type I collagen gels and their interaction with glioma cells. Biomaterials **31**, 5678–5688 (2010)
84. Yarlagadda, P.K., Chandrasekharan, M., Shyan, J.Y.: Recent advances and current developments in tissue scaffolding. Biomed. Mater. Eng. **15**, 159–177 (2005)
85. Loh, Q.L., Choong, C.: Three-dimensional scaffolds for tissue engineering applications: role of porosity and pore size. Tissue Eng. Revisions B **19**, 485–502 (2013)
86. Koschwanez, H.E., Reichert, W.M.: Textured and porous materials. In: Ratner, B.D., Hoffman, A.S., Schoen, F.J., Lemons, J.E. (eds.) Biomaterials Science, 3rd edn, chap I.2.15. Academic Press, New York (2013)

87. Salzmann, D.L., Kleinert, L.B., Berman, S.S., Williams, S.K.: The effects of porosity on endothelialization of ePTFE implanted in subcutaneous and adipose tissue. J. Biomed. Mater. Res. **34**, 463–476 (1997)
88. Sharkawy, A.A., Klitzman, B., Truskey, G.A., Reichert, W.M.: Engineering the tissue which encapsulates subcutaneous implants. II. Plasma-tissue exchange properties. J. Biomed. Mater. Res. **40**, 586–597 (1998)
89. Sharkawy, A.A., Klitzman, B., Truskey, G.A., Reichert, W.M.: Engineering the tissue which encapsulates subcutaneous implants. I. Diffusion properties. J. Biomed. Mater. Res. **37**, 401–412 (1997)
90. Ward, W.K., Slobodzian, E.P., Tiekotter, K.L., Wood, M.D.: The effect of microgeometry, implant thickness and polyurethane chemistry on the foreign body response to subcutaneous implants. Biomaterials **23**, 4185–4192 (2002)
91. Dhandayuthapani, B., Yoshida, Y., Maekawa, T., Kumar, D.S.: Polymeric scaffolds in tissue engineering application: a review. Int. J. Polymer Sci. Article ID **290602**, 1–19 (2011)
92. Yang, S., Leong, K.F., Du, Z., Chua, C.K.: The design of scaffolds for use in tissue engineering. Part I. Traditional factors. Tissue Eng. **7**, 679–689 (2001)
93. Chang, H.I., Wang, Y.: Cell responses to surface and architecture of tissue engineering scaffolds. In: Eberli D (ed.) Cells and Biomaterials, Chap 27, InTech, Croatia (2011)
94. Yang, J., Shi, G., Bei, J., Wang, S., Cao, Y., Shang, Q., Yang, G., Wang, W.: Fabrication and surface modification of macroporous poly(L-lactic acid) and poly(L-lactic-co-glycolic acid) (70/30) cell scaffolds for human skin fibroblast cell culture. J. Biomed. Mater. Res. **62**, 438–446 (2002)
95. Ashman, A., Moss, M.L.: Implantation of porous polymethylmethacrylate resin for tooth and bone replacement. J. Prosthet. Dent. **37**, 657–665 (1977)
96. De Groot, J.H., De Vrijer, R., Pennings, A.J., Klompmaker, J., Veth, R.P., Jansen, H.W.: Use of porous polyurethanes for meniscal reconstruction and meniscal prostheses. Biomaterials **17**, 163–173 (1996)
97. Yannas, I.V., Lee, E., Orgill, D.P., Skrabut, E.M., Murphy, G.F.: Synthesis and characterization of a model extracellular matrix that induces partial regeneration of adult mammalian skin. Proc. Nat. Acad. Sci. USA **86**, 933–937 (1989)
98. Zeltinger, J., Sherwood, J.K., Graham, D.A., Mueller, R., Griffith, L.G.: Effect of pore size and void fraction on cellular adhesion, proliferation, and matrix deposition. Tissue Eng. **7**, 557–572 (2001)
99. Salem, A.K., Stevens, R., Pearson, R.G., Davies, M.C., Tendler, S.J., Roberts, C.J., Williams, P.M., Shakesheff, K.M.: Interactions of 3T3 fibroblasts and endothelial cells with defined pore features. J. Biomed. Mater. Res. **61**, 212–217 (2002)
100. Lim, J.Y., Liu, X., Vogler, E.A., Donahue, H.J.: Systematic variation in osteoblast adhesion and phenotype with substratum surface characteristics. J. Biomed. Mater. Res. A **68**, 504–512 (2004)
101. Merrett, K., Cornelius, R.M., McClung, W.G., Unsworth, L.D., Sheardown, H.: Surface analysis methods for characterizing polymeric biomaterials. J. Biomater. Sci. Polymer Ed13, 593–621 (2002)
102. Ratner, B.D.: Surface properties and surface characterization of biomaterials. In: Ratner, B.D., Hoffman, A.S., Schoen, F.J., Lemons, J.E. (eds.) Biomaterials Science: An Introduction to Materials in Medicine, 3rd edn. Elsevier Science, Academic Press, New York (2013)
103. Vogler, E.A.: Structure and reactivity of water at biomaterial surfaces. Adv. Colloid Interface Sci. **74**, 69–117 (1998)
104. Vogler E.A (1999) Water and the acute biological response to surfaces. J. Biomater. Sci. Polymer Ed 10_1015-1045
105. Vogler, E.A., Bussian, R.W.: Short-term cell-attachment rates: a surface-sensitive test of cell-substrate compatibility. J. Biomed. Mater. Res. **21**, 1197–1211 (1987)

106. Arima, Y., Iwata, H.: Effect of wettability and surface functional groups on protein adsorption and cell adhesion using well-defined mixed self-assembled monolayers. Biomaterials **28**, 3074–3082 (2007)
107. Goddard, J.M., Hotchkiss, J.H.: Polymer surface modification for the attachment of bioactive compounds. Prog. Polym. Sci. **32**, 698–725 (2007)
108. Healy, K.E., Thomas, C.H., Rezaina, A., Kim, J.E., McKeown, P.J., Lom, B., Hockberger, P.E.: Kinetics of bone cell organization and mineralization on materials with patterned surface chemistry. Biomaterials **17**, 195–208 (1996)
109. Hlady, V., Buijs, J.: Protein adsorption on solid surfaces. Curr. Opin. Biotechnol. **7**, 72–77 (1996)
110. Hlady, V., Buijs, J., Jennissen, H.P.: Methods for studying protein adsorption. Methods Enzymology **309**, 402–429 (1999)
111. Lim, J.Y., Shaughnessy, M.C., Zhou, Z., Noh, H., Vogler, E.A., Donahue, H.J.: Surface energy effects on osteoblast spatial growth and mineralization. Biomaterials **29**, 1776–1784 (2008)
112. Poncin-Epaillard, F., Vrlinic, T., Debarnot, D., Mozeitic, M., Coudrreuse, A., Legeay, G., El Moualij, B., Zorzi, W.: Surface Treatment of Polymeric Materials Controlling the Adhesion of Biomolecules. J. Funct. Biomaterials **3**, 528–543 (2012)
113. Xu, L.C., Siedlecki, C.A.: Effects of surface wettability and contact time on protein adhesion to biomaterial surfaces. Biomaterials **28**, 3273–3283 (2007)
114. Lee, J.H., Khang, G., Lee, J.W., Lee, H.B.: Interaction of different types of cells on polymer surfaces with wettability gradient. J. Colloid Interface Sci. **205**, 323–330 (1998)
115. Lee, J.H., Lee, J.W., Khang, G., Lee, H.B.: Interaction of cells on chargeable functional group gradient surfaces. Biomaterials **18**, 351–358 (1997)
116. Gray, J.J.: The interaction of proteins with solid surfaces. Curr. Opin. Struct. Biol. **14**, 110–115 (2004)
117. Nakanishi, K., Sakiyama, T., Imamura, K.: On the adsorption of proteins on solid surfaces, a common but very complicated phenomenon. J. Biosci. Bioeng. **91**, 233–244 (2001)
118. Rabe, M., Verdes, D., Seeger, S.: Understanding protein adsorption phenomena at solid surfaces. Adv. Colloid Interface Sci. **162**, 87–106 (2011)
119. Ballet, T.L.B., Brechet, Y., Bruckert, F., Weidenhaupt, M.: Protein conformational changes induced by adsorption onto material surfaces: an important issue for biomedical applications of material science. Bull. Pol. Acad. Sci. **58**, 303–315 (2010)
120. Keselowsky, B.G., Collard, D.M., Garcia, A.J.: Surface chemistry modulates focal adhesion composition and signaling through changes in integrin binding. Biomaterials **25**, 5947–5954 (2004)
121. Michael, K.E., Vernekar, V.N., Keselowsky, B.G., Meredith, J.C., Latour, R.A., Garcia, A.J.: Adsorption-induced conformational changes in fibronectin due to interactions with well-defined surface chemistries. Langmuir **19**, 8033–8040 (2003)
122. Schmidt, D., Waldeck, H., Kao, W.: Protein adsorption to biomaterials. In: Puleo, D.A., Bizios, R. (eds.) Biological Interactions on Materials Surfaces. Springer, US (2009)
123. Abraham, G.A., De Queiroz, A.A.A., Román, J.S.: Hydrophilic hybrid IPNs of segmented polyurethanes and copolymers of vinylpyrrolidone for applications in medicine. Biomaterials **22**, 1971–1985 (2001)
124. Anderson, J.M.: Biological Responses to Materials. Annu. Rev. Mater. Res. **31**, 81–110 (2001)
125. Lee, J.H., Khang, G., Lee, J.W., Lee, H.B.: Platelet adhesion onto chargeable functional group gradient surfaces. J. Biomed. Mater. Res. **40**, 180–186 (1998)
126. Wang, Y.-X., Robertson, J., Spillman, W, Jr., Claus, R.: Effects of the chemical structure and the surface properties of polymeric biomaterials on their biocompatibility. Pharm. Res. **21**, 1362–1373 (2004)
127. Barbosa, J.N., Madureira, P., Barbosa, M.A., Aguas, A.P.: The influence of functional groups of self-assembled monolayers on fibrous capsule formation and cell recruitment. J. Biomed. Mater. Res. A **76**, 737–743 (2006)

128. Faucheux, N., Schweiss, R., Lutzow, K., Werner, C., Groth, T.: Self-assembled monolayers with different terminating groups as model substrates for cell adhesion studies. Biomaterials **25**, 2721–2730 (2004)
129. Kamath, S., Bhattacharyya, D., Padukudru, C., Timmons, R.B., Tang, L.: Surface chemistry influences implant-mediated host tissue responses. J. Biomed. Mater. Res. A **86**, 617–626 (2008)
130. Keselowsky, B.G., Collard, D.M., Garcia, A.J.: Integrin binding specificity regulates biomaterial surface chemistry effects on cell differentiation. Proc. Nat. Acad. Sci. USA **102**, 5953–5957 (2005)
131. Kidoaki, S., Matsuda, T.: Adhesion forces of the blood plasma proteins on self-assembled monolayer surfaces of alkanethiolates with different functional groups measured by an atomic force microscope. Langmuir **15**, 7639–7646 (1999)
132. Lan, M.A., Gersbach, C.A., Michael, K.E., Keselowsky, B.G., Garcia, A.J.: Myoblast proliferation and differentiation on fibronectin-coated self-assembled monolayers presenting different surface chemistries. Biomaterials **26**, 4523–4531 (2005)
133. Lorenz, M.R., Holzapfel, V., Musyanovych, A., Nothelfer, K., Walther, P., Frank, H., Landfester, K., Schresenmeier, H., Mailander, V.: Uptake of functionalized, fluorescent-labeled polymeric particles in different cell lines and stem cells. Biomaterials **27**, 2820–2828 (2006)
134. Tang, L., Wu, Y., Timmons, R.B.: Fibrinogen adsorption and host tissue responses to plasma functionalized surfaces. J. Biomed. Mater. Res. **42**, 156–163 (1998)
135. Verena, H., Myriam, L., Clemens Kilian, W., Hubert, S., Katharina, L., Volker, M.: Synthesis and biomedical applications of functionalized fluorescent and magnetic dual reporter nanoparticles as obtained in the miniemulsion process. J. Phys.: Condens. Matter **18**, S2581 (2006)
136. Guney, A., Kara, F., Ozgen, O., Aksoy, E.A., Hasirci, V., Hasirci, N.: Surface Modification of Polymeric Biomaterials. Biomaterials Surface Science. Wiley-VCH Verlag/GmbH & Co KGaA, Weinheim (2013)
137. Hoffman, A.S.: Surface modification of polymers. Chin. J. Polym. Sci. **13**, 195–203 (1995)
138. Ratner, B.D.: Surface modification of polymers: chemical, biological and surface analytical challenges. Biosens. Bioelectron. **10**, 797–804 (1995)
139. Gonçalves, S., Leiros, A., Van Kooten, T., Dourado, F., Rodrigues, L.R.: Physicochemical and biological evaluation of poly(ethylene glycol) methacrylate grafted onto poly(dimethyl siloxane) surfaces for prosthetic devices. Colloids Surf. B Biointerfaces **109**, 228–235 (2013)
140. Lin, P., Lin, C.-W., Mansour, R., Gu, F.: Improving biocompatibility by surface modification techniques on implantable bioelectronics. Biosens. Bioelectron. **47**, 451–460 (2013)
141. Olivier, A., Meyer, F., Raquez, J.-M., Damman, P., Dubois, P.: Surface-initiated controlled polymerization as a convenient method for designing functional polymer brushes: From self-assembled monolayers to patterned surfaces. Prog. Polym. Sci. **37**, 157–181 (2012)
142. Ul Ahad, I., Bartnik, A., Fiedorowicz, H., Kostecki, J., Korczyc, B., Ciach, T., Brabazon, D.: Surface modification of polymers for biocompatibility via exposure to extreme ultraviolet radiation. J. Biomed. Mater. Res. A (2013). doi:10.1002/jbm.a.34958
143. Variola, F., Vetrone, F., Richert, L., Jedrzejowwski, P., Yi, J.H., Zalzal, S., Clair, S., Sarkissian, A., Perepichka, D.F., Wuest, J.D., Rosei, F., Nanci, A.: Improving biocompatibility of implantable metals by nanoscale modification of surfaces: an overview of strategies, fabrication methods, and challenges. Small **5**, 996–1006 (2009)
144. Pascolini, D., Mariotti, S.P.: Global estimates of visual impairment: 2010. Br. J. Ophthalmol. **96**, 614–618 (2012)
145. Chamberlain, M., Baird, P., Dirani, M., Guymer, R.: Unraveling a complex genetic disease: age-related macular degeneration. Surv. Ophthalmol. **51**, 576–586 (2006)
146. Ciulla, T.A., Danis, R.P., Harris, A.: Age-Related macular degeneration: a review of experimental treatments. Surv. Ophthalmol. **43**, 134–146 (1998)

147. Jager, R.D., Mieler, W.F., Miller, J.W.: Age-Related macular degeneration. N. Engl. J. Med. **358**, 2606–2617 (2008)
148. Leeuwen, R., Klaver, C.C., Vingerling, J.R., Hoffman, A., Jong, P.T.: Epidemiology of age-related maculopathy: a review. Eur. J. Epidemiol. **18**, 845–854 (2003)
149. Madonna, R.J.: Age-related macular degeneration. Clin. Eye Vis. Care **9**, 65–69 (1997)
150. Celesia, G.G.D.P.J. Jr.: Anatomy and physiology of the visual system. J. Clin. Neurophysiol. **11**, 482–492 (1994)
151. Edward, D.P.K.L.M.: Anatomy, development, and physiology of the visual system. Pediatr. Clin. North Am. **50**, 1–23 (2003)
152. Remington, L.: Retina. In: Reminggton L. (ed.) Clinical anatomy and physiology of the visual system, 3rd ed., Elsevier, Amstredam (2011)
153. Wassle, H., Boycott, B.B.: Functional architecture of the mammalian retina. Physiol. Rev. **71**, 447–480 (1991)
154. Bhutto, I.L.G.: Understanding age-related macular degeneration (AMD): Relationships between the photoreceptor/retinal pigment epithelium/Bruch's membrane/choriocapillaris complex. Mol. Aspects Med. **33**, 295–317 (2012)
155. Goodwin, P.: Hereditary retinal disease. Current Opinion. Ophthalmology **19**, 255–262 (2008)
156. Hageman, G.S., Marmor, M.F., Yao, X.Y., Johnson, L.V.: The interphotoreceptor matrix mediates primate retinal adhesion. Arch. Ophthalmol. **113**, 655–660 (1985)
157. Hartnett, M.E.: Breakdown of the Retinal Pigmented Epithelium Blood–Retinal Barrier. In: Dartt, D.A., Besharse, J.C., Dana, R. (eds.) Encyclopedia of the Eye. 1st edn. Academic Press, Inc, New York (2010)
158. Hollyfield, J.G., Varner, H.H., Rayborn, M.E., Osterfeld, A.M.: Retinal attachment to the pigment epithelium. Linkage through an extracellular sheath surrounding cone photoreceptors. Retina **9**, 59–68 (1989)
159. Rizzolo, L.J., Peng, S., Luo, Y., Xiao, W.: Retinal pigmented epithelium barrier. Prog. Retinal Eye Res. **30**, 296–323 (2010)
160. Sama, T.: Properties and function of the ocular melanin—a photobiophysical view. J. Photochem. Photobiol. **12**, 215–258 (1992)
161. Strauss, O.: The retinal pigment epithelium in visual function. Physiol. Rev. **85**, 845–881 (2005)
162. Afshari, F.T., Fawcett, J.W.: Improving RPE adhesion to Bruch's membrane. Eye (Lond) **23**, 1890–1893 (2009)
163. Booij, J.C., Baas, D.C., Beisekeeva, J., Gorgels, T.G.M.F., Bergen, A.A.B.: The dynamic nature of Bruch's membrane. Prog. Retinal Eye Res. **29**, 1–18 (2010)
164. Curcio, C.A., Johnson, M.: Structure, function, and pathology of Bruch's Membrane. In: Ryan, S.J., Schachat, A.P., Wilkinson, C.P., Hinton, D.R., Sadda, S.V.R., Wiedemann, P. (eds.) Retina, chap 20, Elsevier Health Sciences (2012)
165. Ferris 3rd, F.L., Fine, S.L., Hyman, L.: Age-related macular degeneration and blindness due to neovascular maculopathy. Arch. Ophthalmol. **102**, 1640–1642 (1984)
166. Campochiaro, P.A., Soloway, P., Ryan, S.J., Miller, J.W.: The pathogenesis of choroidal neovascularization in patients with age-related macular degeneration. Molecular Vision **5**, 34 (1999)
167. Feeney-Burns, L., Burns, R.P., Gao, C.L.: Age-related macular changes in humans over 90 years old. Am. J. Ophthalmol. **109**, 265–278 (1990)
168. Feeney-Burns, L., Hilderbrans, E.S., Eldridge, S.: Aging human RPE: morphometric analysis of macular, equatorial, and peripheral cells. Invest. Ophthalmol. Vis. Sci. **25**, 195–200 (1984)
169. Grunwald, G.B.: Structure and function of the retinal pigment epithelium. In: Jaeger, E.A., Duane, T.D., Tasman, W. (eds.) Duane's Foundations of Clinical Ophthalmology. Lippincott-Raven, Philadelphia (2004)

170. Panda-Jonas, S., Jonas, J.B., Jakobczyk-Zmija, M.: Retinal pigment epithelial cell count, distribution, and correlations in normal human eyes. Am. J. Ophthalmol. **121**, 181–189 (1996)
171. Wing, G.L., Blanchard, G.C., Weiter, J.J.: The topography and age relationship of lipofuscin concentration in the retinal pigment epithelium. Invest. Ophthalmol. Vis. Sci. **17**, 601–607 (1978)
172. Ambati, J., Ambati, B.K., Yoo, S.H., Ianchulev, S., Adamis, A.P.: Age-Related macular degeneration: etiology, pathogenesis, and therapeutic strategies. Surv. Ophthalmol. **48**, 257–293 (2003)
173. Zarbin, M.A.: Current concepts in the pathogenesis of age-related macular degeneration. Arch. Ophthalmol. **122**, 598–614 (2004)
174. Zarbin, M.A.: Retinal pigment epithelium–retina transplantation for retinal degenerative disease. Am. J. Ophthalmol. **146**, 151–153 (2008)
175. Nag, T.C., Wadhwa, S.: Ultrastructure of the human retina in aging and various pathological states. Micron **43**, 759–781 (2012)
176. Prasad, P.S., Schwartz, S.D., Hubschman, J.: Age-related macular degeneration: current and novel therapies. Maturitas **66**, 5–5 (2010)
177. Stokkermans, T.J.: Treatment of age-related macular degeneration. Clin. Eye Vis. Care **12**, 15–35 (2000)
178. Tao, S., Young, C., Redenti, S., Zhang, Y., Klassen, H., Desai, T., Young, M.J.: Survival, migration and differentiation of retinal progenitor cells transplanted on micro-machined poly(methyl methacrylate) scaffolds to the subretinal space. Lab Chip **7**, 695–701 (2007)
179. Treharne, A.J., Grossel, M.C., Lotery, A.J., Thomson, H.A.: The chemistry of retinal transplantation: the influence of polymer scaffold properties on retinal cell adhesion and control. Br. J. Ophthalmol. **95**, 768–773 (2011)
180. Binder, S.: Scaffolds for retinal pigment epithelium (RPE) replacement therapy. Br. J. Ophthalmol. **95**, 441–442 (2011)
181. Binder, S., Stanzel, B.V., Krebs, I., Glittenberg, C.: Transplantation of the RPE in AMD. Prog Retinal Eye Res. **26**, 516–554 (2007)
182. Hynes, S.R., Lavik, E.B.: A tissue-engineered approach towards retinal repair: Scaffolds for cell transplantation to the subretinal space. Graefes Arch. Clin. Exp. Ophthalmol. **248**, 763–778 (2010)
183. Imai, H., Honda, S., Kondo, N., Ishibashi, K., Tsukahara, Y., Negi, A.: The upregulation of angiogenic gene expression in cultured retinal pigment epithelial cells grown on type I collagen. Curr. Eye Res. **32**, 903–910 (2007)
184. Neeley, W.L., Redenti, S., Klassen, H., Tao, S., Desai, T., Young, M.J., Langer, R.: A microfabricated scaffold for retinal progenitor cell grafting. Biomaterials **29**, 418–426 (2008)
185. Redenti, S., Neeley, W.L., Rompani, S., Saigal, S., Yang, J., Klassen, H., Langer, R., Young, M.J.: Engineering retinal progenitor cell and scrollable poly(glycerol-sebacate) composites for expansion and subretinal transplantation. Biomaterials **30**, 3405–3414 (2009)
186. Redenti, S., Tao, S., Yang, J., Gu, P., Klassen, H., Saigal, S., Desai, T., Young, M.J.: Retinal tissue engineering using mouse retinal progenitor cells and a novel biodegradable, thin-film poly(e-caprolactone) nanowire scaffold. J. Ocul. Biol., Dis. Inform. **1**, 19–29 (2008)
187. Thumann, G., Hueber, A., Dinslage, S., Schaeffer, F., Yasukawa, T., Kirchhof, B., Yafai, Y., Eichler, W., Bringmann, A., Wiedemann, P.: Characteristics of iris and retinal pigment epithelial cells cultured on collagen type I membranes. Curr. Eye Res. **31**, 241–249 (2006)
188. Tomita, M., Lavik, E., Klassen, H., Zahir, T., Langer, R., Young, M.J.: Biodegradable polymer composite grafts promote the survival and differentiation of retinal progenitor cells. Stem Cells **23**, 1579–1588 (2005)

Chapter 5
Polymers in Orthopaedic Surgery

Catherine G. Ambrose, Braden E. Hartline, Thomas O. Clanton, Walter R. Lowe and William C. McGarvey

Abstract Polymers have been used as biomaterials in Orthopaedic Surgery for decades. Despite reports of complications with some polymeric materials, most are biocompatible and have been used successfully in total joint replacements, for soft tissue reconstruction, for joint fusion, and as fracture fixation devices. In this chapter we will describe the types of polymers used in commercially-available orthopaedic implants, and then give a breakdown by clinical application.

Keywords Orthopaedic implants · Polymeric biomaterials

Abbreviations

PMMA	Poly(methylmethacrylate)
PE	Poly(ethylene)
UHMWPE	Ultra-high molecular weight poly(ethylene)
HXPE	Highly cross-linked PE
PEEK	Poly(etheretherketone)
LPLA	Poly(L-lactide)
DLPLA	Poly(DL-lactide)
LDLPLA	Poly(DL-lactide-*co*-L-lactide)
PGA	Poly(glycolide)
LPLG	Poly(L-lactide-*co*-glycolide)
DLPLG	Poly(DL-lactide-*co*-glycolide)

C.G. Ambrose (✉) · B.E. Hartline · W.R. Lowe · W.C. McGarvey
Department of Orthopaedic Surgery, UTHSC-Houston, 6431 Fannin, Rm 6.154, Houston, TX 77030, USA
e-mail: catherine.g.ambrose@uth.tmc.edu

T.O. Clanton
Steadman Philippon Research Institute, Vail, CO, USA

F. Puoci (ed.), *Advanced Polymers in Medicine*, DOI 10.1007/978-3-319-12478-0_5

Introduction

When selecting a biomaterial for orthopaedic applications, special consideration must be given to the structural properties of the material, since orthopaedic implants must be able to withstand significant and repeated mechanical loads. Ultimate strength, fatigue resistance, and wear are more critical than in other clinical applications since materials used in total joint replacements, fracture fixation plates, and spinal cages must be able to withstand millions of cycles of loading several times body weight. Although metals were the first biomaterials to be used in orthopaedic surgery and are still widely used today, polymers have been used successfully for more than half a century. Currently, polymers are widely used in total joint replacement, sports medicine, spine, and orthopaedic trauma applications. There are many ways to categorize the polymers used in orthopaedics: absorbable versus nonabsorbable, synthetic versus naturally-occurring, commercially-available versus in-research-use only, or by the clinical application. In this chapter we will first discuss the polymers currently used in orthopaedic implants, and then discuss the clinical applications of the polymers in commercial use.

ASTM International publishes several standard specifications that relate specifically to polymers used in medical applications. Table 5.1 gives a list of the ASTM standards that describe the standard specification of polymers used in orthopaedic surgery implants. Similar standards are published by the International Organization for Standardization (ISO), but are not listed here.

Nonabsorbable Polymers

Polymethylmethacrylate

Otto Rohm is credited with the development of perhaps the most widely used polymer in orthopaedic surgery—poly(methylmethacrylate) (PMMA)—in 1901 [1] but the material did not come into widespread use in orthopaedics until Sir John Charnley described its use for bonding prostheses to bone in the early 1960s [2]. A good review of the early work in characterizing PMMA including the evolution of the use in orthopaedics can be found in the article by Dennis Smith where he describes his collaboration with Charnley [3].

PMMA is composed of a powder polymer and a liquid monomer, which is usually mixed in a 2:1 ratio just prior to implantation. The liquid monomer is mainly (approximately 97 %) methylmethacrylate, but also contains an accelerator and a stabilizer [4]. The composition of the powder component varies by brand but contains mainly microspheres of ground PMMA or copolymer with small amounts of radiopaque substances and an initiator. Some formulations also contain a dye or antibiotics. Mixing of the polymer and the monomer creates an exothermic reaction, which can have a necrotic effect on surrounding musculoskeletal tissues. The resulting polymer will progress through several stages during curing, usually reaching

Table 5.1 ASTM standards related to polymeric materials used in orthopaedic surgery

Designation	Title
F451-08	Standard specification for Acrylic Bone Cement
F639-09	Standard specification for Polyethylene Plastics for medical applications
F648-14	Standard specification for Ultra-High-Molecular-Weight Polyethylene Powder and Fabricated Form for surgical implants
F755-99(2011)	Standard specification for selection of Porous Polyethylene for use in surgical implants
F1925-09	Standard specification for Semi-Crystalline Poly(lactide) Polymer and Copolymer Resins for surgical implants
F2026-14	Standard specification for Polyetheretherketone (PEEK) Polymers for surgical implant applications
F2033-12	Standard specification for Total Hip Joint Prosthesis and Hip Endoprosthesis Bearing Materials Made of Metallic, Ceramic, and Polymeric Materials
F2313-10	Standard specification for Poly(glycolide) and Poly(glycolide-co-lactide) Resins for surgical implants with mole fractions greater than or equal to 70 % Glycolide
F2565-13	Standard guide for Extensively Irradiation-Crosslinked Ultra-High Molecular Weight Polyethylene Fabricated Forms for surgical implant applications
F2579-10	Standard specification for Amorphous Poly(lactide) and Poly(lactide-co-glycolide) Resins for surgical implants
F2695-12	Standard specification for ultra-high molecular weight Polyethylene Powder Blended with Alpha-Tocopherol (Vitamin E) and Fabricated Forms for surgical implant applications
F2759-11	Standard guide for assessment of the Ultra High Molecular Weight Polyethylene (UHMWPE) used in Orthopedic and Spinal Devices
F2820-12	Standard specification for Polyetherketoneketone (PEKK) Polymers for surgical implant applications
F2902-12	Standard guide for assessment of Absorbable Polymeric Implants

a workable, dough-like consistency within a few minutes followed by the hardening phase where peak temperatures are reached. There is a published standard that describes the required characteristics of all acrylic bone cements including setting time, material properties, and maximum temperature of polymerization (Table 5.1).

PMMA is strongest in compression and weakest in tension and under shear stresses with the ultimate compressive strength lying between trabecular and cortical bone [5]. The addition of antibiotics to the cement, commonly done to prevent or treat infections, can significantly impair the strength of the cement [5, 6]. There are numerous other factors that can affect the mechanical properties of PMMA including molecular weight, mixing method, and sterilization [7–11].

Despite its widespread and successful use, relatively rare complications have been documented with the use of PMMA in orthopaedic surgery. Tissue necrosis can be caused by the high heat of polymerization or by the chemicals themselves [12, 13]. Bone cement implantation syndrome (BCIS) is usually associated with total hip arthroplasty and can be fatal for the patient. Clinical manifestations include hypoxia, hypotension, cardiac arrhythmias and in some cases cardiovascular collapse [14]. Extravasation of the cement from the site of implantation can lead to a so-called "cement emboli", which although rare is a potentially fatal complication. [15–18] The cement can fail mechanically, leading to loosening of the implant it is meant to stabilize [5, 19, 20] or osteolysis due to the accumulation of wear particulates [21].

Polyethylene

After PMMA, the most commonly used polymer in orthopaedic surgery is polyethylene (PE). For several decades, this material has been the gold standard for bearing surfaces in total joint replacement devices. In general, the type of PE used in total joint replacements is ultra-high molecular weight polyethylene (UHMWPE) or highly cross-linked polyethylene (HXPE) [22]. Implant bearing surfaces are usually machined from ram-extruded bar stock, and then packaged and sterilized prior to shipment. Table 5.2 includes a list of some of the types of stock PE used by orthopaedic implant manufacturers.

The method of sterilization has critical effects on the mechanical properties of PE. Sterilization using gamma radiation produces free-radicals. If oxygen is present, the free-radicals produce chain scission and significant degradation of the mechanical strength of the implant. On the other hand, gamma irradiation without the presence of oxygen results in cross-linking of the polymer chains and can produce implants with improved wear properties [22, 23]. The addition of vitamin E, a natural antioxidant, is also thought to counteract the oxidative degradation of PE, and currently there are commercially-available PE implants containing vitamin E [24].

One of the greatest concerns about the use of PE in joint replacement bearing surfaces is the wear of the material and the effect the wear debris has on the surrounding tissues. For many years, it has been demonstrated that this wear debris leads to osteolysis and loosening of the prosthetic components [21, 25]. Wear of the polyethylene or loosening of the implants, which may be related to wear debris, remains a common reason for revision surgery after total hip [26, 27] or total knee arthroplasty [28].

Polyetheretherketone

Polyethertherketone (PEEK) is a member of the polyaryletherketone (PAEK) family. PEEK possesses excellent chemical and thermal resistance, and its biocompatibility, mechanical wear characteristics and stability under gamma irradiation makes it a good candidate material for orthopaedic implants. PEEK is a relatively ductile material, with a flexural modulus and ultimate tensile strength higher than that of UHMWPE or PMMA. For some applications, chopped carbon fibers are added to reinforce the PEEK material, further increasing it stiffness and strength [29, 30].

Table 5.2 Sample of commercially available polymer products used in orthopaedic surgery

Company	Product type/trade name	Polymer type	Polymer detail
Arthrex	Interference screws	Bioabsorbable	PLLA
Arthrex	Interference screws	Bioabsorbable	70 % PLDLA 30 % Biphasic Calcium Phosphate
Arthrex	Interference screws	Nonabsorbable	PEEK
Arthrex	Tenodesis screws	Bioabsorbable	PLLA
Arthrex	Tenodesis screws	Bioabsorbable	85 % PLLA 15 % β-Tricalcium Phosphate
Arthrex	Tenodesis screws	Nonabsorbable	PEEK
Arthrex	Transfix	Bioabsorbable	PLLA
Arthrex	Transfix	Bioabsorbable	70 % PLDLA 30 % Biphasic Calcium Phosphate
Arthrex	Graftbolt	Bioabsorbable	70 % PLDLA 30 % Biphasic Calcium Phosphate
Arthrex	Graftbolt	Nonabsorbable	PEEK
Arthrex	Compression screw	Bioabsorbable	PLLA
Arthrex	Corkscrew	Bioabsorbable	PLDLA
Arthrex	Corkscrew FT	Bioabsorbable	PLLA
Arthrex	Corkscrew FT	Bioabsorbable	85 % PLLA 15 % β-Tricalcium Phosphate
Arthrex	PushLock	Bioabsorbable	PLLA
Arthrex	PushLock	Bioabsorbable	85 % PLLA 15 % β-Tricalcium Phosphate
Arthrex	PushLock	Nonabsorbable	PEEK
Arthrex	SwiveLock	Bioabsorbable	PLLA
Arthrex	SwiveLock	Bioabsorbable	85 % PLLA 15 % β-Tricalcium Phosphate
Arthrex	SwiveLock	Nonabsorbable	PEEK
Arthrex	FASTak	Bioabsorbable	PLDLA
Arthrex	SutureTak	Bioabsorbable	PLDLA
Arthrex	SutureTak	Bioabsorbable	PLLA
Arthrex	SutureTak	Bioabsorbable	85 % PLLA 15 % β-Tricalcium Phosphate
Arthrex	SutureTak	Nonabsorbable	PEEK
Arthrex	SwiveLock tenodesis	Bioabsorbable	85 % PLLA 15 % β-Tricalcium Phosphate
Arthrex	SwiveLock tenodesis	Nonabsorbable	PEEK
BioMet	Active articulation™ Dual mobility hip	Nonabsorbable	E1® Antiosidant infused PE
DePuy Synthes	Plivios revolution cage for posterior lumbar interbody dusion (PLIF)	Nonabsorbable	PEEK

(continued)

Table 5.2 (continued)

Company	Product type/trade name	Polymer type	Polymer detail
Medtronic	Prevail cervical interbody device	Nonabsorbable	PEEK
Medtronic	Bryan cervical disc	Nonabsorbable	Polyurethane
Small Bones Innovations	STAR™ ankle	Nonabsorbable	UHMWPE
Small Bones Innovations	rHead™ recon	Nonabsorbable	UHMWPE
Small Bones Innovations	RE-MOTION™ total Wrist	Nonabsorbable	UHMWPE
Small Bones Innovations	Avanta CMC	Nonabsorbable	UHMWPE
Smith & Nephew	Healicoil regenesorb	Bioabsorbable	PLGA, β-TCP, Calcium Sulfate
Stryker	Mobile bearing hip™ system	Nonabsorbable	Polyethylene
Stryker	X3 bearing	Nonabsorbable	Polyethylene
Stryker	Crossfire polyethylene	Nonabsorbable	Polyethylene
Stryker	Solar shoulder	Nonabsorbable	UHMWPE
Stryker	Biosteon® Wedge interference screw	Bioabsorbable	25 % Hydroxyapatite (HA), 75 % amorphous PLLA
Stryker	Bioabsorbable interference screw	Bioabsorbable	PLLA
Stryker	BioZip absorbable anchor	Bioabsorbable	PLLA
Stryker	Intraline, Zip, Twinloop, ReelXAnchors	Nonabsorbable	PEEK
Stryker	AVS AL spacer system	Nonabsorbable	PEEK
Synthes	ProDisc	Nonabsorbable	Polyethylene
Zimmer	Conventional polyethylene	Nonabsorbable	GUR 1050 polyethylene resin or bar stock
Zimmer	Sulene®	Nonabsorbable	GUR 1020 polyethylene bar stock
Zimmer	Prolong® Highly crosslinked polyethylene	Nonabsorbable	GUR 1050 polyethylene bar stock
Zimmer	Longevity® Highly crosslinked polyethylene	Nonabsorbable	GUR 1050 polyethylene bar stock
Zimmer	Durasul® Highly crosslinked polyethylene	Nonabsorbable	GUR 1050 polyethylene bar stock/pre-forms
Zimmer	Vivacit-E® Vitamin E highly crosslinked polyethylene	Nonabsorbable	GUR 1020 polyethylene resin, VitE

PEEK lends itself to a variety of commercial processing techniques, including molding, extrusion, injection molding and compression molding, making it attractive to use as an implant material. In 1998, Invibio, LTD, offered PEEK commercially as an implant material [30], which has allowed for increased research into the applicability of this material for orthopaedic trauma, spine and adult reconstruction implants. Currently, the orthopaedic application of PEEK is concentrated in fusion cages (both spine and foot and ankle) [30–33] and for interference screws in sports medicine applications [34–36].

Absorbable Polymers

Bioabsorbable polymers are becoming increasingly popular in orthopaedic surgery and several review articles have been written to describe their use [37–41]. Absorbable implants have several advantages over traditional metallic implants or those made from nonabsorbable polymers. First, absorbable implants reduce stress shielding and the resulting bone weakening since the degradation profile of the material can be optimized to allow a gradual increase in the load transferred to the healing tissue. Second, although there are instances where bioabsorbable implants have had to be removed due to adverse tissue reactions, the incidence of a required second surgery to remove these implants is lower than with metallic implants [42]. Finally, bioabsorbable implants can be manufactured to include drugs or growth factors which are gradually released as the implant degrades, making them function as both a structural component and a drug delivery system [43, 44]. Bioabsorbable implants do have several disadvantages when compared to metallic or nonabsorbable polymeric implants including lower strength, higher cost, and in some cases, a sterile, non-specific inflammatory response.

The most commonly used absorbable polymers used in orthopaedic surgery are those made from polylactide (PLA), polyglycolide (PGA) or combinations of the two. PLA has two isoforms, a D and an L, and is usually listed using the acronyms LPLA or DPLA, or DLPLA if a combination is used. As these polymers degrade into acidic products that are easily eliminated, the host reaction to the implant is usually negligible. However, in cases where the degradation products accumulate, such as in tissues with poor blood flow, the reaction can be severe and may require a second surgery to remove the implant [39]. Many factors affect the degradation of the implant and the resulting biological reaction, including the implant material, implant geometry (surface area to volume ratio), site of implantation, and the method of sterilization.

Resorption of polymers generally occurs in two phases. First, the polymer chains are broken down through hydrolysis and the molecular weight of the polymer drops, followed by loss of mechanical strength and loss of mass in the implant. Second, the implant loses its form and breaks into particles, which are attacked by macrophages and the by products are excreted by the kidneys and lungs [45].

Animal studies indicate that implants made from PGA fully degrade in 3–9 months. Since most instances of adverse tissue response in humans have been reported to occur between 2 weeks and 6 months, this is consistent with the theory that the adverse tissue reaction is related to the accumulation of acidic degradation products during the final stages of implant resorption. The rate of adverse tissue reaction varies but has been reported to be as low as 3 % in trauma applications to as high as 60 % when implants are used for treating wrist fractures [39]. The clinical presentation of the reaction is that of a sterile, non-specific inflammatory response with multinucleated foreign body giant cells seen in histological sections. Polymeric debris is also usually visible both extra- and intra-cellularly and osteolytic lesions are often present.

Implants made from LPLA degrade much more slowly in vivo, taking up to several years. In animal studies the degradation time was shown to be between 2 and 3 years depending on the polymer, and in a few human trials the degradation was reported to take between 10 and 68 months. The reports of adverse tissue reaction to these implants indicate that most reactions occur between 5 months and 5 years, again consistent with the theory that the reactions occur at the final stages of implant degradation, if these reactions are going to occur [39, 40].

In some cases hydroxyapatite or calcium phosphate are added to PGA or PLA implants. The addition of these materials helps to increase the mechanical strength of the implants and is thought to decrease the accumulation of acidic degradation products during polymer resorption, which may decrease the incidence of adverse tissue reactions. Long-term clinical trials are needed to determine if implants made from these materials lead to better patient outcomes.

Applications of Polymers in Orthopaedic Surgery

Table 5.2 contains a partial listing of commercially available polymer products used in orthopaedic surgical procedures. Here we describe the general applications of polymers in orthopaedic surgery.

Joint Replacement

The 1960s hip replacement implant developed by Sir John Charnley resembles many joint replacement implants used today. His prosthesis consisted of a metal femoral component and PE acetabulum, with the implants bonded to the bone using PMMA [46]. The low friction design of the articulating surfaces gave good surgical outcomes and because of this design joint replacement surgeries are considered some of the most successful orthopaedic surgeries [47].

Since PMMA has mechanical properties that are similar to bone, its use in joint replacement devices may allow a more physiologic transfer of loads from the prosthesis to the remaining bone, which may in turn reduce stress-shielding and the resulting bone loss. PMMA stabilizes implants within the surrounding bone, reducing unwanted micromotions and can act as a load damper [5].

PE remains the workhorse of joint replacement liners as it functions as a low-friction implant articulating surface. There have been many adaptations and

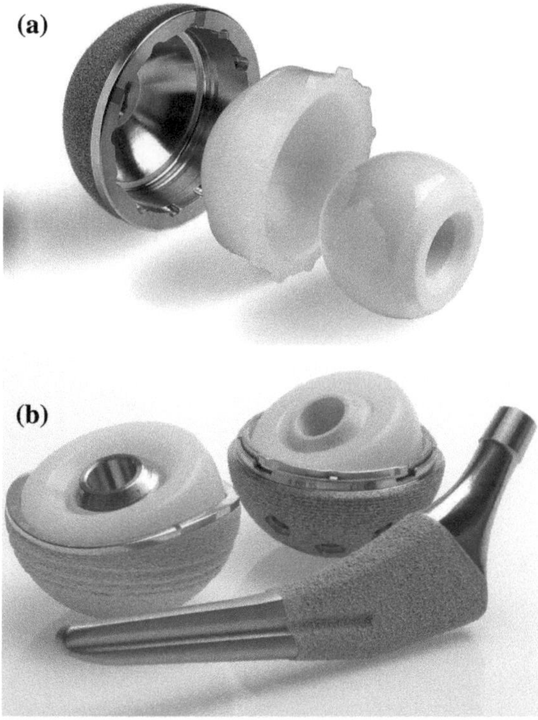

Fig. 5.1 Example total hip replacement systems. **a** is the Continuum™ Acetabular System made by Zimmer. In this example the liner, made from highly-crosslinked polyethylene, is shown positioned between a porous metal acetabular cup and a ceramic femoral head. **b** shows the ADM™ and MDM™ acetabular systems with an Acolade II™ femoral stem made by Stryker. Highly-crosslinked polyethylene liners are shown between both metal and ceramic femoral heads and the metal acetabular cups

modifications made to PE over the years in attempts to improve its wear properties. Today's highly cross-linked PE provides a durable low friction surface between metal surfaces of hip, knee, shoulder, and ankle arthroplasty implants (Figs. 5.1 and 5.2).

Particle formation from arthroplasty implants can lead to complications in the post-operative period. It has been shown that wear particles from implants induce a systemic reaction that stimulates an immune response to the implants and joint. This immune reaction brings activated macrophages into the joint that medicate a process of osteolysis and bone resorption from the implants [25]. The end product of this devastating complication is implant failure and revision arthroplasty surgery. Ideal implants have minimal to no wear particle formation and therefore would not stimulate the immune response that causes failure.

Although some commercially available systems for spinal disc replacement are metal-on-metal or metal-on-ceramic systems, there are commercially available systems with either polyurethane or PE articulating surfaces. The review article by Cason gives a good overview of the implant systems available for cervical disc replacement [48] and discusses the existing evidence for their use. The 2013 Cochrane Review by Jacobs describes the available evidence for lumbar disc replacement systems [49]. Both reviews suggest that the evidence for or against these devices is limited and further long-term randomized clinical trials are needed to fully evaluate them.

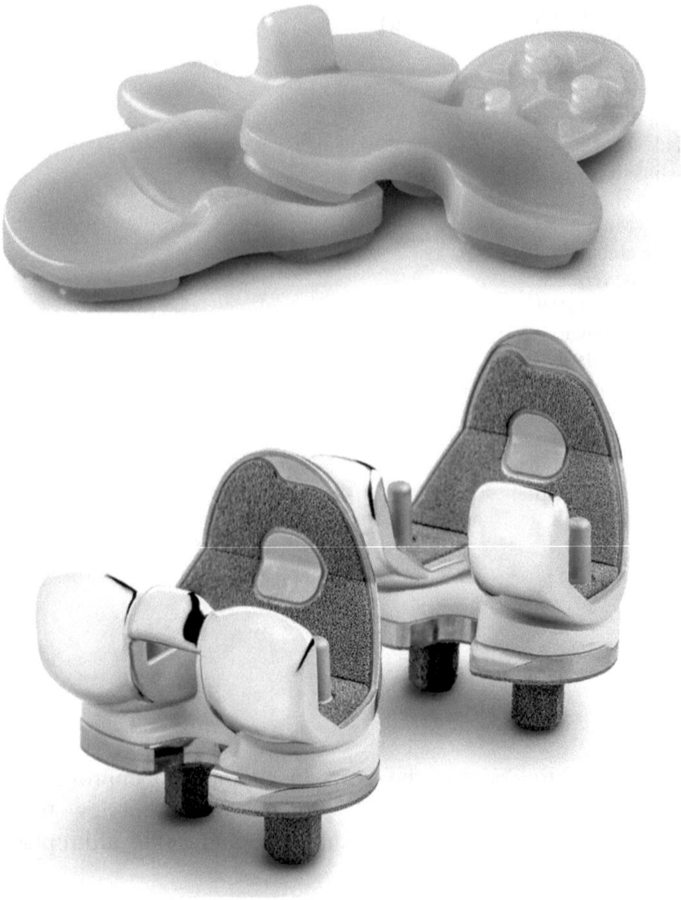

Fig. 5.2 Example total knee replacement system. The *top portion* of the figure highlights the polyethylene components available for the Persona™ personalized knee system manufactured by Zimmer, which includes both the tibia trays and the patellar resurfacing components. These liners are made from highly-crosslinked polyethylene with vitamin E added. In the *bottom portion* of the figure tibial trays are shown in their articulating position between the femoral and tibial metal components

Joint Fusion

An alternative approach to treating degenerative joints and the resulting pain is joint fusion. Porous cages are often used in these surgeries to preserve the spacing between the previously articulating bones while allowing for fusion between the segments. Commercially available spine cages using polymers are included in Table 5.2 and some example cages are shown in Figs. 5.3 and 5.4. While there are studies suggesting that the clinical outcomes with polymeric cages are superior to that when metallic cages are used [32] other studies suggest that the differences are not clinically significant [33].

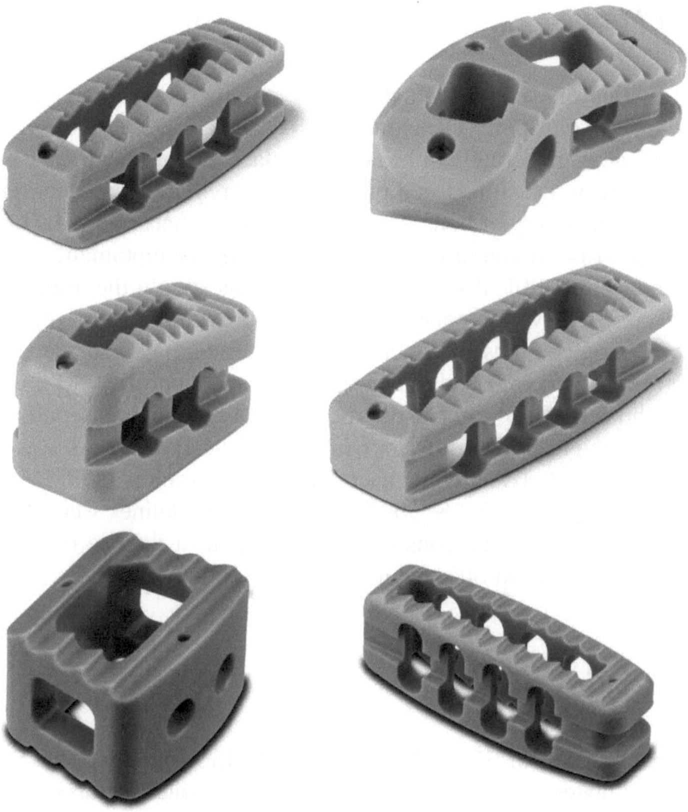

Fig. 5.3 Examples of PEEK cages made by Nuvasive for intervertebral body fusion procedures. The cages are meant to be filled with materials to promote bone fusion, such as bone graft taken from the patient's pelvis

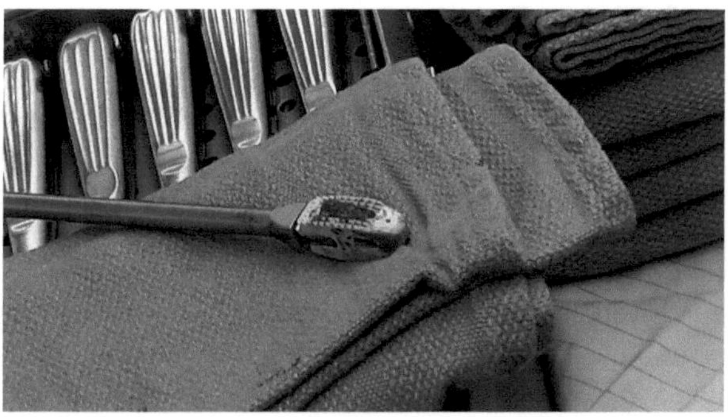

Fig. 5.4 Example of a PEEK cage filled with bone graft ready to be inserted into a patient. In this case the cage is the Opal™ spacer system made by Depuy Synthes

Bone Void Filling

Traumatic injuries or cancer treatment often requires bone resection, which can result in extensive voids in the skeleton. PMMA can be used to fill the voids, but the hope is that tissue engineering will be able to replace the missing bone material with the patient's own tissue. Spinal compression fractures are also a common consequence of traumatic injury or bone degeneration due to cancer or metabolic diseases such as osteoporosis. Although these fractures can be asymptomatic, they can also be painful and lead to difficulty with breathing or digestion if the resulting kyphosis becomes severe. Both vertebroplasty and kyphoplasty surgeries have been used to treat vertebral body compression fractures. These are both percutaneous procedures that aim to restore vertebral body height through injection of PMMA into the collapsed body; however, in kyphoplasty procedures, a balloon is inserted and inflated to restore body height prior to the introduction of the PMMA. As was mentioned previously in Sect. "Polymethylmethacrylate", extravasation of PMMA can lead to adverse consequences [15, 18, 50, 51]. Recently, guidelines were the American Academy of Orthopaedic Surgeons recommends against the use of vertebroplasty for patients with an osteoporotic spinal compression fracture [52].

Fracture Repair

Both absorbable [37, 38, 53] and nonabsorbable [30] polymers have been used to manufacture plates and screws for the fixation of bone fractures [54]. Metallic implant systems are more commonly used however, and are better suited to most applications due to the required mechanical strength needed for these applications [37, 55].

Soft Tissue Repairs

In general, surgery for soft tissue injuries involves either repair or reconstruction of the injured tissue. Intra-substance repairs of injured ligaments and tendons often involve suture fixation and apposition of the injured ligaments. When injuries occur near tendon or ligament insertions or origins, bony fixation constructs are typically used to fix the soft tissue in the anatomic origin or insertion site. Devices employed to repair and reconstruct soft tissues range include both interference screws used to constrain soft tissues within bony drill hole sites and suture anchors that secure soft tissues to bony surfaces with suture material attached to anchors that are fixed into bone.

Interference screws and suture anchors have evolved over time and now come in a variety of sizes, materials and designs (Figs. 5.5 and 5.6). The various

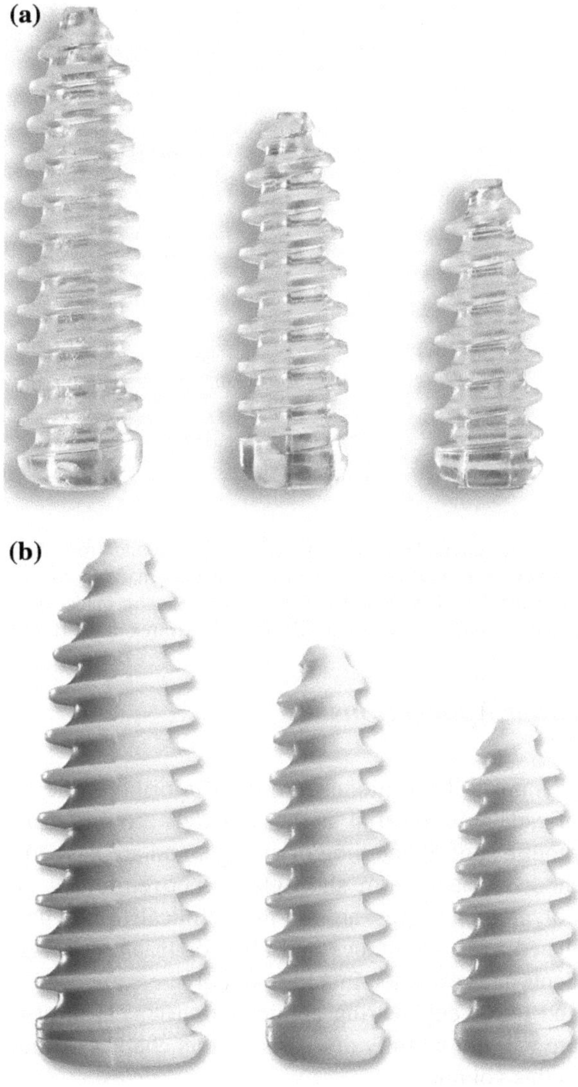

Fig. 5.5 Two example systems of interference screws made by Stryker. **a** shows screws made from PLLA and **b** shows the Biosteon™ screws made from a mixture of PLLA and hydroxyapatite

polymers that are used in these procedures offer advantages and disadvantages over other options of fixation [56–58]. Metal implants have been used for these procedures and still offer the advantage of superior strength and fracture resistance. Polymers are also in frequent use for these soft tissue repair procedures and offer their own advantages. Although complications have been reported with the use of absorbable implants, particularly in shoulder surgery [59, 60], a recent review suggests that there is not a relevant clinical difference in outcomes when either polymeric and metallic implants are used [61].

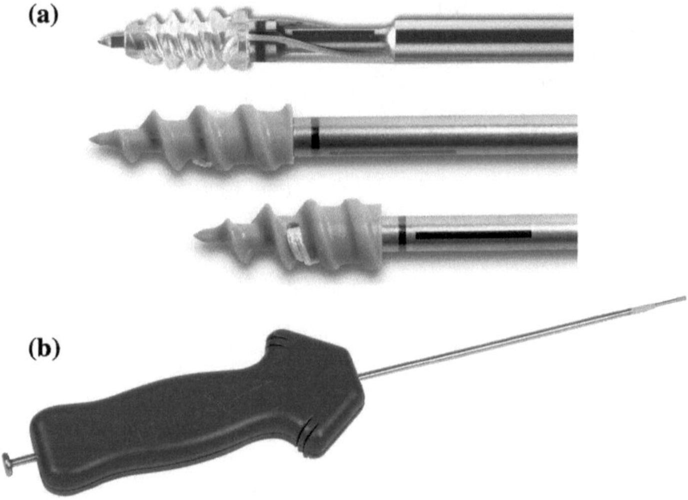

Fig. 5.6 Example suture anchors systems made from polymers. **a** shows both the Biozip™ (PLLA) and Intraline™ (HA-PLLA) anchors made by Stryker. **b** shows the Arthrex PushLock® instrumentation with a BioComposite® anchor made from biphasic calcium phosphate and PLDLA. Anchors are also available from Arthrex made from PLLA or PEEK

Other Applications

Composite bone models are used in orthopaedic research and education in place of cadaveric material as these models are uniform, relatively inexpensive, do not require special handling or storage, and are easy to obtain [62–64] Although these models, made from short-glass fiber-reinforced polyepoxide shells surrounding polyurethane cores, are not used clinically, they have been used in numerous published research studies and also for teaching surgical techniques to medical students and residents. In addition, polymers are used for drug delivery [6, 44, 65–67] and tissue engineering applications [68–71] in orthopaedic surgery. These topics are will not be fully discussed in this chapter as they are covered in other chapters in this volume.

References

1. Rohm, O.: On the polymerization products of acrylic acid. Chemistry (dissertation). University of Tubingen, Tubingen (1901)
2. Charnley, J.: The bonding of prostheses to bone by cement. J. Bone Joint Surg. Br. **46**, 518–529 (1964)
3. Smith, D.C.: The genesis and evolution of acrylic bone cement. Orthop. Clin. North Am. **36**, 1–10 (2005)
4. Jaeblon, T.: Polymethylmethacrylate: properties and contemporary uses in orthopaedics. J. Am. Acad. Orthop. Surg. **18**, 297–305 (2010)

5. Lewis, G.: Properties of acrylic bone cement: state of the art review. J. Biomed. Mater. Res. **38**, 155–182 (1997)
6. Lewis, G.: Properties of antibiotic-loaded acrylic bone cements for use in cemented arthroplasties: a state-of-the-art review. J. Biomed. Mater. Res. B Appl. Biomater. **89**, 558–574 (2009)
7. Harper, E.J., Braden, M., Bonfield, W., et al.: Influence of sterilization upon a range of properties of experimental bone cements. J. Mater. Sci.: Mater. Med. **8**, 849–853 (1997)
8. Lewis, G., Mladsi, S.: Effect of sterilization method on properties of Palacos R acrylic bone cement. Biomaterials **19**, 117–124 (1998)
9. Lewis, G.: Apparent fracture toughness of acrylic bone cement: effect of test specimen configuration and sterilization method. Biomaterials **20**, 69–78 (1999)
10. Graham, J., Pruitt, L., Ries, M., Gundiah, N.: Fracture and fatigue properties of acrylic bone cement: the effects of mixing method, sterilization treatment, and molecular weight. J. Arthroplasty **15**, 1028–1035 (2000)
11. An, Y.H., Alvi, F.I., Kang, Q., et al.: Effects of sterilization on implant mechanical property and biocompatibility. Int. J. Artif. Organs **28**, 1126–1137 (2005)
12. Mjoberg, B., Pettersson, H., Rosenqvist, R., Rydholm, A.: Bone cement, thermal injury and the radiolucent zone. Acta Orthop. Scand. **55**, 597–600 (1984)
13. Urrutia, J., Bono, C.M., Mery, P., Rojas, C.: Early histologic changes following polymethylmethacrylate injection (vertebroplasty) in rabbit lumbar vertebrae. Spine **33**, 877–882 (2008)
14. Donaldson, A.J., Thomson, H.E., Harper, N.J., Kenny, N.W.: Bone cement implantation syndrome. Br. J. Anaesth. **102**, 12–22 (2009)
15. Chen, Y.J., Tan, T.S., Chen, W.H., et al.: Intradural cement leakage: a devastatingly rare complication of vertebroplasty. Spine **31**, E379–E382 (2006)
16. Zhang, J.D., Poffyn, B., Sys, G., Uyttendaele, D.: Comparison of vertebroplasty and kyphoplasty for complications. Orthop. Surg. **3**, 158–160 (2011)
17. Wang, L., Gardner, A.W., Kwek, E.B., Naidu, G.R.: Retrograde cement arteriovenogram of nutrient vessels following hemiarthroplasty of the hip. Acta Orthop. Belg. **78**, 431–435 (2012)
18. Corcos, G., Dbjay, J., Mastier, C., et al.: Cement leakage in percutaneous vertebroplasty for spinal metastases: a retrospective evaluation of incidence and risk factors. Spine **39**, E332–E338 (2014)
19. Krause, W., Mathis, R.S.: Fatigue properties of acrylic bone cements: review of the literature. J. Biomed. Mater. Res. **22**, 37–53 (1988)
20. Cuckler, J.M.: If hip implant retrievals could speak, what would they tell us? J. Bone Joint Surg. Br. **94**, 11–13 (2012)
21. Goodman, S.: Wear particulate and osteolysis. Orthop. Clin. North. Am. **36**(1), 41–48 (2005)
22. Rajpura, A., Kendoff, D., Board, T.N.: The current state of bearing surfaces in total hip replacement. Bone Joint J. **96**(2), 147–156 (2014)
23. Gordon, A.C., D'Lima, D.D., Colwell Jr, C.W.: Highly cross-linked polyethylene in total hip arthroplasty. J. Am. Acad. Orthop. Surg. **14**, 511–523 (2006)
24. Oral, E., Muratoglu, O.K.: Vitamin E diffused, highly crosslinked UHMWPE: a review. Int. Orthop. **35**, 215–223 (2011)
25. Goodman, S.B., Gibon, E., Yao, Z.: The basic science of periprosthetic osteolysis. Instr. Course Lect. **62**, 201–206 (2013)
26. Ulrich, S.D., Seyler, T.M., Bennett, D., et al.: Total hip arthroplasties: what are the reasons for revision? Int. Orthop. **32**, 597–604 (2008)
27. Bozic, K.J., Kurtz, S.M., Lau, E., et al.: The epidemiology of revision total hip arthroplasty in the United States. J. Bone Joint Surg. Am. **91**, 128–133 (2009)
28. Bozic, K.J., Kurtz, S.M., Lau, E., et al.: The epidemiology of revision total knee arthroplasty in the United States. Clin. Orthop. Relat. Res. **468**, 45–51 (2010)
29. Eschbach, L.: Nonresorbable polymers in bone surgery. Injury **31**(Suppl 4), 22–27 (2000)
30. Kurtz, S.M., Devine, J.N.: PEEK biomaterials in trauma, orthopedic, and spinal implants. Biomaterials **28**, 4845–4869 (2007)
31. Nino Gomez, D., Eslava, S., Federico, A., et al.: Use of poly(ether ether ketone) cages in foot and ankle surgery. Foot Ankle Clin. **17**, 449–457 (2012)

32. Chen, Y., Wang, X., Lu, X., et al.: Comparison of titanium and polyetheretherketone (PEEK) cages in the surgical treatment of multilevel cervical spondylotic myelopathy: a prospective, randomized, control study with over 7-year follow-up. Eur. Spine J. **22**, 1539–1546 (2013)
33. Kersten, R.F., van Gaalen, S.M., de Gast, A., Oner, F.C.: Polyetheretherketone (PEEK) cages in cervical applications: a systematic review. Spine J.: Official J. North Am. Spine Soc. (2013)
34. Barber, F.A., Herbert, M.A., Beavis, R.C., Barrera Oro, F.: Suture anchor materials, eyelets, and designs: update 2008. Arthroscopy **24**, 859–867 (2008)
35. Barber, F.A., Herbert, M.A., Hapa, O., et al.: Biomechanical analysis of pullout strengths of rotator cuff and glenoid anchors: 2011 update. Arthroscopy **27**, 895–905 (2011)
36. Uzumcugil, O., Yalcinkaya, M., Ozturkmen, Y., et al.: Effect of PEEK polymer on tunnel widening after hamstring ACL reconstruction. Orthopedics **35**, e654–e659 (2012)
37. Gogolewski, S.: Bioresorbable polymers in trauma and bone surgery. Injury **31**(Suppl 4), 28–32 (2000)
38. Rokkanen, P.U., Bostman, O., Hirvensalo, E., et al.: Bioabsorbable fixation in orthopaedic surgery and traumatology. Biomaterials **21**, 2607–2613 (2000)
39. Ambrose, C.G., Clanton, T.O.: Bioabsorbable implants: review of clinical experience in orthopedic surgery. Ann. Biomed. Eng. **32**, 171–177 (2004)
40. Kontakis, G.M., Pagkalos, J.E., Tosounidis, T.I., et al.: Bioabsorbable materials in orthopaedics. Acta Orthop. Belg. **73**, 159–169 (2007)
41. Mukherjee, D.P., Pietrzak, W.S.: Bioabsorbable fixation: scientific, technical, and clinical concepts. J Craniofac. Surg. **22**, 679–689 (2011)
42. Bostman, O.M.: Metallic or absorbable fracture fixation devices: a cost minimization analysis. Clin. Orthop. Relat. Res. **329**, 233–239 (1996)
43. Nair, L.S., Laurencin, C.T.: Polymers as biomaterials for tissue engineering and controlled drug delivery. Adv. Biochem. Eng. Biotechnol. **102**, 47–90 (2006)
44. Kluin, O.S., van der Mei, H.C., Busscher, H.J., Neut, D.: Biodegradable vs non-biodegradable antibiotic delivery devices in the treatment of osteomyelitis. Expert Opin. Drug Deliv. **10**, 341–351 (2013)
45. Ciccone 2nd, W.J., Motz, C., Bentley, C., Tasto, J.P.: Bioabsorbable implants in orthopaedics: new developments and clinical applications. J. Am. Acad. Orthop. Surg. **9**, 280–288 (2001)
46. Knight, S.R., Aujla, R., Biswas, S.P.: Total hip arthroplasty—over 100 years of operative history. Orthop. Rev. **3**, e16 (2011)
47. Callaghan, J.J., Albright, J.C., Goetz, D.D., et al.: Charnley total hip arthroplasty with cement minimum twenty-five-year follow-up. J. Bone Joint Surg. Am. **82**(4), 487–497 (2000)
48. Cason, G.W., Herkowitz, H.N.: Cervical intervertebral disc replacement. J. Bone Joint Surg. Am. **95**, 279–285 (2013)
49. Jacobs, W., Van der Gaag, N.A., Tuschel, A., et al. Total disc replacement for chronic back pain in the presence of disc degeneration. Cochrane Database Syst. Rev. **9,** CD008326 (2012)
50. Abdul-Jalil, Y., Bartels, J., Alberti, O., Becker, R.: Delayed presentation of pulmonary polymethylmethacrylate emboli after percutaneous vertebroplasty. Spine **32**, E589–E593 (2007)
51. Bose, R., Choi, J.W.: Successful percutaneous retrieval of methyl methacrylate orthopedic cement embolism from the pulmonary artery. Cathet. Cardiovasc. Interv. **76**, 198–201 (2010)
52. Esses, S.I., McGuire, R., Jenkins, J., et al.: American academy of orthopaedic surgeons clinical practice guideline on: the treatment of osteoporotic spinal compression fractures. J. Bone Joint Surg. Am. **93**, 1934–1936 (2011)
53. Waris, E., Konttinen, Y.T., Ashammakhi, N., et al.: Bioabsorbable fixation devices in trauma and bone surgery: current clinical standing. Expert Rev. Med. Devices **1**, 229–240 (2004)
54. Yetkin, H., Senkoylu, A.: Biomaterials in orthopaedic surgery and traumatology. Technol. Health Care **10**, 173–175 (2002)
55. Cotic, M., Vogt, S., Hinterwimmer, S., et al. A matched-pair comparison of two different locking plates for valgus-producing medial open-wedge high tibial osteotomy: peek-carbon composite plate versus titanium plate. Knee Surg. Sports Traumatol. Arthrosc. 1–9 (2014)
56. Alan Barber, F., Boothby, M.H., Richards, D.P.: New sutures and suture anchors in sports medicine. Sports Med. Arthrosc. **14**, 177–184 (2006)

57. Gunja, N.J., Athanasiou, K.A.: Biodegradable materials in arthroscopy. Sports Med. Arthrosc. **14**, 112–119 (2006)
58. Denard, P.J., Burkhart, S.S.: The evolution of suture anchors in arthroscopic rotator cuff repair. Arthroscopy **29**, 1589–1595 (2013)
59. Dhawan, A., Ghodadra, N., Karas, V., et al.: Complications of bioabsorbable suture anchors in the shoulder. Am. J. Sports Med. **40**, 1424–1430 (2012)
60. McCarty 3rd, L.P., Buss, D.D., Datta, M.W., et al.: Complications observed following labral or rotator cuff repair with use of poly-L-lactic acid implants. J. Bone Joint Surg. Am. **95**, 507–511 (2013)
61. Papalia, R., Franceschi, F., Diaz Balzani, L., et al. The arthroscopic treatment of shoulder instability: bioabsorbable and standard metallic anchors produce equivalent clinical results. Arthroscopy (2014)
62. Gardner, M.P., Chong, A.C., Pollock, A.G., Wooley, P.H.: Mechanical evaluation of large-size fourth-generation composite femur and tibia models. Ann. Biomed. Eng. **38**, 613–620 (2010)
63. Grover, P., Albert, C., Wang, M., Harris, G.F. Mechanical characterization of fourth generation composite humerus. Proc. Inst. Mech. Eng. Part H J. Eng. Med. 225, 1169–1176 (2011)
64. Elfar, J., Menorca, R.M., Reed, J.D., Stanbury, S.: Composite bone models in orthopaedic surgery research and education. J. Am. Acad. Orthop. Surg. **22**, 111–120 (2014)
65. Saito, N., Murakami, N., Takahashi, J., et al.: Synthetic biodegradable polymers as drug delivery systems for bone morphogenetic proteins. Adv. Drug Deliv. Rev. **57**, 1037–1048 (2005)
66. Tan, H.L., Lin, W.T., Tang, T.T.: The use of antimicrobial-impregnated PMMA to manage periprosthetic infections: controversial issues and the latest developments. Int. J. Artif. Organs **35**, 832–839 (2012)
67. Ambrose, C.G., Clyburn, T.A., Mika, J., et al.: Evaluation of antibiotic-impregnated microspheres for the prevention of implant-associated orthopaedic infections. J. Bone Joint Surg. Am. **96**, 128–134 (2014)
68. Fedorovich, N.E., Alblas, J., de Wijn, J.R., et al.: Hydrogels as extracellular matrices for skeletal tissue engineering: state-of-the-art and novel application in organ printing. Tissue Eng. **13**, 1905–1925 (2007)
69. Spiller, K.L., Maher, S.A., Lowman, A.M.: Hydrogels for the repair of articular cartilage defects. Tissue Eng. Part B, Rev. **17**, 281–299 (2011)
70. Kosuge, D., Khan, W.S., Haddad, B., Marsh, D.: Biomaterials and scaffolds in bone and musculoskeletal engineering. Curr. Stem Cell Res. Ther. **8**, 185–191 (2013)
71. Raftery, R., O'Brien, F.J., Cryan, S.A. Chitosan for gene delivery and orthopedic tissue engineering applications. Molecules (Basel, Switzerland) 18(5), 5611–5647 (2013)

Chapter 6
Polymers in Ophthalmology

Javier Adrián Calles, José Bermúdez, Enrique Vallés, Daniel Allemandi and Santiago Palma

Abstract Ophthalmological sciences are disciplines focused in the health of the eyes and related structures, as well as vision, visual systems, and vision information processing in humans; dealing with the anatomy, physiology and diseases of the eye. Along time a wide variety of materials, including metals, ceramics and polymers, have been developed and used in different ophthalmic applications. Although, modern ophthalmic devices and drug platforms are made with polymeric materials. Applications of polymers in ophthalmology include vitreous replacement fluids, contact lenses, intraocular lenses, artificial orbital walls, artificial corneas, artificial lacrimal ducts, glaucoma drainage devices, viscoelastic replacements, drug delivery systems, sclera buckles, retinal tacks and adhesives, and ocular endotamponades. Both synthetic and natural polymeric biomaterials are used in ophthalmological applications, although in the lasts years most efforts were focused in natural and biocompatible materials, such as gelatin, hyaluronan, chitosan, gums, etc.; developing, tablets, films, suspensions, nanosystems, inserts, etc. This chapter attempts to offers an insight into the importance of polymers in the design and development of pharmaceuticals platforms used in ocular therapeutics.

Keywords Ophthalmology · Polymers · Inserts · Hydrogels · Microparticles · Nanoparticles · Drug delivery

---

J.A. Calles (✉) · E. Vallés
PLAPIQUI-CONICET, Universidad Nacional del Sur, Bahía Blanca, Argentina,
Camino "La Carrindanga" - Km 7, Casilla de Correo 717, 8000 Bahía Blanca, Argentina
e-mail: jcalles@plapiqui.edu.ar

J.A. Calles
Department. Biology, Biochemistry and Pharmacy, Universidad Nacional del Sur, Bahía Blanca, Argentina

J. Bermúdez
INIQUI-CONICET, Universidad Nacional de Salta, Salta, Argentina

D. Allemandi · S. Palma
UNITEFA-CONICET, Universidad Nacional de Córdoba, Córdoba, Argentina

F. Puoci (ed.), *Advanced Polymers in Medicine*, DOI 10.1007/978-3-319-12478-0_6

Abbreviations

MC	Methylcellulose
HEC	Hydroxyethylcellulose
HPC	Hydroxypropycellulose
HPMC	Hydroxypropylmethylcellulose
CMC Na	Sodium carboxymethylcellulose
PVA	Poly(vinyl alcohol)
SH	Sodium hyaluronate
AUC	Area under the curve
HEMA	Hydroxy ethyl metacrylate
PVP	Polyvinyl pyrrolidone
EGDM	Ethylene glycol dimethacrylic acid
DDS	Drug delivery system
PLA	Polylactic acid
PGA	Polyglycolic acid
PLGA	Copolymer polylactic-co-glycolic acid
NEs	Nanoemulsions
PEO	Polyethylene oxide
PPO	Polypropylene oxide

Introduction

Ophthalmic drug delivery is one of the most interesting and challenging endeavors facing the pharmaceutical scientist. Over the past decade, the understanding of ocular physiopathology and pharmacokinetic and pharmacodynamic parameters of ophthalmic drugs has increased markedly and resulted in the development of new drugs and drug delivery systems for the human eye. The move from traditional ophthalmic dosage forms toward more sophisticated drug delivery systems has been slow. This is due to the fact that certain prerequisites are necessary for ophthalmic formulations which impose certain limitations to the formulator. These include sterility, absence of local toxicity, tolerance, ease of dispensing, antimicrobial preservation for multidose formulations, and iso-osmolarity for aqueous-based formulations. On the other hand, the development of drug treatments for diseases of the retina and posterior tissues of the eye have been slow. Among the principal causes for this, the technical difficulty in delivering drugs to the back of the eye seems to be the most important. Most of the drugs used in ophthalmology had initially been developed for other applications and subsequently found to be useful in ophthalmology. All these factors have limited the access to the market of innovative ophthalmic modified-release formulations. One potential reason for this is economics. Even worse, many potentially effective drugs languish on the laboratory shelves of pharmaceutical companies for lack of safe and efficacious formulations. This problem is critical in the eye due to the great differences and variety of tissues that need to be targeted according to the involved therapy and the significant barriers for penetration of foreign or exogenous compounds through ocular mucosa. After topical instillation of an eye drop, the drug is subject to a number of very efficient elimination mechanisms such as drainage, binding to proteins, normal tear turnover, induced tear production, and nonproductive absorption via the conjunctiva. Typically, the effective period of time for drug absorption is about 90s due to the rapid removal of drug from the precorneal area. Besides, the cornea is poorly permeable to both hydrophilic and hydrophobic compounds. As a result, only approximately 10 % or less of the topically applied dose can be absorbed into the anterior segment of the eye. Basically, the two major barriers found in ocular drug delivery are (a) short residence time in the precorneal area and (b) poor permeability of the cornea. For example, various efforts have been made to prolong the drug solution residence time via vehicle modification [1, 2], bioadhesives [3], inserts [4]. A successful design of a drug delivery system, therefore, requires an integrated knowledge of the drug molecule properties and effective formulation strategies in order to overcome the constraints offered by the ocular route of administration.

There is a clear need for ophthalmic products able to offer more therapeutic benefits than those derived from simple solutions/suspensions. Another important aspect of drug delivery is "targeting." To maximize efficacy and safety, drugs need to be directed as best as possible to a specific tissue or cell type once ocular penetration has been achieved. In certain circumstances, the drug delivery systems can be designed in order to achieve this goal. The development of the nanotechnology oriented to the design of drug delivery systems offers new possibilities for the improvement of the treatment of ocular diseases. Particularly, the potential use of nanoparticles became one the most attractive alternative for this objective.

The final goal of drug delivery system is to achieve and maintain therapeutic concentrations of the drug at the site of action along sufficient time to produce a beneficial effect. A secondary aim is to avoid exposing eye's tissues to high enough drug concentrations able to cause unacceptable side effects. In the design of a drug delivery system intended for ophthalmic administration an equilibrium must be kept among the limitations imposed by the physicochemical properties of the drugs, the limitations imposed by the anatomy and disease state of the eye, and the dosing requirements of the drug for that particular disease.

A significant challenge to the formulator is to circumvent the protective barriers of the eye without causing permanent tissue damage. Development of more sensitive diagnostic techniques as well as novel therapeutic agents leads to the design of ocular delivery systems with higher therapeutic efficacy. Although being useful formulations several decades ago, conventional ophthalmic dosages forms such as solution, suspension, and ointment no longer constitute an optimal therapy for these indications. Therefore, nowadays a lot of attention is paid to the development of the pharmaceutical system in addition to efficiency of the drug itself.

Although many drugs can be safely delivered by mean of eye drops, the efficiency of the treatment depends on patient compliance. Non-compliance is a major problem, especially in poorly educated patients and patients who are required to apply drops frequently. Lack of compliance frequently results in suboptimal therapeutics, which may lead to blindness depending on the pathology.

The dosing of patients suffering chronic conditions or motor problems is very complicated since an adequate schedule of administration of eye drops is very hard to complete.

However, the next decade promises great strides in therapy for many poorly treated or untreatable ocular diseases with any drug treatment. For new medications to be used effectively, and for those now available to provide maximal benefit, improvements in ocular drug delivery are essential.

This new type of ophthalmic formulations has to possess well defined properties in order to meet biopharmaceutical requirements such as be capable of delivering the effective ocular drug concentrations along an extended period of time (without inducing systemic side effects), user friendly, and exempt of side effects such as blurring, irritation, or foreign-body sensation.

Many attempts have been made to develop practical approaches to the modified delivery of drugs. The reason for the high demand for developing novel options for delivery of drugs to the eye is based on the need to progress from drug delivery concerns discovered in earlier research on topically administered drugs.

The unique anatomy and physiology of the eye offer many challenges to develope effective ophthalmic drug delivery systems, but the knowledge in this field is rapidly expanding. Systems range from simple solutions to novel delivery systems such as biodegradable polymeric systems, corneal collagen shields, iontophoresis, and viral and non viral gene delivery systems, to name a few. An increase in our understanding of ocular drug absorption and disposition mechanisms has led to the development of many of these new systems.

The aim of this Chapter is to describe the various polymeric systems used to achieve prolonged contact time of drugs with the cornea and increase their bioavailability. Advantages and shortcomings of the different systems are discussed, as well as their characteristics and their in vivo applications.

Anatomophysiological Aspects in Ocular Drug Therapy

The eye is the organ of vision; it receives and encodes external light stimuli that are then sent through the optic nerve to the occipital lobe of the brain where images are processed. To achieve this, the eye requires some independence and protection from the external environment, in order to maintain their structures unchanged. However, this feature makes it an organ difficult to reach for certain types of drugs.

The eyeball (Fig. 6.1) is composed of three compartments, front to back: (i) anterior chamber, (ii) posterior chamber and (iii) vitreous chamber. It also has three concentric layers from outside to inside they are: (i) outer fibrous tunic, (ii) vascular tunic and (iii) retina.

The fibrous layer is composed of a rear opaque part, the sclera, and anterior and transparent, the cornea. The cornea is the transparent frontal window of the

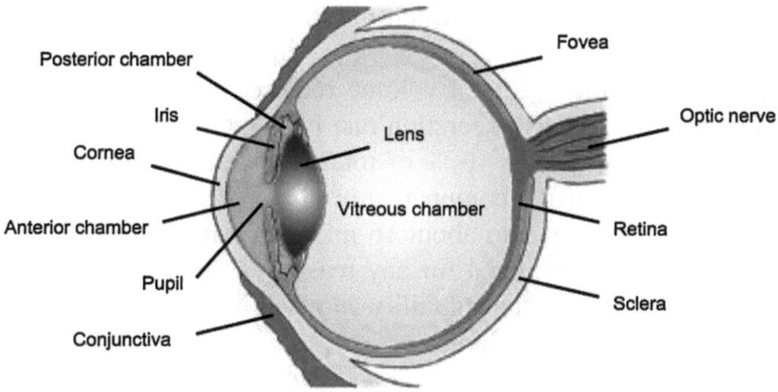

Fig. 6.1 Eyeball anatomy

eye, is formed by several layers: an outer hydrophobic epithelium of about 50 μm thick delimited by the Bowman's layer, followed by the hydrophilic stromal layer and finally, the thin Descemet's membrane and the endothelium. The intact corneal epithelium permeability is very low, due to its polylaminated non-keratinized structure with zonulaocludens joints (tight junctions) between the cells of the outer layer. This structure has a protective function and exclude any movement of solutes (resulting consequently in exclusion of hydrophilic drugs with low lipophilicity or large molecular sizes) except those that occur through the apical and basal plasma membranes of surface epithelial cells [5]. The vascular tunic is formed, from back to front, by the choroid, ciliar body and iris, which form a continuous structure. The ciliary body, has several important functions, including the active secretion of aqueous humor. Much of the volume secreted goes through the trabecular meshwork to Schlemm's canal, leaving the eye through the episcleral veins [6]. Here there is a blood-aqueous barrier formed by tight junctions between epithelial cells of the non-pigmented ciliary processes along with not fenestrated vessels of the iris, limiting the systemic all access of drugs. Finally, the retinal pigment epithelium also forms a blood-retinal barrier to accessing components that may come from systemic circulation.

Whereas the dosage form most widely used in topical ocular treatment are the eye drops (conjunctivitis, dry eye syndrome, glaucoma, iritis (anterior uveitis), keratitis); there are other parameters of ocular surface that affect pharmacotherapy, including: lower conjunctival sac capacity, blinking, tear secretion and tear drainage.

When the lower eyelid is carried forward gently with your fingers the lower conjunctival sac forms a funnel-shaped reservoir that can accommodate the instilled formulation, but the conjunctival surface cannot accommodate a larger volume than 25 μL if added quickly. When the eyelid returns to its normal position conjunctival sac capacity is reduced to less than 10 μL.

Blinking is one me the most important defense mechanisms of the eye. The blink reflex is usually fast enough to anticipate a strange body approaching at high speed to the eye. Flicker is also essential in the reformation of the tear film and activates the pump mechanism by which the tears drain. Blink rate in humans is 15–20 per minute.

Under normal baseline, the total volume required to cover the eye surface is approximately 6–8 μL, the tear secretion rate is about 1.2 μL/min and the rate of lacrimal turnover per minute is 16 % of total tear volume. However in stimulus conditions, by irritation of the conjunctiva or cornea reflects, tearing occurs. The volume of the tear film grows to about 16 ml, with a range between 5 and 6 μL [7]. Thus reflex tearing stimulated for any reason, including many parameters of eye drop formulation to enhance solubility and stability of the dosage form, cause an accelerated drop instilled washing.

The tear leaves the surface of the eye and eyelids before going to the lacrimal sac before draining to the nasolacrimal duct. In addition much of the tear film is removed by evaporation or absorption at lacrimal sac level. When blinking is prevented, tear accumulation occur, leading to spill to the skin of the eyelids and cheeks [8]. Some studies have shown that the drainage of the instilled solution is the main cause of the loss of drug in the precorneal area [9].

In response to this problem a growing interest in research related to pharmaceutical technology has been generated. A lot of work has been done on solving inherent problems of drug release, administered dose and site of action in order to design new drug delivery platforms. The design of this new group of pharmaceutical forms has focused primarily on the use of polymers as base material.

Systems for Ocular Controlled Drug Delivery Currently Investigated

Hydrogels

Hydrogels are water-swollen, cross-linked polymeric structures produced by the simple polymerization reaction of one or more monomers or by association of bonds such as hydrogen bonds and strong van der Waals interactions between chains. These systems exist in a state between rigid solids and liquid and this feature sets them apart from other forms of matter. Presently, a huge number of synthetic hydrogels is known. Hydrogels and viscous solutions, based upon the addition of hydrocolloids to simpler aqueous solutions, are the most common formulations. There is no clear cut frontier between very viscous solutions and gels in terms of biopharmaceutical results. According to Plazonnet et al. [10], aqueous gels are at the upper limit of viscous preparations, and they are formed when high molecular weight polymers or high polymer concentrations are incorporated in the formulations.

Currently, two groups of hydrogels are distinguished, namely preformed and in situ forming gels. The preformed gels can be defined mainly as hydrogels which do not undergo further modification after administration, whereas in situ gelling systems can be described as viscous liquids or suspensions that, upon exposure to physiological eye conditions (ionic strength, temperature or pH), will shift to a gel phase. Preformed gels are administered in the same way as an ointment, which is less convenient for the patient than the instillation of a viscous drop. The most common polymers used in viscous solutions are cellulose derivatives, carbomers, polysaccharides, and, recently, hyaluronic acid. The advantage offered by this last product depends upon the active ingredient and the formulation environment [11]. Polyvinyl alcohol and polyvinyl pyrolidone are also used in ophthalmic drugs. Gels permit longer residence time in the precorneal area than viscous solutions. This has encouraged researchers to work on formulations that would be (viscous) solutions in the drug vials but would gel in the conjunctival cul-de-sac. The polymers chosen to prepare ophthalmic hydrogels should meet some specific rheological characteristics. It is generally well accepted that the instillation of a formulation should influence tear behavior as little as possible. Because tears have a pseudoplastic behavior, pseudoplastic vehicles would be more suitable than Newtonian formulations, which have a constant viscosity independent of the shear rate. Pseudoplastic solutions exhibit decreased viscosity with increasing shear rate, thereby offering lowered viscosity during blinking and stability of the tear film during fixation.

A large amount of today's research is focused on the so-called 'smart' or 'intelligent' hydrogels. A representative of this interesting class of hydrogels is a polymer system with a defined phase transition capable of abruptly swelling to many times its original size or collapsing into a compact mass when stimulated externally [12]. Smart hydrogels react in response to an external stimulus in a manner similar to many living organisms rather than to non-living organic matter [13].

The improvement in residence time of ophthalmic semisolid hydrogels is primarily based on an increase in ocular residence time as a result of a reduction in drainage rate through enhanced viscosity and mucoadhesive properties.

Preformed Hydrogels

Preformed hydrogels for topical administration in the eye can be based on natural, synthetic, or semisynthetic polymers.

Cellulose Derivatives. The pioneering group of polymers used as components of ophthalmic preformed hydrogels is the family of cellulosic derivatives. Because pure cellulose is not water soluble due to its relatively high crystallinity, cellulosic derivatives have been used for a long time as viscosifiers in collyria. Methylcellulose (MC) (Fig. 6.2) was first introduced in ophthalmic formulations in the 1940s as a mean of decreasing their fluidity [14]. Since then, cellulosic polymers have been extensively studied in human, [15–17] as well as in veterinary medicine [16, 18–20], for ocular administration. The cellulosic derivatives most commonly used in ophthalmology are: (1) Methylcellulose, (2) Hydroxyethylcellulose (HEC), (3) Hydroxypropycellulose (HPC), (4) Hydroxypropylmethylcellulose (HPMC) and (5) Sodium carboxymethylcellulose (CMC Na).

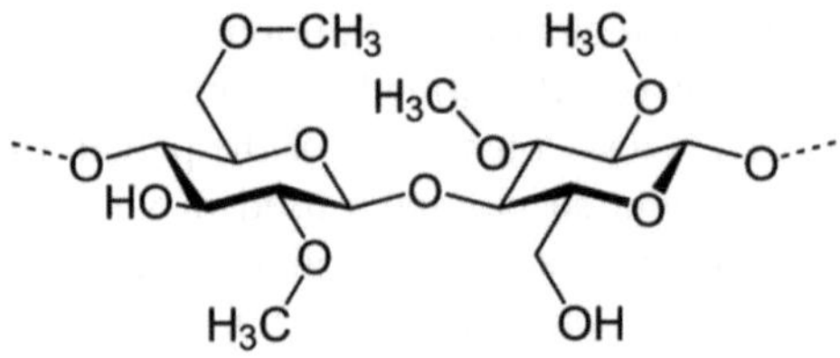

Fig. 6.2 Methylcellulose monomer

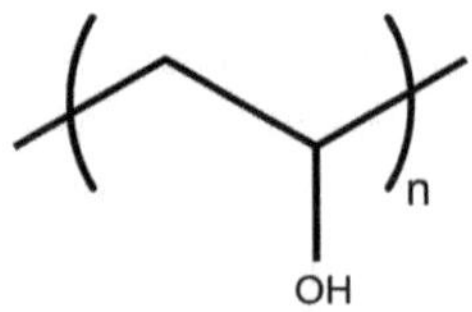

Fig. 6.3 Poly(vinyl alcohol) monomer

The boundary between viscous solutions and gels for cellulosic derivatives is particularly difficult to define, because data regarding the hydrocolloid concentration or the viscosity of the final formulation are not always available. These cellulosic polymers appear in several currently available commercial preparations such as Adsorbotear® (Alcon, Fort Worth, Texas), Lacril® (AUergan, Irvine, California) and Celluvisc® (AUergan, Irvine, California).

Subsequent advances in the polymers field with respect to ocular drug delivery have led to the use of poly(vinyl alcohol) (PVA); sodium hyaluronate, and carbomer, which often give better results [21–24] than celluloses. On the other hand cellulose-based hydrogels are still in focus for ophthalmical applications as ocular bandage [25].

Poly(vinyl alcohol). Scientific interest has been directed toward using other viscosifying agents. Poly(vinyl alcohol) (PVA) is a synthetic polymer commercially obtained by polymerization of vinylacetate to poly(vinyl acetate) (Fig. 6.3) and subsequent hydrolysis to PVA [26]. Polyvinyl alcohol was introduced in the early 1960's as a mean to increase solution viscosity and, hence, prolong precorneal residence time. The presence of PVA in ophthalmic preparations has been shown to significantly delay precorneal drainage of topically applied formulations and to increase drug bioavailability as well as pharmacological effects such as miotic response to pilocarpine exposure when compared with conventional saline [27]. Some commercial products, particularly for the treatment of dry eye, are based on PVA, including HypoTearse® (IOLAB Corp., Claremont, California) and Liquifilm® (Allergan, Irvine, California).

Sodium Hyaluronate. The actual trend in ocular delivery is to use sodium salt of hyaluronic acid (SH). The SH is a high molecular weight biological polymer composed of repeating disaccharide units of glucuronic acid and n-acetylglucosamine (Fig. 6.4), a specific ultrapure fraction being patented as Healon (Kabi Pharmacia, Sweden) by Balazs [28] in 1979. The HS is a natural polysaccharide found in skin, connective tissues, umbilical cord, vitreous body and aqueous humor. The main advantages of SH are its excellent biocompatibility, mucoadhesiveness as well as its pseudoplastic and viscoelastic behavior. Its use

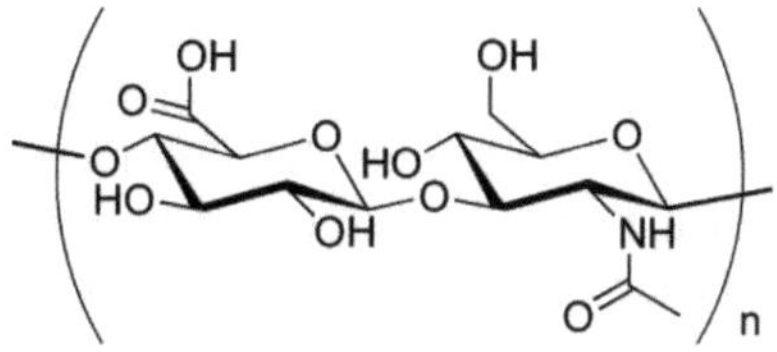

Fig. 6.4 Hyaluronic acid monomer

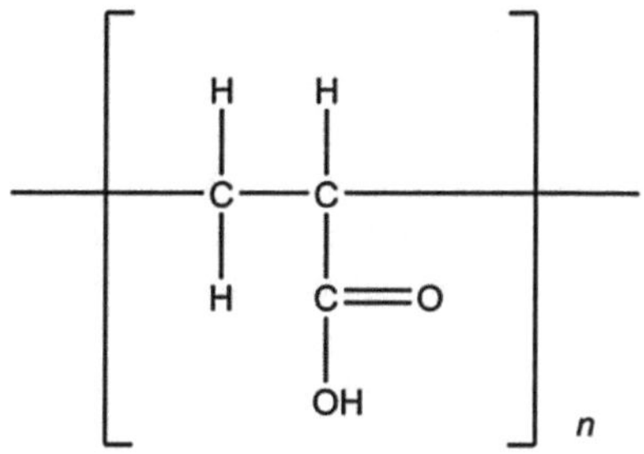

Fig. 6.5 Poly(acrylic acid) monomer

as a vehicle in ocular drug delivery has been extensively reviewed by Bernatchez et al. [29]. This polysaccharide is frequently proposed as a vehicle of choice in tear substitutes since it has been reported to possess a desirable protective effect against damage caused by benzalkonium chloride, a compound commonly added as a preservative in multiple dosage forms [30]. An extended residence time is one of the factors used to select artificial tears for the therapy of KCS (Keratoconjunctivitissicca), being effective in reducing common symptoms such as blurring vision, pain and photophobia. A further advantage of SH in this application is its pseudoplastic behavior. The ability of SH to prolong drug release by increasing precorneal drug residence time has been studied (mostly in animals) for several ophthalmic compounds such as pilocarpine [31–33] or, more recently, gentamicin [34]. Some commercial products containing SH are currently available being mostly indicated (for example Healon® and Viscoat®) for use as surgical aids in anterior segment procedures such as cataract extraction or intraocular lens implantation rather than for topical administration.

New efforts were directed to use this material in novel ophthalmic drug delivery platforms; recent reports in scientific literature propose the SH as solid bioadhesivedrug delivery system. Crosslinked SH films loaded with timolol maleate were successfully used to reduce intra ocular pressure in normotensive rabbits, prolonging the hypotensive effect for longer than commercial timolol maleate eye drops [35].

Carbomer. Cross-linked poly (acrylic acid) (Fig. 6.5) of high molecular weight, commercially available as Carbopol® (B.F. Goodrich Chemical Company, Cleveland, Ohio), is widely used in ophthalmology to enhance precorneal retention to the eye. The superiority of Carbopol over simple saline and suspensions in enhancing precorneal residence time [36] and drug bioavailability [37, 38] has been demonstrated by several authors. Preparation of Carbopol hydrogels is simply based on the dispersion of the polymer in water at room temperature, followed by a neutralization process with agents such as sodium hydroxide, triethanolamine, or directly with active basic compounds. The maximal viscosity is obtained at neutral pH. Carbopol offers the advantage of exhibiting excellent mucoadhesive properties when compared with others polymers (e.g., cellulose derivatives, PVA and SH). The efficacy of Carbopol in enhancing precorneal residence time has been extensively studied by incorporating tracers such as sodium fluorescein [39] or active compounds such as pilocarpine or prednisolone [24, 38, 40]. A large number of commercial ophthalmic preparations contain Carbopol, including tear substitutes such as Lacrigel® (Europhta, Monaco), Lacrinorm® (Chauvin, Montpellier, France) or formulations containing active compounds such as Iduviran® (Chauvin, Montpellier, France) and Pilopine® (Alcon, Fort Worth, Texas).

Other polymers. Other natural or synthetic polymers have also been evaluated as potential vehicles to prolong the residence time of drugs at the surface of the eye but are currently being further investigated, such as xanthan gum or chitosan are currently under investigation for topical administration. An important difference between the two polymers is the anionic character of xanthan gum, whereas chitosan exhibits positive charges. Xanthan gum has been proposed as a material for artificial tears preparations [41] as well as vehicle for drug delivery [42, 43]. Evaluating transcorneal delivery of pilocarpine from several ophthalmic formulations, Saettone et al. [44] demonstrated that the presence of 1.5 % of xanthan gum induced a significant improvement of the pharmacokinetic parameters of the drug such as area under the curve (AUC), half-life time of elimination and the mean residence time in aqueous humor. Chitosan is emerging as a polymer of interest for ophthalmic use [45–47]. Formulations based on the concept of mucoadhesion (Fig. 6.6) have been investigated to overcome the rapid elimination of instilled ophthalmic solutions. They appear less viscous than those based on traditional viscolizers. The possible advantage of chitosan over xanthan gum lies in the presence of positive charges at physiological pH on the sugar backbone of chitosan, which are supposed to interact with the negative charges of the mucus, thereby conferring a bioadhesive property to this polysaccharide. Therefore, chitosan has attracted attention for topical ophthalmic applications, for example, promising results have been obtained demonstrating

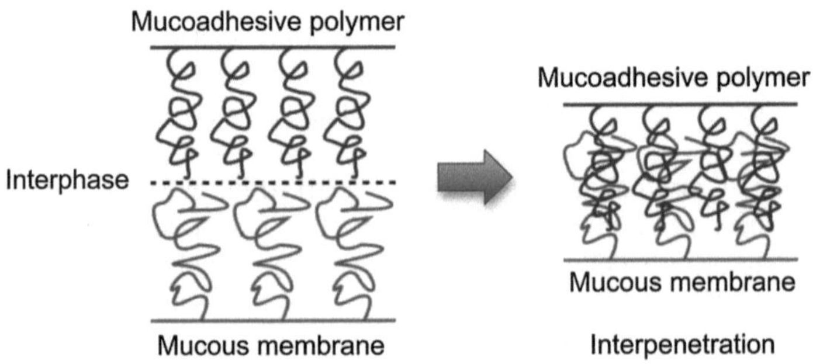

Fig. 6.6 Polymer-mucous membrane chains interpenetration in mucoadhesion phenomena

that chitosan formulations remained significantly longer on the corneal surface when compared with a conventional commercial solution [48].

In Situ Forming Gels

The use of preformed hydrogels still has drawbacks that can limit their interest for ophthalmic drug delivery or as tear substitutes. They do not allow accurate and reproducible administration of quantities of drugs and, after administration, they often produce blurred vision, crusting of eyelids, and lachrymation. A new approach is to try to combine advantages of both, solutions and gels, such as accuracy and facility of administration of the former and prolonged residence time of the latter. Thus, in situ hydrogels can be instilled as eye drops and undergo an immediate gelation when in contact with the eye.

"Smart" hydrogels or stimuli-sensitive hydrogels or in situ forming (Fig. 6.7), are very different from inert hydrogels in that they can "sense" changes in environmental properties such as pH and temperature and respond by increasing or decreasing their degree of swelling. These sensing capabilities are attractive in many biomedical applications. The volume-changing behavior of "smart" hydrogels is particularly useful in drug-delivery applications as drug release can be desirably triggered upon environmental changes [49–51]. Temperature responsiveness is particularly useful for in situ formation of drug-delivery devices since it allows handling of the formulation in the sol-phase at room temperature and solidification of the carrier upon injection [52]. Stimuli-responsive hydrogels, especially those sensitive to temperature and pH, are attractive because these factors are variables that change in typical physiological, biological and chemical systems. Product(s) using the gellan gum technology [53], and with polymer associations like those published by the University of Nebraska researchers [54, 55], and Smart Gel® technology [56] are examples of technologies that use this approach. This field of intricately entangled polymers seems promising since new "patentable" entities might be obtained through in-depth studies of associations of well-established products.

In situ forming gels influenced by ionic strength. Ionic-strength-responsive polymers undergo their phase transitions, resulting from the different concentration of salts (e.g., ionic strength). Gellan gum is an anionic polysaccharide

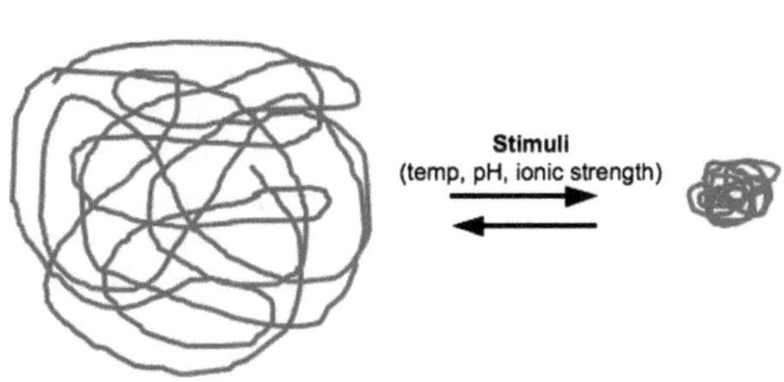

Fig. 6.7 Stimuli-sensitive hydrogels

produced by the bacterium Pseudomonas elodea [57] which, when dispersed in aqueous solutions, undergoes a liquid-gel transition under the influence of an increase in ionic strength [58]. The acetylated form is commercially available as Gelrite® (Kelco Division of Merck and Co, USA). The sol-gel transition process is induced by the presence of monovalent or divalent ions such as Na^{+} and Ca^{2+}. Some other parameters influence the phase transition, e.g., the concentration of polysaccharide, the temperature of the preparation, and the nature and the concentration of cations. Exceptional rheological properties of gellan gum such as thixotropy, pseudoplasticity, and thermoplasticity [59] are further advantages for its use in ophthalmology: the fluidity of the solution can be increased simply by shaking or slightly warming the preparation. The gellation increases proportionally to the amount of either monovalent or divalent cations present in the lacrimal fluid and in vitro experiments have demonstrated that divalent cations are more efficient in promoting sol-gel transition than monovalent ions. However, the in vivo conditions (i.e. the concentration of sodium in tears) is sufficient to induce the gellation process. Recently two other natural polymers believed to be able to form in situ gels by interacting with the lachrymal fluid have been evaluated as potential adjuvants in ophthalmic formulations [60, 61]. Carrageenans, a group of water soluble sulphated galactans extracted from red seaweed, showed similar features to gellan gum regarding their rheological behavior, gelling properties [62], and tolerance. This suggested that they could be interesting polymers for prolonging the residence time of topical ocular formulations [60]. Furthermore, the authors suggested that since these compounds are strong polyelectrolytes, they will have an identical gelling mechanism to gellan gum. Some alginates, rich in guluronic acid residues, have been demonstrated to exhibit reversible liquid-gel transition after administration and to be efficient in reducing intraocular pressure when carrying pilocarpine [61]. Also, alginate-pectine combinations and thiolated pectines were studied. Thiolation of pectin was observed to result in an increase in the gelling behavior, viscosity, and bioadhesive strength; combination of pectin and sodium alginate demonstrated good in vitro release characteristics [63].

In situ forming gels influenced by temperature. The volume-changing behavior of "smart" hydrogels is particularly useful in drug-delivery applications as drug release can be desirably triggered upon environmental changes [49–51]. Temperature responsiveness is particularly useful for in situ formation of drug-delivery devices since it allows handling of the formulation in the sol-phase at room temperature and solidification of the carrier upon injection [52]. These hydrogels are liquid at room temperature (20–25 °C) and undergo gelation when in contact with body fluids (35–37 °C), due to an increase in temperature. Different thermal setting gels have been described in the literature, including for example acrylic acid copolymers [43, 64] and N-isopropylacrylamide derivatives [65]. However, specific requirements inherent to ophthalmic administration such as tolerance have limited the choice of such polymers. Poloxamers, commercially available as Pluronic® (BASF-Wyandotte, USA), are the most commonly used thermal setting polymers in ophthalmology owing to their low toxicity, mucomimetic properties and optical clarity. They are formed by a central hydrophobic part (polyoxypropylene) surrounded by hydrophilic part (ethylene oxide). Their concentration is chosen in accordance with the desired liquid-gel transition [66]. At concentrations above 20 % w/w, poloxamers exhibit the phenomenon of reverse thermal gellation, that is, gelling upon warming up from ambient to body temperature [67]. Interestingly, the temperature of transition of poloxamers can be modulated by adding solutes or polymers such as poly(ethylene glycols) [68] or cellulosic derivatives such as MC or HPMC to the formulation. The mucomimetic property of poloxamers is supposed to be due to their hydrophobic and hydrophilic sequences simulating mucin action by adsorption of the aqueous layer of tears on the hydrophobic epithelium. However, the disadvantage of poloxamers as compared to Gelrite® lies in their mechanism of gellation. In fact, since sol-gel transition takes place as the temperature increases, accidental gellation during conservation may occur. A new attractive thermal sensitive hydrogel, Smart Hydrogel® composed of a polymeric network of poly (acrylic acid) and poloxamer, has been described by Gilchrist et al. [69]. Owing to their protective and mucomimetic action, poloxamers have also been evaluated for the treatment of dry eye [70]. Poloxamers have also been widely investigated as ocular drug delivery systems. Miller and Donovan [71] reported enhanced activity of pilocarpine in poloxamers 407 gels when compared with a simple solution, whereas Dumortier et al. [72] have shown that a thermoreversible gel does not improve the kinetic profile of morphine over a reference solution. Despite all the promising results obtained with thermoreversible gels, it remains an important drawback associated with the use of these hydrogels; the risk of gelling before administration by an increase in the ambient temperature during packaging or storage.

In situ forming gels influenced by pH. All the pH-sensitive polymers contain pendant acidic or basic groups either accept or release protons in response to changes in environmental pH. The polymers with a large number of ionisable groups are known as polyelectrolytes. Swelling of the hydrogel increases as the external pH increases in the case of weakly acidic (anionic) groups, but decreases if the polymer contains weakly basic (cationic) groups [73].

pH-sensitive hydrogels are composed of polymer chain networks crosslinked to each other and surrounded by a salt solution. A change in the pH of the solution surrounding the gel will initiate a physical process of either gel swelling or deswelling. The physical process, in general, is not instantaneous, and modelling the gel swelling/deswelling rate helps us to have a thorough understanding of the gel dynamics. This is particularly important when hydrogels are used in controlled drug-delivery devices, where the drug is released during the swelling process.

Pseudo-latexes have been defined by El-Aasser [74] as artificial latices obtained by the dispersion of a pre-existing polymer in an aqueous medium. Such systems correspond to low viscosity aqueous dispersions, which can undergo spontaneous coagulation in the conjunctival cul-de-sac owing to an increase of the local pH. The massive swelling of the particles is due to the neutralization of the acid groups contained in the polymer chain. The increase in viscosity is by several orders of magnitude [75]. In situ gelling pseudo-latexes can be prepared by two manufacturing processes; the solvent evaporation process [76] and the salting out process [77].

The uses of new technologies were recently combined to developnovel pH triggered polymeric nanoparticulate in situ gel for ophthalmic delivery of acetazolamide to enhance conjunctival permeation and precorneal residence time of the formulation. Nanoparticles were developed by nanoprecipitation method and exhibited significantly higher ex vivo transcorneal ACZ permeation than eye drops and ACZ suspension [78]. Similar findings were also described for a fluconazole pH triggered nanoemulsified in situ ophthalmic gel [79].

Inserts

This section is devoted to solid devices delivering drugs to the anterior segment of the eye that are denoted by the general name insert, originating from the Latin *inserere*, to introduce. Ophthalmic inserts are defined as preparations with a solid or semisolid consistency, whose size and shape are especially designed for ophthalmic application (i.e. rods or shields) [80]. These inserts are placed in the lower fornix and, less frequently, in the upper fornix, or on the cornea. They are usually composed of a polymeric vehicle containing the drug and are mainly used for topical therapy.

Ophthalmic inserts have been, and continue to be, in fashion in research and development laboratories, which is testified by abundant literature [81, 82]. The insert is probably the oldest ophthalmic formulation. Historically, the first solid medication precursors of the present insoluble inserts, were described in the 19th century. They consisted of squares of dry filter paper, previously impregnated with drug solutions (e.g., atropine sulfate, pilocarpine hydrochloride) [83], small sections were cut and applied under the eyelid. However, although the British Pharmacopoeia 1948 described an atropine in gelatin "wafer", and notwithstanding all the formulation possibilities as well as the modulation of biopharmaceutical properties that inserts permit, the insert market never took off. This was apparently caused by incompatibility between the product-insert and the user-patient, particularly in the elderly; difficulty of insertion by the patient and foreign-body sensation. Besides the initial discomfort upon administration, other potential disadvantages arising from their solid state are, possible movement around the eye, occasional inadvertent loss during sleep or while rubbing the eyes, interference with vision and difficult placement (and removal for insoluble devices) [84]. Most of the ongoing research is therefore dedicated to improving ocular retention and to ensure an easy placement, while reducing the foreign body sensation in the eye. Two products, AlzaOcusert® [85] and Merck Lacrisert® [86], have been marketed, although Ocusert is no longer sold. Ocusert was an insoluble delicate sandwich technology filled with sufficient pilocarpine for 1 week's use, whereas Lacrisert is a soluble minirod of hydroxypropyl cellulose, nonmedicated and dissolving within 24 h to treat dry-eye syndromes [86]. Other inserts are more like implants to be placed in the eye tissues by surgery and are not within the present scope of this Chapter.

Ophthalmic inserts are generally classified according to their solubility behavior and their possible biodegradability.

Soluble Inserts

Soluble inserts are the most frequently investigated class of ophthalmic inserts. Their main advantage relies on their complete solubility compared with their insoluble counterparts, so that they do not need to be removed from the eye after deposition. The major problems of these soluble inserts are the rapid penetration of the lacrimal fluid into the device, the blurred vision caused by the solubilization of insert components and the glassy constitution of the insert increasing the risk of expulsion. They are usually divided into two categories according to their polymer composition. The first type is based on natural polymers whereas the second is derived from synthetic or semisynthetic polymers.

Natural polymers. Natural polymers include collagen, which was the first ophthalmic insert excipient described in the literature. Inserts containing collagen were first developed by Fyodorov [87, 88] as corneal bandages following surgical operations and eye disease. Later, collagen shields as drug carriers were suggested by Bloomfield et al. [89]. As described for contact lenses, the therapeutic agents are generally absorbed by soaking the collagen shield in a solution containing the drug and, once placed in the eye, the drug is gradually released from the interstices between the collagen molecules, as the collagen dissolves. Accordingly, the residence time of drugs [90] such as antibacterials, [91, 92] anti-inflammatory agents [93, 94] antivirals [95] or combination drugs [96] was increased when compared to traditional eye drops. However, as observed for contact lenses, most drugs are released quite rapidly by a diffusion process, whereas dissolution requires a much longer time.

Solid Precorneal Inserts (Collagen Shields). Collagen shields were first introduced by Fyodorov in 1984 for use as a bandage contact lens following radial keratotomy and photorefractive surgery [97]. Collagen shields are manufactured from porcine scleral tissue and commercially available (Bio-Cor, Bausch & Lomb) with three dissolution times of 12, 24, and 72 h, depending on the level of collagen cross-linking induced during the manufacture process. Bloomfield et al. [89] were the first to suggest that collagen might provide a suitable carrier for sustained ocular drug delivery. They showed that wafer shaped collagen inserts impregnated with gentamicin produced higher levels of drug in the tear film and tissue in the rabbit eye compared to drops, ointment, or subconjunctival injection. They appeared useful as a delivery system for anti-infective agents and might possibly be of interest for some other drugs. Hydrophilic drugs are entrapped within the collagen matrix when the dry shield is soaked in aqueous solution of the drug whereas water-insoluble drugs are incorporated into the shield during the manufacturing process. When compared with intensive topical treatment, collagen shields have been found superior with regard to the delivery of different antibiotics and antifungal agents in the rabbit model [91, 98, 99]. In experimental bacterial keratitis in animal models, the enhanced drug delivery ability of collagen shield was translated to enhanced bacterial eradication [92, 100–102]. Improved results were reported also for the delivery of anti-inflammatory agents by collagen shields [93, 94, 103].

The main advantages of collagen shields over contact lenses is their solubility. For this reason they do not need to be removed. However, collagen may cause an inflammatory response in the ocular tissues. Also, if shields are not used in association with antibacterials, a secondary infection may occur [95]. Nowadays, these devices have the further disadvantage of not being well accepted by the authorities, because of possible prion-based infection. Furthermore, the complexity of the manufacturing process and the resulting blurred vision are serious drawbacks that have curbed the enthusiasm raised during the development of corneal shields. Corneal shield self-administration is also difficult for the average user and their positioning should be monitored since they can be easily dislocated.

Another interesting approach is Gelfoam©, which is made of absorbable gelatin sponge USP. It can be inserted in the conjunctival pouch in the form of small disks (e.g., 4 mm in diameter and 0.5 mm thick) impregnated with drug solutions. They have been shown to improve the management of pupillary dilation in humans as well as the delivery of pilocarpine [104–106].

Synthetic and semisynthetic polymers. Ophthalmic inserts containing synthetic, i.e. PVA [107, 108] and semisynthetic, i.e. cellulose based [108–110] polymers, are extensively described in the literature. This stems in part from their advantage of being based in products well adapted for ophthalmic use and their ease of manufacture by conventional methods, including extrusion [110], compression [111] and compression molding [112]. Ethylcellulose, a hydrophobic polymer, can be incorporated in the formulation to decrease insert deformation, and therefore prevent blurred vision [113]. Regarding the risk of expulsion, several authors have incorporated carbomer, which, at low concentrations, is strong, but well-tolerated bioadhesive polymer.

Lacrisert® is a soluble insert that was successfully commercialized by Merck Sharp and Dohme in 1981 [87]. The device weighs 5 mg, measures 1.27 mm in diameter with a length of 3.5 mm, and is composed of HPC and is useful in the treatment of dry eye syndrome.

Insoluble Inserts

Insoluble inserts can be classified into two categories: reservoir and matrix systems.

Reservoir inserts. Reservoir inserts consist of a central reservoir of drug enclosed in a specially designed semipermeable or microporous membranes which allow the drug to diffuse from the reservoir at a precisely determined rate in a zero order release fashion. Reservoir controlled release systems may be manufactured in a wide range of geometries including conventional tablets/pellets, laminated films and other defined shapes, (e.g., hemispheres, cylinders, rods). Similarly there are a number of methods by which these systems may be produced. For example pellets, spheres and tablets may be coated with an insoluble polymeric coating using conventional spray/film coating techniques, e.g., pan coating, air suspension coating. Alternatively, planar (laminated) drug delivery systems, e.g., transdermal patches, are manufactured using extrusion or film casting techniques. All reservoir systems share a common design, namely the drug core is housed within a polymeric barrier. The choice of the composition of the polymeric membrane is performed according to the physicochemical properties of the drug, particularly the ability of the therapeutic agent to diffuse through the polymer coating at the appropriate rate, the chosen manufacture method and the proposed route of administration to the patient. Reservoir inserts based on an osmotic release mechanism of the drug are mostly described in the patent literature, however in vivo tests on such technologies are rarely reported [80]. These types of ocular delivery systems are generally made up of a unique central reservoir surrounded by a peripheral component [114]. The peripheral part of these osmotic inserts comprises in all cases of a covering film made of an insoluble semipermeable polymer.

Ocusert® (developed by Alza Corporation, Palo Alto, California) is undoubtedly the most extensively described insoluble insert in the literature [115, 116]. The delivery of therapeutic agents to the eye for the treatment of disorders of the eye, (e.g., glaucoma), using conventional drug delivery systems, e.g., drops, ointments, is an inefficient process. This is primarily due to the rapid clearance of drugs from the surface of the eye due to blinking and tear flow. One method by which the efficiency of ocular drug delivery may be improved is through the use of polymeric implants that are implanted under the lower cul-de-sac of the eye [117]. The Ocusert represents one such example that has been designed to release either 20 $\mu g\ h^{-1}$ or 40 $\mu g\ h^{-1}$ of a therapeutic agent (pilocarpine) for a seven day period following implantation. In design terms the Ocusert is flat, flexible elliptical device which consists of a pilocarpine reservoir comprising alginic acid, which is surrounded on both sides by a membrane of ethylene-vinyl acetate copolymer. These layers act as the rate controlling membranes. The device is encircled by a retaining ring impregnated with titanium dioxide. Drug release from this delivery system occurs by diffusion. Initially lachrymal (tear) fluid diffuses through the rate controlling membranes and enters into the inner (alginate) matrix at which stage dissolution of pilocarpine occurs. Now in the molecular state, pilocarpine diffuses from the region of high concentration (the drug-containing matrix) to the lachrymal fluid through the rate controlling membrane. Recent clinical studies were done to compare the efficacy and safety of a new ocular insert versus conventional mydriasis in cataract surgery. Mydriasert® (Laboratories Théa, Clermont-Ferrand) is a tropicamide and phenylephrine insert, formulated with ammonio methacrylate copolymer, polyacrylate dispersion and ethylcellulose as excipients. The researchers concluded that the effect of the Mydriasert insert was similar to conventional mydriatic agents. Pupil size was restored to normal faster when using the Mydriasert insert compared with conventional mydriatic agents for pupil dilation. Another advantage of the insert is that this method requires only two simple maneuvers, one to insert and one to withdraw the device, thus reducing patients' discomfort and saving time for the nursing staff, compared to having to administer drops to patients every 15 min [118].

Matrix inserts. The matrix insoluble inserts are typically represented by the contact lenses. The initial use of contact lenses was for vision correction. Its use has been extended to drug delivery devices by presoaking them in drug solutions. The main advantage of this system is the possibility of correcting vision and releasing drug simultaneously. Contact lenses are composed of a hydrophilic polymer which swells by absorbing water. The swelling, caused by the osmotic pressure of the polymer segments, is opposed by the elastic restoring forces arising along the chains as they are stretched until a final swelling (equilibrium) is reached. Refojo [119] has proposed classifying contact lenses according to five groups, namely rigid, semi-rigid, elastomeric, soft hydrophilic and biopolymeric. Soft hydrophilic contact lenses were developed for prolonged release of drugs such as pilocarpine [120], chloramphenicol and tetracycline [121], and prednisolone sodium phosphate [122]. This type contact lenses are better tolerated on ocular surface than collagen shields. The most commonly used polymer in the composition of these types of lenses is hydroxy ethyl metacrylate (HEMA) copolymerized with polyvinyl pyrrolidone (PVP) or ethylene glycol dimethacrylic acid (EGDM). PVP is used to increase water retention, while EGDM is used to decrease the water of hydration.

The main drawback of a contact lens as a therapeutic lens is their high cost of manufacture, and the low drug-loading capacity, which is not sufficient to build up a therapeutic concentration in the eye for most drugs [123]. Besides, these devices are insoluble, hence they need to be removed from the eye after treatment. For hydrophilic contact lenses, evidence has shown that the drug-loading capacity can deliver a drug amount, which is equivalent to only a small fraction of the dose that can be delivered by topical drug instillation [124]. Indeed, this Drug Delivery System (DDS) is barely represented in the modern array of ocular DDS [125]. Disposable contact lenses have been commercially available for many years, and the continued progress made in polymer chemistry should facilitate the development of this type of ocular insert.

Actually new concepts in drug loaded contact lenses is investigated. Diverse polymers properties discussed in this chapter were combined in temperature sensitive contact lenses. Authors focuses on dispersing timolol encapsulating highly crosslinked nanoparticles in contact lenses to increase the duration of drug release to about 2–4 weeks. The highly crosslinked particles were prepared from monomers with multivinyl functionalities such as ethylene glycol dimethacrylate and propoxylatedglyceryltriacylate. In vitro release studies exhibited drug release profiles compatible with a first order reaction model with a temperature dependent rate constant [126].

Biodegradable Inserts

In recent years, systems that control and prolong the action of therapeutic agents have grown in importance with the development of biodegradable polymers. There are stringent requirements, the drug delivery for the ocular route should be sterile, isotonic, and nonirritant. There are no available marketable sterile ophthalmic products based on these systems. Biodegradable polymers are the polymers of choice for retinal drug delivery. The drug release from biodegradable polymeric devices depends on several factors: the molecular weight of the polymers, the monomer composition, and drug loading [127]. These polymers provide the advantage of being degraded and eliminated from the body thus avoiding the risk of toxic accumulation or the need for intervention to eliminate them. Lactic acid and glycolic acids are biodegradable, and they are produced and eliminated by the body. These polymers decompose into carbon dioxide and water. Polylactic acid (PLA) and polyglycolic acid (PGA) and their copolymer polylactic-co-glycolic acid (PLGA) are among the most widely used biodegradable polymers. They are approved for human use by worldwide health authorities and are degraded to nontoxic compounds (lactic acid and glycolic acid, respectively) following hydrolysis and enzymatic cleavage. These polymers undergo bulk erosion and drug diffusion may change according to the erosion rate of the polymer matrix. The great advantage of these inserts is the possibility of modulating their erosion rate by modifying their final structure during synthesis, and by addition of anionic or cationic surfactants. Thus, drug burst phenomena are likely to occur depending on the MW and chemical structure of the polymers. PGA for example is not an appropriate candidate for prolonged controlled DDS as it is highly sensitive to hydrolysis. However, erodible systems can have significantly variable erosion rates based on individual patient physiology and lachrymation patterns. In some cases, the degradation products or residual solvents used during the polymer preparation can cause inflammatory reaction. In conclusion, the majority of therapeutic agents can be delivered using inserts which are a promising alternative administration route, because of their various advantages compared with classical dosage forms. In contrast, other biodegradable polymers like polyorthoester and polyanhydride undergo surface erosion, and subsequently the drug release from such systems depends on the extent of the surface area. However, only few of these compounds have been commercialized. This can be attributed to the reluctance of ophthalmologists and patients to replace the traditional ophthalmic solutions as well as the cost and the need to train both the prescribers and the patients to place the inserts correctly in the eyes. In the future, the use of ophthalmic inserts will certainly increase because of the development of new polymers, the emergence of new drugs having short biological half-lives or systemic side effects, and the need to improve the efficacy of ophthalmic treatments by ensuring an effective drug concentration in the eye for several days.

In another interesting approaches, a composite collagen hydrogel containing protein-encapsulated alginate microspheres was developed for ocular applications using bovine serum albumin. Sustained release of bovine serum albumin was achieved during an 11 day period in neutral phosphate buffer [128]. Also, micro- and nanostructured poly(caprolactone) films were studied in terms of ocular tolerance and structural integrity while residing in rabbit's eye, exhibiting acceptable results [129].

Dispersed Systems

Dispersed systems based on liposomes, nanoparticles, or nanocapsules have been extensively studied for potential ophthalmic use [130–132]. The development of marketable products based on these nanoproducts has been challenging but a definitive technology has not yet been established. The major issues for this type of delivery system include: percentage of dispersed phase/entrapment coefficient problem (i.e. how much of the active ingredient will be present in a drop of the final product), stability and shelf life, antimicrobial preservation, tolerance of the used surfactants, and, last but not least, large-scale manufacture of sterile preparations. Beyond the problem of the entrapment percentage of the active pharmaceutical ingredient, the retention of these particles in the conjunctival pouch is a key consideration. This retention must be effective in providing an extended source of active drug and to allow the drug to leak out from the dispersed phase before the instilled formulation is drained away from the precorneal area.

Liposomes

While these systems exceed the chapter topic, a brief description of them will be done because of their relevance in scientific literature related to ocular treatment.

Liposomes (Fig. 6.8) are microscopic vesicles composed of alternating aqueous compartments and lipid bilayers (mainly phospholipids and cholesterol). The efficacy of liposomes in ophthalmic therapy depends on several parameters, including (1) the drug encapsulation efficiency, (2) the size and the charge of the vesicles, (3) the distribution of the drug in the liposomes, (4) the stability of the liposomes after instillation, (5) the residence time of the liposomes in the conjunctival sac, and finally, (6) the affinity of the liposomes with the cornea [131]. Of these, a major factor affecting ocular drug bioavailability is the unstability of liposomes to the proteins in the conjunctival sac. Liposomes and other types of colloidal drug

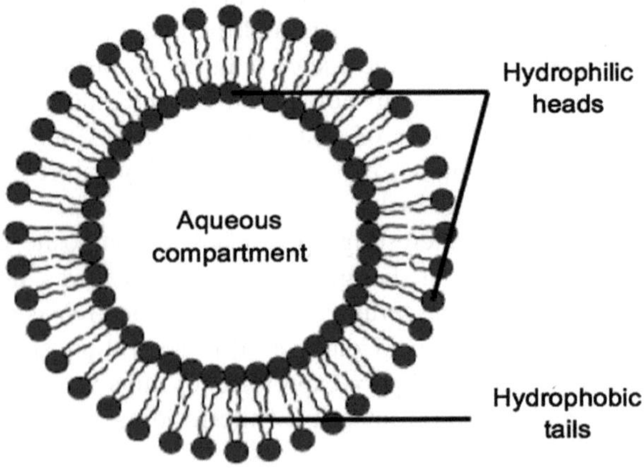

Fig. 6.8 Liposome

carriers offer at least some potential in relation to ocular drug delivery, since they can be used to generate a sustained release, and also a prolonged retention of the drug in intraocular cell populations. The use of liposomes as ocular delivery systems was first reported by Smolin et al. [133] and Schaeffer and Krohn [134]. A central strategy of the use of liposomes in ocular drug delivery based on liposomes has been to improve the adhesion between the liposomes and the cornea. This can be achieved in different ways, including: (1) Ganglioside-containing liposomes together with wheat ger agglutinin, a lectin binding to both the cornea and gangliosides, (2) Liposomes coated with antibodies to components in the corneal surface, and (3) Liposomes coated with mucoadhesive polymers.

One of the major constraints of the ocular route of delivery is the very low residence time of a drug in the ocular cavity, leading to a subsequent reduction in the bioavailability of therapeutic moieties. Charge and vesicular size are important parameters that affect the biodistribution of liposomes. Law et al. [135] reported a higher corneal uptake of positively charged liposomal acyclovir. Also Seyfoddin and Al-Kassas found faster permeation through excised cornea indicating potential enhanced corneal penetration properties for acyclovir nanostructured lipid carriers [136].

New formulations of polymeric and lipid nanoparticles are currently in development. The non-biodegradable positively-charged polymer Eudragit® RS 100 and semi-solid lipid excipient Gelucire® 44/14 were used as a vehicle, the cationic lipid octadecylamine was used as a cationic agent; obtaining successfully a pilocarpine HCl system for ocular application [137].

Microparticles and Nanoparticles

Microparticles and nanoparticles are colloidal drug carriers in the micrometer and submicrometer range, which have been evaluated for ophthalmic drug delivery purposes over the past 15 years. Micro- or nanoparticles are divided in two groups, micro- or nanospheres and micro- or nanocapsules. Microspheres are monolithic particles possessing a porous or solid polymer matrix, whereas microcapsules consist of a polymeric membrane surrounding a solid or a liquid drug reservoir [138]. Practically, the term nanoparticles is applied to nanospheres and nanocapsules because it is often difficult to determine if they are real capsules or matrix-type particles. The active compound can be dissolved, trapped, encapsulated, adsorbed or linked to these colloidal systems [138]. Nanocapsules can be used to increase the accessibility of drugs to the receptors localized in specific areas. They can serve as vehicles for use in the treatment of ophthalmic pathologies, because increased corneal penetration and prolonged therapeutic response have been achieved for some drugs [139]. Another drug used as eyedrops, pilocarpine, was encapsulated in polyisobutylcyanoacrylate nanocapsules incorporated in a Pluronic F127 gel [140]. The formulation increased the contact time of the drug with the absorbing tissue in the eye and improved ocular bioavailability. The principal materials used so far to prepare colloidal systems for ophthalmic drug delivery have been synthetic biodegradable polymers belonging to the group of poly(alkyl cyanoacrylate). These polymers can be degraded following two concomitant metabolization pathways, which are the erosion of the polymer backbone leading to the formation of formaldehyde [141] or the cleavage of the ester inducing the formation of a water-soluble polymer backbone and the corresponding alcohol [142]. The potential of microparticulate formulations has been described but, as of today, they are not frequently employed as part of ophthalmic vehicles [143, 144].

Indomethacin in vitro corneal penetration was evaluated using nanocapsules as drug carriers [145]. The transcorneal flux of the drug through isolated rabbit cornea showed a considerable increase of 4–5 times the penetration rate of the nanoencapsulated drug compared to commercial eyedrops. In addition, PCL nanocapsules containing indomethacin were coated with chitosan, poly(l-lysine), or both in order to combine the features of nanocapsules with the advantages of a cationic mucoadhesivecoating [146]. Chitosan-coated nanocapsules provided an optimal corneal penetration of indomethacin and displayed good ocular tolerance. Promising findings were also reported for optimized celecoxib loaded bioadhesive cationic chitosan or anionic alginate nanoparticles. All formulations possessed pH and viscosity values compatible with the eye and uniform drug contents. In vitro release data showed a sustained release without any burst effect then followed by Higuchi non-Fickian diffusion mechanism. The results of in vitro cell toxicity revealed that all prepared formulations were non-toxic, with percentage cell viability ranging from 89.9 to 97.7 % [147].

Microemulsions and Nanoemulsions

Microemulsions might be systems of future interest, with the basic caveats concerning sterile manufacturing, long-term stability, patient tolerance vis-a`-vis any surfactant, and the difficulty to adequately preserve a biphasic system. The O/W Nanoemulsions (NEs) can also be used for ocular delivery to improve corneal penetration or sustain the pharmacological effect of drugs [148, 149]. These emulsions could be advantageous because they are supposed to diminish vision-blurring effects [150]. These NEs can prolong the release of the drug and sustain the pharmacological effect of drugs in the eye following ocular application [151]. Muchtar et al. [148] and Navech et al. [149] showed the application of NEs to prolong the response of antiglaucomatous drugs applied to rabbits.

Micelles

In micellar systems, nonpolar molecules are solubilized within the internal micelle hydrophobic core, polar molecules are adsorbed on the micelle surface and substances with intermediate polarity are distributed along surfactant molecules in intermediate positions. Micellar ocular DDS should be based on nontoxic and non-irritant materials and should be stable enough to achieve a reasonable shelf life.

Attention should be paid to the CMC of detergents used for micellar assembly, since high CMC often renders them toxic and irritant to ocular tissues. The nonionic triblock copolymer polyethylene oxide–polypropylene oxide–polyethylene oxide (PEO–PPO–PEO) has been widely used in medicine and has shown low toxicity. The potential of a micellar carrier for topical ocular delivery using pilocarpine as a model drug was evaluated in another study [152]. Micellar solution of pilocarpine for topical ocular delivery was prepared by a simple method of drug dissolution within an aqueous solution of a surface-active high molecular weight triblock copolymer, Pluronic F127. For this purpose, an aqueous solution of Pluronic F127 was prepared in concentrations above the CMC, where the copolymer is supposed to form micelles.

Cyclodextrin-based formulations (Fig. 6.9) should not be missed by ophthalmic drug development groups [153, 154]. Their typical domain of use would be sparingly soluble drugs, e.g., sulfonamides inhibiting carbonic anhydrase for the treatment of glaucoma [155] or steroids against inflammation [156]. However, their action might be equivocal in some cases: a cyclodextrin solution of L 671,152 (dorzolamide hydrochloride, a topically active sulfonamide) induced—in rabbits—intraocular levels lower than the corresponding suspension. On the other hand auspicious results were reported for other inhibiting carbonic anhydrase drug (acetazolamide) in hydroxypropyl-ß-cyclodextrin (Fig. 6.10) formulations.

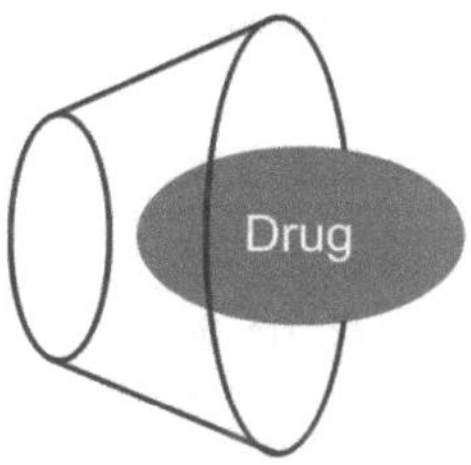

Fig. 6.9 Cyclodextrin-drug complex

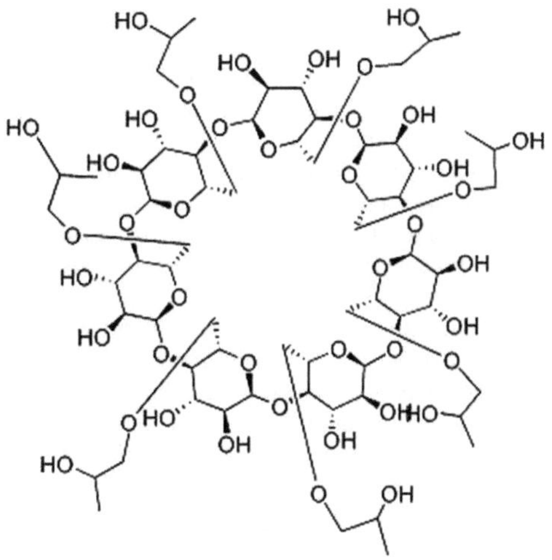

Fig. 6.10 Hydroxypropyl-ß-cyclodextrin

Hydroxypropyl-ß-cyclodextrin–acetazolamide–triethanolamine ternary complexes, showed better results in terms of in vitro corneal permeability and in vivo intraocular pressure reduction, in comparison with acetazolamide–triethanolamine complexes [157].

Conclusions

The eye presents unique challenges to the delivery of drugs. When the demand for sustained delivery to the target tissue is coupled with the desire to avoid systemic exposure, circumstances are ripe for creative approaches. Pharmaceutical research and development provides a pathway to achieve this, but it is governed by available technology, innovations, and regulatory constraints. Importantly, the cost of the finished product must be bearable by the individuals and/or communities who will use the product, and it has to be economically viable for the manufacturer. In the future, the use of ophthalmic drug delivery systems will certainly increase because of the development of new polymers, the emergence of new drugs having short biological half-lives or systemic side effects and the need to improve the efficacy of ophthalmic treatments by ensuring an effective drug concentration in the eye for several days.

References

1. Sieg, J.W., Robinson, J.R.: Vehicle effects on ocular drug bioavailability i: evaluation of fluorometholone. J. Pharm. Sci. **64**(6), 931–936 (1975)
2. Patton, T.F., Robinson, J.R.: Ocular evaluation of polyvinyl alcohol vehicle in rabbits. J. Pharm. Sci. **64**(8), 1312–1316 (1975)
3. Robinson, J.R., Mlynek, G.M.: Bioadhesive and phase-change polymers for ocular drug delivery. Adv. Drug. Deliv. Rev. **16**, 45–50 (1975)
4. Salminen, L., et al.: Prolonged pulse-entry of pilocarpine with a soluble drug insert. Graefes. Arch. Clin. Exp. Ophthalmol. **221**(2), 96–99 (1983)
5. Wilson, C.G., et al.: Structure and physiological functions. In: Touitou, E., Barry, B.W. (eds.) Enhancement in Drug Delivery. pp. 473–487. (2007)
6. Snell, R.S., Lemp, M.A.: Clinical Anatomy of the Eye, 2nd edn, p. 423. Blackwell Science, Malden (1998)
7. Norn, M.S.: Tear secretion in normal eyes. estimated by a new method: the lacrimal streak dilution test. Acta. Ophthalmol. (Copenh) **43**(4), 567–573 (1965)
8. Records, R.E: The tear film. In: Tasman, W., Jaeger, E.A.(eds.) Duane's Foundations of Clinical Ophthalmology, Lippincott Williams & Wilkins, Philadelphia (2005)
9. Patton, T.F., Robinson, J.R.: Quantitative precorneal disposition of topically applied pilocarpine nitrate in rabbit eyes. J. Pharm. Sci. **65**(9), 1295–1301 (1976)
10. Plazonnet, B., et al.: Pharmacokinetics and biopharmaceutical aspects of some anti-glaucoma drugs. In: Saettone, M.F., Bucci, M., Speiser, P. (eds.) Ophthalmic Drug Delivery; Biopharmaceutical, Technological and Clinical Aspects, pp. 117–139. Liviana Press/ Springer Verlag, Padova/New york (1987)
11. Gurny, R., Ibrahim, H., Buri, P.: The development and use of in situ formed gels, triggered by pH. In: Edman, P. (ed.) Biopharmaceutics of Ocular Drug Delivery, pp. 81–90. CRC Press, Florida (1993)

12. Tanaka, T.: Collapse of gels and the critical endpoint. Phys. Rev. Lett. **40**(12), 820–823 (1978)
13. Ahn, S.-K., et al.: Stimuli-responsive polymer gels. Soft. Matter. **4**(6), 1151–1157 (2008)
14. Swan, K.C.: Use of methyl cellulose in ophthalmology. Arch. Ophthalmol. **33**(5), 378–380 (1945)
15. Zaki, I., et al.: A comparison of the effect of viscosity on the precorneal residence of solutions in rabbit and man. J. Pharm. Pharmacol. **38**(6), 463–466 (1986)
16. Tous, S.S., Abd-El Nasser, K.: Acetazolamide topical formulation and ocular effect. STP Pharm Sci. **2**, 125–131 (1992)
17. Grove, J., et al.: The effect of vehicle viscosity on the ocular bioavailability of L-653,328. Int. J. Pharm. **66**(1–3), 23–28 (1990)
18. Ludwig, A., Van Ooteghem, M.: Influence of viscolysers on the residence of ophthalmic solutions evaluated by slit lamp fluorophotometry. STP. Pharma. Sci. **2**, 81–87 (1992)
19. Mueller, W.H., Deardorff, D.L.: Ophthalmic vehicles: the effect of methylcellulose on the penetration of homatropine hydrobromide through the cornea. J. Am. Pharm. Assoc. (Baltim) **45**(5), 334–341 (1956)
20. Haas, J.S., Merrill, D.L.: The effect of methyl-cellulose on responses to solutions of pilocarpine. Am. J. Ophthalmol. **54**, 21–24 (1962)
21. Hardberger, R., Hanna, C., Boyd, C.M.: Effects of drug vehicles on ocular contact time. Arch. Ophthalmol. **93**(1), 42–45 (1975)
22. Schoenwald, R.D., et al.: Inlfuence of high-viscosity vehicles on miotic effect of pilocarpine. J. Pharm. Sci. **67**(9), 1280–1283 (1978)
23. Saettone, M.F., et al.: Polymer effects on ocular bioavailability—the influence of different liquid vehicles on the mydriatic response of tropicamide in humans and rabbits. Int. J. Pharm. **20**, 187–202 (1984)
24. Deshpande, S.G., Shirolkar, S.: Sustained release ophthalmic formulations of pilocarpine. J. Pharm. Pharmacol. **41**(3), 197–200 (1989)
25. Patchan, M., et al.: Synthesis and properties of regenerated cellulose-based hydrogels with high strength and transparency for potential use as an ocular bandage. Mater. Sci. Eng. C. Mater. Biol. Appl. **33**(5), 3069–3076 (2013)
26. Peppas, N.A.: Hydrogels. In: Peppas, N.A.(ed.) Medicine and Pharmacy. CRC Press, Boca Raton (1987)
27. Davies, N.M., et al.: Evaluation of mucoadhesive polymers in ocular drug delivery. I. Viscous solutions. Pharm. Res. **8**(8), 1039–1043 (1991)
28. Balazs, E.A.: Ultrapure hyaluronic acid and the use thereof. US Patent #4,141,973 (1979)
29. Bernatchez, S.F., et al.: Use of hyaluronic acid. In: Edman P.(ed.) Biopharmaceutics of Ocular Drug Delivery, pp. 105–120. CRC Press, Boca Raton (1993)
30. Wysenbeek, Y.S., et al.: The effect of sodium hyaluronate on the corneal epithelium. An ultrastructural study. Invest. Ophthalmol. Vis. Sci. **29**(2), 194–199 (1988)
31. Camber, O., Edman, P., Gurny, R.: Influence of sodium hyaluronate on the meiotic effect of pilocarpine in rabbits. Curr. Eye. Res. **6**(6), 779–784 (1987)
32. Saettone, M.F., et al.: Mucoadhesive ophthalmic vehicles: evaluation of polymeric low-viscosity formulations. J. Ocul. Pharmacol. **10**(1), 83–92 (1994)
33. Saettone, M.F., et al.: Evaluation of muco-adhesive properties and in vivo activity of ophthalmic vehicles based on hyaluronic acid. Int. J. Pharm. **51**, 203–212 (1989)
34. Bernatchez, S.F., Tabatabay, C., Gurny, R.: Sodium hyaluronate 0.25 % used as a vehicle increases the bioavailability of topically administered gentamicin. Graefes. Arch. Clin. Exp. Ophthalmol. **231**(3), 157–161 (1993)
35. Calles, J.A., et al.: Novel bioadhesive hyaluronan-itaconic acid crosslinked films for ocular therapy. Int. J. Pharm. **455**(1–2), 48–56 (2013)
36. Edsman, K., Carlfors, J., Harju, K.: Rheological evaluation and ocular contact time of some carbomer gels for ophthalmic use. Int. J. Pharm. **137**(2), 233–241 (1996)
37. von der Ohe, N., et al.: How can the bioavailability of timolol be enhanced? A pharmacokinetic pilot study of novel hydrogels. Graefes. Arch. Clin. Exp. Ophthalmol. **234**(7), 452–456 (1996)

38. Schoenwald, R.D., Boltralik, J.J.: A bioavailability comparison in rabbits of two steroids formulated as high-viscosity gels and reference aqueous preparations. Invest. Ophthalmol. Vis. Sci. **18**(1), 61–66 (1979)
39. Ludwig, A., Unlu, N., van Ooteghem, M.: Evaluation of viscous ophthalmic vehicles containing carbomer by slit-lamp fluorophotometry in humans. Int. J. Pharm. **61**(1–2), 15–25 (1990)
40. Saettone, M.F., et al.: Semisolid ophthalmic vehicles III. An evaluation of four organic hydrogels containing pilocarpine. Int. J. Pharm. **31**, 261–270 (1986)
41. Amin, P.D., Bhogte, C.P., Deshpande, M.A.: Studies on gel tears. Drug. Dev. Ind. Pharm. **22**(7), 735–739 (1996)
42. Meseguer, G., et al.: Gamma scintigraphic study of precorneal drainage and assessment of miotic response in rabbits of various ophthalmic formulations containing pilocarpine. Int. J. Pharm. **95**(1–3), 229–234 (1993)
43. Albasini, M., Ludwig, A.: Evaluation of polysaccharides intended for ophthalmic use in ocular dosage forms. Farmaco (Societa chimica italiana: 1989) **50**(9), 633–642 (1995)
44. Burgalassi, S., Chetoni, P., Saettone, M.F.: Hydrogels for ocular delivery of pilocarpine: preliminary evaluation in rabbits of the influence of viscosity and of drug solubility. Eur. J. Pharm. Biopham. **42**, 385–392 (1996)
45. Felt, O., Buri, P., Gurny, R.: Chitosan: a unique polysaccharide for drug delivery. Drug. Dev. Ind. Pharm. **24**(11), 979–993 (1998)
46. Felt, O., et al.: Topical use of chitosan in ophthalmology: tolerance assessment and evaluation of precorneal retention. Int. J. Pharm. **180**(2), 185–193 (1999)
47. Felt, O., et al.: Chitosan as tear substitute: a wetting agent endowed with antimicrobial efficacy. J. Ocul. Pharmacol. Ther. **16**(3), 261–270 (2000)
48. Felt, O., Buri, P., Gumy, R.: Ocular bioavailability of tobramycin after topical administration of formulations based on polysaccharide. In: 2nd International Symposium on Experimental Clinical Ocular Pharmacology and Pharmaceutics (1997)
49. Qiu, Y., Park, K.: Environment-sensitive hydrogels for drug delivery. Adv. Drug. Deliv. Rev. **53**(3), 321–339 (2001)
50. Ron, E.S., Bromberg, L.E.: Temperature-responsive gels and thermogelling polymer matrices for protein and peptide delivery. Adv. Drug. Deliv. Rev. **31**(3), 197–221 (1998)
51. Kost, J., Langer, R.: Responsive polymeric delivery systems. Adv. Drug. Deliv. Rev. **46**(1–3), 125–148 (2001)
52. Ruel-Gariepy, E., Leroux, J.C.: In situ-forming hydrogels—review of temperature-sensitive systems. Eur. J. Pharm. Biopharm. **58**(2), 409–426 (2004)
53. Mazuel, C., Friteyre, M.C.: Ophthalmological composition of the type which undergoes liquid-gel phase transition, Google Patents (1989)
54. Kumar, S., Haglund, B.O., Himmelstein, K.J.: In situ-forming gels for ophthalmic drug delivery. J. Ocul. Pharmacol. **10**(1), 47–56 (1994)
55. Kumar, S., Himmelstein, K.J.: Modification of in situ gelling behavior of carbopol solutions by hydroxypropyl methylcellulose. J. Pharm. Sci. **84**(3), 344–348 (1995)
56. Ron, E.S.: Smart gel: a new thermogelling polymer mixture for drug delivery. Proceedings in international symposium of Controlled Rel Bioactive Materials. **23**, 23–24 (1996)
57. Zimmer, A.K., Zerbe, H., Kreuter, J.: Evaluation of pilocarpine-loaded albumin particles as drug delivery systems for controlled delivery in the eye I. in vitro and in vivo characterisation. J. Controlled. Release. **32**(1), 57–70 (1994)
58. Zimmer, A.K., et al.: Evaluation of pilocarpine-loaded albumin particles as controlled drug delivery systems for the eye. II. co-administration with bioadhesive and viscous polymers. J. Controlled. Release. **33**(1), 31–46 (1995)
59. Deasy, P.B., Quigley, K.J.: Rheological evaluation of deacetylated gellan gum (gelrite) for pharmaceutical use. Int. J. Pharm. **73**(2), 117–123 (1991)
60. Verschueren, E., Van Santvliet, L., Ludwig, A.: Evaluation of various carrageenans as ophthalmic viscolysers. S.T.P. Pharma. Sci. **6**, 203–210 (1996)
61. Cohen, S., et al.: A novel in situ-forming ophthalmic drug delivery system from alginates undergoing gelation in the eye. J. Controlled. Release. **44**(2–3), 201–208 (1997)

62. Kang, K.S., et al.: Agar-like polysaccharide produced by a pseudomonas species: production and basic properties. Appl. Environ. Microbiol. **43**(5), 1086–1091 (1982)
63. Mittal, N., Kaur, G.: In situ gelling ophthalmic drug delivery system: Formulation and evaluation. J. Appl. Polym. Sci. **131**(2) (2014)
64. Hoffman, A.S., Afrassiabi, A., Dong, L.C.: Thermally reversible hydrogels: II. delivery and selective removal of substances from aqueous solutions. J. Controlled. Release. **4**, 213–222 (1986)
65. Hoffman, A.S.: Applications of thermally reversible polymers and hydrogels in therapeutics and diagnostics. J. Controlled. Release. **6**(1), 297–305 (1987)
66. Bermudez, J.M., et al.: Challenges and opportunities in polymer technology applied to veterinary medicine. J. Vet. Pharmacol. Ther. **37**(2), 105–124 (2014)
67. Gilbert, J.C., et al.: The behaviour of Pluronic F127 in aqueous solution studied using fluorescent probes. Int. J. Pharm. **40**, 93–99 (1987)
68. Gilbert, J.C., et al.: The effect of solutes and polymers on the gelation properties of pluronic F-127 solutions for controlled drug delivery. J. Controlled. Release. **5**(2), 113–118 (1987)
69. Gilchrist, P., et al.: The precorneal residence of a thermally sensitive hydrogel. In: 137th British Pharmaceutical Conference Scarborough (1997)
70. Waring, G.O., Harris, R.R.: Double-masked evaluation of a poloxamer artificial tear in keratoconjunctivitis. In: Leopold, L.H., Burns, B.P. (eds.) Symposium on Ocular Therapy, pp. 127–140. Wiley, New York (1979)
71. Miller, S.C., Donovan, M.D.: Effect of Poloxamer 407 gel on the mitotic activity of pilocarpine nitrate in rabbits. Int. J. Pharm. **12**, 147–152 (1982)
72. Dumortier, G., et al.: Comparison between a thermoreversible gel and an insert in order to prolong the systemic absorption of morphine after ocular administration. S.T.P. Pharma. Sci. **2**, 111–117 (1992)
73. Zhang, R., et al.: A novel pH- and ionic-strength-sensitive carboxy methyl dextran hydrogel. Biomaterials **26**(22), 4677–4683 (2005)
74. El-Aasser, M.S.: Formation of polymer latexes by direct emulsification. Advances in emulsion polymerization and latex technology. In: 10th Annual Short Coarse (1979)
75. Ibrahim, H., et al.: Concept and development of ophthalmic pseudolatexes triggered by pH. Int. J. Pharm. **77**, 211–219 (1991)
76. Gumy, R., et al.: Recent developments in controlled drug delivery to the eye. In: Proceedings in International Symposium Controlled Rel Bioactive Materials (1985)
77. Ibrahim, H., et al.: Aqueous nanodispersions prepared by a salting-out process. Int. J. Pharm. **87**(1–3), 239–246 (1992)
78. Singh, J., Chhabra, G., Pathak, K.: Development of acetazolamide-loaded, pH-triggered polymeric nanoparticulate in situ gel for sustained ocular delivery: in vitro. ex vivo evaluation and pharmacodynamic study. Drug Dev. Ind. Pharm. **40**(9), 1223–1232 (2014)
79. Pathak, M.K., Chhabra, G., Pathak, K.: Design and development of a novel pH triggered nanoemulsified in-situ ophthalmic gel of fluconazole: ex-vivo transcorneal permeation, corneal toxicity and irritation testing. Drug. Dev. Ind. Pharm. **39**(5), 780–790 (2013)
80. Gurtler, F., Gurny, R.: Patent literature review of ophthalmic inserts. Drug. Dev. Ind. Pharm. **21**, 1–18 (1995)
81. Maichuk, Y.F.: Ophthalmic drug inserts. Invest. Ophthalmol. **14**, 87–90 (1975)
82. Friedrich, S.W., et al.: Pharmacokinetic differences between ocular inserts and eyedrops. J. Ocul. Pharmacol. Ther. **12**(1), 5–18 (1996)
83. Saettone, M.F.: Solid polymeric inserts/disks as drug delivery devices. In: Edman, P. (ed.) Biopharmaceutics of Ocular Drug Delivery, pp. 61–67. CRC Press, London (1993)
84. Saettone, M.F., Salminen, L.: Ocular inserts for topical delivery. Adv. Drug. Del. Rev. **16**, 95–106 (1995)
85. Urquhart, J.: Development of ocusert pilocarpine ocular therapeutic systems. In: Robinson J.R. (ed) Ophthalmic Drug Delivery Systems, pp. 105–108. American Pharmaceutical Association, Washington DC (1980)
86. Katz, I.M.: Shaped ophthalmic inserts for treating dry eye syndrome, Google Patents (1982)

87. Bawa, R.: Ocular inserts. In: Mitra, A.K. (ed.) Ophthalmic Drug Delivery Systems, pp. 223–260. Dekker, New York (1993)
88. Fyodorov, S.N., et al.: Ophthalmological collagen coverings, Google Patents (1990)
89. Bloomfield, S.E., et al.: Soluble gentamicin ophthalmic inserts as a drug delivery system. Arch. Ophthalmol. **96**(5), 885–887 (1978)
90. Friedberg, M.L., Pleyer, U., Mondino, B.J.: Device drug delivery to the eye. Collagen shields, iontophoresis, and pumps. Ophthalmology **98**(5), 725–732 (1991)
91. Phinney, R.B., et al.: Collagen-shield delivery of gentamicin and vancomycin. Arch. Ophthalmol. **106**(11), 1599–1604 (1988)
92. Sawusch, M.R., et al.: Use of collagen corneal shields in the treatment of bacterial keratitis. Am. J. Ophthalmol. **106**(3), 279–281 (1988)
93. Hwang, D.G., et al.: Collagen shield enhancement of topical dexamethasone penetration. Arch. Ophthalmol. **107**(9), 1375–1380 (1989)
94. Sawusch, M.R., O'Brien, T.P., Updegraff, S.A.: Collagen corneal shields enhance penetration of topical prednisolone acetate. J. Cataract. Refract. Surg. **15**(6), 625–628 (1989)
95. Gussler, J.R., et al.: Collagen shield delivery of trifluorothymidine. J. Cataract. Refract. Surg. **16**(6), 719–722 (1990)
96. Milani, J.K., et al.: Collagen shields impregnated with gentamicin-dexamethasone as a potential drug delivery device. Am. J. Ophthalmol. **116**(5), 622–627 (1993)
97. Fyodorov, S.N.: Efficiency of collagen covers: application in cases in keratotomy. In: Fydorov, S.N. (ed.) Eye Microsurgery, Research Institute of Eye Microsurgery, Moscow (1984)
98. O'Brien, T.P., et al.: Use of collagen corneal shields versus soft contact lenses to enhance penetration of topical tobramycin. J. Cataract. Refract. Surg. **14**(5), 505–507 (1988)
99. Pleyer, U., et al.: Use of collagen shields containing amphotericin B in the treatment of experimental Candida albicans-induced keratomycosis in rabbits. Am. J. Ophthalmol. **113**(3), 303–308 (1992)
100. Hobden, J.A., et al.: Treatment of experimental Pseudomonas keratitis using collagen shields containing tobramycin. Arch. Ophthalmol. **106**(11), 1605–1607 (1988)
101. Silbiger, J., Stern, G.A.: Evaluation of corneal collagen shields as a drug delivery device for the treatment of experimental Pseudomonas keratitis. Ophthalmology **99**(6), 889–892 (1992)
102. Callegan, M.C., et al.: Efficacy of tobramycin drops applied to collagen shields for experimental staphylococcal keratitis. Curr. Eye. Res. **13**(12), 875–878 (1994)
103. Chen, Y.F., et al.: Cyclosporine-containing collagen shields suppress corneal allograft rejection. Am. J. Ophthalmol. **109**(2), 132–137 (1990)
104. Simamora, P., et al.: Controlled delivery of pilocarpine. 2. In-vivo evaluation of Gelfoam device. Int. J. Pharm. **170**, 209–214 (1998)
105. Lee, Y.C., et al.: Formulation and in vivo evaluation of ocular insert containing phenylephrine and tropicamide. Int. J. Pharm. **182**(1), 121–126 (1999)
106. Negvesky, G.J., et al.: Ocular gelfoam disc-applicator for pupillary dilation in humans. J. Ocul. Pharmacol. Ther. **16**(4), 311–315 (2000)
107. Saettone, M.F., et al.: Controlled release of pilocarpine from coated polymeric ophthalmic inserts prepared by extrusion. Int. J. Pharm. **86**, 159–166 (1992)
108. Attia, M.A., Kassem, M.A., Safwat, S.M.: In vivo performance of [3H]dexamethasone ophthalmic film delivery systems in the rabbit eye. Int. J. Pharm. **47**(1–3), 21–30 (1988)
109. Kaga, Y., et al.: Ultraviolet-hardenable adhesive, Google Patents (1992)
110. Gurtler, F., et al.: Long-acting soluble bioadhesive ophthalmic drug insert (BODI) containing gentamicin for veterinary use: optimization and clinical investigation. J. Controlled. Release. **33**(2), 231–236 (1995)
111. Saettone, M.F., et al.: Application of the compression technique to the manufacture of pilocarpine inserts. Acta. Pharm. Technol. **1**, 15–19 (1990)
112. Harwood, R.J., Schwartz, J.B.: Drug release from compression molded films: preliminary studies with pilocarpine. Drug. Dev. Ind. Pharm. **8**(5), 663–682 (1982)

113. Baeyens, V., et al.: Optimized release of dexamethasone and gentamicin from a soluble ocular insert for the treatment of external ophthalmic infections. J. Controlled. Release. **52**(1–2), 215–220 (1998)
114. Gale, R.M., Ben-Dor, M., Keller, N.: Ocular therapeutic system for dispensing a medication formulation, Google Patents (1980)
115. Robinson, J.R.: Ocular drug delivery: mechanism(s) of corneal drug transport and mucoadhesive delivery systems. STP. Pharm. Sci. **5**(12), 839–846 (1989)
116. Drance, S.M., Mitchell, D.W., Schulzer, M.: The duration of action of pilocarpine ocusert on intraocular pressure in man. Can. J. Ophthalmol. **10**(4), 450–452 (1975)
117. Chien, Y.W.: Novel Drug Delivery Systems. Marcel Dekker, New York (1992)
118. Torron, C., et al.: Use of a new ocular insert versus conventional mydriasis in cataract surgery. Biomed. Res. Int. p. 849349 (2013)
119. Refojo, M.F.: Polymers in contact lenses: an overview. Curr. Eye. Res. **4**(6), 719–723 (1985)
120. Maddox, Y.T., Bernstein, H.N.: An evaluation of the Bionite hydrophilic contact lens for use in a drug delivery system. Ann. Ophthalmol. **4**(9), 789–790 (1972)
121. Praus, R., et al.: Hydrophilic contact lenses as a new therapeutic approach for the topical use of chloramphenicol and tetracycline. Ophthalmologica **165**(1), 62–70 (1972)
122. Hull, D.S., Edelhauser, H.F., Hyndiuk, R.A.: Ocular penetration of prednisolone and the hydrophilic contact lens. Arch. Ophthalmol. **92**(5), 413–416 (1974)
123. Wajs, G., Meslard, J.C.: Release of therapeutic agents from contact lenses. Crit. Rev. Ther. Drug. Carrier. Syst. **2**(3), 275–289 (1986)
124. Weiner, A.L.: Polymeric drug delivery systems for the eye. In: Domb, A.J. (ed.) Polymeric Site-Specific Pharmacotherapy, pp. 315–346. Wiley, Chichester (1994)
125. McMahon, T.T., Zadnik, K.: Twenty-five years of contact lenses: the impact on the cornea and ophthalmic practice. Cornea **19**(5), 730–740 (2000)
126. Jung, H.J., Chauhan, A.: Temperature sensitive contact lenses for triggered ophthalmic drug delivery. Biomaterials **33**(7), 2289–2300 (2012)
127. Kimura, H., Ogura, Y.: Biodegradable polymers for ocular drug delivery. Ophthalmologica **215**(3), 143–155 (2001)
128. Liu, W., Griffith, M., Li, F.: Alginate microsphere-collagen composite hydrogel for ocular drug delivery and implantation. J. Mater. Sci. Mater. Med. **19**(11), 3365–3371 (2008)
129. Bernards, D.A., et al.: Ocular biocompatibility and structural integrity of micro- and nano-structured poly(caprolactone) films. J. Ocul. Pharmacol. Ther. **29**(2), 249–257 (2013)
130. Gurny, R., Boye, T., Ibrahim, H.: Ocular therapy with nanoparticulate systems for controlled drug delivery. J. Controlled. Release. **2**, 353–361 (1985)
131. Lee, V.H., et al.: Ocular drug bioavailability from topically applied liposomes. Surv. Ophthalmol. **29**(5), 335–348 (1985)
132. Marchal-Heussler, L., et al.: Poly(epsilon-caprolactone) nanocapsules in carteolol ophthalmic delivery. Pharm. Res. **10**(3), 386–390 (1993)
133. Smolin, G., et al.: Idoxuridine-liposome therapy for herpes simplex keratitis. Am. J. Ophthalmol. **91**(2), 220–225 (1981)
134. Schaeffer, H.E., Krohn, D.L.: Liposomes in topical drug delivery. Invest. Ophthalmol. Vis. Sci. **22**(2), 220–227 (1982)
135. Law, S.L., Huang, K.J., Chiang, C.H.: Acyclovir-containing liposomes for potential ocular delivery. Corneal penetration and absorption. J. Controlled. Release. **63**(1–2), 135–140 (2000)
136. Seyfoddin, A., Al-Kassas, R.: Development of solid lipid nanoparticles and nanostructured lipid carriers for improving ocular delivery of acyclovir. Drug. Dev. Ind. Pharm. **39**(4), 508–519 (2013)
137. Lutfi, G., Muzeyyen, D.: Preparation and characterization of polymeric and lipid nanoparticles of pilocarpine HCl for ocular application. Pharm. Dev. Technol. **18**(3), 701–709 (2013)
138. Zimmer, A., Kreuter, J.: Microspheres and nanoparticles used in ocular delivery systems. Adv. Drug. Deliv. Rev. **16**(1), 61–73 (1995)
139. Losa, C., et al.: Design of new formulations for topical ocular administration: polymeric nanocapsules containing metipranolol. Pharm. Res. **10**(1), 80–87 (1993)

140. Desai, S.D., Blanchard, J.: Pluronic F127-based ocular delivery system containing biodegradable polyisobutylcyanoacrylate nanocapsules of pilocarpine. Drug. Deliv. **7**(4), 201–207 (2000)
141. Vezin, W.R., Florence, A.T.: Diffusion of small molecules in poly-N-alkyl cyanoacrylates [proceedings]. J. Pharm. Pharmacol. **30**(Suppl), 2P (1978)
142. Lenaerts, V., et al.: Degradation of poly (isobutyl cyanoacrylate) nanoparticles. Biomaterials **5**(2), 65–68 (1984)
143. Joshi, A.: Microparticulates for ophthalmic drug delivery. J. Ocul. Pharmacol. **10**(1), 29–45 (1994)
144. Genta, I., et al.: Bioadhesive microspheres for ophthalmic administration of acyclovir. J. Pharm. Pharmacol. **49**(8), 737–742 (1997)
145. Calvo, P., et al.: Polyester nanocapsules as new topical ocular delivery systems for cyclosporin A. Pharm. Res. **13**(2), 311–315 (1996)
146. Calvo, P., Vila-Jato, J.L., Alonso, M.A.J.: Evaluation of cationic polymer-coated nanocapsules as ocular drug carriers. Int. J. Pharm. **153**(1), 41–50 (1997)
147. Ibrahim, M.M., et al.: Natural bioadhesive biodegradable nanoparticles-based topical ophthalmic formulations for sustained celecoxib release. J. Pharm. Tech. Drug. Res. **2**(1), 7 (2013)
148. Muchtar, S., et al.: A submicron emulsion as ocular vehicle for delta-8-tetrahydrocannabinol: effect on intraocular pressure in rabbits. Ophthalmic. Res. **24**(3), 142–149 (1992)
149. Naveh, N., Muchtar, S., Benita, S.: Pilocarpine incorporated into a submicron emulsion vehicle causes an unexpectedly prolonged ocular hypotensive effect in rabbits. J. Ocul. Pharmacol. **10**(3), 509–520 (1994)
150. Schulz, M.B., Daniels, R.: Hydroxypropylmethylcellulose (HPMC) as emulsifier for submicron emulsions: influence of molecular weight and substitution type on the droplet size after high-pressure homogenization. Eur. J. Pharm. Biopharm. **49**(3), 231–236 (2000)
151. Hagigit, T., et al.: The influence of cationic lipid type on in-vitro release kinetic profiles of antisense oligonucleotide from cationic nanoemulsions. Eur. J. Pharm. Biopharm. **70**(1), 248–259 (2008)
152. Pepic, I., Jalsenjak, N., Jalsenjak, I.: Micellar solutions of triblock copolymer surfactants with pilocarpine. Int. J. Pharm. **272**(1–2), 57–64 (2004)
153. Loftssona, T., Jarvinen, T.: Cyclodextrins in ophthalmic drug delivery. Adv. Drug. Deliv. Rev. **36**(1), 59–79 (1999)
154. Bibby, D.C., Davies, N.M., Tucker, I.G.: Mechanisms by which cyclodextrins modify drug release from polymeric drug delivery systems. Int. J. Pharm. **197**(1), 1–11 (2000)
155. Gudmundsdottir, E., et al.: Methazolamide 1 % in cyclodextrin solution lowers IOP in human ocular hypertension. Invest. Ophthalmol. Vis. Sci. **41**(11), 3552–3554 (2000)
156. Kristinsson, J.K., et al.: Dexamethasone-cyclodextrin-polymer co-complexes in aqueous eye drops. Aqueous humor pharmacokinetics in humans. Invest. Ophthalmol. Vis. Sci. **37**(6), 1199–1203 (1996)
157. Palma, S.D., et al.: An efficient ternary complex of acetazolamide with HP-ss-CD and TEA for topical ocular administration. J. Controlled. Release. **138**(1), 24–31 (2009)

Chapter 7
Polymers in Tissue Engineering

Rebecca L. Heise, B. Adam Blakeney and Robert A. Pouliot

Abstract The landscape of polymer selection and processing techniques is constantly evolving in the field of tissue engineering and regenerative medicine. This chapter will cover new advances in polymers that are used to regenerate functional tissues used to repair or replace tissues lost to age, disease, injury, or congenital defect. The focus will be on new processing techniques and the incorporation of biologics or drug delivery to enhance cellular response and ingrowth into the polymers that will create a more functional tissue replacement by engineering the polymer tissue interface. Special emphasis is placed on new frontiers in tissue engineering the lung and liver.

Abbreviations

CT	Computer aided X-ray tomography
E′	Storage modulus
E″	Loss modulus
ECM	Extracellular matrix
ELISA	Enzyme linked immunoabsorbant assay
HAG	Hydroxyethyl methacrylate-alginate-gelatin
MGLA	Modified gelatin sponges with lactobionic acid
PCL	Poly(carprolactone)
PCL-U4U	Polycaprolactone bisurea

R.L. Heise (✉) · R.A. Pouliot
Department of Biomedical Engineering, Virginia Commonwealth University, Richmond, VA, USA
e-mail: rlheise@vcu.edu

R.L. Heise · B. Adam Blakeney
Department of Physiology and Biophysics, Virginia Commonwealth University, Richmond, VA, USA

F. Puoci (ed.), *Advanced Polymers in Medicine*, DOI 10.1007/978-3-319-12478-0_7

PDMS	Polydimethysiloxane
PEG	Poly ethylene glycol
PLA	Poly lactic acid
PLGA	Poly lactic co-glycolic acid
PLLA	Poly-l lactic acid
TLR4	Toll-like receptor 4

Introduction

While there are many polymeric biomaterials used in medical applications, many of which are covered in other chapters of this textbook, we will limit our focus to tissue engineered polymer containing constructs that either 1. Contain a polymeric scaffold + cells prior to implantation or 2. Contain a polymeric scaffold with a bioactive factor to elicit native cellular recruitment into the scaffold or drug delivery to form a functional tissue replacement. This book chapter is not meant to be all encompassing. Rather, it is to provide an up to date view of the status of new breakthroughs and in the field of polymers in tissue engineering. This chapter focuses on aspects important to the engineering and design of polymeric biomaterials for use in functional tissue regeneration.

Market reports estimate a steadily increasing market for tissue engineered products through 2016 at an $85 billion dollar market worldwide. While some polymers + cell products have been on the market for over a decade (mostly in the wound healing arena), there are emerging areas wherein more polymeric tissue engineering products will likely move to the marketplace. These emerging areas are likely in tissue engineered blood vessels, neurological regeneration, and hydbrid assist devices for the lung or liver. The general concepts of tissue engineering with polymers are shifting focus from the polymeric scaffolds to not merely be a structure, but to become an active template to guide cellular growth and differentiation. This emerging understanding of cellular signaling in response to polymeric matrices is shaping the field of tissue engineering. Material science technology advances in arenas of three dimensional bioprinting, new hybrid biopolymers, and complex microfluidics will also continue to shape the field.

Polymer Processing Techniques to Mimic Tissue Architecture and Strength

Proper tissue growth, function, and adaptation have as much to do with the architecture of the extracellular matrix as it does with the cells that populate the tissue. Skin without elasticity is a strait-jacket. A lung without branching bronchi is a wet paper bag. Bone without intricately-connected canals through concentric layers of hydroxyapatite and buttressed by trabeculae is a ceramic coffee cup waiting to be smashed. The biological polymers which form the shape and scaffold of the organ cells are not merely blank shelves; the very architecture and mechanical properties of the polymer scaffold signal the cells on them to perform specific tasks and grow to a specific form within the confines of a specific scaffold. When the scaffold architecture fails to contain the cells on them, free-floating blobs of bio-matter can form thrombi, cysts, or tumors. When the scaffold mechanical properties fail to fit the requirements of function, the cells react by reacting with inflammation or scarring that destroy the function. And when mal-processed scaffolds fail to provide the proper signals to the attaching integrins of the cell, the health and shape of the cells deteriorate in like-step with the engineered organ as a whole.

This section addresses the current polymer processing techniques used to create engineered extracellular matrix (ECM) for cells that provide the appropriate architecture and mechanical properties for cells, while maintaining the appropriate embedded cell-signaling molecules. Each material and processing method (gelation, heat or high voltage extruding, printing, or biological formation) each have their own strengths and weaknesses. We will also briefly cover current strategies in accounting for material processing weaknesses by combining techniques.

Hydrogel Polymers with Self-Assembled Nanostructure

The versatility of hydrogels makes them one of the most popularly studied and medically applied polymers in the tissue engineering field. Hydrogels, which are polymers suspended in water, are apt for perfusing with hydrophilic nutrients and growth factors that will diffuse to the residing cells. Because the material is often processed from an aqueous state, they can be physiologically safe for suspended cells during and after the processing of the material which takes it from viscous fluid to gel. The hydrophilic diffusion and aqueous beginnings of this polymer make it uniquely suited for encapsulating cells deep within the scaffold from the initial constitution of the polymer. The ability to be injected also give hydrogels a unique advantage over numerous polymers in clinical applications where surgery would like to be avoided.

However, it is worth noting that although numerous organs have a soft and flexible consistency, only a few tissues (such as bone marrow or the nucleus pulposus of the intervertebral disc) have mechanical properties comparable to hydrogels. When compared to most tissues, hydrogels have numerous mechanical compatibility issues which are related the material's fabrication and processing. Hydrogels can break apart due to stresses such as compression or sheering, their ability to degrade has to be balanced to their physiological function, their ability to diffuse nutrients and factors is difficult to regulate, and controlling those factors often sacrifice biological functions. The mechanical properties of hydrogels are measured with storage modulus $\mathbf{E'}$, the amount of energy a gel can store as elasticity without permanent deformation, and the loss modulus $\mathbf{E''}$, the energy dissipated as heat. For example, a sheep's nucleus pulposus has a mean storage modulus of $E' = 64{,}000$ Pa, and a loss modulus of $E'' = 23{,}000$ Pa [1]. A gel with the bare minimum of practical use has a storage modulus of at least E′ > 1 Pa [2]. To address those issues, there are various molecular designs and hydrogel processing techniques.

Picking-up on one of nature's own methods of assembly, self-assembling peptides are amino acid sequences which use the charges of the side groups to attract another strand and form strong van der Waal interactions. One of the simplest strategies is to use strands of alternating sequences of hydrophobic and hydrophilic amino acids which form β-sheets [3, 4], one of the major secondary structures in a protein. Repeating sequences of peptides can also form bonds with itself to form α-helices hydrogels [5]. Peptides can also be tethered with other non-amino segments, such as hydrophobic carbon chains, to form polar molecules with a hydrophobic and hydrophilic side. These amphiphilic molecules assemble in a similar fashion to a micelle or liposome and form hydrophilic fibers with hydrophobic cores [6]. With peptide-based gels, modifying the amino acid sequence affects the inter-molecular bonds. For example, basic physics tells us that positive charges are attracted to negative charges, and vice versa. Positively charged amino acids such as Arginine (R) and Lysine (K) are patterned with negatively charged residues such as Aspartic Acid (D) and Glutamic Acid (E) on the same or differing peptides. Varying the quantity and pattern of repeating ionic amino acid residues will change the mechanical properties [7]; however, longer peptides does not necessarily mean stronger peptides [8] so a proper balance between interacting molecules and unwieldy size must be struck. Much like varying the quantity of charged amino acid residues, varying the length of the hydrophobic and hydrophilic components of an amphiphilic molecule will change the degree of interaction between molecules, and vary the mechanical properties and structure of the hydrogel [9, 10]. The concentration of the peptide in solution will also affect the amount of molecular interaction, and thus an increase in peptide concentration will usually increase the storage modulus of a hydrogel [4, 11]. Because hydrogels initially start as a suspension of molecules in a viscous solution, the final result is usually a haphazard arrangement of fibers and molecules distributed by Brownian motion. One molecular level is to use electromagnetic fields to process the material. Peptide hydrogel fibers have been shown to align along a magnetic field [12]. This provides physical cues at the molecular level to proliferating cells.

The degree of interaction between peptides is also affected by the ionic environment. Changing the pH [4] or concentration of ionic salts [13] in solution will also affect the inter-molecular bonds between the peptides, modifying the mechanical properties of the hydrogel. A simple demonstration of this principle is the isoelectric point of a protein, where at a particular pH a peptide will lose charge (like and repulsive charges) and aggregate together. Temperature also affects the mechanical properties of gels. Not only can gelation be induced by change in temperature, the temperature at which gelation is induced (by alternative means such as pH or concentration) affects that mechanical properties of the material [14].

In most biological circumstances, a physiological pH, ionic balance, and temperature is needed for cell culture in a hydrogel. So while this usually doesn't affect tissue culture, which is usually at physiologic conditions, this is important to remember when you are testing mechanical properties outside the culture environment.

Chemical cross-linkers and photo-sensitive chemical processes can also cross-link peptide hydrogels to initiate gelation and strengthen bonds. Ultraviolet light breaks peptide and other bonds which then re-form, but the biological function of the modified material must be tested due to the random nature with which the bonds are broken. Chemicals such as gluteraldehyde are strong cross-linking agents with a known toxicity, and thus alternative "natural" cross-linkers such as transglutaminase and genipin are being investigated [15].

By modulating properties such as temperature and pH to maintain the solution-state, the concentration of the hydrogel's solutes can be increased without inducing gelation. The temperature or pH can then be modified back to the desired state, and the hydrogel formation will have a concentration or property that may not have otherwise been attainable. However, the process should be careful not to permanently denature the peptide during heating or changing pH, as the molecular or biomechanical properties may not be what were expected if the peptides are damaged by high temperature or variation from neutral pH. Another strategy for inducing gelation is mixing different combinations of similar peptides. A peptide sequence with a biological function may not be conducive to forming a gel, but when combined with a similar peptide with stronger mechanical properties the combination can have intermediate qualities in mechanics [2] and biological activity.

Spun, Extruded, and Crosslinked Polymers with Arranged Nanostructure

Even though most natural biological polymers are microscopic, with dimensions on the order of nanometers, they often assemble into a macroscopic structure that can be seen with the naked eye. The connective tissue of muscle, tendons, cartilage, and skin can appear stringy when stretched and teased apart. Even bone, lung, nerve, and other tissue have apparent millimeter-scale structures which belie the fact that their true functional units are really much smaller.

Extrusion and spinning are material processing methods that long-predates micron-level materials engineering. The simplest example of extrusion is pushing dough through a press to create strings of noodle-like polymers. Spinning is best exemplified by exerting centripetal force on melted sugar to form cotton candy. In both examples, there is a force pushing the material in one direction (either a press, a spinner, or even an electromagnetic force), and another force pulling the opposite direction (the mold or molecular forces). When a balance is achieved between those pushing and pulling forces, the material forms a fiber which can resemble the stringy material found in tissue. These macro-scale materials can very closely match the topography and mechanical properties of biological tissue, including porosity for the diffusing nutrients and isotropic or anisotropic strength (force-bearing in single or multiple directions). The modern challenge of tissue-targeted polymer engineering is incorporating the unseen physical cues of nano-scale components (such as collagen fibers) of the milli-scale materials (a collagen fibril). Beyond the mechanical properties, incorporating biological components are also challenging; the solvents and environments used to process the polymers for extrusion and spinning can be corrosive to the organic material. Synthetic polymers are also fundamentally problematic because the most common and versatile polymers are almost exclusively hydrophobic, a property which cells and other biological components respond to poorly. Fortunately, there are strategies to overcome those issues and more-closely mimic natural tissue.

Electrospinning

Electrospinning as a material fabrication process has existed for decades to create a densely-woven mesh of fibers. What makes this process unique is that the fiber diameters achieved by electrospinning are much smaller, down to several nanometers in diameter, compared to other synthetic polymer synthesis methods. New and creative means to applying the electrospinning process has led to numerous potential applications for tissue engineering. The process resembles extrusion in that the material in solution is usually pressed out of a syringe before forming a fiber. However, the process of using a syringe is optional (for example, rolling drums of polymer can be used for mass-production methods [16]), because the true material "extrusion" comes from the electromagnetic force on the solution which pulls molecules out of solution and towards a collection site. As the solvent evaporates around the solute, the molecules of the polymer pull with it a chain of polymer which forms the deposited fibers at the collection site. If there is too much electric force, too little molecular attraction between the solute molecules, too much distance for the polymer to travel, or not enough polymer at the site where the solution is being charged, the fiber becomes discontinuous or just deposits as droplets at the collection site. The rate at which polymer is placed into the field of electricity (often controlled by a syringe pump), the distance between polymer source and collection, and the environmental conditions such as temperature and humidity all affect the mechanical properties of the electrospun fibers [17]. The type of polymer, the solvent, and the concentration vary greatly. The method of collecting the fibers serve as one of the final processing steps for electrospinning which determines mechanical properties, and these methods vary greatly.

The classical method of collecting electrospun fibers is to place a grounded sheet of metal opposite the charged source with the polymer. This creates a dense, isotropic (all-directional), mat of fibers. This structure tends to lack space between the fibers, and important feature if cell migration into the material is desired, but strategies such as adding dissolvable fibers [18, 19], leaching inorganic salts [20, 21] or other particulates [22], or even jets of air [23] at the site of collection mechanically create some space for residents cells on the material to grow into. However, while many human tissues have significant thickness and require a length and depth of cells on an extracellular matrix, it is important to consider that many tissues (such as epithelial cell-based tissue) are single-layered, and a basement membrane which isn't penetrable by cells is important for proper morphology of attached cells [24].

Collection doesn't have to be a static process. By rotating the collector in the axis perpendicular to the incoming fiber at increasing velocities, the direction of the fibers collected increase in their alignment perpendicular to the axis of rotation [25]. Put simply: the faster the collector rotates towards the polymer source, the more aligned the collected fibers are in the direction of rotation. This is key for a number of tissues that have anisotropic (single-directed) properties such as connective tissue and nerves, as the direction the fibers are arranged serve as the guide for the proliferating and extending cells [26, 27].

When processing the electrospun fibers into suitable scaffolding for cell culture, the forces don't have to be applied as the fibers come to rest. Strategies for manipulating the fibers mid-air have been devised to create more complex structures. Manipulation of the electric field by using curved collection plates and point-probes can create turbulence as the fibers approaches the collection site, causing the electrospun fibers to tangle before coming to rest [28]. The result is a material which is not packed as tightly as sheets of fibers and resembles a cotton ball. Air-collecting electrospun fibers can also produce aligned scaffold between conductive points [29] or directed by a combination of blower and electric fields to a non-conductive target [30].

The fibers themselves can be modified significantly in the way they are processed. The emulsion of immiscible liquids which are then electrospun creates fibers with a core of one type and a surface of another type. If the internal material is dissolvable, it creates a hollow core [31]. And additives to the polymer do not have to be removed. Blends of inorganic and organic material, which can be purified [32] or heterogenous extracellular matrix components [33], can add bioactive components for interacting cells or change the material's mechanical and chemical properties.

The choice of material for any materials processing method can lead to a dilemma with the choice of solvent. In electrospinning, the polarity (polar or non-polar), relative permittivity (or dielectric permittivity, the force between two points in a material), conductivity, and viscosity affect the fiber diameter of the final product [34, 35]. Materials such as polycaprolactone, poly-lactic acid, and poly-ethylene oxide are generally very soluble in any organic solvent, but more complex or organic materials such as collagen may have a smaller range of acceptable solvents [36], and the types of solvents used may be harsher on the material's final biological composition. While there are some examples of non-toxic solvents used for biological materials [37], any solvent should be fully dried via desiccation or other means to ensure the removal of solvent. Sterilization procedures, whether it is ethanol washing or other biochemical processes, should also consider the effects on the final material's mechanical and biological properties [38, 39].

Extruding and Printing

Melt extrusion is a cost-effective means of producing a number of structures, and for applications in science and medicine melt extrusion is useful in pharmacology with drug delivery [40, 41]. However, achieving the nano-scale detail in architecture is difficult with this method compared to other processes, but there are other advantages. With the explosion of affordable home desktop 3D printing options (either home-made or commercial), it was inevitable that tissue engineering applications would be found. But even before the recent advances, the paper-thin process of ink printing was just as applicable when printing sheets of cells. Synthetic materials can be printed as melted extrusions or powders with binder. Printing biomaterials with or without cells involves computer-controlled positioning of a nozzle connected to a material source composed of liquid or hydrogel and guided to a target either by gravity and charge (such as in Fluorescent-Assisted Cell Sorting) or by laser (remember that photons can impart a force). The end result is controlled positioning of biomaterial and/or cells in a pattern that can mimic the tissue of choice. Two challenges facing this method is what would be expected from any type of prototypical printer: accuracy and resolution. Also, because natural tissue is interconnected, connecting the individual depositions of biomaterial to accurately impart mechanical properties is another challenge to be tackled.

Creating an anatomically-shaped scaffold is relatively simple for a 3D printer. A computer-aided X-ray tomography (CT) of a patient's bone can be converted to a 3D model and replicated as porous melt-extruded polycaprolactone [42] in a day. Fortunately, materials such as porous PCL has similar mechanical properties (compressive modulus and yield strength) to trabecular bone [43]. Because bone tissue grows heals itself when set properly, bone tissue engineering appears relatively forgiving of shortcomings in nano-structural material characteristics. Powders deposited by a 3D printer can also create shapes that are bioactive and have a range of mechanical properties dependent on the pore sizes and structures created; however, the ceramic-like materials powders such as calcium phosphate often produced tend to be very brittle and not suited for load-bearing [44]. Improvements to the flexural strength and bioactive properties in printing of calcium phosphate powders has been made by adding collagen and an emulsifier to the binder [45].

Biologically Generated Polymers

Synthetic materials and the processing that goes with it give the tissue engineer a degree of control over the process; however, there are still many things that cells construct better than our best designed equipment. Decellularized tissues have been used as implants for bone, tendons, ligaments, and heart valves for many years now. Some grafts are wholly-accepted by the body and incorporate the patient's cells. Other grafts, such as heart valves, have to be processed in a way that destroys the biological signaling in order to serve their mechanical function and never integrate into the recipient. Using decellularized organs as the biopolymer for tissue engineering come with a number of advantages: the remaining polymer is mechanically and morphologically similar to the original organ, the polymer has bio-active molecules matching what the native tissue would expect.

However, the availability of human-sourced tissue is limited and potentially controversial, and animal sources can have important differences compared to their human counter-parts.

Tissues are decellularized using a several different approaches, sometimes in combination with one another, which effectively remove the overwhelming majority of all cells and cellular material from the extracellular matrix architecture. These techniques include the use physical techniques such as snap freezing or mechanical agitation, and chemical techniques such as using ionic or non-ionic detergents, zwitterionic detergents, basic or acidic solutions, and hypotonic or hypertonic solutions [1]. Depending on the methods used the leftover scaffold will retain mechanical components (elastin, collagen), natural binding sites, and growth factors in different quantities; some decellularization methods are better at retaining certain components over others [1–3]. Equally important to the methods or solutions used for decellularization is the process used to expose the intact tissue. Tissues composed of complex architecture or expansive vasculature will most likely benefit from a perfusion decellularization system where the vasculature is perfused with detergent as well. This works especially well with lung decellularization where the pulmonary artery as well as the trachea can be cannulated [4, 5]. Thin tissues such as bladder or skin can be decellularized using an immersion process where the tissue is suspended in the decellularization solution [6]. Thick tissues or organs can be decellularized using immersion processes as well; however they must first be cut into thin strips. Both immersion and perfusion techniques can benefit from constant flow or agitation provided from a decellularization bioreactor [4, 7].

To exploit the biochemical benefit from naturally-derived polymers, it isn't always necessary to wholesale incorporate the entire molecule. Specific peptide sequences from laminin such as RGD [46–49] and YIGSR [46, 48, 50] or from elastin like VAPG [51] have been isolated as cell-interacting sequences. These molecules can be chemically tethered to synthetic polymers by means such as carbodiimide chemistry [46], click chemistry [50], or custom-designed by synthesizing peptides with Fmoc chemistry [2]. Biologically derived polymers don't have to be for cell attachment, but for other enzymatic processes such as degradation if cell-regulated metalloproteinase cleavage is desired [2, 8]. While this doesn't directly affect the mechanical properties or architecture of a polymer scaffold, it does allow for greater biological activity of polymers that may have desired mechanical and architectural features you can't achieve with biologically-derived polymers.

Combining Techniques

It is unlikely that a single solution can be found to solve the problems of tissue engineering. Our own organic tissue is not merely deposited by cells, but requires techniques to compartmentalize the material, mechanical and biological signals to direct the orientation, and particularly arranged charges within specific environments to induce assembly of the raw biological material. A truly biomimetic approach to tissue engineering involves incorporating multiple polymer processing techniques to form the desired shape, micro-architecture, strength, and cell interaction needed to form tissue just as nature intended.

For example, while electrospun nanofiberous material of synthetic polymers can be mass produced and have a tune-able properties, they often lack biological motifs and hydrophilic chemistry that a cell is accustomed to. Hydrogels and biological polymers can be much more similar to the cell's native environment, but far more difficult to tune mechanically. However, by coating an electrospun scaffold with peptides in hydrogels new biological properties are given to the electrospun scaffold, and new mechanical properties are given to what was originally just a hydrogel material [48].

While decellularized organs to produce ECM provide ready-made scaffolding, the end result might not be the ideal material for the purposes. Instead of a porous organ, a hydrogel encapsulating the cells may be more feasible for culture. However, taking an example from hydrogel synthesis and processing, ECM after processing by proteases can reform as a hydrogel, providing the cell-interactive motifs and growth factors of normally-decellularized ECM [52].

The use of a method for fabricating a material doesn't have to be used exclusively for fabrication. While 3D printing is known for producing a material or object from the ground-up, the method can also be used to print on and over other materials. An example of this is using a 3D printer to deposit hydrogels onto a mold, and then use the printer to apply cells [53].

Fusing the spatial customization of 3D printing with the fiber diameters of electrospinning, short-range high-voltage polymer extruding through a computer-controlled nozzle across a high voltage electrical field can create customizable micro-fiber structures with controlled pore sizes [54, 55]. While not quite yet at a level where printed nano-resolution structures are a reality, innovative ideas are marching towards that goal.

Processing a material to mimic tissue architecture and strength requires planning at the material composition phase, the scaffold synthesis phase, the sterilization phase, and even the cell impregnation and attachment phase. While this section provides an overview of the considerations and processes available, a thorough understanding of the architecture of the tissue of you want to create, and a grasp of the biological necessities needed for those cells, are the most critical pieces of knowledge needed when performing your own research to determine what you need to do to produce the appropriately processed biomaterial.

Polymers as Cell Scaffolds

The perfect polymer structure shaped exactly like organ tissue down to an angstrom-level of detail is completely worthless if the cell does not respond to the material. A cell has integrins, cadherins, cytoskeletons, growth factor receptors, and more components that respond to the environment around them. If the cell feels that the polymers surrounding it do not properly engage its chemo-mechanical sensors, then that cell will respond either by changing itself or dying. Cells do have the capacity to shape their own environment and produce collagen, integrins, elastin, fibronectin, or their own growth factors to shape their environment and the surrounding cells. Unfortunately, the cell's process of adapting itself and its environment to better suit itself is often permanent, changing the cell so that it cannot re-adapt itself to a better environment and form the functional tissue which it was intended to be.

This section will address the various responses cells have to polymers and their architecture. We will address the polymer's biochemistry, mechanical force, and nano-scale features that cells can detect and adapt as a result. We will also note that every tissue has differences, and this means in different tissue engineering techniques for different cell and tissue types.

Cell Response to Polymers

"Putting lipstick on a pig" is a clever idiom that drives home an important point: it is much more difficult to make something attractive if you start with something very unattractive. While synthetic polymers such as polycaprolactone, poly-lactic acid, or almost anything with "poly" on it, is often easier and cheaper to synthesize, process, and shape, there are numerous considerations that are negative for the living cell. First, these easy-to-process polymers are often hydrophobic, which means that the cell membrane and its outward-facing hydrophilic molecules will be repelled by the polymer surface. Second, these polymers are repeating blocks of the same molecule which has little familiarity or meaning to the cells exposed to them. A cell on the surface is just as likely to see these polymers as a foreign object rather than a structure fit to become an organ.

Early scaffold designs with materials such as polycaprolactone focused on the cell's ability to penetrate a scaffold's porous network and proliferate, and for certain cells such as fibroblasts and the periosteal cells used to coating bone this was all that was needed to produce impressive results [56]. However, the addition of natural polymers such as collagen [57] or synthetic peptides nanofibers that coat hydrophobic polymers [48] were shown to improve the proliferative properties of the scaffold over bare polymer. Mesenchymal stem cells cultured in pro-chondrogenic media on electrospun nanofibers made with a blend of polycaprolactone and ECM derived from cultured MSCs expressed more pro-chondrogenic gene activity [58]. While the physical and mechanical architecture of scaffolds is critical, if the cell can't properly attach to the polymer used then the engineering is all for naught. While a strategy to improve interaction between cells and synthetic ECM involves wholesale addition of components such as collagen and elastin or heterogeneous ECM, more targeted strategies involve the functional modification of polymers with cell-responsive amino acid sequences. Laminin-derived RGD and YIGSR for cells such as cardiac muscle showed greater adhesion and contractile fiber expression [46], and elastin-derived VAPG appears to be selective for smooth muscle [51].

Cell Response to Polymer Architecture and Mechanical Properties

Building a house on a foundation of sand is a bad idea for an obvious reason: it washes away. But assuming the house is far away from the ocean, the inevitable result is that parts of the frame, or skeleton, of the house will lack a structure to rest on and shift, resulting in the movement and cracking of any wall or shelf or portrait lying on that part of the frame. The extracellular matrix of tissue is both a foundation and a frame: it serves as the foundation for cells upon which rest their cytoskeleton, and it serves as the direction and structure of the organ tissue upon which the organ's features are patterned and positioned. A solid and firm foundation for certain tissues' cells makes sense: bone is hard and firm, a liver or a pancreas is a mechanically static organs, and kidneys don't go anywhere (unless you are giving one away). However, unlike a house, many organs exist in a constant state of movement and tension: lungs and bladders expand and contract, blood vessels and neurons stretch with the movement of our body, muscles and tendons pull on our bones, and even bone responds to the muscles' site of tension by forming tubercles. Function does manifest form in a cell's response to polymer scaffolds, and with this knowledge mechanical properties and architecture is being engineered into new polymer designs not just to mimic the target organ tissue, but because the cells require it for proper development.

Fibers are emphasized in tissue engineering because the collagen and elastin proteins that cells reside on are fibers. The evolutionary reason for this is likely out of convenience, as the building blocks of all life (amino acids, nucleic acids, carbohydrates) arrange themselves as either single or branched chain polymers. Architecturally, fibers are the logical scaffold component because they provide physical directional cues, size differences, mechanical force direction, and differences in density of packing for porosity. Cells have biochemical means (known or apparent) to detect or affect each of those parameters.

Architecture

Fiber arrangement is a critical cue for cell growth patterns. We know that mesenchymal cells [59, 60], neurons [29, 61], smooth muscle [62], even breast cancer cells [63], and likely other cells types grow along an axis cued by the substrate they grow upon. Cells which form solid tissue possess integrins, membrane-bound composed of two subunits (α and β) that bind to particular amino acid sequences found on the ECM components. Integrins are biochemically linked to a number of cell signaling pathways, but physically they are attached to α-actinin or talin and/or vinculin, which then links it to the cell's thin filament actin which is a critical regulator of cell shape. This serves as a biochemical and physical link to the scaffold on the outside [64], and cell with mutations causing deficits in the binding capabilities between actin and vinculin demonstrate cell spreading deficits [65].

Cells not only grow and align their cytoskeleton in the direction they are pointed, but they also express genes and produce proteins because of their alignment (or lack thereof). For neurons, fiber alignment increases the expression of a myelin-specific gene for the neural-insulating Schwann cells [66] and increases pro-neuron gene expression in stem cells [50]. For bone tissue engineering, aligned fibers increases cell-to-cell junctions [67] and osteogenic markers for mineralization [67, 68]. Endothelial cells, which form the inner walls of blood vessels and capillaries, increase the expression of cell-to-cell connecting cadherins and are less likely to detach under fluid shearing [69]. It is important to note that the cells which benefit from fiber alignment are cells that require alignment of some sort. Using grooved culture plates, it was shown that fibroblasts are more responsive in their growth to designed culture templates than epithelial cells [70]. This is sensible because epithelial tissue like skin, lung, and GI are regularly enduring forces in all directions. While most tissue (such as bone) will receive force perpendicular to their normal axis of alignment, those tissue often rely on inherent material properties to bend and not break. Bone, muscle, and vessels are designed for pulling and shearing forces in a particular direction, and their axis of orientation is sensible for that purpose therefore their cellular biochemistry to respond to directionality.

Fiber diameter is also an important component to tissue engineered architecture which cells respond to. Collagen starts as a trimer tropocollagen fibril 1.5 nm in diameter, but bundles into fibrils with diameters from 10 to 500 nm apparent under SEM, and further bundles into macroscopic fibers up to 100 μm in diameter [71]. How the cell responds to fiber diameter depends on the cell type, but the size of collagen fiber bundles give us a hint as to what the threshold is. Endothelial cells cultured on fibers with diameters of 300 and 1,200 nm proliferated more than endothelial cells cultured on fiber mats greater than 7 μm [72]. Bone marrow derived mesenchymal cells expressed more markers for several ECM materials when cultured on 300 nm diameter fibers compares to 2.3 μm diameter fibers [60]. Smaller does seem to be better, and this would correlate with the diameter of collagen fibrils, but an exception seems to be neurite extensions from neurons, which did not extend as far on 300 nm diameter fibers compared to 800+ nm diameter fibers [73]. This leaves plenty of room for theorizing as to what a cell is looking for in its foundation, but it is likely different for every cell and tissue type, and some logical inferences will likely help in this exploration. For cells that are looking to cover area, such as epithelial and endothelial cells, their basement membranes and densely packed and impenetrable (unless those cells become cancerous and metastatic). For cells like neurons reaching around and between tissue to find organ, the topology and architecture for their scaffolds will likely serve that purpose better. And as new techniques for scaffold design create smaller details, a critical eye towards how the material or its breakdown products could potentially mimic irritant ultrafine particulate matter (<100 nm) and upset immune modulators should be considered [74].

Mechanical Properties

We use the mechano-sensitive biochemistry of cells daily. Although our brain interprets mechanical properties through special force-sensitive neurons, individual muscle cells also detect tension and will grow or atrophy in response. Non-muscle cells do their own force and tension sensing, and respond to the firmness or softness of their substrate by the mechanical forces transduced through ECM-binding integrins to the internal proteins such as talin, vinculin, paxillin, actin and myosin [75]. Tension through these proteins result in phosphorylation of these proteins and activation of downstream pathways [76, 77]. The degree to which cells can sense mechanical resistance can be quite sensitive: mesenchymal stem cells will spread out and flatten over a firm surface (as determined by cytoskeletal actin staining), but place a soft gel over the surface and the degree to which the cell stays compact and rounded correlates with the thickness of the gel with a sensitivity of approximately 20 μm before the cell struggles to sense the hard surface below [78]. Spreading is fine for cells the need to cover a surface or an injury, but cardiac myocytes demonstrate that they have better organized contractile fibers and more calcium stores for contraction [79], although there does appear to be a threshold for the degree of stiffness which best functionally controls cardiac myocytes [80]. Bone remodeling is an example of cells that respond to create their environment, proliferating on hard surfaces, and mineralizing softer material [81].

When testing these properties in designed scaffolds, do take note that varying one property can affect the other. Fiber diameter, polymer types, and additives can affect the mechanical properties such as strength and density of the scaffold, and it can be difficult to tease out which of these is the cause of the phenotype change in the cell [72]. These measurement techniques are outlined in Sect. "Polymer material properties and functional tissue replacement".

Hidden Cell-Modulating Molecules in Polymers

Before polymer customization and scaffold design was an important part of what is now called tissue engineering, biologists and physiologists were trying to elucidate the molecules animal tissue needed to grow. The original tissue engineering was determining what to coat a dish with for the cells to attach and to add extracts of blood for the proper growth factors. Diligent research developed pre-treated plastics for attachment and an assortment of growth mediums specific for cell types. Standards for tissue culture techniques allowed for experimentation with the substrates these cells were grown upon. As the field matures and tissue engineering combines synthetic processes with natural processes and polymers, we are discovering that our own native polymers have growth factors of their own, separate from the traditional soluble factors.

Collagen is a significant component of the extracellular matrix, and breakdown of the ECM inevitably releases collagen fragments. These fragments could have implications that should be considered when designing a polymer scaffold with these components. Collagen 6A3 when expressed leads to the loss of contact-inhibited growth [82], and soluble collagen 1 encourages pancreatic cancer spread and migration in a similar fashion to pro-cancer myofibroblasts [83]. Laminin $\chi 2$ chain, a component of a cell-adhesive ligand for integrins important in modulating cell attachment and migration, can also activate the epidermal growth factor receptor when processed and solubilized [84, 85]. Hyaluronan can also be released from ECM breakdown; hyaluronan serve as a potent immune signaling molecule through TLR4 [86], and as a pro-fibrotic agent via CD44 on the cell surface [87].

The inherent cell-modulating peptides and molecules in a polymer scaffold can also mimic the pathology they come from. Whole-lung of mice treated with pro-fibrotic agents and then homogenized and used as a coating over synthetic polymer nanofibers induced pro-fibrotic gene expression in bone marrow-derived cells [88]. This research does not specify whether the causative agent in the lung homogenate is trapped soluble factors or a change in the composition of the ECM, but it does highlight that not all ECM is alike, even between the same organ. Changes in the ECM's composition affect the way cells respond.

It is very difficult to control for every possible circumstance in material, synthetic or naturally-derived. It is important to be aware of what can happen, and consider the possibilities if cells do not respond to an environment as expected. Considerations for polymer effects need not be limited to influencing the cells they are designed to contain. For example, the inclusion of polyphenols into polymer coatings scavenge free radicals and prevent immune destruction of implanted cells such as sensitive pancreatic beta islet cells [89]. Having a strong knowledge of the biology of your scaffold, your cell, and any factor that can interact with it will help lead to an effective and medically feasible design.

Polymers as Cell Scaffolds Beyond Regenerative Medicine

As scientific knowledge advances, we are running out of simple solutions to serious diseases and problems. Most research into the physiology of a disease state relies on a model to experiment upon without actually running sacrificial experiments on ailing patients. Where a tissue culture doesn't quite meet our needs, a mouse or larger mammal might suit the purposes (with some ethical questions and serious monetary costs) but at the expense of losing the control of a culture and the subtle differences between primate and rodent biology. This is where polymers as cell scaffolds and tissue engineering techniques can make an immediate impact in medicine before the regulations and hurdles of product development are met and crossed for human medical consumption. Human tissue engineered in realistic models can provide the native response of our own species in a life-like environment. Short of a whole human, these types of models can give a more realistic picture of cell-level human physiology. The three-dimensional design of scaffolds better allows for determining how tumor cell-to-matrix interactions work compared to tissue culture [90]. Scaffolds with depth and thickness provide a better model for angiogenesis [91], a potentially powerful target in many solid tumor treatments. Like any other cell, cancer responds to mechanical cues, both tension [92] and fiber direction [63], which serves as another potential target considering. While it is important to use appropriate cell types specific for the pathology being investigated, the use of fibrotic lung ECM with a tissue-engineered polymer to induce fibrotic characteristics in mesenchymal cells [88] is a potential model for pulmonary fibrosis that allows for a degree of control that is difficult to match in a mouse model.

As with any research, the way you design and control your experiment will determine the insight you can get. With polymer scaffold design, you create avenues of research that can be controlled far better than live models, yet can provide a closer picture to reality than by remaining inside a glass dish. Many advances in tissue engineering will provide the most benefit to human health by providing a more-accurate in vitro testing platform.

Polymers as Drug or Growth Factor Delivery for Tissue Regeneration

Polymers have a dynamic range of applications and are essential to the design and innovation of the next generation of drug delivery, release, and targeting systems. Polymers as drug delivery systems exploit the capability to tailor their properties by modifying the components, method of assembly, or mechanism of release. These are important concepts such as the physical and material properties, solubility, biodegradability, drug release kinetics, and ability to sense and respond to environmental conditions/stimuli. Some of the main polymer systems used in drug delivery include polymeric micelles for drug delivery, dendrimers, hydrogels, and other scaffolds or implants. This section will discuss important concepts in design of polymers for drug delivery, specific polymer drug delivery systems, and approaches for drug delivery to clinical targets in tissue regeneration.

Important Concepts in Drug Delivery in Tissue Engineering

The *physical* and *mechanical properties* of drug delivery systems are essential in matching the needs of the target. For example, one useful property of macromolecules used in drug delivery for cancer is that they have the passive ability to accumulate in tumors due to increased accumulation of serum due to leaky vasculature in the tumor and decreased lymphatic drainage [93]. Other important physical properties include: ability to mimic the tissue stiffness, implants without corners, carriers small enough to cross membranes, or even large enough to keep them out of certain tissues.

Biodegradability and compatibility are important considerations for drug delivery system. For a polymer to be *biodegradable* it requires there to be hydrolytically or proteolytically breakable bonds in the backbone or as a cross linker. Degradation reactions are often non-linear because the degradation products of the polymer are acidic and catalyze an increase in degradation [94]. One major advantage of polymer bound drug conjugates is their increased blood circulation time resulting from their ability to escape filtration by the kidney. The potential downfall of escaping kidney filtration is over exposure of the drug to the body. However, carriers are often biodegradable in serum conditions, and the time before the polymer is broken down can be controlled through its design. Drug delivery vehicles in solution or as an implant need to be easily broken down to prevent accumulation and a chronic inflammatory response [95]. If the vehicle is non-toxic and degradable, new tissue will readily heal. However if the vehicle is non-degradable or inert, it could be contained in a fibrous capsule by the body [95]. Biodegradability can also be used as a mechanism for controlling drug release over time, for example systems using poly lactic acid (PLA) and poly lactic co-glycolic acid (PLGA) allow the designer to determine the degradation time based on the ratio of lactide and glycolide polymer components [96]. An additional consideration when designing biodegradable polymers is that the degradation products should be non-toxic and small enough to be cleared through natural mechanisms. Products that are not cleared could build up in tissues and cause toxic or inflammatory reactions [94]. Toxicity assessment is detailed in Sect. "Polymer material properties and functional tissue replacement".

Control over the release kinetics of drugs from polymer drug delivery systems is paramount in design. Regulation of drug release is the most important separation from traditional drug delivery in which the drug levels in the blood or tissue increases during administration, peak, and then decline rapidly making it difficult to navigate between toxic or ineffective levels of the drug in vivo [97]. Release kinetics can be controlled by the system used sequester the drug, the polymer components, the amount of drug in the delivery vehicle, and environmental conditions. Controlled release systems improve the effectiveness of delivery by modifying the release profile of the drug, ability to cross biological barriers, bio distribution, clearance, and stability [98]. This level of control is especially useful when the natural distribution of the drug would cause side effect by interaction with non-target tissues and if normal administration does not allow the drug to reach its site of activity due to degradation [98].

An especially exciting research thrust is in the area of responsive or externally regulated delivery systems in which the polymer system containing the drug can be manipulated to increase release, pulse release, or stop release in response to a stimulus. Systems using this strategy are increasingly being referred to as smart scaffolds. Stimuli include temperature, pH, magnetic modulation, ultrasonic waves, or electrical stimulation [7, 9–12]. Smart polymers could provide unique solutions to old some of the most difficult challenges such as cancer drug delivery, specific tissue targeting, and direct control drug release [99].

Polymer Delivery Systems

Polymeric Micelles

Polymeric micelles are made up of hydrophilic and hydrophobic block copolymers in the form of a sphere in which the hydrophobic portions form the core and the hydrophilic regions form the shell. The hydrophobic structures in the middle of the micelles act as a reservoir for drugs, proteins, or DNA while the hydrophilic shell acts as an interface with the biologic environment. This allows for the solubility of otherwise non-soluble payloads [100].

Micelle-forming polymer drug conjugates are used to directly incorporate and stabilize a drug onto the polymer. The drug is attached to functional groups on the polymer backbone by hydrolysable chemical bonds. Depending on the number and location of functional groups single or multiple drug molecules can be attached to each micellar unit [100].

Instead of chemical attachment, drugs or growth factors can be sequestered in micellar nano-containers through hydrophobic interactions or hydrogen bonds with the polymer backbone. Several methods of encapsulation are used to incorporate drugs into micelle nano-containers. In the *dialysis method* the block polymers and drug are dissolved in an organic solvent and dialysis against water is used to gradually replace the organic solvent with water. The replacement with water causes the self-association of the block polymers resulting in the encapsulation of the drug within the micelle core. Non-loaded drug is removed through the dialysis bag while the drug loaded micelles are trapped inside [100, 101]. The *oil/water emulsion method* uses a selective solvent for the core polymers (hydrophobic) of pre-prepared micelles, and then drug dissolved in organic solvent is added to the micelle solution with agitation. The organic solvent is evaporated from the solution resulting in the encapsulation of the drug in the micelles [100]. The *solvent evaporation method* is performed by combining the drug and polymer in a volatile organic solvent followed by the complete evaporation of the solvent and resulting in a polymer and drug film. This and aqueous phase is then added to the film and agitated resulting in the encapsulation of the drug. While this method has scale-up advantage it can only be used in conjunction with block-polymer films that have high hydrophilic lipophilic balance values so it can be readily reconstituted in aqueous solution [100, 101]. The *co-solvent evaporation method* uses a volatile, water miscible, organic solvent to dissolve the drug and polymer. Encapsulation through self-assembly is caused by the addition of an aqueous phase followed by evaporation of the organic phase [100]. The final method for forming micelle nano-containers is the *freeze drying method*. This utilizes a freeze dryable organic solvent to dissolve the polymer and drug components, and then the solution is mixed with water and then freeze dried. Isotonic aqueous solution is added to the freeze dried product to create the drug encapsulated micelles. This method is useful for scale up, however the insolubility of some block polymers in freeze dryable organic solvent limits it uses [100].

Therapeutic drug molecules that carry charge can be delivered using polyion complex molecules in which drugs are incorporated into the micelle through electrostatic charge interactions between polymers and oppositely charged drugs/molecule. The association of the drug with the core-forming block polymer cause the self-assembly of polyion complex micelle [100].

Polymeric micelles have the potential to be useful for drug delivery as they can be tailored to specify biological destination, increase specificity to a certain organ/tissue, or make them responsive to a certain condition or stimulus [100]. Drug can be released from copolymer-drug conjugate micelles via two mechanisms; micellar disassociation and drug cleavage or water penetration into the micelle followed by drug diffusion form the micelle. Drug release from micellar nano-containers occurs solely through diffusion from the hydrophobic core, while polyion complex micelles release drug molecules though ion exchange. Polymeric Micelles are useful because they allow solubilization of hydrophobic drugs which allow them to deliver some of the most challenging molecules [102]. The relatively small size of the complexes, stability, and ability to be tailored for drug of choice make polymer micelles effective for drug delivery [100, 102].

Dendrimers

Dendrimers are a growing class of macromolecules which are known for their highly branched architecture and extensive surface functionality. Dendrimers are complex molecules and have a set architecture consisting of an interior core where branching will begin, and interior layer including several generations of repeating branched polymer units, and exterior layer attached to the outermost branched generations. These structures are often created by well-controlled reaction steps that contribute new molecules onto each layer resulting in a globular or spherical shape with 1–20 nm as the diameter range [103, 104]. Dendrimers benefit from unique properties including uniform size, extensive branching, water solubility, and multivalency that make them interesting prospects for many drug delivery applications.

Classically, there are two main methods for synthesizing dendrimers, the *divergent method*: growth originates from a core site and perpetuates radially branch by branch, and the *convergent growth process*: several dendrons are reacted with a multifunctional core to obtain the final dendrimer [103]. The divergent growth method begins with a core which is reacted with protecting branching sites. The protected groups are then removed and the free active sites are ready to react with an additional layer of branched polymers. The reaction is iterated until the desired size (branching) is obtained. The divergent method requires extensive monomer loading and chromatographic separation however is preferred method of many large scale producers. If the divergent growth method could be described as "inward-out", conversely the convergent growth process could be described as "outward-in". Convergent growth starts with what will become the outermost layer units and systematically works in by linking outermost units with monomers. Once optimal dendrimer size is obtained the massive branches are attached to a common core molecule resulting in a complete dendrimer [103]. The convergent growth process has the benefits of minimizing side reactions and the ability to control precise molecular weight and specific functional groups locations, as well as being easier to purify in the early stages. However this method is limited to production of lower order dendrimers and suffers from low yield when synthesizing larger structures [103].

Additional approaches have been developed and studied that build upon the major methods and address their disadvantages. The Hypercores and Branched

Monomers' growth method focuses on the speed of the dendrimer reactions. This method uses the pre-assembly of oligomeric units which can be combined to give dendrimers in fewer steps and/or higher yields. The Double exponential growth method allows for both divergent and convergent growth from a single starting material. The products are convergent and divergent trimers protected and repeated again for exponential growth. *Lego chemistry* uses highly functionalized cores and branched monomers to prepare phosphorus dendrimers. The method allows multiplication of terminal surface groups from 48 to 250 in just one step requiring minimum volume of solvent, easy purification, and environmentally non-hazardous byproducts. *Click chemistry* allows for dendrimers with multiple surface groups to be obtained with high purity and excellent yield [103, 104].

Dendrimers have been celebrated for their potential as a drug delivery tool due to their highly controlled branched and functionalized architecture, water solubility, nano-size, biocompatibility, ability to control peripheral charge (polyvalency), and drug release kinetics [103–106]. Dendrimers can be immediately introduced to blood circulation and can be absorbed across various epithelial barriers, although ideally design includes specific tissue targeting to increase therapeutic effect and decrease toxicity of free drugs in non-target organs [105].

Hydrogels

Hydrogels are defined as polymeric networks with a three dimensional architecture with the ability to absorb and sequester large amounts of water or biologic medium due to the presence of hydrophilic groups [107]. The hydrogel network can be hydrated to varying degrees depending on the environment and polymer composition. Commonly, hydrogels exhibit physical properties similar to actual tissues including low interfacial tension between the sequestered fluids and their environment. Additionally, instead of dissolving in an aqueous environment hydrogels tend to show a swelling behavior resulting from crosslinking in the structure. Crosslinks are classified as either physical or chemical and are the result of colvalent bonds, hydrogen bonds, van der Waals interactions, and physical entanglements [107]. Hydrogels can often be readily tailored to control mechanical properties, release kinetics, and degradation rate. Additionally, a class of "smart" hydrogels can be designed to respond to environmental cues to increase or decrease drug release through a specific, physical or chemical, stimuli/gradient [107]. Modern hydrogel research with respect to biologic use first started in 1960 and in the last decade the number of publications discussing the topic has increased exponentially. Recent advances and interest in using "smart" polymer systems is also driving research in the field [108].

Hydrogel use hinges on the polymers used in the system as well the the technique for formation and cross linking. *Chemical crosslinking* is effective at making mechanically stable hydrogels, the chemical crosslinking agents used in the process are often toxic and could have unwanted reactions with the bioactive agents in the gel [109]. Chemical cross linking methods include cross linking by radical polymerization, chemical reaction of complementary groups, with aldehydes, with addition reactions, using condensation reactions, using high energy radiation, and using enzymes [109]. *Physical cross-linking* methods are growing in popularity because they don't require chemical agents that would need to be removed or that could potentially damage the delivered drug or substance. Physical cross linking methods include cross linking by ionic reactions, crosslinking by crystallization, using block and graft copolymers, hydrogen bonds, and protein interactions [109].

Some hydrogels have the ability to *self-assemble* under certain conditions, such as specific temperature and pH conditions. Injectable co-polymer hydrogels with this ability can be used to encapsulate drugs or cells for treatment of otherwise difficult to reach locations by injecting the solution to the site of action and then allowing the gel to form at body temperature and pH [110, 111]. Some polymer complexes that can be used in this capacity include PEG/polyester copolymers, polyphosphazenes, polypeptides, chitosan among others [112, 113].

In addition to synthetic injectable hydrogels, extracellular matrix hydrogels have been derived from decellularized tissues such as cardiac, dermis, adipose, bladder, and lungs [114–117]. These hydrogels are processed from the isolated extracellular matrix scaffold remaining after tissue decellularization usually including the natural polymer and proteins that make up every tissue. These scaffolds are also thought to sequester some of the naturally bound growth factors from the specific tissue type allowing them to be particularly bioactive in a regenerative role. Naturally derived ECM hydrogels benefit from an more compatible interface with the tissue, the ability to form gels at physiological conditions for inject ability, and has pro-regenerative degradation productions [118, 119]. In addition to delivering growth factors these gels have been used to deliver cells and other drugs through encapsulation.

Implants for Tissue Regeneration

In addition to standalone drug delivery systems such as hydrogels, polymeric micelles, and dendrimers whose main focus is drug delivery, polymers can be incorporated into larger implants or scaffolds and drug delivery may even be a secondary mechanism of the system. An example of this is a joint implant with a polymeric coating that elutes inflammation reducing drugs to help with healing/rejection, or an electrospun vascular graft that has bound growth factors to stimulate endothelial growth or angiogenesis [120]. Drugs can be coated onto polymers for direct dilution from of the surface, bound to functional groups on the polymers, or sequestered in the polymer structure itself. Drug eluting scaffolds can be used effectively for long term.

One class of scaffolds that can be used as a surface or implantable drug delivery scaffold system are created using *electrospinning* technique. This process, as described in Sect. "Polymer processing techniques to mimic tissue architecture and strength" can be used to create porous nanofiber scaffold from a variety of polymer substrates and has the potential to be combined with therapeutic drugs for a sustained release of the molecule when the scaffold is implanted in vivo [121]. The process can be controlled to create scaffolds with a range of fiber sizes, orientation, and porosity to effect drug release profile [121]. Electrospinning for drug delivery has applications in wound healing, long term treatment of heart and vascular disorders, and cancer treatment among others [122]. Electrospinning can be done using both naturally derived and synthetic fibers, as an emerging technique in scaffold design it may overcome current limitations with drug or growth factor delivery [120, 123].

Polymer Coatings are another example of a secondary purpose drug delivery system, were they are used in conjunction with a main implant, such as a stent, joint replacement, or other permanent implant [124]. Coating like this can be used to attenuate negative interactions between the implant interface and the tissue, and even promote tissue ingrowth into the implant. Bone ingrowth into knee, hip, or other replacements is one huge application for these coatings. The main reasons that orthopaedic implants fail is because of bacterial infection, chronic inflammation, and limited bone integration with the implant [125].

Polymer Material Properties and Functional Tissue Replacement

Classical tissue engineering follows the paradigm cells + scaffold = tissue replacement. In order for tissue replacement to occur, the polymeric scaffold must degrade. There are two common degradation mechanisms of polymeric materials in the body: swelling/dissolution and chain scission. In swelling/dissolution, hydrophilic domains of the material swell and dissolve in the body. In the chain scission, primary bonds of the polymer are broken through hydrolysis or oxidation. Polymeric properties that influence hydrolysis are the reactivity of groups in polymer backbone, extent of inter-chain bonding, and amount of water present. In chain scission by oxidation, reactive oxygen species attack and break covalent bonds. The three steps to oxidative chain scission are initiation, propagation, and termination. The extent of oxidation depends upon the number of susceptible domains in the polymer. Typically, lower molecular weight polymers and those that are not heavily crosslinked will have faster degradation due to fewer secondary and tertiary interactions. Polymeric materials for use in tissue engineering may be designed to have inherent domains for intentional hydrolysis or enzymatic degradation.

Biomaterials paradigms for designing polymers for functional tissue replacement follow criteria believed to be good for cellular ingrowth and formation of functional tissue. The criteria often followed for material properties that may be tailored for specific tissue types are 1. Polymer degradation rate 2. Polymer fiber diameter 3. Polymer pore size 4. Polymer hydrophilicty/hydrophobicity 5. Polymer mechanical properties (often influenced by numbers 1–4). Discussion of each of these criteria in specific tissue engineering examples and techniques for measurement follows.

Polymer Degradation Rate

Depending on the tissue to be engineered, and the approach chosen for processing the polymer, the degradation rate may be the most important factor when choosing a polymer for tissue engineering. One goal of classical tissue engineering is for the scaffold to degrade as it is replaced with regenerated tissue [126]. For example, if you are engineering a functional tissue replacement for skin, you may want to choose a polymer or polymer combination whose degradation rate will match the typical wound healing timeframe for proper tissue influx [127]. When properly designed, polymer scaffold degradation may be associated with remodeling of the collagen network in engineered polycaprolactone bisurea (PCL-U4U) thermoplastic elastomer scaffolds by human saphenous vein vascular derived cells [128]. In these PCL-U4U scaffolds, the vascular derived cells followed the orientation of the remodeled fiber architecture. For tissue engineering architecture that you do not expect to be replaced by the patient's own tissue, such as a heart valve or dental implant, you will want to choose a polymer with little to no biodegradation. The stability of the polymer in vivo is an incredibly important variable to ensure long term effectiveness of the engineered tissue.

Polymer degradation rate may be measured in vitro or in vivo, with in vivo testing being the most reliable. A typical degradation test in vitro would involve first obtaining an accurate weight of the engineered polymer. Next, the engineered polymer tissue is placed in a saline bath at 37 °C. Samples may be taken from the saline bath over time and analyzed for the polymer concentration in the bath using mass spectrometry or other chemical analysis. At the end of a set period, the polymer will be taken out of the bath and a final weight will be obtained. This in vitro technique has limitations. The first limitation is that the simple degradation measurement does not take into account any cellular or metabolic activity. The second limitation is that the weight analysis does not take into account any swelling or increase in water weight of the polymer. Another in vitro technique that may be used is similar degradation measurements with the addition of cells + media. However, this technique cannot replicate the complex in vivo environment. The most common in vivo degradation test is to perform a subcutaneous implant of the polymeric material in the side flank of a mouse. Mice may be euthanized at various time points and the area may be assessed histologically for degradation of the polymeric material. This in vivo testing will provide basic information about how an immune response and tissue environment may affect polymer degradation. However, this side flank model may not be adequate in assessing the degradation of polymers used to engineer tissues that undergo large or repeated mechanical loads. The side flank model is often a needed first step towards assessing polymer degradation. Further degradation testing is usually necessary in vivo in models that mimic the disease or injury for which a functional tissue replacement is needed.

Polymer Fiber Diameter

Polymeric fiber diameter is important for several reasons in tissue engineering, some of which are discussed earlier in this chapter. The fiber diameter will play a large role in both the cellular infiltration into the scaffold and the mechanical properties of the scaffold. In order to engineer functional tissue replacements for structures that have high amounts of fibrillar collagen, the polymeric fiber diameter is increasingly important. Such tissue structures include tendon, heart valves, the urinary bladder, vascular grafts, or ligaments among others. These are typically tissues that undergo large changes in mechanical forces and must have the structural fortitude for these load bearing situations. Fiber diameter may also play a role in the immune or foreign body response of cells to the polymeric scaffold. One study showed that fiber diameter in the nanometer scale caused a pro-regeneration response of macrophages, while a larger fiber diameter in the micrometer scale caused a pro-inflammatory response of macrophages to the poly-l lactic acid (PLLA) scaffolds [129].

Polymer fiber diameter will depend upon the type of polymer or polymer blend used and the technique of polymer processing. These techniques are outlined in Sect. "Polymer processing techniques to mimic tissue architecture and strength". Polymer fiber diameters are most adequately measured with imaging based technology. For example, in a poly-l lactic acid (PLLA) electrospun polymer scaffold, fiber diameter is commonly measured by first performing scanning electron microscopy followed by image analysis and statistics to calculate average fiber diameter size. The image analysis technique may also work well for other polymer processing techniques such as hydrogel formations and woven scaffolds.

Polymer Pore Size

The easiest way for a cell to penetrate the scaffold material and form a three-dimensional engineered tissue is through large interconnected pores. Cells will range from 5 to 50 μm and can squeeze themselves through pores ranging from 3 to 20 μm. Many factors will influence whether or not a cell will penetrate the pore including nutrient availability, growth factor or cytokine recruitment, and cell phenotype. While these biological factors may be engineered into the polymer or cell choice, the physical factor of pore size will usually be altered through processing techniques.

The pore size measurement may be done with image analysis, similar to that described above for polymer fiber diameter. However, this imaging based technique may not be adequate for polymers with three dimensional and non-uniform pores. A measure of porosity may instead be adequate using an liquid exclusion porosimetry measurement [130]. In liquid exclusion porosimetry, the scaffold is immersed in pure ethanol or other solvent that will disperse throughout the polymeric scaffold under a non-reacting gas pressure. The differential pressure required to displace the wetting liquid is related to pore diameter by the Washburn equation [Eq. (7.1)], which states that higher pressure is required to remove liquid from smaller pores:

$$p = 4\gamma \cos\ \theta / D \tag{7.1}$$

where p is the differential pressure across the length of the pore, D is the pore diameter, γ is the surface tension of the wetting liquid; and θ is the contact angle of the wetting liquid with the sample [130]. The volume of the liquid flowing out of the membrane is collected and weighed in an analytical balance. This volume corresponds to the flow-through pore volume within the scaffold. This technique works well for electrospun polymeric scaffolds; however, it may be replaced with simpler gravimetric analysis for other scaffold formations.

Polymer Hydrophilicty/Hydrophobicity

Polymer degradation by hydrolysis will be governed by the amount of water present in the formulation. The degradation rate is thus influenced by the hydrophobicity of the polymeric side chains and their ability to take on water. The hydrophobicity of the polymeric structure must strike a balance with the optimal hydrophobicity needed for protein adsorption and cellular attachment. In order for cells to adhere to a polymeric scaffold, the scaffold must be hydrophilic. However, many of the polymers utilized for scaffold fabrication are highly hydrophobic. Thus, surface modifications or pre-wetting the scaffold with a solvent is typically needed for successful cell adherence.

Testing for hydrophilicty/hydrophobicity is most commonly performed by calculating the contact angle of a water droplet on the surface of the material. The more hydrophobic the polymer is, the greater angle will be formed between the water droplet and the surface. For example, a material with a contact angle of 90° will be more hydrophobic compared to one with a contact angle of 30°. Contact angles may be measured using imaging and standard image analysis tools or physically measured with a goniometer.

Polymer Biomechanical Properties

The biomechanical properties of the polymer used in tissue engineering are an important factor in ensuring durability of the tissue engineered structure. The biomechanical properties must be understood at the time of implant and throughout degradation of the polymer as it is filled in with regenerated tissue. For example, if a polymer is utilized to repair a defect in a mineralized, load bearing tissue, such as bone, the tissue engineered polymer construct must be able to withstand the loads during healing. If a polymeric scaffold is used in a vascular graft repair, it must be able to withstand the shear stress environment under pulsatile flow. A clear understanding of the mechanical profile of the material and the mechanical environment at the location of the implant is necessary for a successful engineered tissue.

Common tests for biomechanical properties include traditional uniaxial testing, biaxial testing, three-point bending, compression, or torsion tests. In all of these modes of mechanical testing, the viscoelastic (or time dependent) nature of the polymer must be assessed. Biomechanical tests need to be performed on the polymer alone, the polymer + cells, and explanted tissues from animal studies. Each of these sample groups can be compared to the biomechanical properties of the native tissue that is to be replaced. These tests are often utilized in combination with finite element analysis and computational simulations to fully understand the biomechanical properties of the engineered tissue. Many experts in the field believe the mechanical tests to be the ultimate measure of a tissue engineered polymer. However, in vivo testing in relevant animal models is likely the best measure prior to use in patients.

Other Important Considerations in the Design of Biodegradable Polymers for Functional Tissue Replacement

Polymer scaffolds of conventional tissue engineering techniques must not only degrade at a kinetic rate appropriate for tissue replacement, the scaffolds must also serve as templates to engineer the proper cellular niche for cellular differentiation into a pro-regenerative phenotype. Growth factors or other additive factors may be added to the polymer scaffold for release. These growth factors or other drugs will provide a favorable cellular microenvironment and/or may serve to recruit cells to the site for regeneration. Growth factor or drug release is measured similarly to in vitro degradation rate tests as described above. Growth factor release may be assayed in sampling buffer from the scaffold at various time points via enzyme linked immunoabsorbant assay (ELISA). Many new advances in the synthesis of polymers as degradable cellular templates are being reported daily; however, few have made it to market.

As with any polymeric material that interfaces with the body, the acute and chronic toxicity of the polymer and its degradation byproducts must be taken into consideration. The best way to examine acute and chronic toxicity is through an animal model. For example, in the rat, acute toxicity would be measured within the first 24 h of implantation. Chronic toxicity would be assessed at 90 days post implantation, which corresponds to 10 % of the animal's lifespan. Toxicity is commonly assessed by material tracking in vivo through X-ray, MRI, or other non-invasive in vivo imaging such as IVIS (Perkin Elmer). At the end of the time duration, histological analysis is performed to ensure that the material causes minimal cell death at the site of implantation. For a tissue engineered implant containing a polymeric biomaterial to be safe and effective, chronic toxicity must be eliminated.

Polymers for Engineering Complex Architectures Such as the Lung and Liver

Several different polymers are utilized in order to engineer tissues with complex tissue architectures and highly specialized cell function. The focus of this section will be on the lung and liver. Both the lung and liver are organs with high need of replacement due to fibrotic disease or other dysfunction. There is high unmet demand for donor lungs and livers. Tissue engineering strategies may either fully replace the lung or liver or may be employed in assist devices to replicate function until a donor organ is available. This section will highlight the course of research in polymeric based tissue engineering the lung and liver. The state of the art in tissue engineering these two organs has followed a similar course of development as follows: polymers for structured cellular transplantation, the use of combined synthetic and naturally-derived polymer approaches to large structures, the use of decellularized tissues, and the use of polymers in assist devices.

Polymer Sponges or Hydrogels for Structured Cellular Transplantation

The basic paradigm for engineering polymeric structures for cellular transplant in the lung and liver is to utilize a hydrogel or sponge structure with either adult differentiated cells or progenitor cells. In both the lung and the liver, these polymer-cell structures have shown great success in vitro. Additionally, in vivo animal studies show promising results of cellular survival and functional differentiation.

Although the liver has some regenerative ability, there is a large need for liver transplantation due to cirrhosis, drug toxicity, or congenital defect. Tissue engineering functional liver units has been a focus for many years as a potential source for liver replacement. The first examples of functional transplantable liver-like structures used prevascularized, non-degradable polyvinyl alcohol sponges to accommodate transplanted hep-atocytes with limited success [131, 132]. Modified gelatin sponges with lactobionic acid (MGLA) have also been used to support mouse hepatocyte growth [133]. Microhydrogels made of fibrinogen attached to poly(ethylene glycol) (PEG)-diacrylate side chains were used as a cell carrier for intravascular transplantation of hepatocytes in a rat model [134]. Another naturally derived material, silk fibroin, has been utilized in several tissue engineering approaches. Silk fibroin is a naturally-derived material which has high molecular weight organic polymers characterized by repetitive hydrophobic and hydrophilic peptide sequences. Silk fibroin assembles into regular structures during materials formation and can be considered as nature's equivalent to synthetic block copolymers [135]. Due to its polymeric nature, silk fibroin has been utilized in a cryogel to support hepatocyte growth with aims for future transplantation [136]. A cryogel is a porous hydrogel formed from polymerization under low temperature

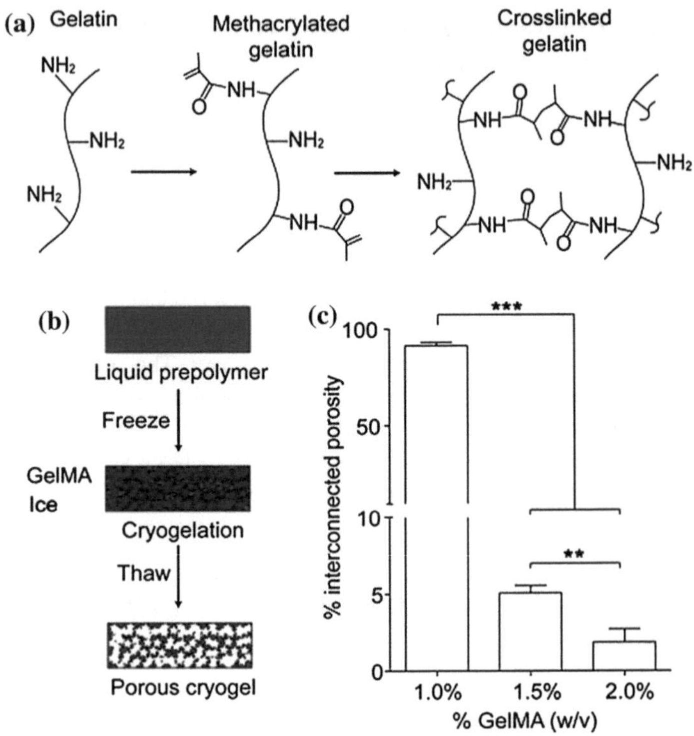

Fig. 7.1 Preparation and assessment of gelatin cryogel. **a** Schematic of GelMA synthesis and crosslinking. Pendant methacrylate groups are added primarily to the free amines of gelatin by reaction with methacrylic anhydride. Free radical polymerization results in crosslink formation between methacrylate groups. **b** Cryopolymerization of methacrylated gelatin. Freezing of methacrylated gelatin in the presence of radical initiators (APS and TEMED) allows polymerization to occur in the partially frozen state (cryopolymerization). Ice crystals formed during the freezing process and thawing after cryopolymerization results in the formation of a hydrogel with micron-scale pores. **c** Volume of interconnected pores in gelatin cryogels (normalized to total gel volume). Values represent mean and standard deviation ($n = 10$). Data were compared using ANOVA with Bonferroni's post-hoc test (**$p < 0.01$, ***$p < 0.001$). Reproduced from [163]

conditions. The ice crystals that form allow for highly interconnected pores within the hydrogel. Preparation and assessment of a gelatin hydrogel with methacrylated crosslinking is shown in Fig. 7.1.

In the lung, similar approaches have been employed focusing on naturally-derived polymers alone or in combination with synthetic scaffolds. Gelfoam sponges are commercially available surgical devices that are derived from porcine skin gelatin (Pfizer.com). Gelfoam sponges are water-insoluble and capable of absorbing up to 45 times their weight (Pfizer). Gelfoam sponges have been utilized to grow lung organotypic structures in vitro [137, 138]. Additionally, Gelfoam sponges seeded with fetal rat lung cells were viable in the adult animal lung for up to 35 days with neovascularization apparent [139]. Other hydrogels with natural and synthetic components have been used to engineer pulmonary cell structures. The natural components of these are typically either gelatin or Matrigel. Gelatin is a low-cost, non-immunogenic natural material derived from collagen. Matrigel is a product from Corning Life Sciences that is a gelatinous extracellular matrix mixture made from mouse sarcoma cell secreted matrix. These two naturally-derived materials have been used in vitro and in vivo animal models extensively. Additionally, gelatin has been used in numerous human applications, which makes it an appealing polymer for new tissue engineered products. Gelatin in the form of a three-dimensional microbubble scaffold was used to provide the proper cellular microenvironment for differentiation of mouse pulmonary stem cells into alveolar pneumocytes [140]. Similarly, hydroxyethyl methacrylate-alginate-gelatin (HAG) hydrogels have been employed as three-dimensional structures for lung epithelial cell growth [141]. Additionally, three-dimensional structures for alveolar cell growth using matrigel hydrogel and synthetic polymer scaffolds of poly-lactic-co-glycolic acid (PLGA) and poly-L-lactic-acid (PLLA) fabricated into porous foams and nanofibrous matrices have been used successfully in vitro [142]. Engineering the cellular microenvironment for progenitor cell differentiation will likely continue to be the focus of new polymer formulations in lung and liver cell delivery.

Naturally-Derived and Synthetic Polymer Strategies for Larger Pulmonary and Hepatic Structures

While hydrogels or sponges have been examined for cell transplant for the parenchyma of the liver or lung, more traditional tissue engineering approaches have been utilized for some of the larger structures such as bile ducts, trachea, or bronchioles. These traditional tissue engineering approaches utilize scaffold materials made from naturally-derived and/or synthetic polymers and have been implanted with some success in vivo in both humans and in animal models.

In the liver, there have been few attempts to re-create functional liver structures using polymeric biomaterials in the context of engineering the bile duct or liver capsule. Three dimensional stacked polycarbonate membranes with hepatocytes showed functional liver units in vitro [143]. Functional liver units were also observed using micropatterned Poly(ethylene glycol)-poly(DL-lactide) and lactosylated poly(DL-lactide) electrospun fibrous mats [144]. For larger structures, like the bile duct or vascular structures, polymers may be formed into sheets and then tube structures. The bile duct was successfully replaced in an animal study using polycaprolactone and polylactic acid reinforced with polyglycolic acid fibers in a tube structure [145]. Continuing advances in synthetic polymer processing, such as three-dimensional printing and micropatterning, will improve the field of engineering larger liver structures such as the bile duct.

In the lung, tissue engineering strategies have been employed to engineer larger airway structures such as the trachea, main stem bronchi, and bronchiole. In 2008, the first transplantation of a tissue-engineered trachea in a human being

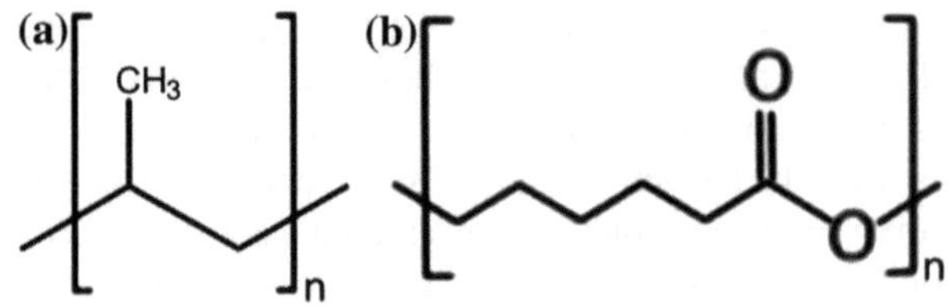

Fig. 7.2 Chemical formulas for **a** Polypropylene and **b** Polycaprolactone

was done to replace an end-staged left main bronchus with malacia in a 30-year-old woman. The implanted trachea was engineered from a decellularized cadaveric trachea seeded with autologous epithelial cells and mesenchymal stem cell-derived chondrocytes [146]. Five years post implantation, the tissue engineered trachea remained viable and patent with stenting needed in the native trachea near the implant [147]. This initial success advanced the field of clinical applications of tissue engineered airways (Fig. 7.2).

New advances and improvements on tissue engineered trachea involve synthetic and natural combination polymer strategies. Polypropylene meshes with collagen and/or poly(L-lactic-acid-co-e-caprolactone) coating have been used in an animal model for replacement of the left main stem bronchi [148, 149]. Greater success was achieved utilizing the poly (L-lactic-acid-co-e-caprolactone) coating for epithelial regeneration. Other success has been reported in a rabbit model where tissue engineered tracheas were formed from articular cartilage matrix and chondrocytes [150]. New advances in 3D printing polymers have been harnessed for applications to the airway. A half-pipe polycaprolactone 3D printed trachea seeded with mesenchymal stromal cells in a fibrin matrix was implanted into a rabbit model with initial success of regenerated epithelium [151]. Tissue engineering polymer approaches for the large airways have gained momentum due to the ease of fabrication and implantation. However, smaller airways, termed bronchioles, have been attempted for in vitro understanding of small airway diseases such as asthma with the eventual goal of a functional tissue engineered lung. For the bronchiole, a type I collagen gel seeded with fibroblasts, epithelial cells, and airway smooth muscle cells was engineered utilizing a pulsatile flow bioreactor [152]. Similarly, another study cites tubular bronchiole structures engineered using airway smooth muscle tubular structure collagen pulsatile flow [153]. The engineering of these smaller airway structures highlights the need for advances in bioreactor technology to go hand in hand with the advances in polymeric biomaterials. A true tissue engineered lung will likely utilize a combination approach of polymeric materials, the proper cell choices, and proper in vitro conditioning.

Vascularization and the Mechanical Environment

Vascularization is often the limiting factor in tissue engineering complex three dimensional tissues for lung and liver replacement. Both hepatocytes and pulmonary epithelium have high oxygen needs, so the design of polymeric structures must allow for a highly vascularized system. Furthermore, the blood supply is crucial in both of these systems to maintain functionality. The liver's main function is to filter the blood coming from the digestive tract, and the lung's main function is to allow for gas exchange in the blood to occur. This functionality, while seemingly obvious to include, is non-trivial when engineering three dimensional structures for replacement of liver and lung. Several strategies have been employed to improve oxygenation of cells grown in vitro including the addition of perfluorcarbons and the bubbling of oxygen through the culture media.

In addition to the flows from the vasculature, the mechanical environment of the three-dimensional construct must be taken into account. When engineering a portal triad for the liver, the shear forces in the bile duct must also be considered in the design. Furthermore in the lung, a very complex mechanical environment exists as the lung is constantly distended and relaxed. The polymeric structures used to engineer the lung must have large elastic recoil in order to withstand this repeated deformation. Due to the complex mechanical environment and vascularization structure of the lung and liver, decellularized organs may provide the best natural polymeric scaffolding material.

Decellularized Organs

Decellularized organs from human cadavers or animal sources provide the structural architecture necessary for complex three dimensional tissues. Key natural polymers, proteins, and structural components remaining in decellularized organs are collagen types I–IV, elastin, fibronectin, and laminin. Depending on the mode of decellularization (as described in Sect. "Biologically Generated Polymers"), many active growth factors and cytokines may also be present in the matrix.

Lung decellularization has had successes in animal implantation [154]. Several other studies have examined effects of decellularization processes on matrix architecture and strength [155, 156]. Lung decellularization leaves the complex architecture of the lung airways and alveoli with the vascular network available for repopulation with endothelial cells (Fig. 7.3). Repopulation of decellularized lung matrix with progenitor cells and subsequent differentiation into lung phenotypes shows that the decellularized lung matrix provides a hospitable environment for regeneration [157]. Although there has been much progress in the field of decellularized lung scaffolds, it remains unclear what the proper cellular choices are for recapitulating proper lung function and air-tight gas exchange.

Liver structure/function relationship is paramount in engineering hepatic units. To retain the complex structure/function relationship, decellularized livers have also been utilized for repopulation and transplantation into in vivo models [158, 159]. Using the decellularized livers as scaffolds causes the proper cellular spatial distribution that is so difficult to achieve using other polymeric scaffold fabrication techniques. As with the lung, similar issues remain to be worked out in whole organ liver tissue engineering. These issues include clotting, cell choice, cell fate, and long term functionality of the organ.

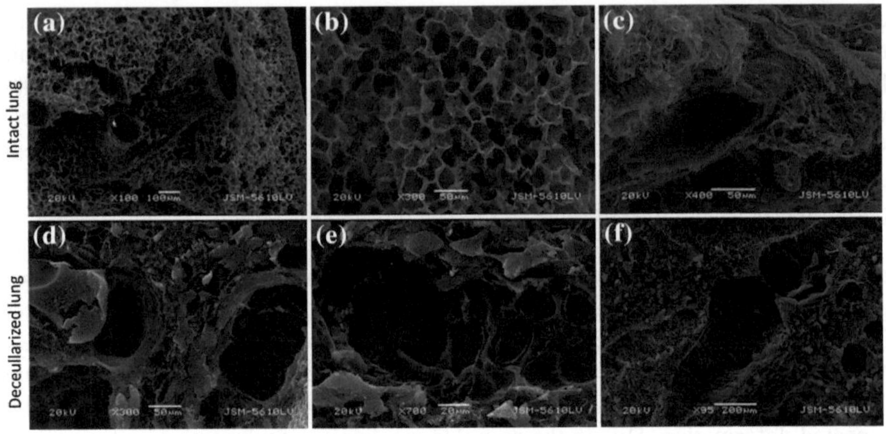

Fig. 7.3 Intact and decellularized mouse lung shows retention of pulmonary structures. **a** and **d** show larger airways, **b** and **e** show alveoli, **c** and **f** show blood vessels

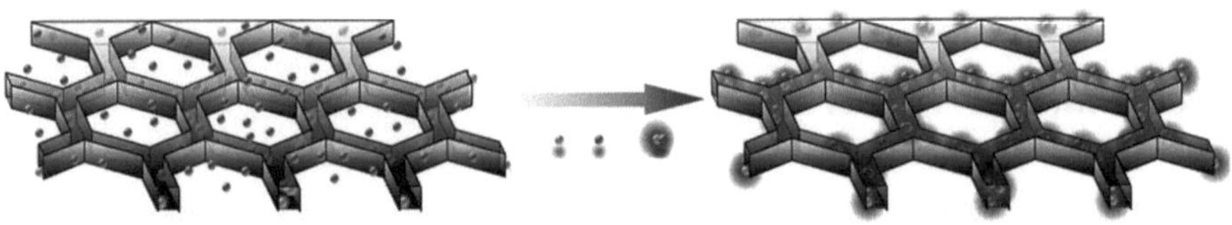

Fig. 7.4 Bio-inspired 3D liver detoxification device. Polydiacetylene nanoparticles (*green*) are installed in poly(ethylene glycol) diacrylate hydrogel matrix (*grey*) with liver-mimetic 3D structure fabricated by 3D printing. The nanoparticles attract, capture and sense toxins (*red*), while the 3D matrix with modified liver lobule structure allows toxins to be trapped efficiently. This biomimetic 3D detoxifier has promising clinical application for detoxification by collecting and removing toxins. Reproduced from [164]

Assist Technologies

Due to the complexity and remaining issues in engineering replacement organs for lungs and livers, "lab on a chip" approaches have been utilized to engineer assist devices. The assist devices can provide essential replacement of function that is missing even in decellularized organs. These assist devices are meant to perform the function of the lung or liver as either a bridge to transplant or as a permanent assist technology. The majority of assist devices are fabricated using soft photolithography or three dimensional printing. In the former, polydimethysiloxane (PDMS) is typically the polymer of choice because it can be poured into a photolithographic mold. The PDMS is often coated with a naturally-derived extracellular matrix protein such as collagen or fibronecin. Cells are then placed within the channels to perform function [160, 161]. With 3D printing, the polymer choice is broadened such that any polymer that can be put into solution at a viscosity matching the printer nozzle may be utilized. For the liver, polymers have been used as the structural components of assist devices as well as to perform function by capturing toxins (Fig. 7.4).

In the lung, endothelial cells and ECM proteins have been added to polymeric tubes for enhanced gas exchange in extracorporeal membrane oxygenation devices [162]. There will continue to be a future push toward incorporating tissue engineered external devices to avoid coagulation and better prognosis for assist or hybrid technologies.

References

1. Leahy, J.C., Hukins, D.W.: Viscoelastic properties of the nucleus pulposus of the intervertebral disk in compression. J. Mater. Sci. Mater. Med. **12**, 689–692 (2001)
2. Anderson, J.M., Andukuri, A., Lim, D.J., Jun, H.-W.: Modulating the gelation properties of self-assembling peptide amphiphiles. ACS Nano **3**, 3447–3454 (2009). doi:10.1021/nn900884n
3. Holmes, T.C., de Lacalle, S., Su, X., et al.: Extensive neurite outgrowth and active synapse formation on self-assembling peptide scaffolds. Proc. Natl. Acad. Sci. USA **97**, 6728–6733 (2000)
4. Mujeeb, A., Miller, A.F., Saiani, A., Gough, J.E.: Self-assembled octapeptide scaffolds for in vitro chondrocyte culture. Acta Biomater. **9**, 4609–4617 (2013). doi:10.1016/j.actbio.2012.08.044
5. Banwell, E.F., Abelardo, E.S., Adams, D.J., et al.: Rational design and application of responsive alpha-helical peptide hydrogels. Nat. Mater. **8**, 596–600 (2009). doi:10.1038/nmat2479
6. Jun, H.-W., Paramonov, S.E., Dong, H., et al.: Tuning the mechanical and bioresponsive properties of peptide-amphiphile nanofiber networks. J. Biomater. Sci. Polym. Ed. **19**, 665–676 (2008). doi:10.1163/156856208784089625
7. Kopecek, J., Yang, J.: Peptide-directed self-assembly of hydrogels. Acta Biomater. **5**, 805–816 (2009). doi:10.1016/j.actbio.2008.10.001
8. Chau, Y., Luo, Y., Cheung, A.C.Y., et al.: Incorporation of a matrix metalloproteinase-sensitive substrate into self-assembling peptides—a model for biofunctional scaffolds. Biomaterials **29**, 1713–1719 (2008). doi:10.1016/j.biomaterials.2007.11.046
9. Han, S., Cao, S., Wang, Y., et al.: Self-assembly of short peptide amphiphiles: the cooperative effect of hydrophobic interaction and hydrogen bonding. Chem. Weinh. Bergstr. Ger. **17**, 13095–13102 (2011). doi:10.1002/chem.201101970
10. Xu, X.-D., Jin, Y., Liu, Y., et al.: Self-assembly behavior of peptide amphiphiles (PAs) with different length of hydrophobic alkyl tails. Colloids Surf. B Biointerfaces **81**, 329–335 (2010). doi:10.1016/j.colsurfb.2010.07.027
11. Stendahl, J.C., Rao, M.S., Guler, M.O., Stupp, S.I.: Intermolecular forces in the self-assembly of peptide amphiphile nanofibers. Adv. Funct. Mater. **16**, 499–508 (2006). doi:10.1002/adfm.200500161
12. Löwik, D.W.P.M., Shklyarevskiy, I.O., Ruizendaal, L., et al.: A highly ordered material from magnetically aligned peptide amphiphile nanofiber assemblies. Adv. Mater. **19**, 1191–1195 (2007). doi:10.1002/adma.200602295
13. Feng, Y., Taraban, M., Yu, Y.B.: The effect of ionic strength on the mechanical, structural and transport properties of peptide hydrogels. Soft Matter. **8**, 11723–11731 (2012). doi:10.1039/C2SM26572A
14. Ramachandran, S., Taraban, M.B., Trewhella, J., et al.: Effect of temperature during assembly on the structure and mechanical properties of peptide-based materials. Biomacromolecules **11**, 1502–1506 (2010). doi:10.1021/bm100138m
15. Yunoki, S., Ohyabu, Y., Hatayama, H.: Temperature-responsive gelation of type I collagen solutions involving fibril formation and genipin crosslinking as a potential injectable hydrogel. Int. J. Biomater. (2013). doi:10.1155/2013/620765

16. Alamein, M.A., Stephens, S., Liu, Q., et al.: Mass production of nanofibrous extracellular matrix with controlled 3D morphology for large-scale soft tissue regeneration. Tissue Eng. Part C Methods **19**, 458–472 (2012). doi:10.1089/ten.tec.2012.0417
17. Pham, Q.P., Sharma, U., Mikos, A.G.: Electrospinning of polymeric nanofibers for tissue engineering applications: a review. Tissue Eng. **12**, 1197–1211 (2006). doi:10.1089/ten.2006.12.1197
18. Baker, B.M., Gee, A.O., Metter, R.B., et al.: The potential to improve cell infiltration in composite fiber-aligned electrospun scaffolds by the selective removal of sacrificial fibers. Biomaterials **29**, 2348–2358 (2008). doi:10.1016/j.biomaterials.2008.01.032
19. Lee, S., Cho, S., Kim, M., et al.: Highly moldable electrospun clay-like fluffy nanofibers for three-dimensional scaffolds. ACS Appl. Mater. Interfaces **6**, 1082–1091 (2014). doi:10.1021/am404627r
20. Kim, T.G., Chung, H.J., Park, T.G.: Macroporous and nanofibrous hyaluronic acid/collagen hybrid scaffold fabricated by concurrent electrospinning and deposition/leaching of salt particles. Acta Biomater. **4**, 1611–1619 (2008). doi:10.1016/j.actbio.2008.06.008
21. Nam, J., Huang, Y., Agarwal, S., Lannutti, J.: Improved cellular infiltration in electrospun fiber via engineered porosity. Tissue Eng. **13**, 2249–2257 (2007). doi:10.1089/ten.2006.0306
22. Schneider, O.D., Loher, S., Brunner, T.J., et al.: Cotton wool-like nanocomposite biomaterials prepared by electrospinning: in vitro bioactivity and osteogenic differentiation of human mesenchymal stem cells. J. Biomed. Mater. Res. B Appl. Biomater. **84**, 350–362 (2008). doi:10.1002/jbm.b.30878
23. McClure, M.J., Wolfe, P.S., Simpson, D.G., et al.: The use of air-flow impedance to control fiber deposition patterns during electrospinning. Biomaterials **33**, 771–779 (2012). doi:10.1016/j.biomaterials.2011.10.011
24. McHugh, K.J., Tao, S.L., Saint-Geniez, M.: A novel porous scaffold fabrication technique for epithelial and endothelial tissue engineering. J. Mater. Sci. Mater. Med. **24**, 1659–1670 (2013). doi:10.1007/s10856-013-4934-1
25. Thomas, V., Jose, M.V., Chowdhury, S., et al.: Mechano-morphological studies of aligned nanofibrous scaffolds of polycaprolactone fabricated by electrospinning. J. Biomater. Sci. Polym. Ed. **17**, 969–984 (2006)
26. Bashur, C.A., Shaffer, R.D., Dahlgren, L.A., et al.: Effect of fiber diameter and alignment of electrospun polyurethane meshes on mesenchymal progenitor cells. Tissue Eng. Part A **15**, 2435–2445 (2009). doi:10.1089/ten.tea.2008.0295
27. Wang, H.B., Mullins, M.E., Cregg, J.M., et al.: Varying the diameter of aligned electrospun fibers alters neurite outgrowth and Schwann cell migration. Acta Biomater. **6**, 2970–2978 (2010). doi:10.1016/j.actbio.2010.02.020
28. Blakeney, B.A., Tambralli, A., Anderson, J.M., et al.: Cell infiltration and growth in a low density, uncompressed three-dimensional electrospun nanofibrous scaffold. Biomaterials **32**, 1583–1590 (2011). doi:10.1016/j.biomaterials.2010.10.056
29. Jha, B.S., Colello, R.J., Bowman, J.R., et al.: Two pole air gap electrospinning: Fabrication of highly aligned, three-dimensional scaffolds for nerve reconstruction. Acta Biomater. **7**, 203–215 (2011). doi:10.1016/j.actbio.2010.08.004
30. Kim, G.H., Yoon, H.: A direct-electrospinning process by combined electric field and air-blowing system for nanofibrous wound-dressings. Appl. Phys. A **90**, 389–394 (2008). doi:10.1007/s00339-007-4330-0
31. Li, D., Xia, Y.: Direct fabrication of composite and ceramic hollow nanofibers by electrospinning. Nano Lett. **4**, 933–938 (2004). doi:10.1021/nl049590f
32. Klossner, R.R., Queen, H.A., Coughlin, A.J., Krause, W.E.: Correlation of chitosan's rheological properties and its ability to electrospin. Biomacromolecules **9**, 2947–2953 (2008). doi:10.1021/bm800738u
33. Francis, M.P., Sachs, P.C., Madurantakam, P.A., et al.: Electrospinning adipose tissue-derived extracellular matrix for adipose stem cell culture. J. Biomed. Mater. Res. A **100**, 1716–1724 (2012). doi:10.1002/jbm.a.34126

34. Guarino, V., Cirillo, V., Taddei, P., et al.: Tuning size scale and crystallinity of PCL electrospun fibres via solvent permittivity to address hMSC response. Macromol. Biosci. **11**, 1694–1705 (2011). doi:10.1002/mabi.201100204
35. Nakano, A., Miki, N., Hishida, K., Hotta, A.: Solution parameters for the fabrication of thinner silicone fibers by electrospinning. Phys. Rev. E: Stat., Nonlin, Soft Matter Phys. **86**, 011801 (2012)
36. Matthews, J.A., Wnek, G.E., Simpson, D.G., Bowlin, G.L.: Electrospinning of collagen nanofibers. Biomacromolecules **3**, 232–238 (2002)
37. Jiang, Q., Reddy, N., Zhang, S., et al.: Water-stable electrospun collagen fibers from a non-toxic solvent and crosslinking system. J. Biomed. Mater. Res. A **101**, 1237–1247 (2013). doi:10.1002/jbm.a.34422
38. Braghirolli, D.I., Steffens, D., Quintiliano, K., et al.: The effect of sterilization methods on electronspun poly(lactide-co-glycolide) and subsequent adhesion efficiency of mesenchymal stem cells. J. Biomed. Mater. Res. B Appl. Biomater. **102**, 700–708 (2014). doi:10.1002/jbm.b.33049
39. Rainer, A., Centola, M., Spadaccio, C., et al.: Comparative study of different techniques for the sterilization of poly-L-lactide electrospun microfibers: effectiveness vs. material degradation. Int. J. Artif. Organs **33**, 76–85 (2010)
40. Lang, B., McGinity, J.W., Williams, R.O.: Hot-melt extrusion—basic principles and pharmaceutical applications. Drug Dev. Ind. Pharm. (2014). doi:10.3109/03639045.2013.838577
41. Vynckier, A.-K., Dierickx, L., Voorspoels, J., et al.: Hot-melt co-extrusion: requirements, challenges and opportunities for pharmaceutical applications. J. Pharm. Pharmacol. **66**, 167–179 (2014). doi:10.1111/jphp.12091
42. Temple J.P., Hutton D.L., Hung B.P., et al.: Engineering anatomically shaped vascularized bone grafts with hASCs and 3D-printed PCL scaffolds. J. Biomed. Mater. Res. A n/a–n/a. (2014). doi: 10.1002/jbm.a.35107
43. Williams, J.M., Adewunmi, A., Schek, R.M., et al.: Bone tissue engineering using polycaprolactone scaffolds fabricated via selective laser sintering. Biomaterials **26**, 4817–4827 (2005). doi:10.1016/j.biomaterials.2004.11.057
44. Butscher, A., Bohner, M., Hofmann, S., et al.: Structural and material approaches to bone tissue engineering in powder-based three-dimensional printing. Acta Biomater. **7**, 907–920 (2011). doi:10.1016/j.actbio.2010.09.039
45. Inzana, J.A., Olvera, D., Fuller, S.M., et al.: 3D printing of composite calcium phosphate and collagen scaffolds for bone regeneration. Biomaterials **35**, 4026–4034 (2014). doi:10.1016/j.biomaterials.2014.01.064
46. Yu, J., Lee, A.-R., Lin, W.-H., et al.: Electrospun PLGA fibers incorporated with functionalized biomolecules for cardiac tissue engineering. Tissue Eng. Part A (2014). doi:10.1089/ten.TEA.2013.0008
47. Tsai, W.-B., Chen, Y.-R., Liu, H.-L., Lai, J.-Y.: Fabrication of UV-crosslinked chitosan scaffolds with conjugation of RGD peptides for bone tissue engineering. Carbohydr. Polym. **85**, 129–137 (2011). doi:10.1016/j.carbpol.2011.02.003
48. Tambralli, A., Blakeney, B., Anderson, J., et al.: A hybrid biomimetic scaffold composed of electrospun polycaprolactone nanofibers and self-assembled peptide amphiphile nanofibers. Biofabrication **1**, 025001 (2009). doi:10.1088/1758-5082/1/2/025001
49. Mager, M.D., LaPointe, V., Stevens, M.M.: Exploring and exploiting chemistry at the cell surface. Nat. Chem. **3**, 582–589 (2011). doi:10.1038/nchem.1090
50. Callahan, L.A.S., Xie, S., Barker, I.A., et al.: Directed differentiation and neurite extension of mouse embryonic stem cell on aligned poly(lactide) nanofibers functionalized with YIGSR peptide. Biomaterials **34**, 9089–9095 (2013). doi:10.1016/j.biomaterials.2013.08.028
51. Gobin, A.S., West, J.L.: Val-ala-pro-gly, an elastin-derived non-integrin ligand: smooth muscle cell adhesion and specificity. J. Biomed. Mater. Res. A **67**, 255–259 (2003). doi:10.1002/jbm.a.10110
52. Duan, Y., Liu, Z., O'Neill, J., et al.: Hybrid gel composed of native heart matrix and collagen induces cardiac differentiation of human embryonic stem cells without

supplemental growth factors. J. Cardiovasc. Transl. Res. **4**, 605–615 (2011). doi:10.1007/s12265-011-9304-0
53. Tan, Y., Richards, D.J., Trusk, T.C., et al.: 3D printing facilitated scaffold-free tissue unit fabrication. Biofabrication **6**, 024111 (2014). doi:10.1088/1758-5082/6/2/024111
54. Li, J.L., Cai, Y.L., Guo, Y.L., et al.: Fabrication of three-dimensional porous scaffolds with controlled filament orientation and large pore size via an improved E-jetting technique. J. Biomed. Mater. Res. B Appl. Biomater. **102**, 651–658 (2014). doi:10.1002/jbm.b.33043
55. Wei, C., Dong, J.: Direct fabrication of high-resolution three-dimensional polymeric scaffolds using electrohydrodynamic hot jet plotting. J. Micromech. Microeng. **23**, 025017 (2013). doi:10.1088/0960-1317/23/2/025017
56. Hutmacher, D.W., Schantz, T., Zein, I., et al.: Mechanical properties and cell cultural response of polycaprolactone scaffolds designed and fabricated via fused deposition modeling. J. Biomed. Mater. Res. **55**, 203–216 (2001)
57. Reichert, J.C., Heymer, A., Berner, A., et al.: Fabrication of polycaprolactone collagen hydrogel constructs seeded with mesenchymal stem cells for bone regeneration. Biomed. Mater. Bristol Engl. **4**, 065001 (2009). doi:10.1088/1748-6041/4/6/065001
58. Thakkar, S., Ghebes, C.A., Ahmed, M., et al.: Mesenchymal stromal cell-derived extracellular matrix influences gene expression of chondrocytes. Biofabrication **5**, 025003 (2013). doi:10.1088/1758-5082/5/2/025003
59. Thomas, V., Jose, M.V., Chowdhury, S., et al.: Mechano-morphological studies of aligned nanofibrous scaffolds of polycaprolactone fabricated by electrospinning. J. Biomater. Sci. Polym. Ed. **17**, 969–984 (2006)
60. Bashur, C.A., Shaffer, R.D., Dahlgren, L.A., et al.: Effect of fiber diameter and alignment of electrospun polyurethane meshes on mesenchymal progenitor cells. Tissue Eng. Part A **15**, 2435–2445 (2009). doi:10.1089/ten.tea.2008.0295
61. Berns, E.J., Sur, S., Pan, L., et al.: Aligned neurite outgrowth and directed cell migration in self-assembled monodomain gels. Biomaterials **35**, 185–195 (2014). doi:10.1016/j.biomaterials.2013.09.077
62. Morris, G.E., Bridge, J.C., Knox, A.J., et al.: Human airway smooth muscle maintain in situ cell orientation and phenotype when cultured on aligned electrospun scaffolds. Am. J. Physiol. Lung Cell. Mol. Physiol. (2014). doi:10.1152/ajplung.00318.2013
63. Saha, S., Duan, X., Wu, L., et al.: Electrospun fibrous scaffolds promote breast cancer cell alignment and epithelial-mesenchymal transition. Langmuir ACS J. Surf. Colloids **28**, 2028–2034 (2012). doi:10.1021/la203846w
64. Juliano, R.L.: Signal transduction by cell adhesion receptors and the cytoskeleton: functions of integrins, cadherins, selectins, and immunoglobulin-superfamily members. Annu. Rev. Pharmacol. Toxicol. **42**, 283–323 (2002). doi:10.1146/annurev.pharmtox.42.090401.151133
65. Thompson, P.M., Tolbert, C.E., Shen, K., et al.: Identification of an actin binding surface on vinculin that mediates mechanical cell and focal adhesion properties. Struct. Lond. Engl. 1993 **22**, 697–706 (2014). doi:10.1016/j.str.2014.03.002
66. Chew, S.Y., Mi, R., Hoke, A., Leong, K.W.: The effect of the alignment of electrospun fibrous scaffolds on Schwann cell maturation. Biomaterials **29**, 653–661 (2008). doi:10.1016/j.biomaterials.2007.10.025
67. Chang, J.-C., Fujita, S., Tonami, H., et al.: Cell orientation and regulation of cell-cell communication in human mesenchymal stem cells on different patterns of electrospun fibers. Biomed. Mater. Bristol Engl. **8**, 055002 (2013). doi:10.1088/1748-6041/8/5/055002
68. Chen, X., Fu, X., Shi, J., Wang, H.: Regulation of the osteogenesis of pre-osteoblasts by spatial arrangement of electrospun nanofibers in two- and three-dimensional environments. Nanomedicine Nanotechnol. Biol. Med. **9**, 1283–1292 (2013). doi:10.1016/j.nano.2013.04.013
69. Whited, B.M., Rylander, M.N.: The influence of electrospun scaffold topography on endothelial cell morphology, alignment, and adhesion in response to fluid flow. Biotechnol. Bioeng. **111**, 184–195 (2014). doi:10.1002/bit.24995

70. Lücker, P.B., Javaherian, S., Soleas, J.P., et al.: A microgroove patterned multiwell cell culture plate for high-throughput studies of cell alignment. Biotechnol. Bioeng. (2014). doi:10.1002/bit.25298
71. Ushiki, T.: Collagen fibers, reticular fibers and elastic fibers. A comprehensive understanding from a morphological viewpoint. Arch. Histol. Cytol. **65**, 109–126 (2002)
72. Kwon, I.K., Kidoaki, S., Matsuda, T.: Electrospun nano- to microfiber fabrics made of biodegradable copolyesters: structural characteristics, mechanical properties and cell adhesion potential. Biomaterials **26**, 3929–3939 (2005). doi:10.1016/j.biomaterials.2004.10.007
73. Wang, H.B., Mullins, M.E., Cregg, J.M., et al.: Varying the diameter of aligned electrospun fibers alters neurite outgrowth and Schwann cell migration. Acta Biomater. **6**, 2970–2978 (2010). doi:10.1016/j.actbio.2010.02.020
74. Kipen, H.M., Laskin, D.L.: Smaller is not always better: nanotechnology yields nanotoxicology. Am. J. Physiol. Lung. Cell. Mol. Physiol. **289**, L696–L697 (2005). doi:10.1152/ajplung.00277.2005
75. Discher, D.E., Janmey, P., Wang, Y.-L.: Tissue cells feel and respond to the stiffness of their substrate. Science **310**, 1139–1143 (2005). doi:10.1126/science.1116995
76. Smadja-Lamère, N., Boulanger, M.-C., Champagne, C., et al.: JNK-mediated phosphorylation of paxillin in adhesion assembly and tension-induced cell death by the adenovirus death factor E4orf4. J. Biol. Chem. **283**, 34352–34364 (2008). doi:10.1074/jbc.M803364200
77. Pasapera, A.M., Schneider, I.C., Rericha, E., et al.: Myosin II activity regulates vinculin recruitment to focal adhesions through FAK-mediated paxillin phosphorylation. J. Cell Biol. **188**, 877–890 (2010). doi:10.1083/jcb.200906012
78. Buxboim A., Rajagopal K., Brown A.E.X., Discher D.E. How deeply cells feel: methods for thin gels. J. Phys. Condens. Matter. (2010) doi:10.1088/0953-8984/22/19/194116
79. Jacot, J.G., McCulloch, A.D., Omens, J.H.: Substrate stiffness affects the functional maturation of neonatal rat ventricular myocytes. Biophys. J. **95**, 3479–3487 (2008). doi:10.1529/biophysj.107.124545
80. Bhana, B., Iyer, R.K., Chen, W.L.K., et al.: Influence of substrate stiffness on the phenotype of heart cells. Biotechnol. Bioeng. **105**, 1148–1160 (2010). doi:10.1002/bit.22647
81. Mi, H.-Y., Palumbo, S., Jing, X., et al.: Thermoplastic polyurethane/hydroxyapatite electrospun scaffolds for bone tissue engineering: effects of polymer properties and particle size. J. Biomed. Mater. Res. B Appl. Biomater. (2014). doi:10.1002/jbm.b.33122
82. Martianov, I., Cler, E., Duluc, I., et al.: TAF4 inactivation reveals the 3 dimensional growth promoting activities of collagen 6A3. PLoS ONE **9**, e87365 (2014). doi:10.1371/journal.pone.0087365
83. Lu, J., Zhou, S., Siech, M., et al.: Pancreatic stellate cells promote hapto-migration of cancer cells through collagen I-mediated signalling pathway. Br. J. Cancer **110**, 409–420 (2014). doi:10.1038/bjc.2013.706
84. Schenk, S., Hintermann, E., Bilban, M., et al.: Binding to EGF receptor of a laminin-5 EGF-like fragment liberated during MMP-dependent mammary gland involution. J. Cell Biol. **161**, 197–209 (2003). doi:10.1083/jcb.200208145
85. Marinkovich, M.P.: Tumour microenvironment: laminin 332 in squamous-cell carcinoma. Nat. Rev. Cancer **7**, 370–380 (2007). doi:10.1038/nrc2089
86. Muto, J., Morioka, Y., Yamasaki, K., et al.: Hyaluronan digestion controls DC migration from the skin. J. Clin. Invest. **124**, 1309–1319 (2014). doi:10.1172/JCI67947
87. Heise, R.L., Stober, V., Cheluvaraju, C., et al.: Mechanical stretch induces epithelial-mesenchymal transition in alveolar epithelia via hyaluronan activation of innate immunity. J. Biol. Chem. **286**, 17435–17444 (2011). doi:10.1074/jbc.M110.137273
88. Fischer, S.N., Johnson, J.K., Baran, C.P., et al.: Organ-derived coatings on electrospun nanofibers as ex vivo microenvironments. Biomaterials **32**, 538–546 (2011). doi:10.1016/j.biomaterials.2010.08.104
89. Kozlovskaya, V., Zavgorodnya, O., Chen, Y., et al.: Ultrathin polymeric coatings based on hydrogen-bonded polyphenol for protection of pancreatic islet cells. Adv. Funct. Mater. **22**, 3389–3398 (2012). doi:10.1002/adfm.201200138

90. Herrmann, D., Conway, J.R.W., Vennin, C., et al.: Three-dimensional cancer models mimic cell-matrix interactions in the tumour microenvironment. Carcinogenesis (2014). doi:10.1093/carcin/bgu108
91. Chwalek K., Bray L.J., Werner C.: Tissue-engineered 3D tumor angiogenesis models: potential technologies for anti-cancer drug discovery. Adv. Drug Deliv. Rev. (2014). doi: 10.1016/j.addr.2014.05.006
92. Tilghman, R.W., Parsons, J.T.: Focal adhesion kinase as a regulator of cell tension in the progression of cancer. Semin. Cancer Biol. **18**, 45–52 (2008). doi:10.1016/j.semcancer.2007.08.002
93. Larson, N., Ghandehari, H.: Polymeric conjugates for drug delivery. Chem. Mater. **24**, 840–853 (2012). doi:10.1021/cm2031569
94. Liechty, W.B., Kryscio, D.R., Slaughter, B.V., Peppas, N.A.: Polymers for drug delivery systems. Annu. Rev. Chem. Biomol. Eng. **1**, 149–173 (2010). doi:10.1146/annurev-chembioeng-073009-100847
95. Garg T., Singh O., Arora S., Murthy R.S.R.: Scaffold: a novel carrier for cell and drug delivery. Crit. Rev. Ther. Drug Carr. Syst. **29** (2012)
96. Biondi, M., Ungaro, F., Quaglia, F., Netti, P.A.: Controlled drug delivery in tissue engineering. Adv. Drug Deliv. Rev. **60**, 229–242 (2008). doi:10.1016/j.addr.2007.08.038
97. Kost, J., Langer, R.: Responsive polymeric delivery systems. Adv. Drug Deliv. Rev. **64**, 327–341 (2012). doi:10.1016/j.addr.2012.09.014
98. Vilar, G., Tulla-Puche, J., Albericio, F.: Polymers and drug delivery systems. Curr. Drug Deliv. **9**, 367–394 (2012)
99. Brewer, E., Coleman, J., Lowman, A.: Emerging technologies of polymeric nanoparticles in cancer drug delivery. J. Nanomater. **2011**, 1–10 (2011). doi:10.1155/2011/408675
100. Aliabadi, H.M., Lavasanifar, A.: Polymeric micelles for drug delivery. Expert Opin. Drug Deliv. **3**, 139–162 (2006). doi:10.1517/17425247.3.1.139
101. Gaucher, G., Satturwar, P., Jones, M.-C., et al.: Polymeric micelles for oral drug delivery. Eur. J. Pharm. Biopharm. **76**, 147–158 (2010). doi:10.1016/j.ejpb.2010.06.007
102. Croy, S.R., Kwon, G.S.: Polymeric micelles for drug delivery. Curr. Pharm. Des. **12**, 4669–4684 (2006)
103. Nanjwade, B.K., Bechra, H.M., Derkar, G.K., et al.: Dendrimers: emerging polymers for drug-delivery systems. Eur. J. Pharm. Sci. **38**, 185–196 (2009). doi:10.1016/j.ejps.2009.07.008
104. Lallana, E., Fernandez-Trillo, F., Sousa-Herves, A., et al.: Click chemistry with polymers, dendrimers, and hydrogels for drug delivery. Pharm. Res. **29**, 902–921 (2012). doi:10.1007/s11095-012-0683-y
105. Kesharwani, P., Jain, K., Jain, N.K.: Dendrimer as nanocarrier for drug delivery. Prog. Polym. Sci. **39**, 268–307 (2014). doi:10.1016/j.progpolymsci.2013.07.005
106. Svenson, S., Tomalia, D.A.: Dendrimers in biomedical applications—reflections on the field. Adv. Drug Deliv. Rev. **64**, 102–115 (2012). doi:10.1016/j.addr.2012.09.030
107. Hamidi, M., Azadi, A., Rafiei, P.: Hydrogel nanoparticles in drug delivery. Adv. Drug Deliv. Rev. **60**, 1638–1649 (2008). doi:10.1016/j.addr.2008.08.002
108. Lee, S.C., Kwon, I.K., Park, K.: Hydrogels for delivery of bioactive agents: A historical perspective. Adv. Drug Deliv. Rev. **65**, 17–20 (2013). doi:10.1016/j.addr.2012.07.015
109. Hennink, W.E., van Nostrum, C.F.: Novel crosslinking methods to design hydrogels. Adv. Drug Deliv. Rev. **64**, 223–236 (2012). doi:10.1016/j.addr.2012.09.009
110. Matricardi, P., Di Meo, C., Coviello, T., et al.: Interpenetrating polymer networks polysaccharide hydrogels for drug delivery and tissue engineering. Adv. Drug Deliv. Rev. **65**, 1172–1187 (2013). doi:10.1016/j.addr.2013.04.002
111. Zhang, Z., Chen, L., Deng, M., et al.: Biodegradable thermo- and pH-responsive hydrogels for oral drug delivery. J. Polym. Sci. Part Polym. Chem. **49**, 2941–2951 (2011). doi:10.1002/pola.24730
112. Li, Z., Guan, J.: Thermosensitive hydrogels for drug delivery. Expert Opin. Drug Deliv. **8**, 991–1007 (2011). doi:10.1517/17425247.2011.581656

113. Nguyen, M.K., Lee, D.S.: Injectable biodegradable hydrogels. Macromol. Biosci. **10**, 563–579 (2010). doi:10.1002/mabi.200900402
114. Seif-Naraghi, S.B., Horn, D., Schup-Magoffin, P.J., Christman, K.L.: Injectable extracellular matrix derived hydrogel provides a platform for enhanced retention and delivery of a heparin-binding growth factor. Acta Biomater. **8**, 3695–3703 (2012). doi:10.1016/j.actbio.2012.06.030
115. Singelyn, J.M., Sundaramurthy, P., Johnson, T.D., et al.: Catheter-deliverable hydrogel derived from decellularized ventricular extracellular matrix increases endogenous cardiomyocytes and preserves cardiac function post-myocardial infarction. J. Am. Coll. Cardiol. **59**, 751–763 (2012). doi:10.1016/j.jacc.2011.10.888
116. Kwon, J.S., Yoon, S.M., Shim, S.W., et al.: Injectable extracellular matrix hydrogel developed using porcine articular cartilage. Int. J. Pharm. **454**, 183–191 (2013). doi:10.1016/j.ijpharm.2013.06.023
117. Young, D.A., Ibrahim, D.O., Hu, D., Christman, K.L.: Injectable hydrogel scaffold from decellularized human lipoaspirate. Acta Biomater. **7**, 1040–1049 (2011). doi:10.1016/j.actbio.2010.09.035
118. Reing, J.E., Zhang, L., Myers-Irvin, J., et al.: Degradation products of extracellular matrix affect cell migration and proliferation. Tissue Eng. Part A **15**, 605–614 (2008)
119. Brennan, E.P., Reing, J., Chew, D., et al.: Antibacterial activity within degradation products of biological scaffolds composed of extracellular matrix. Tissue Eng. **12**, 2949–2955 (2006). doi:10.1089/ten.2006.12.2949
120. Zhang, G., Suggs, L.J.: Matrices and scaffolds for drug delivery in vascular tissue engineering. Adv. Drug Deliv. Rev. **59**, 360–373 (2007). doi:10.1016/j.addr.2007.03.018
121. Agarwal, S., Wendorff, J.H., Greiner, A.: Use of electrospinning technique for biomedical applications. Polymer **49**, 5603–5621 (2008). doi:10.1016/j.polymer.2008.09.014
122. Thakur, R.A., Florek, C.A., Kohn, J., Michniak, B.B.: Electrospun nanofibrous polymeric scaffold with targeted drug release profiles for potential application as wound dressing. Int. J. Pharm. **364**, 87–93 (2008). doi:10.1016/j.ijpharm.2008.07.033
123. Sokolsky-Papkov, M., Agashi, K., Olaye, A., et al.: Polymer carriers for drug delivery in tissue engineering. Adv. Drug Deliv. Rev. **59**, 187–206 (2007). doi:10.1016/j.addr.2007.04.001
124. Carlyle, W.C., McClain, J.B., Tzafriri, A.R., et al.: Enhanced drug delivery capabilities from stents coated with absorbable polymer and crystalline drug. J. Controlled Release **162**, 561–567 (2012). doi:10.1016/j.jconrel.2012.07.004
125. Gulati, K., Ramakrishnan, S., Aw, M.S., et al.: Biocompatible polymer coating of titania nanotube arrays for improved drug elution and osteoblast adhesion. Acta Biomater. **8**, 449–456 (2012). doi:10.1016/j.actbio.2011.09.004
126. Langer, R., Vacanti, J.P.: Tissue engineering. Science **260**, 920–926 (1993)
127. Imparato, G., Urciuolo, F., Casale, C., Netti, P.A.: The role of microscaffold properties in controlling the collagen assembly in 3D dermis equivalent using modular tissue engineering. Biomaterials **34**, 7851–7861 (2013). doi:10.1016/j.biomaterials.2013.06.062
128. De Jonge, N., Foolen, J., Brugmans, M.C.P., et al.: Degree of scaffold degradation influences collagen (re)orientation in engineered tissues. Tissue Eng. Part A **20**, 1747–1757 (2013). doi:10.1089/ten.tea.2013.0517
129. Saino, E., Focarete, M.L., Gualandi, C., et al.: Effect of electrospun fiber diameter and alignment on macrophage activation and secretion of proinflammatory cytokines and chemokines. Biomacromolecules **12**, 1900–1911 (2011). doi:10.1021/bm200248h
130. Cortez Tornello, P.R., Caracciolo, P.C., Cuadrado, T.R., Abraham, G.A.: Structural characterization of electrospun micro/nanofibrous scaffolds by liquid extrusion porosimetry: a comparison with other techniques. Mater. Sci. Eng. C **41**, 335–342 (2014). doi:10.1016/j.msec.2014.04.065
131. Takeda, T., Murphy, S., Uyama, S., et al.: Hepatocyte transplantation in swine using prevascularized polyvinyl alcohol sponges. Tissue Eng. **1**, 253–262 (1995). doi:10.1089/ten.1995.1.253

132. Uyama, S., Kaufmann, P.M., Takeda, T., Vacanti, J.P.: Delivery of whole liver-equivalent hepatocyte mass using polymer devices and hepatotrophic stimulation. Transplantation **55**, 932–935 (1993)
133. Hong, S.R., Lee, Y.M., Akaike, T.: Evaluation of a galactose-carrying gelatin sponge for hepatocytes culture and transplantation. J. Biomed. Mater. Res. A **67A**, 733–741 (2003). doi: 10.1002/jbm.a.10138
134. Saadi, T., Nayshool, O., Carmel, J., et al.: Cellularized biosynthetic micro-hydrogel polymers, for intravascular liver tissue regeneration therapy. Tissue Eng. Part A (2014). doi:10.1089/ten.TEA.2013.0494
135. Hofmann, S., Wong Po Foo, C.T., Rossetti, F., et al.: Silk fibroin as an organic polymer for controlled drug delivery. J. Controlled Release **111**, 219–227 (2006). doi:10.1016/j.jconrel.2005.12.009
136. Kundu, B., Kundu, S.C.: Bio-inspired fabrication of fibroin cryogels from the muga silkworm Antheraea assamensis for liver tissue engineering. Biomed. Mater. Bristol Engl. **8**, 055003 (2013). doi:10.1088/1748-6041/8/5/055003
137. Simpson, L.L., Tanswell, A.K., Joneja, M.G.: Epithelial cell differentiation in organotypic cultures of fetal rat lung. Am. J. Anat. **172**, 31–40 (1985). doi:10.1002/aja.1001720103
138. Xu, J., Liu, M., Post, M.: Differential regulation of extracellular matrix molecules by mechanical strain of fetal lung cells. Am. J. Physiol. Lung Cell Mol. Physiol. **276**, L728–L735 (1999)
139. Andrade, C.F., Wong, A.P., Waddell, T.K., et al.: Cell-based tissue engineering for lung regeneration. Am. J. Physiol. Lung Cell Mol. Physiol. **292**, L510–L518 (2007). doi:10.1152/ajplung.00175.2006
140. Ling, T.-Y., Liu, Y.-L., Huang, Y.-K., et al.: Differentiation of lung stem/progenitor cells into alveolar pneumocytes and induction of angiogenesis within a 3D gelatin—Microbubble scaffold. Biomaterials **35**, 5660–5669 (2014). doi:10.1016/j.biomaterials.2014.03.074
141. Singh, D., Zo, S.M., Kumar, A., Han, S.S.: Engineering three-dimensional macroporous hydroxyethyl methacrylate-alginate-gelatin cryogel for growth and proliferation of lung epithelial cells. J. Biomater. Sci. Polym. Ed. **24**, 1343–1359 (2013). doi:10.1080/09205063.2012.759505
142. Mondrinos, M.J., Koutzaki, S., Jiwanmall, E., et al.: Engineering three-dimensional pulmonary tissue constructs. Tissue Eng. **12**, 717–728 (2006). doi:10.1089/ten.2006.12.717
143. Sudo, R., Mitaka, T., Ikeda, M., Tanishita, K.: Reconstruction of 3D stacked-up structures by rat small hepatocytes on microporous membranes. FASEB J. (2005). doi:10.1096/fj.04-3269fje
144. Liu, Y., Li, H., Yan, S., et al.: Hepatocyte cocultures with endothelial cells and fibroblasts on micropatterned fibrous mats to promote liver-specific functions and capillary formation capabilities. Biomacromolecules **15**, 1044–1054 (2014). doi:10.1021/bm401926k
145. Miyazawa, M., Torii, T., Toshimitsu, Y., et al.: A tissue-engineered artificial bile duct grown to resemble the native bile duct. Am. J. Transplant. **5**, 1541–1547 (2005). doi:10.1111/j.1600-6143.2005.00845.x
146. Macchiarini, P., Jungebluth, P., Go, T., et al.: Clinical transplantation of a tissue-engineered airway. Lancet **372**, 2023–2030 (2008). doi:10.1016/S0140-6736(08)61598-6
147. Gonfiotti, A., Jaus, M.O., Barale, D., et al.: The first tissue-engineered airway transplantation: 5-year follow-up results. Lancet **383**, 238–244 (2014). doi:10.1016/S0140-6736(13)62033-4
148. Sato, T., Tao, H., Araki, M., et al.: Replacement of the left main bronchus with a tissue-engineered prosthesis in a canine model. Ann. Thorac. Surg. **86**, 422–428 (2008). doi:10.1016/j.athoracsur.2008.04.015
149. Sato, T., Araki, M., Nakajima, N., et al.: Biodegradable polymer coating promotes the epithelization of tissue-engineered airway prostheses. J. Thorac. Cardiovasc. Surg. **139**, 26–31 (2010). doi:10.1016/j.jtcvs.2009.04.006

150. Shin, Y.S., Lee, B.H., Choi, J.W., et al.: Tissue-engineered tracheal reconstruction using chondrocyte seeded on a porcine cartilage-derived substance scaffold. Int. J. Pediatr. Otorhinolaryngol. **78**, 32–38 (2014). doi:10.1016/j.ijporl.2013.10.014
151. Chang, J.W., Park, S.A., Park, J.-K., et al.: Tissue-engineered tracheal reconstruction using three-dimensionally printed artificial tracheal graft: preliminary report. Artif. Organs **38**, E95–E105 (2014). doi:10.1111/aor.12310
152. Miller, C., George, S., Niklason, L.: Developing a tissue-engineered model of the human bronchiole. J. Tissue Eng. Regen. Med. **4**, 619–627 (2010). doi:10.1002/term.277
153. Ghezzi, C.E., Risse, P.-A., Marelli, B., et al.: An airway smooth muscle cell niche under physiological pulsatile flow culture using a tubular dense collagen construct. Biomaterials **34**, 1954–1966 (2013). doi:10.1016/j.biomaterials.2012.11.025
154. Price, A.P., England, K.A., Matson, A.M., et al.: Development of a decellularized lung bioreactor system for bioengineering the lung: the matrix reloaded. Tissue Eng. Part A **16**, 2581–2591 (2010). doi:10.1089/ten.tea.2009.0659
155. Bonvillain, R.W., Danchuk, S., Sullivan, D.E., et al.: A nonhuman primate model of lung regeneration: detergent-mediated decellularization and initial in vitro recellularization with mesenchymal stem cells. Tissue Eng. Part A **18**, 2437–2452 (2012). doi:10.1089/ten.tea.2011.0594
156. Petersen, T.H., Calle, E.A., Colehour, M.B., Niklason, L.E.: Matrix composition and mechanics of decellularized lung scaffolds. Cells Tissues Organs **195**, 222–231 (2012). doi:10.1159/000324896
157. Ghaedi, M., Calle, E.A., Mendez, J.J., et al.: Human iPS cellâ€“derived alveolar epithelium repopulates lung extracellular matrix. J. Clin. Invest. **123**, 4950–4962 (2013). doi:10.1172/JCI68793
158. Uygun, B.E., Soto-Gutierrez, A., Yagi, H., et al.: Organ reengineering through development of a transplantable recellularized liver graft using decellularized liver matrix. Nat. Med. **16**, 814–820 (2010). doi:10.1038/nm.2170
159. Barakat, O., Abbasi, S., Rodriguez, G., et al.: Use of decellularized porcine liver for engineering humanized liver organ. J. Surg. Res. **173**, e11–e25 (2012). doi:10.1016/j.jss.2011.09.033
160. Huh, D., Matthews, B.D., Mammoto, A., et al.: Reconstituting organ-level lung functions on a chip. Science **328**, 1662–1668 (2010). doi:10.1126/science.1188302
161. Lee, J., Kim, S.H., Kim, Y.-C., et al.: Fabrication and characterization of microfluidic liver-on-a-chip using microsomal enzymes. Enzyme Microb. Technol. **53**, 159–164 (2013). doi:10.1016/j.enzmictec.2013.02.015
162. Cornelissen, C.G., Dietrich, M., Gromann, K., et al.: Fibronectin coating of oxygenator membranes enhances endothelial cell attachment. Biomed. Eng. **12**, 7 (2013). doi:10.1186/1475-925X-12-7
163. Koshy, S.T., Ferrante, T.C., Lewin, S.A., Mooney, D.J.: Injectable, porous, and cell-responsive gelatin cryogels. Biomaterials **35**, 2477–2487 (2014). doi:10.1016/j.biomaterials.2013.11.044
164. Gou, M., Qu, X., Zhu, W., et al.: Bio-inspired detoxification using 3D-printed hydrogel nanocomposites. Nat. Commun. (2014). doi:10.1038/ncomms4774

[illegible] Tissue engineered tracheal reconstruction using [illegible] cartilage-derived substance scaffold. Int J Pediatr Otorhinolaryngol 78 [illegible] doi:10.1016/j.ijporl.2013.10.015

[illegible]

[illegible]

Chapter 8
Polymers for Surgery

Shuko Suzuki and Yoshito Ikada

Abstract During surgery, tissue injuries occur intentionally and unintentionally. Intentional injuries include scission of skin to secure the operation area and resection of diseased tissues and organs, whereas accidental injuries can also occur presumably due to mechanical contact of devices and surgeon's gloves with patient's internal organs and tissues. Bioabsorbable polymers have been tremendously contributed to surgical applications for healing those injuries. They include surgical sealants, anti-adhesion barriers, fixation devices, and sutures. This chapter provides a detailed view on surgical bioabsorbable polymeric products that are commercially available as well as the activity of their current research and developments.

Keywords Sealants · Adhesives · Hemostatic agents · Tissue adhesion barriers · Sutures

Abbreviations

AAc	Acrylic acid
CMC	Carboxymethyl cellulose
DHA	Dihydroxyacetone
DMA	Dopamine methacrylamide
DOPA	3,4-dihydroxy-L-phenylalanine

S. Suzuki (✉)
Queensland Eye Institute, 140 Melbourne Street,
South Brisbane QLD 4101, Australia
e-mail: Shuko.Suzuki@qei.org.au

Y. Ikada
Emeritus Professor of Kyoto University, 53 Kawara-cho Shogoin,
Sakyo-ku, Kyoto 606-8507, Japan
e-mail: yyikada@wd5.so-net.ne.jp

F. Puoci (ed.), *Advanced Polymers in Medicine*, DOI 10.1007/978-3-319-12478-0_8

FDA Food and drug administration
GRF Gelatin-resorcinol-formaldehyde
HA Hyaluronic acid
MEA Methoxyethyl acrylate
MPEG Methoxypoly(ethylene glycol)
NHS N-hydroxysuccinimide
PCL Poly(ε-caprolactone)
PEG Poly(ethylene glycol)
PEO Poly(ethylene oxide)
PGA Polyglycolide
PGLA Poly(glycolide-*co*-L-lactide)
PGS Poly(glycerol sebacate)
PLLA Poly(L-lactide)
PVA Poly(vinyl alcohol)
PVP Polyvinylpyrrolidone
TAD Tartaric acid derivative
TMC Trimethylene carbonate

Introduction

During surgery, tissue injuries occur that include scission of skin to secure the operation area and resection of diseased tissues and organs. In addition, unintentional injuries can also occur presumably due to mechanical contact of devices and surgeon's gloves with patient's internal organs and tissues. To repair these injuries, bioabsorbable polymers are most suitable since their function is required only during or for a few days after surgery and a second surgery for their retrieval is not necessary. Clinical applications of bioabsorbable polymers are listed in Table 8.1.

Table 8.1 Clinical applications of bioabsorbable polymers

Function	Purpose	Examples
Binding	Fixation	Fractured bone fixation
	Adhesion	Adhesion of tissue pieces
Closure	Suturing	Tissue approximation and vascular and intestinal anastomosis
	Covering	Wound cover
	Sealing	Topical hemostasis and air leakage
	Occlusion	Vascular embolization
Separation	Isolation	Organ protection
	Contact inhibition	Adhesion prevention
Scaffold	Cellular proliferation	Tissue and organ regeneration
	Tissue guide	Nerve reunion
Capsulation	Controlled drug delivery system	Sustained drug release

Both synthetic and natural biodegradable polymers have been used as surgical materials, and these polymers degrade in the body through hydrolysis or enzymes, respectively. Synthetic polymers are mainly homopolymers or copolymers of poly(α-hydroxyacid)s. Natural polymers include proteins, such as collagen, gelatin, albumin and fibrin, and polysaccharides, such as hyaluronic acid, chitosan and chitin. Alternatively, water soluble polymers, such as carboxymethyl cellulose (i.e. natural polymer) and poly(ethylene glycol) (PEG) (i.e. synthetic polymer), have also been used that are not degradable but are absorbable in the body.

This chapter covers polymeric medical devices that are essential for surgical operation focusing in particular on bioabsorbable devices. Since some of these devices such as bone fixatives and drug delivery systems are covered in details in other chapters, bioabsorbable polymers used as sealants/adhesives/hemostatic agents, anti-adhesive barriers, and sutures are discussed. It is beyond the scope of this chapter to comprehensively cover all the research in this rapidly expanding area. Instead, the focus is on commercially available products and some recent research.

Sealants/Adhesives/Hemostatic Agents Against Bleeding and Other Types of Leakage

Surgical adhesives/sealants have been widely used in surgery to prevent air leaks (from holes in diseased soft tissues such as lung), liquid leaks (including hemostasis, as for oozing), and as adhesives (to bond two separate tissues, but very rarely). They have many advantages over traditional techniques (i.e. sutures and staples) such as reducing both operative time and physical load on patients. Sealants/adhesives are often liquids and cure when applied to form a firm gel. Ideally, they should be rapidly curable even in the presence of water, as pliable as soft tissues when cured, and bioabsorbable in the body. Three main types are available for these materials; naturally-derived (such as fibrin glue), semi-synthetic (such as naturally-derived polymer—aldehyde based), and synthetic (such as cyanoacrylates and PEG).

Requirements for these surgical sealants/adhesives are listed in Table 8.2 [1]. As they are applied to the human body, they must be safe, nontoxic, and free from risk of infectious transmission. They should be bioabsorbable and not persist long as a foreign body. The sealants (i.e. solutions that are applied and form a gel)

Table 8.2 Requirements for these surgical sealants/adhesives

1. In situ curable from the liquid state through polymerization, chemical cross-linking, or solvent evaporation
2. Rapidly curable under wet physiological conditions
3. Strongly bondable to tissue
4. Nontoxic agents and degradation products
5. As tough and pliable as natural tissues
6. Bioabsorbable

as well as their degradation products must be safe. In addition, they must not hinder the natural healing process. Commercial products of these materials and recent research in surgical sealants/adhesives/hemostatic agents are discussed in this section. This is a fast growing area as can be seen from various recent reviews [2–5], and we will not cover all the products and research studies. Several commercially available products are listed in Table 8.3.

Naturally-Derived Sealants/Adhesives/Hemostatic Agents

Fibrin Glue

Fibrin glue is based on the natural clotting process, as shown in Fig. 8.1. It consists of two component systems; one contains human fibrinogen, Factor XIII, fibronectin, and fibrinolysis inhibitor, while the other contains human thrombin and calcium chloride (Table 8.4). When two solutions are mixed, thrombin promotes the conversion of fibrinogen to soluble fibrin molecules, as well as activates factor XIII. Fibrin molecules subsequently assemble into a fibrin clot and are stabilised by the activated factor XIII. Aprotinin is a basic pancreatic trypsin inhibitor which is added to commercial fibrin glues to yield delayed fibrinolysis of clots. The fibrin clot is degraded by physiologic fibrinolysis over a two-week period [6]. The concentration of fibrinogen determines the strength of the fibrin clot, and the amount of thrombin controls the rate of clot network formation. For application, two solutions are set in a dural-chamber delivery system with or without a spraying device. A fibrin clot is formed within 30 s when the components are applied at the site of injury. The process of preparation requires constant warming and stirring, which takes around 20–30 min.

Fibrin glue has many advantages such as acceptable biocompatibility, biodegradability, injectability, and in situ-producible scaffolds for tissue regeneration. Successful clinical application of fibrin glue has been demonstrated in many surgical fields (Table 8.5) [7–9]. Cardiovascular surgery is the most common among them, and its major purpose is hemostasis and suture hole sealing. Fibrin glue is also highly effective as a tissue sealant in cases of diffuse, low-pressure bleeding such as coronary vein bleeding, right-ventricle/pulmonary-artery conduits, and right-ventricular patches.

On the contrary, some clinical applications have shown no effects of fibrin glue such as for reducing drain output or in facilitating early functional recovery in total knee arthroplasty [10] and seroma formation after breast surgery [11]. There are several disadvantages, such as the risk of viral infection due to human- and animal blood-derived products, low strength, and rapid loss of strength [12]. It also requires long preparation time and operator skill, and is quite expensive, at approximately $100–150/ml of fibrinogen.

Many technical efforts have been made to improve its low adhesive strength, especially in situations like sealing of needle holes. Methods of application include

Table 8.3 Commercially-available sealants, adhesives, and hemostatic agents

	Main composition	Manufacturer	Trade name	Introduced/ Approved year	Degradation/ Absorption time
Sealants/Adhesives	Fibrinogen and thrombin from human pooled plasma	Baxter	Tisseel, Artiss	1998	2 weeks
		Johnson & Johnson	Evicel	2006	2 weeks
		Aventis Behring	Beriplast	1980s	2 weeks
	PEG-NHS and trilysine	Confluent surgical	DuraSeal, DuraSeal Xact	2003	4–8 weeks
	PEG-NHS and PEG-SH	Baxter	CoSeal	2001	4 weeks
	PEG[a], triethanolamine and eosin Y	Ethicon	AdvaSeal	1998	1–2 months
	Human serum albumin and PEG-NHS	BARD	Progel	2010	<1 month
	Bovine serum albumin and polyaldehyde	Tenaxis Medical	ArterX vascular sealant	2013	>12–24 months[b]
	Gelatin, resorcinol, formaldehyde and glutaraldehyde	Cardial	GRF glue	1979	>24 months
	Bovine albumin and glutaraldehyde	CryoLife	BioGlue	1999	<24 months
	Octyl-2-cyanoacrylate	Colure Medical	Dermabond[c]	1998	–
	n-Butyl-2-cyanoacrylate	B.Braun	Histoacryl[c]	1968	–
		COVIDIEN	Indermil[c]	1996	–
	Blend of n-butyl and 2-octyl cyanoacrylates	Advanced Medical Solutions	LiquiBand[c]	1999	–
	(PVA)-(AAc)-(AAc-NHS) and PGLA	Tissuemed	TissuePatch3, TissuePatch	2007	<12 weeks[d]

(continued)

Table 8.3 (continued)

	Main composition	Manufacturer	Trade name	Introduced/ Approved year	Degradation/ Absorption time
Hemostatic Agents (Stand-alone)	Gelatin	Pfizer	Gelfoam	1945	4 weeks
	Oxidized cellulose	Ethicon	Surgicel	1942	7–14 days
	Collagen	Bard	Abiten	1970	8 weeks
	Chitosan	HemCon Medical	HemCon[e], ChitoFlex[e]	2002, 2007	–
(Combination)	Fibrinogen, thrombin and collagen fleece	Nycomed Arzneimittel	TachoComb	1990	16–20 weeks
	Thrombin and gelatin particles	Baxter	FloSeal	1999	6–8 weeks
	PEG, trilysine and oxidized cellulose backing	COVIDIEN	Veriset	N/A[f]	N/A[f]

PEG poly(ethylene glycol), *NHS* N-hydroxysuccinimide, *PVA* poly(vinyl alcohol), *AAc* acrylic acid, *PGLA* poly(glycolide-*co*-L-lactide)
[a]Copolymer of PEG and oligotriethylene carbonate with acrylate ester end caps
[b]Significant absorption occurs by 12 months, and continues beyond 24 months
[c]The sealant is topical application to the skin only and comes off from skin after 7–10 days
[d]PGLA degrades within 12 weeks, but the terpolymer remains at this time point
[e]The product is not to be left within the body cavity
[f]Data not available

Fig. 8.1 Fibrin clot formation from fibrinogen

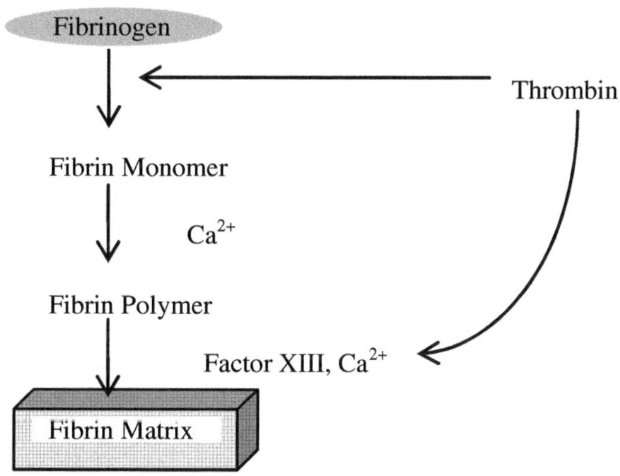

Table 8.4 Compositions of fibrin glues

Components	Concentration	Origin
Fibrinogen (clottable)	80–120 g/l	Human plasma
Factor XIII (activity)	10–30 IU/ml	Human plasma or human placenta
Fibronectin (antigen)	5–20 g/l	Human plasma
Thrombin (activity)	300–600 NIH-U/ml	Human plasma or bovine plasma
Aprotinin	3,000 KIU/ml	Bovine lung
Calcium chloride	40–60 mM	Inorganic

Table 8.5 Clinical applications of fibrin glue

Cardiovascular surgery	Hemostasis of bleeding from mediastinum and small blood vessels, reinforcement of suture line, sealing of vascular grafts and anastomoses
Thoracic surgery	Sealing of air leaks from raw lung surface, and pulmonary and bronchial staple lines
Gynecologic surgery	Anastomosis of fallopian tube, adhesion of peritoneum
Plastic surgery	Closure of skin wound, attachment of skin grafts, fixation of tissue flaps
Orthopaedic surgery	Fixation of bone fragments, hemostasis during total knee arthroplasty
Urologic surgery	Anastomosis of urinary tube and adhesion of kidney, pelvis renalis, and ureter

a separate dripping method using two separate syringes, a simultaneous dripping method using a syringe applicator, and a spray method using a spray applicator. Although the spray method exhibits the strongest sealing effect due to homogeneous application resulting in complete mixing of the two components [13–15], adhesive strength is still not adequate for control of local bleeding in the clinical setting. The rub-and-spray method consists of rubbing the fibrinogen solution onto the needle holes with a finger and then spraying the two solutions using an application nozzle. This technique has been experimentally and clinically found to be effective in cardiovascular surgery [16, 17].

For application in pulmonary surgeries, surgeons have often found that fibrin sealant does not effectively seal air leakages. To overcome this problem, the application of fibrin glue in combination with a polyglycolide (PGA) sheet (Neoveil, Gunze Corp, Kyoto, Japan) has been developed and shown to have clinical effectiveness [18–21]. The PGA sheet is a soft non-woven fabric, which is flexible, easily shaped to reconstruct complex shapes, and highly compatible with fibrin glue. It is degraded by hydrolysis and bioabsorbed in about 15 weeks. The PGA sheet retains fibrin glue that otherwise would run down from the rough site of application. The combination of PGA fabric and fibrin glue has been shown to improve adhesive strength and resistance to air/water leakage. This technique has been expanded to other applications including neurosurgery and gastroenterological surgery [22–27].

Fibrin Glue Sheet

TachoComb® (CSL Behring, PA, USA) is a ready-to-use hemostatic sheet, consisting of equine collagen fleece with surface coating of fibrin agents (human fibrinogen, bovine thrombin, and bovine aprotinin). Further development of TachoComb® is TachoSil®, and their compositions are shown in Table 8.6. The products do not require any preparation or conditioning, and can be immediately applied directly to traumatized tissues, in contrast to the liquid application of fibrin glue. When the coating of collagen fleece comes in contact with fluids (i.e. normal saline, body fluid, or a bleeding surface), the components dissolve and diffuse into the cavities and begin to react. The collagen fleece helps to tamponade the wound and keeps the coagulation components in the region of bleeding. It requires 3–5 min of pressing till the area is sealed. It is mechanically stable and can be used for the treatment of diffuse bleeding of the thoracic wall. The adhesive strength is much higher than that of fibrin glue, since dried fibrinogen and thrombin will form a highly concentrated gel when a small amount of surface water is used from the site of application.

Table 8.6 Active compositions of TachoComb® and TachoSil® (/cm^2 sheet)

TachoComb	TachoSil
Fibrinogen (human, 5.5 mg)	Fibrinogen (human, 5.5 mg)
Thrombin (bovine, 1.38 IU)	Thrombin (human, 2.0 IU)
Aprotinin (bovine, 128 KIU)	
Collagen fleece (equine, 1.65 mg)	Collagen fleece (equine, 2.1 mg)

The application of fibrin glue sheet was reviewed for 408 patients with hemorrhagic risk factors or operations associated with an expected increase in bleeding [28]. The operations were performed on various organs, such as the liver, vascular system, heart, spleen, thorax, and kidney, and the results supported the efficacy and safety of TachoSil® as a hemostatic agent. Other recent clinical studies have demonstrated efficacies of Tachosil® in hepatobiliary and pancreatic surgeries [29–31] and lymph node dissection [32]. Tachosil® Fibrin glue sheet has also been used as a dural substitute, and a clinical study of 288 patients revealed no superficial or deep wound infections or aseptic meningitis [33].

Gelatin—Thrombin Hemostasis

FloSeal® (Baxter Healthcare Corporation, Fremont, CA, USA) consists of cross-linked gelatin granules and human thrombin (Thrombin-JMI®, a sterile freeze-dried powder, Jones Pharma, Inc., Bristol, VA, USA). Bovine-derived gelatin is cross-linked with glutaraldehyde and ground to 500–600 μm sized particle. Prior to use, the thrombin is reconstituted with saline and added to the gelatin matrix component in the operating suite.

When applied to a bleeding site, the gelatin granules swell by 10–20 % within 10 min, reducing blood flow and providing tamponade. It can conform to irregular wound shapes. The high concentration of thrombin reacts with fibrinogen and forms a reinforced clot around the gelatin matrix. Unreacted granules can be removed with gentle irrigation or suction. The granules in the clot are bioabsorbed by the body in 6–8 weeks. Unlike fibrin glue, this agent only works in the presence of blood [34, 35]. FloSeal® has been widely used in various surgical operations [36], and its application in neurosurgery has also been reviewed [37].

Other Types of Natural Physical Hemostatic Agents

Various types of biodegradable hemostatic agents are currently available. These include gelatin foams, collagen microfibrillar, fibrillar/knitted oxidized cellulose, and chitosan sponges (Table 8.3). These hemostatic agents have often been applied to aid to cease hemorrhage mechanically when surgeons compress the bleeding points. They can absorb fluid up to several times of their own weight and are useful in the situation of heavier bleeding. Despite their clinical successes as hemostatic agents, there are some disadvantages, such as weak adherence to wet tissues, complications from the expanded materials pressing nerves in surrounding tissues against hard tissue, confusions of the presence of passive hemostatic agents in subsequent diagnostic images with a tumor or abscess, and prolonged residual products causing foreign body reaction that lead to granuloma formation [38].

Semi-synthetic Sealants/Adhesives/Hemostatic Agents

Gelatin-Based Glue

Gelatin-resorcinol-formaldehyde (GRF glue, Cardial, Techinopole, Sainte-Etienne, France) is composed of two types of solutions, GR solution (gelatin and resorcinol) and F-activator (formaldehyde and glutaraldehyde). Formaldehyde and glutaraldehyde react not only with gelatin and resorcinol, but may also react with amino groups of tissues, creating bonding between the resulting gel and the tissue. The proposed chemical structures of these components and their reaction scheme are shown in Fig. 8.2.

Since the introduction of GRF in 1979 for acute aortic dissection [39], it has been widely used except in the United States. In acute type A aortic dissection, the survival of patients depends on immediate diagnosis and emergent surgical intervention. Without surgery, the mortality rate is 38 % in the first day and up to 90 % after 2 weeks. The clinical use of GRF is problematic due to continued controversy concerning the possible carcinogenicity and mutagenicity of formaldehyde. It has

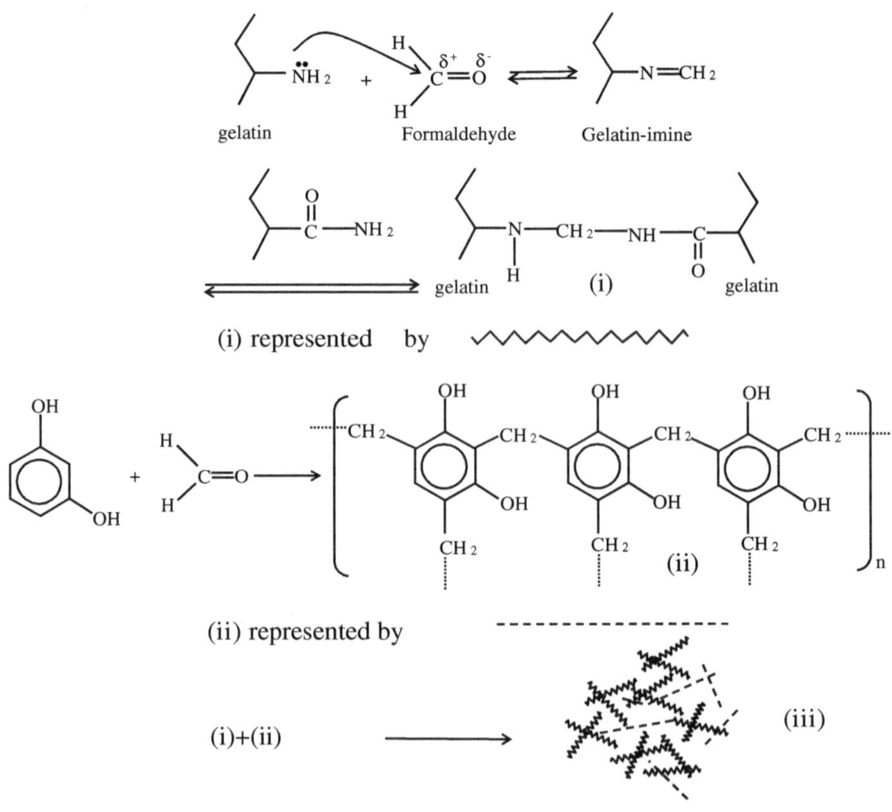

Fig. 8.2 Reaction scheme for gelatin-resorcinol-formaldehyde (*GRF*) glue

been reported that long-term exposure of formaldehyde in embalming practice and in the funeral industry is significantly associated with increased risk for mortality from myeloid leukemia [40].

Efforts have been made to eliminate formaldehyde from the composition of GRF and to replace it with glutaraldehyde alone or glyoxal. However, these attempts were unsuccessful, as its bonding was reduced and affected the efficacy of the product, though greater durability was observed in vivo. By reducing the formaldehyde concentration and mixing with glutaraldehyde, high initial strength and increased durability were achieved [41]. Conflicting data are found in the literature on the effect of GRF glue in aortic surgery. Long-term stability of the dissected, GRF-treated aorta has been reported, whereas other studies found late adverse events such as distal embolization [42–44].

Albumin-Based Glue

In BioGlue® (CryoLife, Inc., Kennesaw, GA, USA), stoichiometrically equivalent doses of bovine serum albumin (45 % solution) and glutaraldehyde (10 % solution) are mixed in a custom cartridge delivery system [45]. It has been used in cardiac, vascular, pulmonary, and soft tissue repairs. The major applications include sealing around suture lines and staples in large blood vessels such as the aorta and femoral arteries. In comparison to fibrin glue, BioGlue® has high adhesive strength to tissues and is much stiffer [46], as well as has longer degradation time (Table 8.3).

In 2007, Zehr reported detailed techniques of application for the use of BioGlue® in a variety of cardiovascular surgical cases and found that BioGlue® was safe and effective when used properly [47]. In a clinical study involving 151 patients undergoing cardiac and vascular repair procedures, anastomotic bleeding was significantly reduced in the Bioglue® group (18.8 %, n = 76) compared with the control group (42.9 %, $p < 0.001$, n = 75). The use of pledgets was reduced in the BioGlue® group (26.2 %) compared with the control group (35.9 %, $p = 0.047$) [48]. In application in thoracic surgery, a randomized, controlled trial of the effectiveness of BioGlue® was carried out in 52 patients being treated for alveolar air leaks [49]. Surgical treatment with BioGlue® exhibited statistically significant effectiveness in all categories compared to the control group (surgical treatment only). Despite its success in clinical studies, the toxicity of unreacted and leached glutaraldehyde and the dense postoperative gel structure have been the concerns and have limited the application of BioGlue®. Fürst et al. investigated the release of glutaraldehyde from BioGlue® and its toxicity in vitro and in vivo [50]. It was found that 100–200 μg/mL of glutaraldehyde was released from 1 mL of gelled BioGlue® into 5 mL of saline, and the supernatant exhibited cytotoxicity in cultured human embryonic fibroblasts (MRC5) and mouse myoblasts (C1C12).

Progel® (Neomend, Inc., Irvine, CA, USA) is based on human serum albumin and PEG disuccinimidyl succinate as a cross-linker. This product is approved by FDA for intraoperative use during pulmonary resection. A review of preclinical and clinical studies demonstrated the efficacy and safety of this product [51].

Another recently approved albumin-based product is ArterX® vascular sealant (Tenaxis Medical, Mountain View, CA, USA), which is composed of bovine serum albumin and polyaldehyde, for use as a sealant around anastomotic sites of synthetic arterial bypass grafts and patches. A randomized prospective multicentre trail, involving 331 anastomotic sites in 217 patients, was undertaken comparing ArterX® vascular sealant with Gelfoam® Plus (i.e. control group), and showed no difference in safety [52]. The operation time was significantly less in the ArterX® vascular sealant group compared with the control group.

Lysine-Based Glue

TissuGlu® (Cohera Medical, Pittsburgh, PA, USA) is a lysine-derived urethane adhesive which cures in the presence of moisture. This is applied to the abdominal wall prior to closure of the abdominoplasty flap to reduce wound drainage and seroma formation. The safety and efficacy of TissuGlu® have been demonstrated in preclinical and clinical studies [53, 54].

Oxidized Cellulose-Based Hemostatic Agent

Veriset™ (COVIDIEN, Inc., Mansfield, MA, USA) is a topical hemostatic agent which is a combination of an oxidized cellulose backing and self-adhesive hydrogel consisting of PEG and trilysine. This ready-to-use hemostatic patch has been clinically compared with TachoSil® in the management of diffuse bleeding after hepatic surgery ($n = 50$) [55]. They found that the median time to hemostasis in the Veriset™ group was faster than that of the control group (1 vs. 3 min, $p < 0.001$).

Synthetic Sealants/Adhesives

Cyanoacrylates

Cyanoacrylates are monomers containing esters of cyanoacrylic acid. Various homologues of cyanoacrylate adhesive have been studied including methyl, ethyl, isobutyl, isohexyl, and octyl cyanoaclylates. These monomers rapidly polymerize when in contact with water or hydroxyl groups on the actual surface being glued [56]. These create strong and flexible films as sealants to bond apposed wound skin edges. Use of these topical skin adhesives is faster and less painful than that of suturing. The skin edges are held in apposition and cyanoacrylate is applied in layers along the entire length of the wound. It is recommended by the manufacturers that a total of three layers of the glue is applied. Spontaneous release of heat occurs as the polymer forms. The agent remains adherent to the skin for approximately 7–10 days while the wound heals, and comes off as the superficial layers of skin exfoliate.

Cyanoacrylates have been used mainly for external surfaces as tissue adhesives for surgical and traumatic wound repair, due to their toxicity.

The shorter chain esters may be more toxic either directly or through their degradation products, which are cyanacrylates and formaldehyde. The degradation products accumulate in tissues and produce acute and chronic inflammation. In contrast, longer alkyl chains (e.g. 10 carbons) are less toxic. In addition, the shorter chain esters such as butyl cyanoacrylate have been used only for small low-tension lacerations and incisions due to its poor tensile strength and brittleness, whereas octyl cyanoacrylate yields stronger and more flexible adhesives [57]. In an animal model, various commercially available cyanoacrylate products have been compared for wound bursting strengths immediately after closure and 1 and 2 days after [58]. Dermabond® (Colure Medical Corporation, Raleigh, NC, USA), which consists of octyl 2-cyanoacrylate, was significantly stronger and more flexible than all the cyanoacrylate-based adhesives tested at all time points of measurement.

Surface application of Dermabond® has been shown to be very successful. A randomized, control trial showed that the wounds closed by Dermabond® had no noticeable differences in subjective cosmetic results and was associated with complications at 3 months postoperatively, compared with wounds closed using monofilament sutures. Adhesives also had the advantage of much faster operative time than traditional suturing. A randomized controlled trail of Liquiband® Surgical S (Advanced Medical Solutions, Devon, UK), which is a blend of n-butyl and 2-octyl cyanoacrylates, and sutures for closure of laparoscopic wounds showed closure with Liquiband® was significantly faster by mean of 2 min [59]. In addition, the use of skin adhesives has shown to reduce surgical site infections from some specific bacterial agents [60, 61].

PEG-Based Sealants

PEG-based sealants are flexible and firmly adherent even on wet tissues. These hydrogels also have the ability to prevent adhesions. DuraSeal™ (Confluent Surgical Inc., Waltham, MA, USA) is one such product developed for watertight closure after dural suturing. Two solutions, PEG-ester and trilysine amine, are mixed together and sprayed on the site of treatment (Fig. 8.3). They rapidly react via electrophilic nucleation reaction and form an elastic hydrogel. A multicentre, prospective randomized trial involving 237 patients was performed to evaluate the safety of DuraSeal™ as a dural sealant in cranial surgery [62]. DuraSeal™ was found to be similarly safe as commonly used dural sealing techniques, and demonstrated faster preparation and application times than other techniques.

CoSeal® (Baxter, Fremont, CA, USA) is another PEG-based hydrogel that is used in vascular reconstructions to achieve adjunctive hemostasis by mechanically sealing the region of leakage. Tetrafunctional succinimdylglutaryl PEG macromer (PEG-NHS) reacts with a thiol PEG macromer (PEG-SH) and protein to form a dimer, which leads to the formation of cross-linked polymers (Fig. 8.4). It polymerizes in ~5 s. The hydrogel swells approximately 400 % over 24 h. A randomized, controlled trial was performed to evaluate the efficacy of CoSeal®

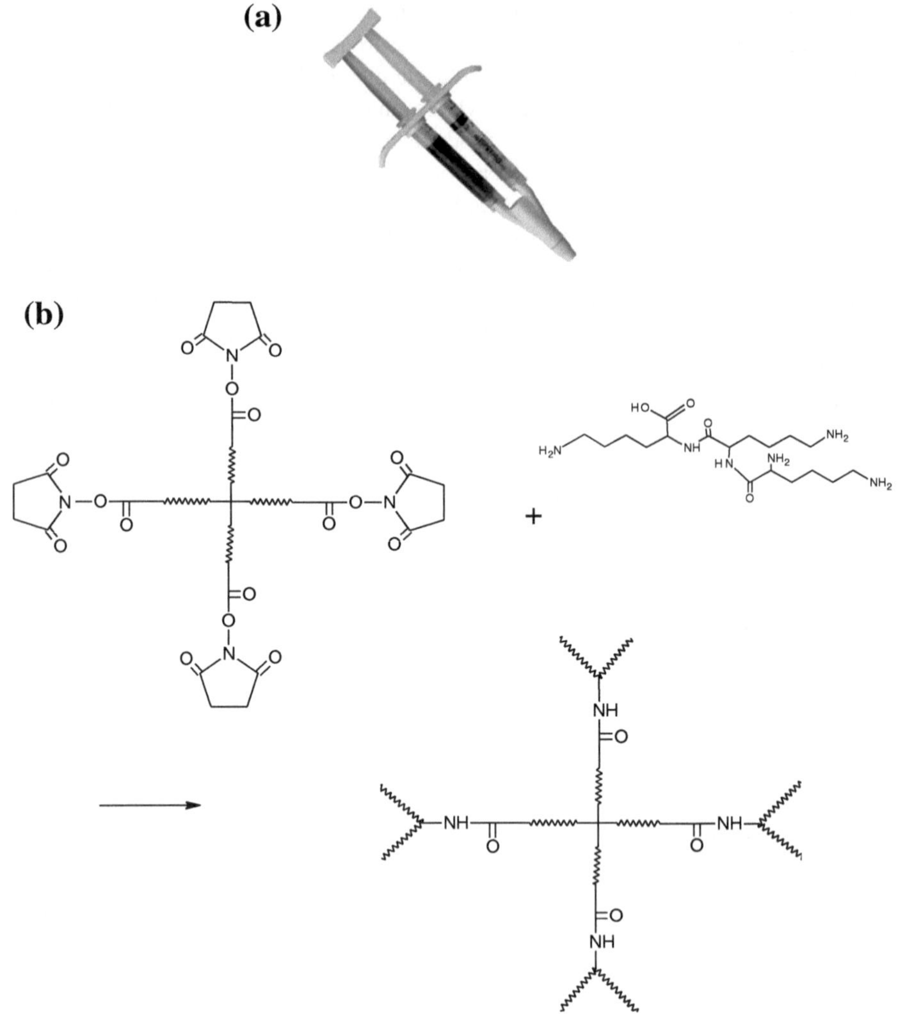

Fig. 8.3 **a** DuraSeal^{TM} applicator and **b** reaction scheme for DuraSeal^{TM}

for anastomotic suture hole bleeding and compare it to Gelfoam® (Upjohn, Kalamazoo, Mich)/Thrombin [63]. One hundred forty-eight patients scheduled for implantation of polytetrafluoroethylene (PTFE) grafts were randomly treated with either CoSeal® (n = 74) or control (n = 74). The efficacy of CoSeal® was equivalent to that of Gelfoam®/Thrombin. Clinical studies have also demonstrated the efficacy of CoSeal® in the anastomotic closure of aortic procedures [64] and preventing prolonged air leaks after lung resection [65].

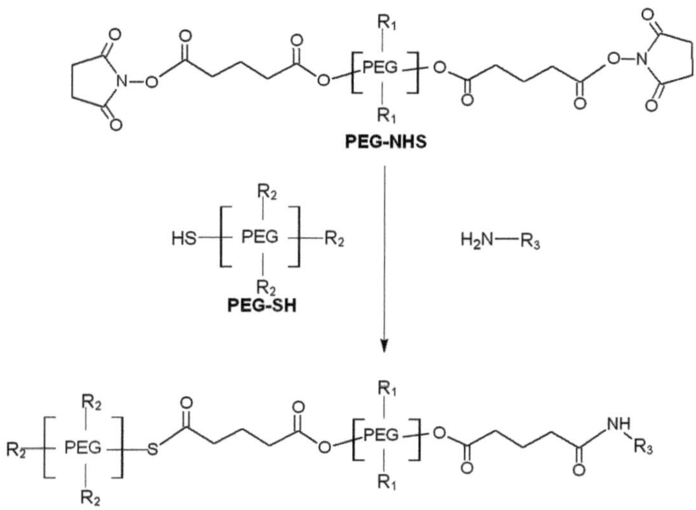

Fig. 8.4 Reaction scheme for CoSeal®

AdvaSeal™ (Ethicon Inc, Johnson & Johnson Medical KK, NJ, USA) is based on photo-polymerization of two aqueous solutions consisting of PEG and oligotriethylene carbonate with acrylate ester end caps, in the presence of triethanolamine and eosin Y as a photo-initiator, using visible light from a xenon arc lamp. It has been clinically used for sealing of pulmonary air leakage in Europe [66, 67].

Synthetic Adhesive Sheet

TissuePatch3™ (Tissuemed Ltd., Leeds, UK) is a synthetic, bioabsorbable self-adhesive film that has been developed to prevent air and liquid leaks in surgery. It consists of adhesive terpolymer (61 %) and poly(lactide-*co*-glycolide) (33.5 %). The terpolymer contains three components: polyvinylpyrrolidone (PVP), acrylic acid (AAc), and acrylic acid/N-hydroxysuccinimide (AAc-NHS), which confer the properties of water solubility, electrostatic interaction, and covalent bonding potential, respectively [68]. The chemical structure of terpolymer is shown in Fig. 8.5. No preparatory step is required and it adheres within 30 s of application. The efficacy of TissuePatch3 was clinically evaluated for sealing of air leakage after lung surgery [69]. It was found that 80 % of patients (12 of 15 patients) became air leakage-free at the end of the surgical procedure. No device-related adverse events were observed. The new generation product, TissuePatch™, has been investigated for alveolar air leak prevention in vitro [70], as well as in the management of chyle leak in major neck surgery [71].

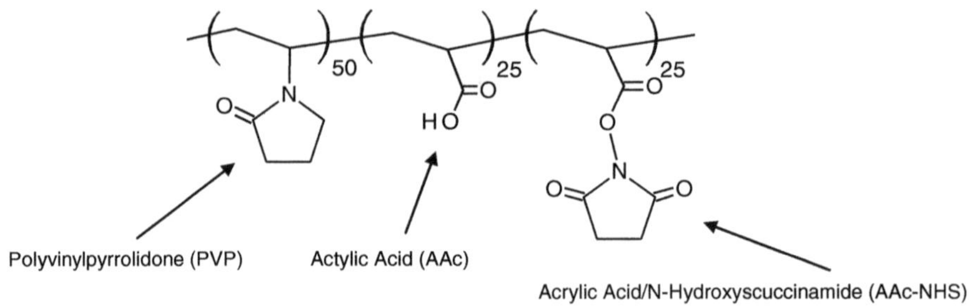

Fig. 8.5 Terpolymer of TissuePatch™

Recent Developments

Albumin-Based Sealant

Taguchi et al. developed biological glues combining an organic acid derivative and proteins such as collagen, gelatin, and human serum albumin. The active ester groups of the organic acid derivative react with amino groups of not only proteins of glue but also applied tissue surfaces. Citric acid derivative was used as a cross-linking agent. Citric acid, which is the source of citric acid derivative, is metabolized in the tricarboxylic acid cycle in the mitochondria. Although gels consisting of citric acid derivative and collagen or human serum albumin have exhibited sufficient bonding strength in vitro and insignificant toxicity, both required comparatively long periods of time to reach a certain bonding strength. To reduce the bonding time, tartaric acid derivative (TAD) was used as a cross-linking agent and the bonding strengths of glues (TAD-A) developed by reacting different concentrations of TAD (0.1, 0.3 and 0.5 mmol) and human serum albumin (44 w/w%) were compared with those of fibrin glue and GRF [72]. The bonding strengths of glues increased with the increasing TAD concentration, and even the lowest TAD glue exhibited significantly higher bonding strength than fibrin glue. The bonding strengths of glues with 0.3 and 0.5 mmol TAD were significantly higher than that of GRF. When the glue was implanted subcutaneously in mice to investigate the inflammatory reaction in surrounding tissues, the glue with low TAD concentrations (0.1 and 0.2 mmol) exhibited very mild inflammation, whereas the 0.3 and 0.5 mmol TAD gels were associated with moderate inflammation, possibly due to the local acidification by N-hydroxysuccinimide, which separates from carboxyl groups after the cross-linking reaction.

Fibrin-Based Sealant

Fibrinogen has been rapidly photo-cross-linked in the presence of ruthenium as the trisbipyridyl complex and the oxidant ammonium or sodium persulfate by light to yield high-molecular-weight products that have strong in vitro adhesive properties [73]. A mixture of fibrinogen (150 mg/mL), 2 mM $Ru^{II}(bpy)_3Cl_2$, and 20 mM sodium persulfate was prepared, and applied immediately to wounds, followed by illumination with a 600 W tungsten-halide light source at 150 mm for 20 s [73]. The sealant was well tolerated and persisted up to 8 weeks but completely dissolved by 18 weeks with minimal inflammatory response. The photo-cross-linked fibrinogen sealed skin incisions in rats, and as an arterial hemostat in pig, it stopped bleeding within 20 s of application.

Gelatin-Based Sealant

Different cross-linking types of gelatin-based glues have been developed. One of such is the sealant consisting of gelatin and glutaraldehyde as a cross-linking agent [74]. The glue consisting of 23 wt% gelatin and 0.12 wt% glutaraldehyde exhibited more than 90 % degradation in 7 days when implanted subcutaneously in rats, and the bonding strength was much higher than that of fibrin glue. The gelatin glue was applied with or without rubbing in with fingers to seal the needle hole on the PTFE vascular graft (Gore-Tex®). The water pressure in the graft was increased and the burst pressure was measured when water leakage occurred. The burst pressure of the gelatin glue applied with rubbing was found to be 400 mmHg, while that of fibrin glue was 200 mmHg. The high viscosity of gelatin solution also prevents leakage through suture line needle-holes, which is often a problem with the low viscosity of serum albumin in Bioglue® [75].

Various gelatins, such as porcine type A (~300 g Bloom), bovine type B (~225 g Bloom) and cold water fish gelatin (~60 kDa), were photo-cross-linked and evaluated in vitro and in vivo for a pulmonary sealant in an animal study [76]. As previously described for photo-cross-linking of fibrinogen, gelatin was also rapidly cross-linked using blue light, a ruthenium catalyst, and a persulfate oxidant. The adhesive strength of porcine gelatin was similar to that of photo-polymerized fibrinogen and approximately 5 times higher than that of the commercial fibrin glue. The maximum adhesion strength was reached within 30 s, but with a light-emitting diode (LED) lamp high adhesive strength was achieved instantaneously. The photo-polymerized porcine gelatin swelled substantially with increase in weight of 240 % within 24 h. To reduce swelling, the gelatin was derivatized to increase content of phenolic (Tyr-like) residues using Bolton-Hunter reagent (N-succinimidyl-3-[4-hydroxy]propionate), and thus to increase its cross-linking density after polymerization. The resultant gel increased the elastic modulus (stiffness) approximately 5-fold, and reduced its swelling to less than 10 % at 24 h. In an animal study, the photo-polymerized gelatin effectively sealed a wound in lung tissue from blood and air leakage, and was not cytotoxic and did not produce any inflammatory response.

PEG-Based Sealant

PEG/dextran aldehyde was developed as biocompatible tissue adhesive [77]. It consisted of a relatively short-chain PEG polymer (linear PEG of 2 kDa or 8-arm PEG of 10 kDa) containing amine-terminated groups, and dextran containing aldehyde groups. Aldehyde to amine ratios of 1, 3, and 10 were examined for linear and star-PEG-based constructs. The adhesive forces of these polymers were determined by the number of aldehyde groups within the gel and reached saturation at a dextran aldehyde content of ~20 wt%. Cytotoxicity and proliferation of 3T3 rat fibroblast tests revealed that PEG/dextran was significantly less cytotoxic than octyl cyanoacrylate. The higher-molecular-weight dextran aldehyde exhibited lower cytotoxicity as well as higher cell proliferation [77].

A topical hemostatic agent comprised of polycarbonate of dihydroxyacetone (pDHA) and methoxypoly(ethylene glycol) (MPEG) was studied by Henderson et al. [78]. DHA is the fifth metabolite of glucose as it is metabolized to pyruvic acid. Polymerized sequence of dihydroxyacetone was PEGylated (MPEG-pDHA). The edge of rat liver was cut and treated with MPEG-pDHA (50 mg), normal saline (0.5 ml), or Instat^{TM} (50 mg). The MPEG-pDHA had significantly decreased bleeding time (97 s) and total blood loss (1.35 g) compared to those with normal saline (464 s and 3.83 g) and Instat^{TM} (165 s and 2.04 g).

Chitosan-Based Sealant

Chitosan, which is an inexpensive and widely available material, has been investigated for its usefulness as a hemostatic material because it is cationic and antimicrobial, but it may not be effective for severe wounds. Photo-cross-linkable chitosan molecules which contain both lactose moieties and photoactive azide groups (Az-CH-LA) have been developed. The Az-CH-LA hydrogel was combined with a chitosan sponge (PCM-S), and its hemostatic efficacy was compared with that of TachoComb® in a heparinized rat model [79]. Even under heparinized condition, the bleeding time and blood loss of the PCM-S group were significantly lower than those of the TachoComb® group. In another study, the photo-curable chitosan was evaluated as an adhesive for peripheral nerve anastomosis to restore continuity to severed peripheral nerves [80]. Photo-chemical tissue bonding has been utilized for the adhesion of chitosan film [81]. In this technique, a solution of rose bengal is applied between two tissue edges and the area is irradiated with a green light to cross-link collagen fibers with minimal heat production. The resulting adhesive strength of the film to intestine was 15 ± 2 kPa, and the average temperature of the adhesive increased from 26 °C to only 32 °C during laser exposure [81].

Dowling et al. [82] developed a chitosan-based amphiphilic biopolymer that exhibits clotting ability in the presence of blood by self-assembly that is readily reversible by introducing a sugar-based supramolecule. First, chitosan was hydrophobically modified by attaching a small number of hydrophobic tails to the backbone (hm-chitosan). The hydrophobes from the chitosan anchor into the hydrophobic interior of blood cell membranes, connecting them into a gel network which can halt the flow of blood. The reaction is not affected by heparinization of blood. To reverse the gel into a sol, α-cyclodextrin, a supramolecular compound with an inner hydrophobic pocket, is added. The strong affinity of α-cyclodextrin for hydrophobes causes these polymer moieties to unhook from the cell membranes and bind to α-cyclodextrin. The initial blood gel based on 0.25 wt% hm-chitosan exhibits an elastic, gel-like response, whereas addition of 3 wt% α-cyclodextrin results in a viscous liquid response. Preliminary tests with small and large animal-injury models demonstrated its increased efficacy at achieving hemostasis.

Polysaccharide-Based Sealant

Adhesives made of aldehyded polysaccharides and ε-poly(L-lysine), which are anti-bacterial additives for medical use and food, have been investigated for use in sutureless amniotic membrane transplantation [83]. The adhesive gel is prepared using a syringe-like container with two cylinders, one with 2 ml of 14 % aldehyded dextran (Mw 75 kDa) solution and the other with 2 mL of 7 % ε-poly(L-lysine) (Mw 4 kDa) solution containing 2 % acetic anhydride. The acetic anhydride concentration added to the ε-poly(L-lysine) solution determines the gelation time. The gel formed by cross-linking via Schiff base in about 30 s at 37 °C and degrades within 4 days in vivo. The bonding strength of the glue was 4 times that of commercial fibrin glue and almost no cytotoxicity was observed. The efficacy of the glue in fixing amniotic membrane without suturing for ocular surface reconstruction was evaluated in an animal model. The sutureless amniotic membrane placement using the adhesive was safely and successfully performed onto a rabbit sclera surface.

Natural Adhesives/Sealants

Mussel-derived adhesive protein is known to be the most powerful natural adhesive, and has both flexibility and elasticity [84, 85]. In 1981, Waite and Tanzer discovered 3,4-dihydroxy-L-phenylalanine (DOPA) as a key component for the wet-resistant adhesion of mussel adhesive proteins [86]. Non-toxic and non-immunogenic effects of mussel proteins have been reported [87–89]. More interestingly, it maintains its adhesion in wet environment, and adheres to virtually any types of synthetic and natural surfaces [90]. However, expensive extraction, which requires 10,000 mussels to obtain 1 g of one type of adhesive proteins, and unsuccessful large-scale production limit its practical applications [84].

DOPA has been used to increase the adhesion strength of PEG-based sealant [91]. Adhesive consisting of star PEG amine and linear dextran aldehyde was developed, but after swelling of the gel the strength of adhesion to soft tissues significantly decreased. Incorporation of DOPA into the PEG: dextran sealant was investigated to determine enhancement of post-swelling sealant performance. Homogeneous solutions of DOPA and lyophilized dextran aldehyde were dialyzed against water followed by freeze-drying. The PEG: dextran doped with 3 mM DOPA aldehyde swelled 50 % less, had 3-fold greater stiffness and 50 % greater functional adhesive strength than the neat hydrogel. Increasing the DOPA concentration to 11 mM decreased the swelling and mitigated loss of properties with hydration, but reduced the initial functional adhesive strength, material modulus, and biocompatibility.

Dermal exudate from *Notaden bennetti* frogs, another natural adhesive, was investigated for medical use [92]. The exudate rapidly forms a protein-based pressure-sensitive adhesive that functions well in wet environments. The glue implanted subcutaneously in mice was bioabsorbed and exhibited no long-term adverse effects. The non-protein components of the frog glue caused local and transient necrosis, although they did not contribute to the adhesive properties of the glue. The glue could bond severed cartilage tissue both ex vivo and in vivo.

The hemostatic characteristics of keratin derived from human hair were investigated using a rabbit model of lethal liver injury [93]. Keratin was extracted from human hair, and the protein solution was concentrated to 20 wt% using a rotary evaporation system prior to surgery and exposed to air overnight to form a cross-linked hydrogel. The keratin gel exhibited adhesion to the tissue, and when deposited onto the bleeding surface of liver it was sufficiently adhesive and absorbed blood and became more adherent within a few minutes. The keratin gel demonstrated efficacy in arresting hemorrhage and improving survivability similar to those of two commercial products, QuickClot® and HemCon®. The gel was non-toxic and non-immunogenic.

Gecko-inspired tissue adhesive, which mimics the nanotopography of gecko feet, was investigated to determine its adhesive properties in a dry environment without chemical glue. However, for tissue adhesive application, the surface should be optimized to adhere on a wet surface. Lee et al. investigated the synthetic gecko-adhesive surface, which is effective under water due to reversible non-covalent bonding to inorganic surfaces, by coating the surface with a DOPA mimetic polymer, poly(dopamine methacrylamide-*co*-methoxyethyl acrylate) (poly(DMA-*co*-MEA)) [85]. This copolymer was synthesized by free-radical polymerization with the adhesive monomer, DMA, which accounts for 17 % of this copolymer by weight. Electron beam lithography was used to create an array of holes in a poly(methyl methacrylate) thin film and poly(dimethyl siloxane) was cast onto the master and cured to create gecko-foot-mimetic nanopillar arrays. Finally, the surface was coated with poly(DMA-*co*-MEA). Atomic force microscopy was used to measure the adhesive force of each pillar. Coating with the muscle-mimetic polymer increased its wet adhesive force nearly 15-fold. Another study modified the surface of poly(glycerol-*co*-sebacate acrylate), which is a tough biodegradable elastomer, to mimic the nanotopography of gecko feet and coated with a oxidized dextran with aldehylde groups [94]. Tissue adhesion was optimized by varying the dimensions of the nanoscale pillars, including the ratio of tip diameter to pitch and the ratio of tip diameter to base diameter. Coating of these nano-molded pillars of biodegradable elastomers with a thin layer of oxidized dextran with aldehylde groups significantly increased interfacial adhesive strength on porcine intestine tissue in vitro and in the rat abdominal subfascial tissue in an in vivo environment.

Barriers to Prevent Tissue Adhesion

Postoperative adhesions of internal organs to each other by formation of fibrous tissue have often been observed during cardiac, thoracic, abdominal, pelvic, and gynecologic surgeries. It is thought that postoperative adhesions occur in 90 % of patients who undergo major abdominal surgery and over 55 % of women undergoing pelvic surgery [95]. Although it is asymptomatic in the majority of patients, tissue adhesion can cause serious post-surgical complications, such as small-bowel obstruction (SBO), infertility, chronic abdominal pain, and difficulty of second operation. Postoperative adhesion has been reported to be responsible for 60–70 % of cases of SBO and 15–40 % of infertilities due to prevention of the ovum pick-up mechanism and gamete transport.

Several recent reviews have extensively covered prevention of adhesions [96, 97]. Cause of adhesion is as follow: fibrin deposition in the surgical area occurs within hours of surgery and this is either resorbed or becomes organized into fibrous adhesions. Tissue injury and inflammatory response are two specific risk factors that lead further organization of fibrin into adhesion. In the ischemic injuries, adhesions form to supply blood to the devascuarized organ. Inflammatory response due to contamination of the foreign materials such as talcum powder and sutures, as well as bacterial infection, has been associated with adhesion formation. Strategies of prevention of adhesions can be grouped into four categories: general principles, surgical techniques, chemical agents, and mechanical barriers [98].

Anti-adhesive materials have been developed to prevent tissue adhesion by providing a physical barrier between an injured site and the adjacent tissues. Although several non-absorbable synthetic materials such as silicone and PTFE have been shown to be effective, bioabsorbable materials are preferred because of the lack of necessity of secondary surgery to remove non-absorbable materials and the lack of need to consider long-term biocompatibility such as encapsulation of the material, which will also evoke tissue adhesion. Moreover, non-absorbable synthetic materials have been shown to form adhesions on long-term application [99]. A wide variety of substances and materials have been used over the years. Commercially available anti-adhesive products are summarized in Table 8.7.

Solutions

Crystalloid solutions, such as Ringer's solution and plain saline, have been commonly used to prevent adhesions in the abdominal cavity after surgery. In addition to its mechanical effect of separation of raw peritoneal surfaces, it dilutes fibrin and fibrinous exudates released from injured tissues [98]. These fluids are absorbed from the peritoneal cavity at an estimated rate of 35 ml/h, and at least 5 L are needed to cover the first 6 postoperative days. However, such a large

Table 8.7 Commercial products used for preventing adhesion

Structure	Main composition	Manufacturer	Trade name	Introduced/approved year	Degradation/absorption time
Solution	32 % dextran 70	Medisan Pharmaceuticals	Hyskon	1970	5–7 days
	4 % icodextrin solution	Baxter Healthcare	Adept	2006	3–4 days
	0.5 % ferric hyaluronate	Lifecore Biomedical	Intergel[a]	2001	1 week
Gel	PVA and CMC	Aesculap AG & Co	A-Part Gel	–	3–4 weeks
	HA and CMC	Genzyme Corporation	Sepracoat[b]	1996	1 week
	PEO and CMC	Ethicon	Intercoat	2002	<1 months
	PEG-NHS and PEG-NH_2	COVIDIEN	SprayGel	2001	3 weeks
	PEG-NHS and trilysine	COVIDIEN	SprayShield	2008	1 week
	PEG-NHS and PEG-SH	Angiotech Pharmaceuticals	Adhibit	2002	4 weeks
Sheet	ePTFE	Gore-Tex	Preclude[c]	1990s	Non degradable
	HA and CMC	Genzyme Corporation	Seprafilm	1996	1 week
	Oxidized cellulose	Johnson & Johnson	Interceed	1989	4 weeks
	Polylactide	MAST Biosurgery	SurgiWrap, CardioWrap	2001, 2003	6 months
	PLLA and PEG	SyntheMed	REPEL-CV	2007	4 weeks
	Porcine type I collagen	Biom'Up	Cova CARD, Cova ABDO	2009	6 months

PVA poly(vinyl alcohol), *CMC* carboxymethyl cellulose, *HA* hyaluronic acid, *PEO* poly(ethylene oxide), *PEG* poly(ethylene glycol), *NHS* N-hydroxysuccinimide, *PLLA* poly(L-lactide)

[a]Withdrawn in 2003

[b]Withdrawn in 1997

[c]Discontinued since 2011

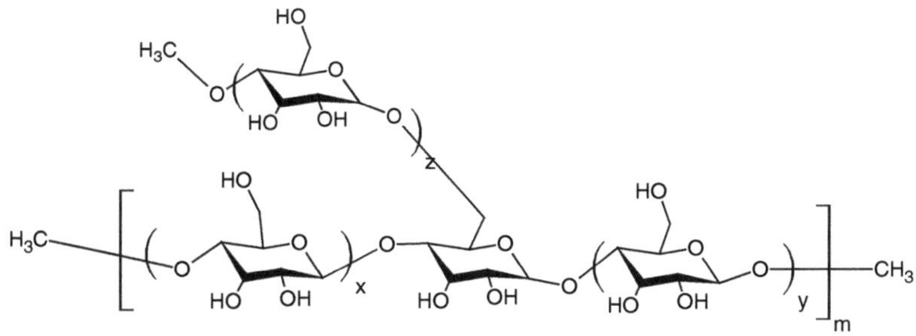

Fig. 8.6 Chemical structure of Adept® (Icodextrin)

amount will increase the risk of infection, fluid overload with pulmonary edema, and leakage at puncture sites. In an attempt to prolong the period of instillate persistence inside the peritoneal cavity, more viscous solutions have been investigated. Hyskon™ (Medisan Pharmaceuticals Inc., Piscataway, NJ, USA) is a solution of 32 % dextran 70 and available in the USA. Hyskon™ is left in the abdominal cavity to prevent sticking by causing tissue to literally slide around freely. Clinical studies of use of Hyskon™ have revealed mixed results. Although use of Hyskon™ exhibited fewer and less severe adhesions than Ringer solution, another study reported no difference between these groups [100]. Side-effects have also been reported, such as vulvar edema, leg edema, pleural effusion, coagulopathy, and rarely allergic response [101–106]. It is hardly used today.

Adept® (Baxter Healthcare, Deerfield, IL, USA) is a 4 % solution of icodextrin, an α-1,4-linked glucose polymer produced by hydrolysis of cornstarch (Fig. 8.6). It is used as an irrigant fluid throughout surgery, and at the end of surgery 1 L is instilled and left in the peritoneal cavity. A randomized study of laparoscopic gynecologic surgery reported that instillation of Adept® decreased adhesion formation and reformation compared to lactated Ringer solution instillation [107]. Intergel® (Lifecore Biomedical, Inc, Chaska, MN, USA) contains 0.5 % cross-linked hyaluronic acid (HA) with ferric ion (Fe). The reaction scheme and the ideal structure of the Fe-HA network are shown in Fig. 8.7. It reduced the extent of adhesion formation following abdominal surgery. Although significant reduction in adhesion formation was observed in a randomized clinical trial [108], a high rate of postoperative complications, including post-operative infection and even death, was reported following the use of Intergel®, and the manufacturer voluntarily recalled Intergel® in 2003 after receiving a warning from FDA [109].

Gels

Gels have been developed for site-specific adhesion prevention devices that can be easily delivered during laparoscopy, since using sheets and films via laparoscopy is challenging. FlowGel® (Angiotech Pharmaceuticals Inc., Vancouver,

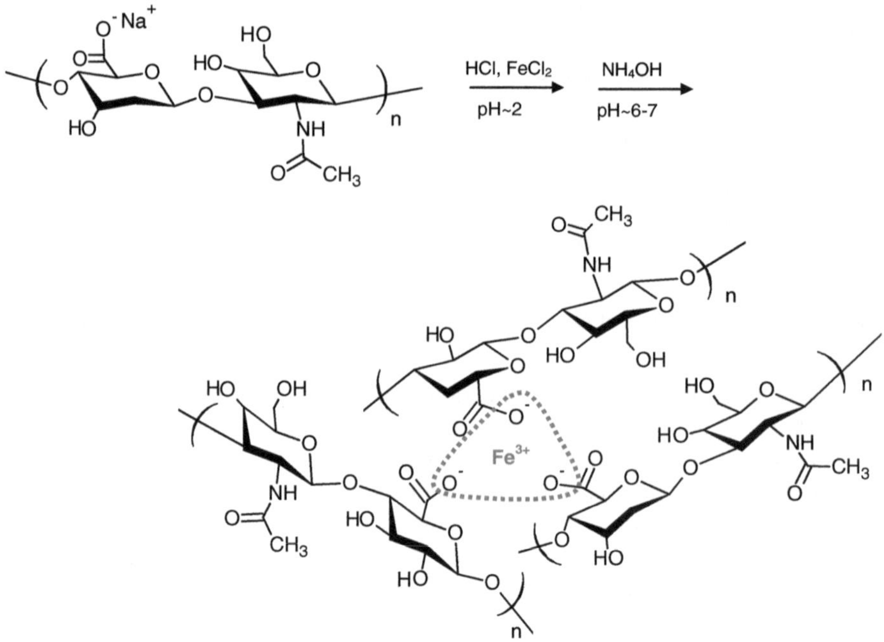

Fig. 8.7 Reaction scheme for the formation of and the idealized structure of the iron-cross-linked hyaluronic acid (Fe-HA) hydrogel

BC, USA) consists of Poloxamer 407, which is a surfactant with the ability for reversible conversion from liquid state at room temperature to a gel form at body temperature [110]. A-Part® gel is a bioabsorbable transparent gel composed of poly(vinyl alcohol) (PVA) and carboxymethyl cellulose (CMC) [111]. Material characteristics such as viscosity and adherence to the wound were tested with good results [112, 113]. Preclinical data in animal studies revealed high efficacy in adhesion prevention [114, 115], and wound and anastomosis healing were not negatively affected by the application of this gel in animal models [116]. Sepracoat (Genzyme Corp., Cambridge, MA, USA) consists of hyaluronic acid and CMC in a highly viscous gel form. A randomized, controlled trial revealed it to be effective, but it did not receive FDA approval, and was withdrawn from the market in 1997. Intercoat® (Ethicon, Somerville, NJ, USA), a viscoelastic gel, is based on poly(ethylene oxide) (PEO) and CMC, which is stabilized with calcium. In a pilot study, 28 patients with pelvic adhesions, tubal occlusion, endometriosis, and/or dermoids were randomized to receive Intercoat® or no treatment after surgery [117]. Second-look surgery was performed 6–10 weeks later. Thirty-four percent of treated adnexa increased in adhesion score, compared to 67 % of the untreated controls.

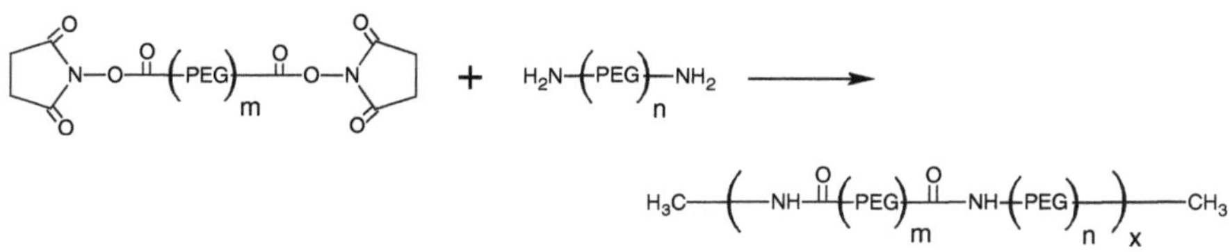

Fig. 8.8 Reaction scheme for the formation of SprayGel™

The following products are poly(ethylene glycol) (PEG)-based precursor liquids that are sprayed onto the surgical site and rapidly cross-link on the target tissue to form a flexible, adherent, bioabsorbable gel barrier. They are indicated for use in both open and laparoscopic abdominopelvic surgical procedures. These products are currently available in Europe, but have not been approved in the USA. SprayGel™ (COVIDIEN, Waltham, MA, USA) consists of PEG ester and PEG amine precursors, which polymerize within seconds of application on tissue (Fig. 8.8). Over the time, the adhesion barrier is hydrolyzed into water-soluble PEG molecules and absorbed into the circulatory system, followed by renal excretion. Clinical studies have shown the effectiveness of SprayGel™ in preventing tissue adhesion [118–120]. The next-generation product of SprayGel™ is called SprayShield™ (COVIDIEN, Waltham, MA, USA), which has been available in Europe since 2008. It consists of PEG ester and trilysine solutions, and is chemically identical to COVIDIEN's DuraSeal™ product. With use of low-molecular-weight trilysine, instead of PEG amine, the final gel formed is anticipated to be better mixed and to react better, and thus more adherent than SprayGel™. Two adhesion barriers, SprayShield™ and SprayGel™, were compared in a laparoscopic porcine model of gynecologic surgery [121]. Both the adhesion barriers demonstrated statistically significant reduction (~50 %) in number of adhesions to the site of injury, while only SprayShield™ demonstrated a statistically significant reduction in adhesion area.

Adhibit™ adhesion prevention gel (Angiotech Pharmaceuticals Inc., Vancouver, BC, Canada) was approved to prevent or reduce post-surgical adhesions during cardiac surgery. It is chemically identical to CoSeal® Surgical Compound. HYAcorp endo gel (Bioscience GmbH, Ransbach-Baumbach, Germany) is available in Europe for reducing the post-surgical adhesion formation in patients undergoing laparoscopic pelvic and hysteroscopic gynaecological surgery. The hyaluronic acid based gel comes in a 10 ml syringe with a special cannular applicator. After the operative site is dried, it is applied in 1–2 mm thick layer of gel. The main component of the gel is cross-linked sodium hyaluronate (20 mg/ml). It also contains sodium hyaluronate (10 mg/ml), and sodium chloride (6.9 mg/ml) in water. The cross-linked sodium hyaluronate degrades slower and hence resulting in a longer duration of effect. The effectiveness of this product has been demonstrated in some animal and clinical studies [122, 123].

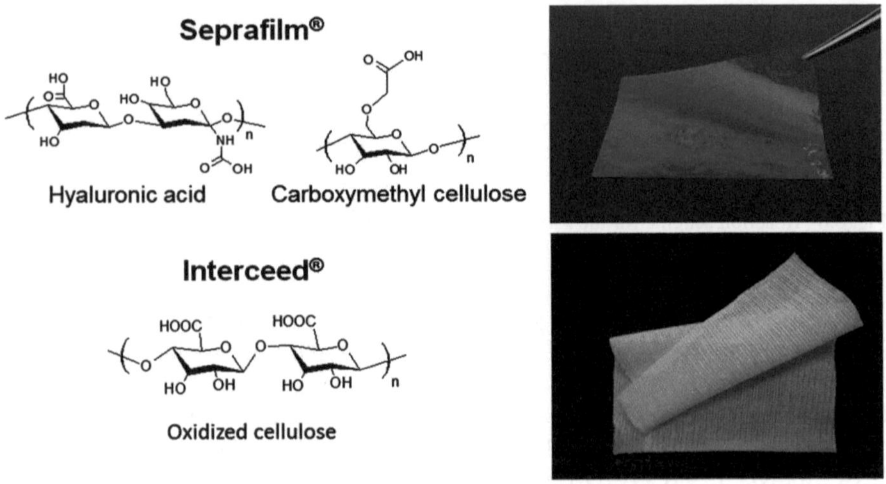

Fig. 8.9 Chemical structures and photographs of Seprafilm® and Interceed®

Sheets

PTFE is a fully fluorinated polymer which is bioinert. Preclude™ (Gore-Tex, W.L. Gore & Associates) is expanded PTFE (ePTFE) non-absorbable permanent membrane. For adhesion prevention, fairly large pieces are needed, and they must be sutured into place as it does not adhere to tissue. Clinical studies have exhibited the effectiveness of this PTFE product [124, 125]. However, adhesion on suture lines and foreign-body reaction due to their prolonged presence make it not preferred. This product was discontinued by the manufacturer since 2011.

Most commonly used bioabsorbable films for adhesion prevention are Seprafilm® (Genzyme Corporation, Cambridge, MA, USA) and Interceed® (Johnson & Johnson, New Brunswick, NJ, USA) (Fig. 8.9). Seprafilm® is a transparent membrane, composed of sodium hyaluronate and CMC. This film adheres to sites of injury by absorbing water from the surrounding region and turns into a hydrophilic gel that separates opposing tissues during the post-operative healing phase. Clinical studies have demonstrated the effectiveness of Seprafilm® [126], but there are concerns regarding a higher incidence of anastomotic leaks in cases in which the film is placed directly around the anastomosis. The use of Seprafilm® in this location is prohibited by instructions provided by the manufacturer. Clinical studies have shown that Seprafilm® reduces abdominal adhesion formation [127, 128] and postoperative small-bowel adhesive obstruction [126, 129–131]. Recent extensive reviews by Diamond et al. demonstrated the safety and efficacy of Seprafilm® in reducing postoperative adhesions in clinical and preclinical studies [132, 133]. Seprafilm® was also clinically evaluated for reduction of pericardial adhesions [134]. However, despite its effectiveness, handling of this film is quite difficult because of its poor mechanical properties and brittleness. Placing this film through a laparoscope is very hard since it easily breaks when bolted. Replacing the film on wet tissue is also difficult.

Another commonly-used bioabsorbable sheet is Interceed® for applications in gynecologic pelvic surgery. It is a knitted fabric of oxidized regenerated cellulose which slowly turns into a gel when placed on tissues. Unlike Seprafilm®, Interceed® is easy to handle and can be placed via laparoscopy. It has been reported that Interceed® prevents tissue adhesion effectively when blood contamination is avoided during application of it [135]. However, as complete blood evacuation is not always possible in clinical situations, surgeons are not keen to use this product. Moreover, increased adhesion formation has been observed when Interceed® is applied to areas where blood accumulation cannot be prevented [136].

CardioWrap® and SurgiWrap® (MAST Biosurgery USA Inc, San Diego, CA, USA) are translucent membranes composed of L-lactide (70) and D,L-lactide (30), and are used for adhesion prevention barriers in cardiovascular and abdominal/pelvic surgeries, respectively. These films can be sutured. A prospective control clinical study was performed to assess the efficacy of SurgiWrap® in preventing adhesion formation in patients undergoing a major colorectal surgery [137]. After the surgery, SurgiWrap® was placed under the midline incision just before closing the abdominal wall for 10 patients. The control group (9 patients) received no treatment. After 14 weeks postoperatively, 5 patients had no adhesion beneath the midline incision in the SurgiWrap® group, in contrast to 0 patients in the control group. The severity of adhesions was significantly lower for the treated group than for the control.

REPEL-CV® (SyntheMed Inc, Iselin, NJ, USA) is composed of a blend of PLLA (52 %) and PEG (47 %). A randomized clinical study was performed to evaluate the efficacy of REPEL-CV® in 142 infants undergoing initial sternotomy for eventual staged palliative cardiac operations [138]. At the time of chest closure, the barrier was applied over the epicardial surface of the heart and fixed in place with four interrupted poly(glycolic acid) sutures ($n = 54$). In the control group ($n = 49$), the chest was closed without the use of any adjuncts. Significantly fewer patients in the REPEL-CV® group had any severe adhesions compared with the control group. There were no statistically significant differences in adverse events between the two groups, indicating no adverse events due to REPEL-CV®.

Cova CARD™ and Cova ABDO™ (Biom'Up, Lyon, France) are CE marked membranes that are made of purified porcine type I collagen membrane. The membrane is cross-linked with an oxidized polysaccharide [139]. In a preclinical study, the efficacy of Cova CARD™ was compared with that of Seprafilm® [140]. Sixteen sheep underwent a sternotomy followed by scratching of the heart surface. When the intensity of adhesion was assessed 4 months postoperatively, Cova CARD™ was found to have been almost totally absorbed, and the adhesion score was significantly lower than that of the Seprafilm® group (1 vs. 3 (score from 1, absence to 3, tight)). There was no adverse inflammatory reaction due to Cova CARD™, and the extent and density of fibrosis were small.

Recent Developments

Fibrin-Based Material

Fibrin sealant has the advantage of decreasing bleeding and increasing the production of plasminogen activator and plasminogen activator inhibitor-1, which may be beneficial in the prevention of adhesion [141]. Fibrin glue has also been shown to reduce adhesion formation onto permanent prosthetic materials such as polypropylene and PTFE in rat and pig models [142–144]. Prevention of adhesion by fibrin glue on a rabbit flexor tendon adhesion model was examined by Feykman et al. [145]. A partial laceration was produced and closed with 5-0 Dexon sutures, and covered with fibrin glue for the experimental group. The operated paw was then immobilized by flexion of the wrist for 3 weeks, or left free for voluntary weight-bearing immediately after surgery. Although the immobilized tendons exhibited no difference in adhesion formation at 6 weeks, the mobile tendons exhibited less adhesion formation in the fibrin glue group than the control.

Gelatin-Based Materials

Gelatin sheets can be cross-linked by thermal, UV, or chemical means, and its degradation can be controlled easily by modifying the degree of cross-linking. A thermally-treated gelatin sheet, which exhibited degradation in 4 weeks, was studied as a pericardial substitute [146, 147]. The gelatin sheet exhibited reduced formation of pleural and pericardial adhesion and inflammatory reaction, compared with the PTFE sheet in a canine model [147]. Despite the effectiveness of the gelatin sheet as a pericardial substitute, there are two considerable drawbacks in its structural properties in the hydrated state: one drawback of the sheet is that it is too malleable to handle, and the other is that it is too low in tensile strength so that it cannot steadily hold sutures to the native pericardium. To overcome these problems, the gelatin sheet was reinforced with bioabsorbable PGA mesh [146]. The modified sheet exhibited ten-fold higher tension of disruption at the suturing margin than the unmodified gelatin sheet (619 ± 141 vs. 62 ± 7 gf). This is similar to that of PTFE. The effectiveness of this reinforced sheet in the prevention of adhesion was confirmed in a canine model.

Bae et al. investigated the anti-adhesion effect of the PVA/gelatin membrane using a rat cecum-side wall abrasion model. The PVA/gelatin membrane was cross-linkd by UV irradiation. The membrane with PVA/gelatin ratio of 10/90 significantly reduced the adhesion extent [148].

Hyaluronic Acid-Based Materials

Vorevolakos et al. [149] synthesized ferric ion-cross-linked networks of HA based on Intergel®, varying the degree of cross-linking, and goniometry, viscometry, and dynamic mechanical analysis were performed. It was found that increasing cross-linking could augment the contact angle, viscosity, storage modulus, and loss modulus, while wetting and lubrication were compromised. It is possible to create materials with mechanical properties softer than or comparable to those of abdominal organs that would be least disruptive to the body.

Synthetic peptides derived from human lactoferrin, PXL01, exhibits an inhibitory effect on the most important hallmarks of scar formation by reducing risk of infection, prohibiting inflammation, and promoting fibrinolysis [150]. The peptide was dissolved in sodium chloride solution and added to 2.5 % HA solution to obtain 1.5–6 mg/ml PXL01 in 1.5 % HA. In vitro release experiments revealed a burst release of PXL01 (approximately 70 %) from the gel within 1 h. The efficacy of PXL01 in HA was evaluated using a sidewall defect-cecum abrasion model and a large bowel anastomosis healing model in rats. At seven days after surgery, PXL01 with the HA gel had significantly reduced adhesion formation in rats.

Chitosan-Based Materials

Several studies have demonstrated anti-adhesive effects of modified chitosan based cross-linked hydrogels. A gel was synthesized from succinyl chitosan and dextran aldehyde, and its efficacy in reducing adhesion formation in the intraperitoneal cavity was evaluated in rat models [151]. The surgical procedure was performed by laparotomy and either cecal abrasion or anastomotic simulation by enterotomy of the cecum with primary closure. After 21 days postoperatively, adhesions were significantly reduced for the treatment group in both the models. There was no adverse effect on wound healing.

The efficacy of in situ cross-linkable hydrogel made from N-carboxyethyl chitosan and oxidized dextran as an adhesion prevention barrier was evaluated in a rat cecal abrasion model and compared to that of Seprafilm® [152]. Both Seprafilm® and 2 % hydrogel significantly decreased adhesion formation compared to the untreated control. The application of hydrogel was easer than that of Seprafilm® and the hydrogel adapted well on complex tissue geometries.

In situ cross-linkable chitosan-hyaluronic acid based hydrogels for preventing postoperative adhesion has been developed [153]. Hyaluronic acid was oxidized with sodium periodate which cleaves carbon-carbon bonds to create aldehyde groups in D-glucuronic acid units of the molecular chain. The solubility of chitosan in neutral aqueous solution was improved by incorporating carboxymethyl groups into chitosan chains. The solutions of modified chitosan and hyaluronic acid were mixed in a volume ratio of 1:1 to prepare the cross-linked hydrogels which is degraded by lysozyme within 2 weeks in vivo. Anti-adhesive effect of this gel was confirmed by rat sidewall defect-cecum abrasion model.

PEG-Based Materials

The efficacy of DuraSeal™ in pericardial adhesion prevention was evaluated with a porcine model [154]. After 6 weeks, all animals exhibited significant pericardial adhesions and there was no significant difference in tenacity, extension, or strength of adhesions between the DuraSeal™ and non-treated sides of the hearts.

Yang et al. investigated the efficacy of injectable poly(ethylene glycol-*b*-ε-caprolactone-*b*-ethylene glycol) (P(EG-*b*-CL-*b*-EG)) triblock copolymer hydrogel in preventing adhesions in rat abdominal and uterine horn adhesion models [155, 156]. This hydrogel was found to be thermosensitive, biocompatible, and bioabsorbable. The hydrogel was a transparent flowing sol at 4 °C, but became a gel in less than 20 s at 37 °C. The reaction was reversible. An adhesion model was created by abrading the peritoneum of the abdominal wall and the uterine horns of rats [155]. The P(EG-*b*-CL-*b*-EG) hydrogel was applied to the injured surfaces. During 12 days postoperatively, none of the animals treated with the hydrogel ($n = 12$) formed adhesions, whereas all the control animals ($n = 12$) exhibited strong adhesions. The hydrogel disappeared in 7–9 days. Similarly, in the study using the rat side wall defect-cecum abrasion model, no animals treated with the hydrogel ($n = 15$) developed adhesions 15 days after operation, whereas all untreated rats ($n = 15$) had severe adhesions [156].

Poly(α-hydroxyacid)s-Based Materials

Niwa et al. investigated the effect of poly(L-lactide) (PLLA) nanosheet as an anti-adhesive barrier in partial hepatectomy [157]. This nanosheet with thickness of 60 nm was prepared by spin-coating a PLLA-dichloromethane solution. The advantage of nanosheet is its excellent bioadhesive properties. The anti-adhesive effect of PLLA nanosheet was examined in combination with Tachocomb® using a rat liver defect model. When the liver wound was covered by Tachocomb® alone, severe adhesion with omentum and/or other parts of the liver was observed. On the other hand, by applying the PLLA nanosheet on top of Tachocomb®, adhesion formation was significantly reduced, presumably by preventing the permeation of oozing blood cells and fibroblasts by the nanosheet.

Another study investigated a multi-functional anti-adhesion barrier composed of a bilayered membrane of P(LA-*b*-EG) and poly(glycolide-*co*-L-lactide) (PGLA) layers carrying multiple drugs [158]. A hydrophilic hemostatic agent, carbazochrome sodium sulfonate, and an anti-infective drug, tinidazole, were incorporated into fibres of P(LA-*b*-EG) (i.e. inner layer) and PGLA (i.e. outer layer), respectively, by dispersing them into polymer solutions before electrospinning. The release of drugs can be adjusted by controlling the swelling behaviour of fibres. Hemostatic and anti-bacterial effects of the membrane were investigated using a rat model and in vitro tests, respectively.

Other Materials

A bioabsorbable film of poly(glycerol sebacate) (PGS) was investigated for prevention of postoperative adhesion in a rat peritoneal adhesion model [159]. This polymer was synthesized by a polycondensation reaction between glycerol and sebacic acid, both of which have FDA approval for use as medical devices. The operated rats were evaluated for adhesions at 3, 5, and 8 weeks postoperatively. Statistically significant reduction (94 %) in adhesion formation rate was observed between the control animals (75 % incidence) and the animals with PGS films (4.8 %).

Gellan gum is a linear anionic extracellular polysaccharide and used as a food additive. It has recently been investigated for medical application because of its biocompatibility. Lee et al. investigated photo-cross-linked gellan gum based film as anti-adhesive barrier [160]. Firstly, to improve the solubility of gellan gum in dimethyl sulfoxide, the sodium ions of gellan gum was exchanged with lipophilic tetrabutylammonium ion. The resulting gellan gum was then reacted with cinnamyl bromide in dimethyl sulfoxide to incorporate photoreactive double bonds. The cast film was then irradiated with UV light to cross-link. The resulting film showed anti-adhesive effects using a rat cecum abrasion model.

Sutures for Wound Closure

After an injury or surgery, a surgical suture is used to hold tissues together. A suture consists of a needle with a length of thread attached. The optimal suture should be easy to handle and have high tensile strength and knot security. It should cause minimal tissue reaction, and its material should resist infection and have good elasticity and plasticity in order to accommodate wound swelling. However, there is no single suture that can fulfill all these criteria. Therefore, a surgeon must choose suture material based on type of surgery that she or he is performing because different tissues have different requirements for suture support (some need only a few days, e.g., muscle, subcutaneous tissue, and skin, while others require weeks or even months, e.g., fascia and tendons). In addition, the healing rates of tissues differ depending on factors such as infection, debility, respiratory problems, obesity, collagen disorders, malnutrition, malignancy, and drugs. Often, the trade-off is tissue handling versus longevity versus healing properties. General classifications of thread material are natural and synthetic, bioabsorbable and non-bioabsorbable, and monofilament and multifilament. Mechanical properties can be further divided in terms of the multiple characteristics of each material, as shown in Table 8.8 [161].

Table 8.8 Suture characteristics

Characteristic	Definition
Coefficient of friction	A suture's relative resistance to being passed through a tissue. A higher coefficient of friction leads to increased local tissue damage. Monofilaments usually have the lowest coefficient of friction
Tensile strength	A suture's ability to resist breakage. The strength of the suture should not be significantly greater than the tissue it is approximating (if the tensile strength is too high, the suture will cut through tissue)
Elasticity	A suture's ability to regain its original length after deformation. Elasticity should be sufficient to accommodate tissue swelling
Memory	A suture's ability to return to its original shape after deformation. Similar to pliability (more memory = less pliability and less knot security)
Cost	A significant issue in today's health care arena. Newer suture materials with precision needles are generally more costly

Originally, sutures were made from biological materials such as catgut and silk. J. Lister first attempted sterilization in the 1860s with "carbolic catgut," and the chromic catgut followed two decades later. Sterile catgut was finally achieved in 1906 with iodine treatment. This became the standard method of suture preparation for nearly half a century. The first synthetic bioabsorbable suture was made from PVA in 1931. Polyesters were developed in the 1950s, and later, the process of radiation sterilization was established for catgut and polyester. Today, most sutures are made of synthetic polymer fibers. Silk and gut sutures are the only materials still–though rarely–in use from ancient times. In fact, gut sutures have been banned in Europe and Japan because of concerns of bovine spongiform encephalopathy.

Non-bioabsorbable Sutures

Non-bioabsorbable sutures are defined by their resistance to degradation by living tissues. They are most useful in percutaneous closures. Synthetic, non-bioabsorbable, monofilament sutures include nylon, polypropylene, and polybutester sutures, while synthetic, non-bioabsorbable, multifilament (braided) sutures are composed of nylon and polyester. Polybutester, developed in 2000, is a block copolymer that contains butylene terephthalate and tetramethylene ether glycol. Metallic fibers such as steel fibers are also used extensively for suturing.

Bioabsorbable Sutures

Bioabsorbable sutures are defined by the loss of most of their strength within 60 days after placement. They provide temporary wound support until the wound heals well enough to withstand normal stress and are used primarily as buried sutures to close the dermis and subcutaneous tissue and reduce wound tension. When the Young's modulus of the thread materials is relatively low, they are processed into monofilament sutures, while multifilament sutures are made of less pliable materials and processed into twisted or braided construction.

Multifilament sutures generally have greater tensile strength and better pliability and flexibility than monofilaments. Multifilament sutures with a high coefficient of friction are more difficult to pass through tissue and cause a greater degree of tissue injury during placement and removal. However, these sutures are easier to handle and manipulate for tying knots. The knots of monofilament sutures are smaller than those of multifilaments. Multifilament sutures have a high degree of capillarity, which is correlated with a tendency to absorb and retain both fluid and bacteria. This may promote infection if bacterial contamination occurs during or shortly after surgery.

Synthetic, bioabsorbable sutures available today are listed in Table 8.9, together with their chemical structure. As can be seen, they are composed of copolymers, except for PGA and poly-*p*-dioxanone. One of the monomers in the copolymers of all sutures is glycolide. The surface of most multifilament sutures is coated to permit easy tissue passage, precise knot placement, and smooth tie-down. The coating materials applied include calcium stearate, poly(ε-caprolactone) (PCL), PGLA (30:70), and poly(CL-*co*-GA). The characteristics of these bioabsorbable sutures are briefly described below.

PGA

This first synthesized bioabsorbable suture has high tensile strength, with a retention of 60 % at day 7, 35 % at day 14, and only 5 % at day 28. Uncoated PGA sutures have good handling and knot security properties, but their high coefficient of friction results in significant tissue drag. Coating with PCL minimizes this drag, but four throws are recommended to ensure secure knots.

PGLA

PGLA is synthesized by means of random ring-opening polymerization of GA and LLA. Depending on the ratio of LLA to GA used for the polymerization, different forms of PGLA can be obtained. Multifilament braided Vicryl® sutures contain 90/10 molar ratio of GA to LLA, and they are coated with 2–10 % of a 50:50 mixture of an amorphous PGLA copolymer of 35/65 mol ratio and calcium stearate. The initial tensile strength of the copolymer suture is slightly greater than that of PGA. The PGLA suture retains 60 % of its tensile strength at day 14 after implantation and only 8 % of its original strength at day 28. Tissue reactivity with PGLA is low, less than that of PGA. The water-repelling quality of the lactide unit may slow the loss of tensile strength, and the bulkiness of the lactide unit leads to rapid bioabsorption of the suture mass once tensile strength is lost. The PGLA sutures are used in general soft tissue approximation and vessel ligation without adverse outcomes and resultant cost savings.

Table 8.9 Commercially-available synthetic absorbable sutures

	Chemical structure	Manufacturer	Trade name	Introduced year	Complete hydrolysis
Multifilament (Braided)	Polyglycolide	COVIDIEN	DEXON II	1970	90–120 days[a]
	Poly(glycolide-*co*-L-lactide) (90:10)	Johnson & Johnson	VICRYL	1974	56–70 days[b]
	Poly(glycolide-*co*-L-lactide) (90:10)	COVIDIEN	Polysorb	1981	
Monofilament	Poly-*p*-dioxanone	Johnson & Johnson	PDS II	1982	180–210 days
	Poly(glycolide-*co*-trimethylene carbonate)	COVIDIEN	Maxon	1985	180–210 days
	Poly(glycolide-*co*-ε-caprolactone)	Johnson & Johnson	Monocryl	1993	91–119 days
	Poly(glycolide-*co*-trimethylene carbonate-co-*p*-dioxanone)	COVIDIEN	Biosyn	1999	90–110 days
	Poly(glycolide-*co*-trimethylene carbonate)	B.Braun	Monosyn	2000	
	Poly(glycolide-*co*-ε-caprolactone-*co*-trimethylene carbonate-*co*-L-lactide)	COVIDIEN	Caprosyn	2002	56 days

[a]42 days for a fast-absorbing poly glycolide suture (Polysyn FA)
[b]35 days for γ-irradiated poly(glycolide-*co*-L-lactide) suture (Vicryl Rapid, 1987)

Poly-*p*-dioxanone

Multifilament sutures such as PGA and PGLA develop a greater amount of friction when penetrating tissues and have a higher risk of infection. Consequently, monofilament sutures made of polydioxanone that had a smooth and soft surface were introduced in the 1980s. Polydioxanone is a colorless, semicrystalline polymer with a very low glass transition temperature, ranging from −10 to 0 °C. In the body, this polymer is broken down into glycoxylate and excreted in the urine or converted into glycine and subsequently into carbon dioxide and water. Although the initial tensile strength of the polydioxanone suture is lower than that of the 2 synthetic multifilament sutures mentioned above, it retains its strength longer. At day 14 after implantation, it has 74 % residual initial strength, 58 % at day 28, and 41 % at week 6. The initial polydioxanone suture was stiff and had poor handling and knot-tying properties, but the newer product (PDS-II) has improved handling capabilities and has replaced the original product. The polydioxanone suture is useful as a buried suture in wounds that require prolonged dermal support and in contaminated wounds or wounds in locations at greater risk for infection. This suture provides extended wound support and elicits only a slight tissue reaction. Polydioxanone is more expensive than PGA and PGLA sutures.

Poly(GA-*co*-TMC)

This type of copolymer is prepared as A–B–A block copolymers in a 2:1 GA:trimethylene carbonate (TMC) ratio, with a GA–TMC center block (B) and pure GA end blocks (A). These materials have better flexibility than pure PGA and are absorbed in approximately 7 months. This copolymer was developed to combine the predictable in vivo performance of a synthetic absorbable suture with the handling characteristics of a monofilament suture. The copolymer has a high initial tensile strength (greater than that of polydioxanone) and retains 81 % of its strength at day 14, 59 % at day 28, and 30 % at week 6. This suture is easier to handle and has greater knot security than the three bioabsorbable sutures mentioned above.

Poly(GA-*co*-CL)

The biodegradability of this copolymer is much higher than that of the polydioxanone suture. The higher rate of degradation of poly(GA-*co*-CL) may be due to its GA content. This copolymer suture has superior pliability despite its monofilament nature, leading to easy handling and tying. Among all bioabsorbable monofilament sutures, this has the highest tensile strength, which is high initially, 50–60 % at day 7, but only 20–30 % at day 14 after implantation. This suture is used for subcuticular closure and is most useful as a buried suture in wounds that do not require prolonged dermal support.

Poly(GA-*co*-TMC-*co*-*p*-dioxanone)

This copolymer suture has greater tensile strength than the PGLA suture 4 weeks after implantation. The handling characteristics and knot security are also superior. Tissue drag and risk of bacterial infection are lower than those of PGLA, similar to the case with monofilament construction. This suture retains 75 % of its initial strength at day 14 and 40 % at day 21.

Poly(GA-*co*-CL-*co*-TMC-*co*-LLA)

This newest synthetic bioabsorbable suture is a rapidly degradable monofilament polyester. When compared with the chromic gut suture, this synthetic suture has high tensile strength, low tissue reactivity, and improved handling characteristics. Its greatest advantage is its rapid rate of bioabsorption. Animal studies indicate that this suture retains a minimum of 50–60 % knot strength at day 5 and a minimum of 20–30 % knot strength at day 10 after implantation. It provides secure wound approximation for 10 days, and all tensile strength is lost by day 21.

Others

Wound infection is considered to be one of the oldest and most common complications in all types of injuries. The presence of foreign materials in a wound has been known to increase the susceptibility of surrounding tissues to wound infection. Suture materials are probably the most important biomaterials in wound infection because the infection begins along or near suture lines. Incorporation of anti-bacterials is used to impart anti-microbial activity to biomaterials. An anti-bacterial form is also available for PGLA and poly(GA-*co*-CL) sutures. The anti-bacterial agent used to coat sutures is triclosan (2,4,4′-trichror-2′-hydroxydiphenyl ether) (Fig. 8.10). This active substance, which is slightly soluble in water, was introduced in 1965. Triclosan inhibits fatty acid biosynthesis and enoylacyl carrier protein reductase, resulting in membrane destabilization. This anti-bacterial agent has been shown to

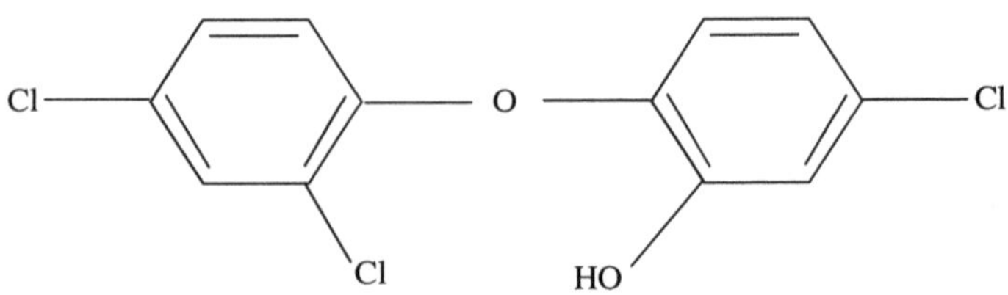

2,4,4′-Trichloro-2′-hydroxydiphenyl ether

Fig. 8.10 Structural formula of triclosan

inhibit colonization on the suture by methicillin-sensitive and methicillin-resistant *Staphylococcus aureus* and *S. epidermis*, *Escherichia coli*, and *Klebsiella pneumoniae*, even after direct in vivo challenge with bacteria. The handling and wound healing characteristics and bioabsorption profile after coating with this non-toxic and non-irritating agent are similar to those with untreated sutures.

A barbed suture, which is self-anchoring with no knots required for wound closure, is manufactured from polydioxanone. This suture consists of axially barbed segments on each side of a mid-point at which the barbs change direction. This wound closure device appears to offer gastrointestinal closure comparable to the poly(GA-*co*-TMC) suture.

One of the major problems in neurosurgery is neuroma formation, which often results in neuropathic pain that can be unbearable for the patient. Neuroma formation can be influenced by the material of suture fibers used in nerve repair. Inhibition of axonal outgrowth accompanied by neuroma formation appears in microsurgical nerve repair as a reaction to common microsuture materials like silk, nylon, or PGA. While nearly every suture material results in granuloma formation, giant cell invasion, and fibrosis, nylon sutures cause less foreign-body reaction than other materials, making them the gold standard in microsurgical nerve repair. Interestingly, recent findings revealed the advantages of spider silk fibers in guiding Schwann cells in nerve regeneration [162, 163]. Therefore, Kuhbier et al. attempted to braid microsutures from native spider silk fibers [164]. Spider silks have proven to possess high anti-microbial properties, which may lead to lower infection rates in peripheral nerve surgery, which is often caused by trauma and leads to septic wound conditions. Additionally, recombinant spider silk has extremely low pyrogenicity, lending further support for its usefulness in trauma surgery where sepsis is common. Both spider silk and nylon are polyamides containing amide bond (−NHCO−) in the main chain. Microsutures braided of native spider dragline silk were manufactured containing either 2×15 or 3×10 single fibers strands. The constructed spider silk sutures had a median thickness of 25 μm, matching the USP definition of 10-0. Maximum load and tensile strength for both spider silk microsutures were significantly more than 2-fold higher than for nylon sutures; the SSR was 1.5-fold higher. All values except elasticity were higher in 3×10 strand sutures than in 2×15 strand sutures but the difference was not significant. With regards to mechanical properties, these sutures were superior to nylon sutures. Since spider silk displays high biocompatibility in nerve regeneration, its usage in microsurgical nerve repair may be considered in the near future.

Conclusions

As demonstrated in this chapter, a variety of bioabsorbable polymers, both natural and synthetic, have been investigated as surgical materials and devices. Sutures have the largest market share among the synthetic bioabsorbable polymer used in medicine. Since different types of monofilament and multifilament sutures with wide range of performance have been fabricated and commercially available, new development in this application is not expected from researchers or sergeants. In contrast, currently available products of sealants/adhesives/hemostatic agents and anti-adhesive barriers still have limitations as discussed. These fields are rapidly growing applications of bioabsorbable polymers.

References

1. Matsuda, S., Ikada, Y.: Glues. In: Bowlin, G.L., Wnek, G. (eds.) Encycropedia of Biomaterials and Biomedical Engineering. Marcel Dekker, NY (2004)
2. Gabay, M., Boucher, B.A.: An essential primer for understanding the role of topical hemostats, surgical sealants, and adhesives for maintaining hemostasis. Pharmacotherapy **33**(9), 935–955 (2013)
3. Spotnitz, W.D., Burks, S.: State-of-the-art review: hemostats, sealants, and adhesives II: update as well as how and when to use the components of the surgical toolbox. Clin. Appl. Thromb. Hemost. **16**(5), 497–514 (2010)
4. Spotnitz, W.D.: Hemostats, sealants, and adhesives: a practical guide for the surgeon. Am. Surg. **78**(12), 1305–1321 (2012)
5. Lodi, D., Iannitti, T., Palmieri, B.: Management of haemostasis in surgery: sealant and glue applications. Blood Coagul. Fibrinolysis **23**(6), 465–472 (2012)
6. Gosain, A.K., Lyon, V.B.: The corrent status of tissue glues: part II For adhesion of soft tissues. Plast. Reconstr. Surg. **110**(6), 1581–1584 (2002)
7. Jackson, M.R.: Fibrin sealants in surgical practice: an overview. Am. J. Surg. **182**, 1S–7S (2001)
8. Morikawa, T.: Tissue sealing. Am. J. Surg. **182**, 29S–35S (2001)
9. Mandell, S.P., Gibran, N.S., Fibrin sealants: surgical hemostat, sealant and adhesive. Expert Opin. Biol. Ther. (2014)
10. Skovgaard, C., Holm, B., Troelsen, A., Lunn, T.H., Gaarn-Larsen, L., Kehlet, H., Husted, H.: No effect of fibrin sealant on drain output or functional recovery following simultaneous bilateral total knee arthroplasty: a randomized, double-blind, placebo-controlled study. Acta Orthop. **84**(2), 153–158 (2013)
11. Miri Bonjar, M.R., Maghsoudi, H., Samnia, R., Saleh, P., Parsafar, F.: Efficacy of fibrin glue on seroma formation after breast surgery. Int. J. Breast Cancer (2012). doi:10.1155/2012/643132
12. Ennker, I.C., Ennker, J., Schoon, H.D., Rimpler, M., Hetzer, R.: Formaldehyde-free collagen glue in experimental lung gluing. Ann. Thorac. Surg. **57**, 1622–1627 (1994)
13. Sawamura, Y., Asaoka, K., Terasaka, S., Tada, M., Uchida, T.: Evaluation of application techniques of fibrin sealant to prevent cerebrospinal fluid leakage: a new device for the application of aerosolized fibrin glue. Neurosurgery **44**(2), 332–337 (1999)
14. Baker, J.W., Spotnitz, W.D., Nolan, S.P., A technique for spray application of fibrin glue during cardiac operations. Ann. Thorac. Surg. **43**(5), 564–565 (1987)
15. Redl, H., Schlag, G., Dinges, H.P.: Methods of fibrin seal application. Thorac. Cardiovasc. Surg. **30**(4), 223–227 (1982)
16. Minato, N., Shimokawa, T., Katayama, Y., Yamada, N., Sakaguchi, M., Itoh, M.: New application method of fibrin glue for more effective hemostasis in cardiovascular surgery: rub-and-spray method. Jpn. J. Thorac. Cardiovasc. Surg. **52**(8), 361–366 (2004)
17. Minato, N., Katayama, Y., Yunoki, J., Kawasaki, H., Satou, H.: Hemostatic effectiveness of a new application method for fibrin glue, the "rub-and-spray method", in emergency aortic surgery for acute aortic dissection. Ann. Thorac. Cardiovasc. Surg. **15**(4), 265–271 (2009)
18. Miyamoto, H., Futagawa, T., Wang, Z., Yamazaki, A., Morio, A., Sonobe, S., Izumi, H., Hosoda, Y., Hata, E.: Fibrin glue and bioabsorbable felt patch for intraoperative intractable air leaks. Jpn. J. Thorac. Cardiovasc. Surg. **51**(6), 232–236 (2003)

19. Yano, S., Tsuiki, H., Kudo, M., Kai, Y., Morioka, M., Takeshima, H., Yumoto, E., Kuratsu, J.: Sellar repair with resorbable polyglactin acid sheet and fibrin glue in endoscopic endonasal transsphenoidal surgery. Surg. Neurol. **67**(1), 59–64 (2007)
20. Itano, H.: The optimal technique for combined application of fibrin sealant and bioabsorbable felt against alveolar air leakage. Eur. J. Cardiothorac. Surg. **33**(3), 457–460 (2008)
21. Ueda, K., Ianaka, T., Li, T.S., Tanaka, N., Hamano, K.: Sutureless pneumostasis using bioabsorbable mesh and glue during major lung resection for cancer: who are the best candidates? J. Thorac. Cardiovasc. Surg. **139**(3), 600–605 (2010)
22. Sugawara, T., Itoh, Y., Hirano, Y., Higashiyama, N., Shimada, Y., Kinouchi, H., Mizoi, K.: Novel dural closure technique using polyglactin acid sheet prevents cerebrospinal fluid leakage after spinal surgery. Neurosurgery **57**(4 Suppl), 290–294 (2005)
23. Hida, K., Yamaguchi, S., Seki, T., Yano, S., Akino, M., Terasaka, S., Uchida, T., Iwasaki, Y.: Nonsuture dural repair using polyglycolic acid mesh and fibrin glue: clinical application to spinal surgery. Surg. Neurol. **65**(2), 136–142 (2006)
24. Terasaka, S., Iwasaki, Y., Shinya, N., Uchida, T.: Fibrin glue and polyglycolic acid nonwoven fabric as a biocompatible dural substitute. Neurosurgery **58**(1), ONS-134–139 (2006)
25. Shimada, Y., Hongo, M., Miyakoshi, N., Sugawara, T., Kasukawa, Y., Ando, S., Ishikawa, Y., Itoi, E.: Dural substitute with polyglycolic acid mesh and fibrin glue for dural repair: technical note and preliminary results. J. Orthop. Sci. **11**(5), 454–458 (2006)
26. Hayashibe, A., Sakamoto, K., Shinbo, M., Makimoto, S., Nakamoto, T.: New method for prevention of bile leakage after hepatic resection. J. Surg. Oncol. **94**(1), 57–60 (2006)
27. Hiura, Y., Takiguchi, S., Yamamoto, K., Kurokawa, Y., Yamasaki, M., Nakajima, K., Miyata, H., Fujiwara, Y., Mori, M., Doki, Y.: Use of fibrin glue sealant with polyglycolic acid sheets to prevent pancreatic fistula formation after laparoscopic-assisted gastrectomy. Surg. Today **43**(5), 527–533 (2013)
28. Haas, S.: The use of a surgical patch coated with human coagulation factors in surgical routine: a multicenter postauthorization surveillance. Clin. Appl. Thromb. Hemost. **12**(4), 445–450 (2006)
29. Simo, K.A., Hanna, E.M., Imagawa, D.K., Iannitti, D.A.: Hemostatic agents in hepatobiliary and pancreas surgery: a review of the literature and critical evaluation of a novel carrier-bound fibrin sealant (TachoSil). ISRN Surg. **2012**, 729086 (2012)
30. Montorsi, M., Zerbi, A., Bassi, C., Capussotti, L., Coppola, R., Sacchi, M.: Italian Tachosil Study Group, Efficacy of an absorbable fibrin sealant patch (TachoSil) after distal pancreatectomy: a multicenter, randomized, controlled trial. Ann. Surg. **256**(5), 853–859 (2012)
31. Zacharias, T., Ferreira, N.: Carrier-bound fibrin sealant compared to oxidized cellulose application after liver resection. HPB (Oxford) **14**(12), 839–847 (2012)
32. Di Monta, G., Caracò, C., Crispo, A., Marone, U., Mozzillo, N.: Collagen sealant patch to reduce lymphatic drainage after lymph node dissection. World J. Surg. Oncol. **10**, 275 (2012)
33. Reddy, M., Schöggl, A., Reddy, B., Holzer, A., Saringer, W., Steiger, C., Matula, C.: Watertightness and effectiveness of a fibrinogen-based collagen fleece (TachoComb®) in neurosurgery. Eur. Surg. **35**(5), 278–281 (2003)
34. Oz, M.C., Rondinone, J.F., Shargill, N.S.: Floseal matrix: new generation topical hemostatic sealant. J. Card. Surg. **18**, 486–493 (2003)
35. Miyamoto, K., Masuda, K., Inoue, N., Okuma, M., Muehleman, C., An, H.S.: Anti-adhesion properties of a thrombin-based hemostatic gelatin in a canine laminectomy model: a biomechanical, biochemical, and histologic study. Spine (Phila Pa 1976) **31**(4), E91–97 (2006)
36. Mayol, J.M., Zapata, C.: Gelatin-thrombin matrix for intraoperative hemostasis in abdomino-pelvic surgery: a systematic review. Surg. Technol. Int. **23**, 23–28 (2013)
37. Yao, H.H., Hong, M.K., Drummond, K.J.: Haemostasis in neurosurgery: what is the evidence for gelatin-thrombin matrix sealant? J. Clin. Neurosci. **20**(3), 349–356 (2013)
38. Samudrala, S.: Topical hemostatic agents in surgery: a surgeon's perspective. AORN J. **88**(3), S2–S11 (2008)
39. Guilmet, D., Bachet, J., Goudot, B., Laurian, C., Gigou, F., et al.: Use of biological glue in acute aortic dissection. Preliminary clinical results with a new surgical techinique. J. Thorac. Cardiovasc. Surg. **77**, 516–521 (1979)

40. Freeman, L.E.B., Blair, A., Lubin, J.H., Stewart, P.A., Hayes, R.B., Hoover, R.N., Hauptmann, M.: Mortality from lymphohematopoietic malignancies among workers in formaldehyde industries: the National Cancer Institute Cohort. J. Natl. Cancer Inst. **101**(10), 751–761 (2009)
41. Bonchek, L.I., Braunwald, N.S.: Experimental evaluation of a cross-linked gelatin adhesive in gastrointestinal surgery. Ann. Surg. **165**(3), 420–424 (1967)
42. Kazui, T., Washiyama, N., Bashar, A.H., Terada, H., Suzuki, K., et al.: Role of biologic glue repair of proximal aortic dissection in the development of early and midterm redissection of the aortic root. Ann. Thorac. Surg. **72**, 509–514 (2001)
43. Fukunaga, S., Karck, M., Harringer, W., Cremer, J., Rhein, C., et al.: The use of gelatin-resorcin-formalin glue in acute aortic dissection type A. Eur. J. Cardiothorac. Surg. **15**, 564–570 (1999)
44. von Oppell, U.O., Karani, Z., Harringer, W., Cremer, J., Rhein, C., et al.: Dissected aortic sinuses repaired with gelatin-resorcin-formaldehyde (GRF) glue are not stable on follow up. J. Heart Valve Dis. **11**, 249–257 (2002)
45. Chao, H.-H., Torchiana, D.F.: BioGlue: albumin/glutaraldehyde sealant in cardiac surgery. J. Card. Surg. **18**, 500–503 (2003)
46. Azadani, A.N., Matthews, P.B., Ge, L., Shen, Y., Jhun, C.S., Guy, T.S., Tseng, E.E.: Mechanical properties of surgical glues used in aortic root replacement. Ann. Thorac. Surg. **87**(4), 1154–1160 (2009)
47. Zehr, K.: Use of bovine albumin-glutaraldehyde glue in cardiovascular surgery. Ann. Thorac. Surg. **84**, 1048–1052 (2007)
48. Coselli, J.S., Bavaria, J.E., Fehrenbacher, J., Stowe, C.L., Macheers, S.K., Gundry, S.R.: Prospective randomized study of a protein-based tissue adhesive used as a hemostatic and structural adjunct in cardiac and vascular anastomotic repair procedures. J. Am. Coll. Surg. **197**(2), 243–252 (2003)
49. Tansley, P., Al-Mulhim, F., Lim, E., Ladas, G., Goldstraw, P.: A prospective, randomized, controlled trial of the effectiveness of BioGlue in treating alveolar air leaks. J. Thorac. Cardiovasc. Surg. **132**(1), 105–112 (2006)
50. Fürst, W., Banerjee, A.: Release of glutaraldehyde from an albumin-glutaraldehyde tissue adhesive causes significant in vitro and in vivo toxicity. Ann. Thorac. Surg. **79**, 1522–1529 (2005)
51. Fuller, C.: Reduction of intraoperative air leaks with progel in pulmonary resection: a comprehensive review. J. Cardiothorac. Surg. **8**, 90 (2013)
52. Stone, W.M., Cull, D.L., Money, S.R.: A randomized prospective multicenter trial of a novel vascular sealant. Ann. Vasc. Surg. **26**(8), 1077–1084 (2012)
53. Gilbert, T.W., Badylak, S.F., Gusenoff, J., Beckman, E.J., Clower, D.M., Daly, P., Rubin, J.P.: Lysine-derived urethane surgical adhesive prevents seroma formation in a canine abdominoplasty model. Plast. Reconstr. Surg. **122**(1), 95–102 (2008)
54. Walgenbach, K.J., Bannasch, H., Kalthoff, S., Rubin, J.P.: Randomized, prospective study of TissuGlu® surgical adhesive in the management of wound drainage following abdominoplasty. Aesthetic Plast. Surg. **36**(3), 491–496 (2012)
55. Öllinger, R., Mihaljevic, A.L., Schuhmacher, C., Bektas, H., Vondran, F., Kleine, M., Sainz-Barriga, M., Weiss, S., Knebel, P., Pratschke, J., Troisi, R.I.: A multicentre, randomized clinical trial comparing the Veriset™ haemostatic patch with fibrin sealant for the management of bleeding during hepatic surgery. HPB (Oxford) **15**(7), 548–558 (2013)
56. Lauto, A., Mawad, D., Foster, L.J.R.: Review: adhesive biomaterials for tissue reconstruction. J. Chem. Tech. Biotech. **83**, 464–472 (2008)
57. Singer, A.J., Thode, H.C.: A review of the literature on octylcyanoacrylate tissue adhesive. Am. J. Surg. **187**, 238–248 (2004)
58. Singer, A.J., Perry, L.C., Allen Jr, R.L.: In vivo study of wound bursting strength and compliance of topical skin adhesives. Acad. Emerg. Med. **15**(12), 1290–1294 (2008)
59. Jan, H., Waters, N., Haines, P., Kent, A.: LiquiBand® Surgical S topical adhesive versus sutures for the closure of laparoscopic wounds. A randomized controlled trial. Gynecol. Surg. **10**, 247–252 (2013)

60. Bookland, M.J., Sukul, V., Connolly, P.J.: Use of a cyanoacrylate skin adhesive to reduce external ventricular drain infection rates. J. Neurosurg. (2014). doi:10.3171/2013.12.JNS13700
61. Ozer, M.T., Sinan, H., Saydam, M., Kilic, A., Akyol, M., Coskun, A.K., Bedir, O., Demibas, S.: Effectiveness of N-butyl cyanoacrylate-based microbial skin sealant on the prevention of surgical site infections. Surg. Infect. (Larchmt) **15**(1), 14–17 (2014)
62. Osbun, J.W., Ellenbogen, R.G., Chesnut, R.M., Chin, L.S., Connolly, P.J., Cosgrove, G.R., Delashaw Jr, J.B., Golfinos, J.G., Greenlee, J.D., Haines, S.J., Jallo, J., Muizelaar, J.P., Nanda, A., Shaffrey, M., Shah, M.V., Tew Jr, J.M., van Loveren, H.R., Weinand, M.E., White, J.A., Wilberger, J.E.: A multicenter, single-blind, prospective randomized trial to evaluate the safety of a polyethylene glycol hydrogel (Duraseal Dural Sealant System) as a dural sealant in cranial surgery. World Neurosurg. **78**(5), 498–504 (2012)
63. Glickman, M., Gheissari, A., Money, S., Martin, J., Ballard, J.L., CoSeal Multicenter Vascular Surgery Study Group: A polymeric sealant inhibits anastomotic suture hole bleeding more rapidly than gelfoam/thrombin: results of a randomized controlled trial. Arch. Surg. **137**(3), 326–331 (2002)
64. Natour, E., Suedkamp, M., Dapunt, O.E.: Assessment of the effect on blood loss and transfusion requirements when adding a polyethylene glycol sealant to the anastomotic closure of aortic procedures: a case-control analysis of 102 patients undergoing Bentall procedures. J. Cardiothorac. Surg. **7**, 105 (2012)
65. Lequaglie, C., Giudice, G., Marasco, R., Morte, A.D., Gallo, M.: Use of a sealant to prevent prolonged air leaks after lung resection: a prospective randomized study. J. Cardiothorac. Surg. **7**, 106 (2012)
66. Ranger, W.R., Halpin, D., Sawhney, A.S., Lyman, M., LoCicero, J.: Pneumostasis of experimental air leaks with a new photopolymerized synthetic tissue sealant. Am. Surgeon **63**, 788–795 (1997)
67. Lyman, M.L., Sawhney, A.S.: Design of a synthetic pneumosealant. Ann. Biomat. **2**, 212 (1996)
68. Thompson, I.: TissuePatch™3 and TissuePatchDural™: a review of constituent materials. Adhesive sealant biomaterials (2009)
69. Mandley, D.: Evaluation of a novel adhesive film for sealing air leaks after lung surgery. Adhesive sealant biomaterials (2009)
70. Zhang, R., Bures, M., Höffler, H.K., Zinne, N., Länger, F., Bisdas, T., Haverich, A., Krüger, M.: TissuePatch™ as a novel synthetic sealant for repair of superficial lung defect: in vitro tests results. Ann. Surg. Innov. Res. **6**(1), 12 (2012)
71. Cheng, L., Lau, C.K., Parker, G.: Use of TissuePatch™ sealant film in the management of chyle leak in major neck surgery. Br. J. Oral. Maxillofac. Surg. **52**(1), 87–89 (2014)
72. Iwasashi, M., Sakane, M., Saito, H., Taguchi, T., Tateishi, T., Ochiai, N.: In vivo evaluation of bonding ability and biocompatibility of a novel biodegradable glue consisting of tartaric acid derivative and human serum albumin. J. Biomed. Mater. Res. A **90**(2), 543–548 (2009)
73. Elvin, C.M., Danon, S.J., Brownlee, A.G., White, J.F., Hickey, M., Liyou, N.E., Edwards, G.A., Ramshaw, J.A., Werkmeister, J.A.: Evaluation of photo-crosslinked fibrinogen as a rapid and strong tissue adhesive. J. Biomed. Mater. Res. A **93**(2), 687–695 (2010)
74. Suzuki, S., Ikada, Y.: Sealing effects of crosslinked gelatin. J. Biomater. Appl. **27**(7), 801–810 (2013)
75. LeMaire, S.A., Carter, S.A., Won, T., Wang, X., Conklin, L.D., Coselli, J.S.: The threat of adhesive embolization: BioGlue leaks through needle holes in aortic tissue and prosthetic grafts. Ann. Thorac. Surg. **80**(1), 106–110 (2005)
76. Elvin, C.M., Vuocolo, T., Brownlee, A.G., Sando, L., Huson, M.G., Liyou, N.E., Stockwell, P.R., Lyons, R.E., Kim, M., Edwards, G.A., Johnson, G., McFarland, G.A., Ramshaw, J.A., Werkmeister, J.A.: A highly elastic tissue sealant based on photopolymerised gelatin. Biomaterials **31**(32), 8323–8331 (2010)
77. Artzi, N., Shazly, T., Crespo, C., Ramos, A.B., Chenault, H.K., Edelman, E.R.: Characterization of star adhesive sealants based on PEG/dextran hydrogels. Macromol. Biosci. **11**(9), 754–765 (2009)

78. Henderson, P.W., Kadouch, D.J., Singh, S.P., Zawaneh, P.N., Weiser, J., Yazdi, S., Weinstein, A., Krotscheck, U., Wechsler, B., Putnam, D., Spector, J.A.: A rapidly resorbable hemostatic biomaterial based on dihydroxyacetone. J. Biomed. Mater. Res. A **93**(2), 776–782 (2010)
79. Horio, T., Ishihara, M., Fujita, M., Kishimoto, S., Kanatani, Y., Ishizuka, T., Nogami, Y., Nakamura, S., Tanaka, Y., Morimoto, Y., Maehara, T.: Effect of photocrosslinkable chitosan hydrogel and its sponges to stop bleeding in a rat liver injury model. Artif. Organs **34**(4), 342–347 (2010)
80. Rickett, T.A., Amoozgar, Z., Tuchek, C.A., Park, J., Yeo, Y., Shi, R.: Rapidly photo-cross-linkable chitosan hydrogel for peripheral neurosurgeries. Biomacromolecules **12**(1), 57–65 (2011)
81. Lauto, A., Mawad, D., Barton, M., Gupta, A., Piller, S.C., Hook, J.: Photochemical tissue bonding with chitosan adhesive films. Biomed. Eng. **9**, 47 (2010)
82. Dowling, M.B., Kumar, R., Keibler, M.A., Hess, J.R., Bochicchio, G.V., Raghavan, S.R.: A self-assembling hydrophobically modified chitosan capable of reversible hemostatic action. Biomaterials **32**(13), 3351–3357 (2011)
83. Takaoka, M., Nakamura, T., Sugai, H., Bentley, A.J., Nakajima, N., Fullwood, N.J., Yokoi, N., Hyon, S.H., Kinoshita, S.: Sutureless amniotic membrane transplantation for ocular surface reconstruction with a chemically defined bioadhesive. Biomaterials **29**(19), 2923–2931 (2008)
84. Cha, H.J., Hwang, D.S., Lim, S.: Development of bioadhesives from marine mussels. Biotechnol. J. **3**, 631–635 (2008)
85. Lee, H., Lee, B.P., Messersmith, P.B.: A reversible wet/dry adhesive inspired by mussels and geckos. Nature **448**, 338–341 (2007)
86. Waite, J.H., Tanzer, M.L.: Polyphenolic substance of mytilus edulis: novel adhesive containing L-Dopa and hydroxyproline. Science **212**(4498), 1038–1040 (1981)
87. Dove, J., Sheridan, P.: Adhesive protein from mussles: possibilities for dentistry, medicine and industry. J. Am. Dent. Assoc. **112**, 879 (1986)
88. Grande, D.A., Pitman, M.I.: The use of adhesives in chodrocyte transplantation surgery: preliminary studies. Bull. Hosp. Jt. Dis. Otrhop. Inst. **48**, 140–148 (1988)
89. Saez, C., Pardo, J., Gutierrez, E., Brito, M., et al.: Immunological studies of the polyphenolic proteins of mussels. Comp. Biochem. Physiol. **98B**, 569–572 (1991)
90. Lee, H., Dellatore, S.M., Miller, W.M., Messersmith, P.B.: Mussel-inspired surface chemistry for multifunctional coatings. Science **318**, 426–430 (2007)
91. Shazly, T.M., Baker, A.B., Naber, J.R., Bon, A., Van Vliet, K.J., Edelman, E.R.: Augmentation of postswelling surgical sealant potential of adhesive hydrogels. J. Biomed. Mater. Res. A **95**(4), 1159–1169 (2010)
92. Graham, L.D., Danon, S.J., Johnson, G., Braybrook, C., Hart, N.K., Varley, R.J., Evans, M.D., McFarland, G.A., Tyler, M.J., Werkmeister, J.A., Ramshaw, J.A.: Biocompatibility and modification of the protein-based adhesive secreted by the Australian frog Notaden bennetti. J. Biomed. Mater. Res. A **93**(2), 429–441 (2010)
93. Aboushwareb, T., Eberli, D., Ward, C., Broda, C., Holcomb, J., Atala, A., Van Dyke, M.: A keratin biomaterial gel hemostat derived from human hair: evaluation in a rabbit model of lethal liver injury. J. Biomed. Mater. Res. B Appl. Biomater. **90**(1), 45–54 (2009)
94. Mahdavi, A., Ferreira, L., Sundback, C., Nichol, J.W., Chan, E.P., Carter, D.J., Bettinger, C.J., Patanavanich, S., Chignozha, L., Ben-Joseph, E., Galakatos, A., Pryor, H., Pomerantseva, I., Masiakos, P.T., Faquin, W., Zumbuehl, A., Hong, S., Borenstein, J., Vacanti, J., Langer, R., Karp, J.M.: A biodegradable and biocompatible gecko-inspired tissue adhesive. Proc. Natl. Acad. Sci. USA **105**(7), 2307–2312 (2008)
95. Liakakos, T., Thomakos, N., Fine, P.M., Dervenis, C., Young, R.L.: Peritoneal adhesions: etiology, pathophysiology, and clinical significance. Recent advances in prevention and management. Dig. Surg. **18**(4), 260–273 (2001)
96. Robertson, D., Lefebvre, G., Leyland, N., Wolfman, W., Allaire, C., Awadalla, A., Best, C., Contestabile, E., Dunn, S., Heywood, M., Leroux, N., Potestio, F., Rittenberg, D., Senikas, V., Soucy, R., Singh, S.: Society of obstetricians and gynaecologists of canada, adhesion prevention in gynaecological surgery. J. Obstet. Gynaecol. Can. **32**(6), 598–608 (2010)

97. Poole, J.H.: Adhesions following cesarean delivery: a review of their occurrence, consequences and preventative management using adhesion barriers. Womens Health (Lond. Engl.) **9**(5), 467–477 (2013)
98. Kamel, R.M.: Prevention of postoperative peritoneal adhesions. Eur. J. Obstet. Gynecol. Reprod. Biol. **150**(2), 111–118 (2010)
99. Novitsky, Y.W., Harrell, A.G., Cristiano, J.A., Paton, B.L., Norton, H.J., Peindl, R.D., Kercher, K.W., Heniford, B.T.: Comparative evaluation of adhesion formation, strength of ingrowth, and textile properties of prosthetic meshes after long-term intra-abdominal implantation in a rabbit. J. Surg. Res. **140**(1), 6–11 (2007)
100. Larsson, B., Lalos, O., Marsk, L., Tronstad, S.E., Bygdeman, M., Pehrson, S., Joelsson, I.: Effect of intraperitoneal instillation of 32 % dextran 70 on postoperative adhesion formation after tubal surgery. Acta Obstet. Gynecol. Scand. **64**(5), 437–441 (1985)
101. Weinans, M.J., Kauer, F.M., Klompmaker, I.J., Wijma, J.: Transient liver function disturbances after the intraperitoneal use of 32 % dextran 70 as adhesion prophylaxis in infertility surgery. Fertil. Steril. **53**(1), 159–161 (1990)
102. Tulandi, T.: Transient edema after intraperitoneal instillation of 32 % dextran 70. A report of five cases. J. Reprod. Med. **32**(6), 472–474 (1987)
103. Sites, C.K., Jensen, B.A., Glock, J.L., Blackman, J.A., Badger, G.J., Johnson, J.V., Brumsted, J.R.: Transvaginal ultrasonographic assessment of hyskon or lactated ringer's solution instillation after laparoscopy: randomized, controlled study. J. Ultrasound Med. **16**(3), 195–199 (1997)
104. Holtz, G., Baker, E., Tsai, C.: Effect of thirty-two per cent dextran 70 on peritoneal adhesion formation and re-formation after lysis. Fertil. Steril. **33**(6), 660–662 (1980)
105. Rose, B.: Safety of Hyskon for routine gynecologic surgery. A case report. J. Reprod. Med. **32**(2) (1987)
106. Ruiz, J.M., Neuwirth, R.F.: The incidence of complications associated with the use of hyskon during hysteroscopy: experience in 1793 consecutive patients. J. Gynecol. Surg. **8**(4), 219–224 (1992)
107. Kossi, J., Gronlund, S., Uotila-Nieminen, M., Crowe, A., Knight, A., Keranen, U.: The effect of 4 % icodextrin solution on adhesiolysis surgery time at the Hartmann's reversal: a pilot, multicentre, randomized control trial vs lactated Ringer's solution. Colorectal Dis. **11**, 168–172 (2008)
108. Johns, D.B., Keyport, G.M., Hoehler, F., diZerega, G.S.: Reduction of postsurgical adhesions with intergel® adhesion prevention solution: a multicenter study of safety and efficacy after conservative gynecologic surgery. Fertil. Steril. **76**(3), 595–604 (2001)
109. FDA: Safety alert—INTERGEL adhesion prevention solution. (2003) Available from: http://www.fda.gov/Safety/MedWatch/SafetyInformation/SafetyAlertsforHumanMedicalProducts/ucm170010.htm
110. Rice, V.M., Shanti, A., Moghissi, K.S., Leach, R.E.: A comparative evaluation of Poloxamer 407 and oxidized regenerated cellulose (Interceed [TC7]) to reduce postoperative adhesion formation in the rat uterine horn model. Fertil. Steril. **59**(4), 901–906 (1993)
111. Weis, C., Odermatt, E.: A-Part Gel—an efficient adheison prevention barrier. J. Biomed. Mater. Res. B Appl. Biomater. **82B**, 174–182 (2006)
112. Weis, C., Odermatt, E.K., Kressler, J., Funke, Z., Wehner, T., Freytag, D.: Poly(vinyl alcohol) membrane for adhesion prevention. J. Biomed. Mater. Res. **70B**, 191–202 (2004)
113. Janigen, B., Weis, C., Odermatt, E.K., Obermaier, R., Hopt, U.T.: The new adhesion prophylaxis membrane A-Part-from in vitro testing to first in vivo results. J. Biomed. Mater. Res. **89B**, 293–299 (2009)
114. Jaenigen, B.M., Weis, C., Odermatt, E.K., Hopt, U.T., Obermaier, R.: The new adhesion prophylaxis membrane A-part–from in vitro testing to first in vivo results. J. Biomed. Mater. Res. B Appl. Biomater. **89**(2), 293–299 (2009)
115. Lang, R.A., Weisgerber, C., Grüntzig, P.M., Weis, C., Odermatt, E.K., Kirschner, M.H.: Polyvinyl alcohol gel prevents adhesion re-formation after adhesiolysis in a rabbit model. J. Surg. Res. **153**(3), 12–16 (2009)

116. Slieker, J.C., Ditzel, M., Harlaar, J.J., Mulder, I.M., Deerenberg, E.B., Bastiaansen-Jenniskens, Y.M., Kleinrensink, G.J., Jeekel, J., Lange, J.F.: Effects of new anti-adhesion polyvinyl alcohol gel on healing of colon anastomoses in rats. Surg. Infect. (Larchmt) **13**(6), 396–400 (2012)
117. Young, P., Johns, A., Templeman, C., Witz, C., Webster, B., Ferland, R., Diamond, M.P., Block, K., diZerega, G.: Reduction of postoperative adhesions after laparoscopic gynecological surgery with Oxiplex/AP Gel: a pilot study. Fertil. Steril. **84**(5), 1450–1456 (2005)
118. Mettler, L., Audebert, A., Lehmann-Willenbrock, E., Jacobs, V.R., Schive, K.: New adhesion prevention concept in gynecological surgery. JSLS **7**(3), 207–209 (2003)
119. Mettler, L., Audebert, A., Lehmann-Willenbrock, E., Schive, K., Jacobs, V.R.: Prospective clinical trial of SprayGel as a barrier to adhesion formation: an interim analysis. J. Am. Assoc. Gynecol. Laparosc. **10**(3), 339–344 (2003)
120. Tjandra, J.J., Chan, M.K.: A sprayable hydrogel adhesion barrier facilitates closure of defunctioning loop ileostomy: a randomized trial. Dis. Colon Rectum. **51**(6), 956–960 (2008)
121. Ferland, R., Campbell, P.K.: Evaluation of SprayShield adhesion barrier system in a porcine model of gynecological surgery. Covidien AG (2008)
122. Mettler, L., Sammur, W., Schollmeyer, T., Alkatout, I.: Cross-linked sodium hyaluronate, an anti-adhesion barrier gel in gynaecological endoscopic surgery. Minim. Invasive Ther. Allied Technol. **22**(5), 260–265 (2013)
123. Mettler, L.: Effect of cross linked sodium hyaluronate in adhesion reduction within the gynecologic surgical window. OJOG **4**, 120–129 (2014)
124. The Myomectomy Adhesion Multicenter Study Group: An expanded polytetrafluoroethylene barrier (Gore-Tex Surgical Membrane) reduces post-myomectomy adhesion formation. Fertil. Steril. **3**(3), 491–493 (1995)
125. Haney, A.F., Hesla, J., Hurst, B.S., Kettel, L.M., Murphy, A.A., Rock, J.A., Rowe, G., Schlaff, W.D.: Expanded polytetrafluoroethylene (Gore-Tex Surgical Membrane) is superior to oxidized regenerated cellulose (Interceed TC7+) in preventing adhesions. Fertil. Steril. **63**(5), 1021–1026 (1995)
126. Kawamura, H., Yokota, R., Yokota, K., Watarai, H., Tsunoda, Y., Yamagami, H., Hata, T., Tanaka, K., Masuko, H., Ishizu, H., Okada, K., Adachi, T., Kondo, Y.: A sodium hyaluronate carboxymethylcellulose bioresorbable membrane prevents postoperative small-bowel adhesive obstruction after distal gastrectomy. Surg. Today **40**, 223–227 (2010)
127. Becker, J.M., Dayton, M.T., Fazio, V.W., Beck, D.E., Stryker, S.J., Wexner, S.D., Wolff, B.G., Roberts, P.L., Smith, L.E., Sweeney, S.A., Moore, M.: Prevention of postoperative abdominal adhesions by a sodium hyaluronate-based bioresorbable membrane: a prospective, randomized, double-blind multicenter study. J. Am. Coll. Surg. **183**(4), 297–306 (1996)
128. Kusunoki, M., Ikeuchi, H., Yanagi, H., Noda, M., Tonouchi, H., Mohri, Y., Uchida, K., Inoue, Y., Kobayashi, M., Miki, C., Yamamura, T.: Bioresorbable hyaluronate-carboxymethylcellulose membrane (Seprafilm) in surgery for rectal carcinoma: a prospective randomized clinical trial. Surg. Today **35**(11), 940–945 (2005)
129. Hayashi, S., Takayama, T., Masuda, H., Kochi, M., Ishii, Y., Matsuda, M., Yamagata, M., Fujii, M.: Bioresorbable membrane to reduce postoperative small bowel obstruction in patients with gastric cancer: a randomized clinical trial. Ann. Surg. **247**(5), 766–770 (2008)
130. Beck, D.E., Cohen, Z., Fleshman, J.W., Kaufman, H.S., van Goor, H., Wolff, B.G., Adhesion Study Group Steering Committee: A prospective, randomized, multicenter, controlled study of the safety of Seprafilm adhesion barrier in abdominopelvic surgery of the intestine. Dis. Colon Rectum. **46**(10), 1310–1319 (2003)
131. Fazio, V.W., Cohen, Z., Fleshman, J.W., van Goor, H., Bauer, J.J., Wolff, B.G., Corman, M., Beart Jr, R.W., Wexner, S.D., Becker, J.M., Monson, J.R., Kaufman, H.S., Beck, D.E., Bailey, H.R., Ludwig, K.A., Stamos, M.J., Darzi, A., Bleday, R., Dorazio, R., Madoff, R.D., Smith, L.E., Gearhart, S., Lillemoe, K., Gohl, J.: Reduction in adhesive small-bowel obstruction by Seprafilm adhesion barrier after intestinal resection. Dis. Colon Rectum. **49**(1), 1–11 (2006)

132. Diamond, M.P., Burns, E.L., Accomando, B., Mian, S., Holmdahl, L.: Seprafilm®adhesion barrier: (1) a review of preclinical, animal, and human investigational studies. Cynecol. Surg. **9**, 237–245 (2012)
133. Diamond, M.P., Burns, E.L., Accomando, B., Mian, S., Holmdahl, L.: Seprafilm® adhesion barrier: (2) a review of the clinical literature on intraabdominal use. Gynecol. Surg. **9**, 247–257 (2012)
134. Walther, T., Rastan, A., Dähnert, I., Falk, V., Jacobs, S., Mohr, F.W., Kostelka, M.: A novel adhesion barrier facilitates reoperations in complex congenital cardiac surgery. J. Thorac. Cardiovasc. Surg. **129**(2), 359–363 (2005)
135. Wiseman, D.M., Trout, J.R., Franklin, R.R., Diamond, M.P.: Metaanalysis of the safety and efficacy of an adhesion barrier (Interceed TC7) in laparotomy. J. Reprod. Med. **44**(4), 325–331 (1999)
136. INTERCEED(TC7) Adhesion Barrier Study Group: Prevention of postsurgical adhesions by INTERCEED(TC7), an absorbable adhesion barrier: a prospective randomized multicenter clinical study. Fertil. Steril. **51**(6), 933–938 (1989)
137. Faerden, A., Reiertsen, O., Marx, A.: The effectiveness of a bioresorbable polymer sheet (SurgiWrap®) in minimizing soft tissue attachments (STA) after major colorectal surgery: a randomized controlled pilot study. MAST Biosurgery from manufactures website. (2006)
138. Lodge, A.J., Wells, W.J., Backer, C.L., O'Brien Jr, J.E., Austin, E.H., Bacha, E.A., Yeh Jr, T., Decampli, W.M., Lavin, P.T., Weinstein, S.: A novel bioresorbable film reduces postoperative adhesions after infant cardiac surgery. Ann. Thorac. Surg. **86**(2), 614–621 (2008)
139. Gagnieu, C.H., Forest, P.O.: In vivo biodegradability and biocompatibility of porcine type I atelocollagen newly crosslinked by oxidized glycogen. Biomed. Mater. Eng. **17**(1), 9–18 (2007)
140. Bel, A., Kachatryan, L., Bruneval, P., Peyrard, S., Gagnieu, C., Fabiani, J.N., Menasché, P.: A new absorbable collagen membrane to reduce adhesions in cardiac surgery. Interact. CardioVasc. Thorac. Surg. **10**(2), 213–216 (2010)
141. Diamond, M.P., Kruger, M., Saed, G.M.: Effect of tisseel on expression of tissue plasminogen activator and plasminogen activator inhibitor-1. Fertil. Steril. **81**, 1657–1664 (2004)
142. Prieto-Díaz-Chávez, E., Medina-Chávez, J.L., Ramírez-Barba, E.J., Trujillo-Hernández, B., Millán-Guerrero, R.O., Vásquez, C.: Reduction of peritoneal adhesion to polypropylene mesh with the application of fibrin glue. Acta Chir. Belg. **108**, 433–437 (2008)
143. Martín-Cartes, J.A., Morales-Conde, S., Suárez-Grau, J.M., Bustos-Jiménez, M., Cadet-Dussort, J.M., López-Bernal, F., Morcillo-Azcárate, J., Tutosaus-Gómez, J.D., Morales-Méndez, S.: Role of fibrin glue in the prevention of peritoneal adhesions in ventral hernia repair. Surg. Today **38**(2), 135–140 (2008)
144. Petter-Puchner, A.H., Walder, N., Redl, H., Schwab, R., Ohlinger, W., Gruber-Blum, S., Fortelny, R.H.: Fibrin sealant (Tissucol) enhances tissue integration of condensed polytetrafluoroethylene meshes and reduces early adhesion formation in experimental intraabdominal peritoneal onlay mesh repair. J. Surg. Res. **150**(2), 190–195 (2008)
145. Frykman, E., Jacobsson, S., Widenfalk, B.: Fibrin sealant in prevention of flexor tendon adhesions: an experimental study in the rabbit. J. Hand. Surg. **18A**, 68–75 (1993)
146. Yoshioka, I., Saiki, Y., Sakuma, K., Iguchi, A., Moriya, T., Ikada, Y., Tabayashi, K.: Bioabsorbable gelatin sheets latticed with polyglycolic acid can eliminate pericardial adhesion. Ann. Thorac. Surg. **84**, 864–870 (2007)
147. Sakuma, K., Iguchi, A., Ikada, Y., Tabayashi, K.: Closure of the pericardium using synthetic bioabsorbable polymers. Ann. Thorac. Surg. **80**, 1835–1840 (2005)
148. Bae, S.H., Son, S.R., Kumar Sakar, S., Nguyen, T.H., Kim, S.W., Min, Y.K., Lee, B.T.: Evaluation of the potential anti-adhesion effect of the PVA/Gelatin membrane. J. Biomed. Mater. Res. B Appl. Biomater. **102**(4), 840–849 (2014)
149. Vorvolakos, K., Isayeva, I.S., Luu, H.-M.D., Patwardhan, D.V., Pollack, S.K.: Ionically cross-linked hyaluronic acid: wetting, lubrication, and viscoelasticity of a modified adhesion barrier gel. Medical Devices Evidence Res. **2011**(4), 1–10 (2010)

150. Nilsson, E., Björn, C., Sjöstrand, V., Lindgren, K., Münnich, M., Mattsby-Baltzer, I., Ivarsson, M.L., Olmarker, K., Mahlapuu, M.: A novel polypeptide derived from human lactoferrin in sodium hyaluronate prevents postsurgical adhesion formation in the rat. Ann. Surg. **250**(6), 1021–1028 (2009)
151. Lauder, C.I., Garcea, G., Strickland, A., Maddern, G.J.: Use of a modified chitosan-dextran gel to prevent peritoneal adhesions in a rat model. J. Surg. Res. (2010) (Epub ahead of print)
152. Falabella, C.A., Melendez, M.M., Weng, L., Chen, W.: Novel macromolecular crosslinking hydrogel to reduce intra-abdominal adhesions. J. Surg. Res. **159**(2), 772–778 (2010)
153. Li, L., Wang, N., Jin, X., Deng, R., Nie, S., Sun, L., Wu, Q., Wei, Y., Gong, C.: Biodegradable and injectable in situ cross-linking chitosan-hyaluronic acid based hydrogels for postoperative adhesion prevention. Biomaterials **35**(12), 3903–3917 (2014)
154. Pätilä, T., Jokinen, J.J., Salminen, J., Kankuri, E., Harjula, A.: Polyglycolic acid glue does not prevent intrapericardial adhesions in a short-term follow-up. J. Surg. Res. **148**(2), 181–184 (2008)
155. Yang, B., Gong, C.Y., Qian, Z.Y., Zhao, X., Li, Z.Y., Zhou, S.T., Qi, X.R., Zhong, Q., Luo, F., Wei, Y.Q.: Prevention of abdominal adhesion formation by thermosensitive PECE-hydrogel in a rat uterine horn model. J. Biomed. Mater. Res. B Appl. Biomater. **96**(1), 57–66 (2011)
156. Yang, B., Gong, C., Zhao, X., Zhou, S., Li, Z., Qi, X., Zhong, Q., Luo, F., Qian, Z.: Preventing postoperative abdominal adhesions in a rat model with PEG-PCL-PEG hydrogel. Int. J. Nanomed. **7**, 547–557 (2012)
157. Niwa, D., Koide, M., Fujie, T., Goda, N., Takeoka, S.: Application of nanosheets as an anti-adhesion barrier in partial hepatectomy. J. Biomed. Mater. Res. B Appl. Biomater. **101**(7), 1251–1258 (2013)
158. Wang, H., Li, M., Hu, J., Wang, C., Xu, S., Han, C.C.: Multiple targeted drugs carrying biodegradable membrane barrier: anti-adhesion, hemostasis, and anti-infection. Biomacromolecules **14**(4), 954–961 (2013)
159. Pryor, H.I., O'Doherty, E., Hart, A., Owens, G., Hoganson, D., Vacanti, J.P., Masiakos, P.T., Sundback, C.A.: Poly(glycerol sebacate) films prevent postoperative adhesions and allow laparoscopic placement. Surgery **146**, 490–497 (2009)
160. Lee, M.W., Tsai, H.F., Wen, S.M., Huang, C.H.: Photocrosslinkable gellan gum film as an anti-adhesion barrier. Carbohydr. Polym. **90**(2), 1132–1138 (2012)
161. Firestone, D.E., Lauder, A.J.: Chemistry and mechanics of commonly used sutures and needles. J. Hand. Surg. Am. **35**, 486–488 (2010)
162. Allmeling, C., Jokuszies, A., Reimers, K., Kall, S., Choi, C.Y., Brandes, G., Kasper, C., Scheper, T., Guggenheim, M., Vogt, P.M.: Spider silk fibres in artificial nerve constructs promote peripheral nerve regeration. Cell Prolif. **41**, 408–420 (2008)
163. Allmeling, C., Jokuszies, A., Reimers, K., Kall, S., Vogt, P.M.: Use of spider silk fibres as an innovative material in a biocompatible artificial nerve coduit. J. Cell Mol. Med. **10**, 770–777 (2006)
164. Kuhbier, J.W., Reimers, K., Kasper, C., Allmeling, C., Hillmer, A., Menger, B., Vogt, P.M., Radtke, C.: First investigation of spider silk as a braided microsurgical suture. J. Biomed. Mater. Res. B Appl. Biomater. **97**, 381–387 (2011)

Chapter 9
Emerging Polymers in Dentistry

Thais Thomé, Maria C.G. Erhardt, Ariene A. Leme, Isra Al Bakri, Ana K. Bedran-Russo and Luiz E. Bertassoni

Abstract Polymers represent the foundation of modern restorative Dentistry. The majority of dental procedures currently utilized in clinical dentistry depend on the close interaction of polymeric materials with dental tissues. In fact, the dental matrix itself is largely constituted of natural polymers, such as collagen fibrils, that constitute the organic matrix of dentin, cementum and bone. In this chapter, several direct restorative materials will be described in light of their polymeric composition and dental application. Particular emphasis will be given to emerging restorative materials, such as new classes of dental adhesives and composite resins. Additionally, we discuss emerging classes of dental polymers, which have been recently utilized to infiltrate demineralized enamel and to assist remineralization of collagen fibrils in carious dentin.

Keywords Resin composite · Dental adhesion · Bonding · Caries · Dentin · Dental polymer

---

Thais Thomé, Maria C.G. Erhardt and Ariene A. Leme have contributed equally to this work.

T. Thomé · M.C.G. Erhardt
Department of Conservative Dentistry, Universidade Federal do Rio Grande do Sul, Porto Alegre, RS 90035-000, Brazil

A.A. Leme · A.K. Bedran-Russo
Department of Restorative Dentistry, College of Dentistry, University of Illinois at Chicago, Chicago, IL 60612, USA

I. Al Bakri · L.E. Bertassoni (✉)
Biomaterials and Bioengineering, Faculty of Dentistry, University of Sydney, Sydney, NSW 2010, Australia
e-mail: luiz.bertassoni@sydney.edu.au

F. Puoci (ed.), *Advanced Polymers in Medicine*, DOI 10.1007/978-3-319-12478-0_9

Abbreviations

PDL	Periodontal ligament
ECM	Extracellular matrix
Bis-GMA	2,2-bis[4-(2-hydroxy-3-methacryloxypropoxy)phenyl]propane
HEMA	Hydroxyethyl methacrylate
TEGDMA	Triethyleneglycol-dimethacrylate
10-MDP	10-methacryloyloxydecyl dihydrogen phosphate monomer
4-MET	4-methacryloxyethyl trimellitic acid
Phenyl-P	2-methacryloxyethyl phenyl hydrogen phosphate
PPD	1-phenyl-1,2-propanedione
Lucerin-TPO	2,4,6-trimethylbenzoyl-diphenylphosphine oxide
BAPO	Bisacylphosphine oxide
DPIHP	Diphenyliodonium hexafluorophosphate
MDPB	12-methacryloyloxydodecylpyridinium bromide
BAC	Benzalkonium chloride
CHX	Chlorhexidine
MMPs	Matrix metalloproteinases
PGs	Proteoglycans
GAG	Glycosaminoglycan
EDC/NHS	1-ethyl-3-[3-dimethylaminopropyl] carbodiimide hydrochloride/n-hydroxysuccinimide
OPACs	Oligomeric proanthocyanidins
PPRF	Prepolymerized resin fillers
QAS	Quaternary ammonium compounds
TCD	Tricyclodecane
SDR	Stress decreasing resin
MMA	Methyl methacrylate
PMMA	Poly(methyl methacrylate)
PILP	Polymer induced liquid precursor
PASP	Poly-L aspartic acid
PGLU	Poly-L-glutamic acid
PVPA	Polyvynilphosphonic acid
PAA	Polyacrylic acid
ACP	Amorphous calcium phosphate

Introduction

Dentistry encompasses a breadth of clinical activities that can range from complex surgical oral maxilofacial reconstructions, preventive treatments against pathological conditions, restorative procedures for treating tooth decay, among a long list of procedures that make up the field of dental sciences. The application of different types of polymers in these procedures is vast, and it can be said that polymers have paved the way for important transitions in clinical dentistry [1].

Like any biological tissue, the tooth complex is essentially constituted of a complex combination of biopolymers [1]. These structures—which include enamel (the outer layer covering the tooth crown), dentin (the tissue immediately underneath the enamel), pulp (the sensory unit and vascular component of the tooth), cementum (the structure covering the root of the tooth), periodontal ligament (PDL-the soft tissue anchoring the root of the tooth), and alveolar bone (the site of anchorage for the tooth in the oral cavity) [2]—present a wide range of biopolymeric building blocks, in the sense that they are composed of proteins with repeating monomeric units having carbon as a structural backbone forming well-defined organic matrices [3].

Biopolymers are present in dental tissues in the form of polynucleotides, 13 or more nucleotide monomers covalently bonded in a chain (i.e. RNA and DNA), which contribute to the genetic make up regulating the functions of odontobalsts and stem cells in the dental pulp [4]. Similarly, polypeptides, which are short polymers of amino acids, form the basic building blocks of the extracellular matrix (ECM) in dentin, alveolar bone, cementum, PDL and pulp in the form of collagen fibrils [1] and elastin (in the pulp and PDL/bone vasculature) [5]. Another example of biopolymers present in the tooth are the polysaccharides that also compose the ECM. These structures are carbohydrate molecules composed of long chains of monosaccharide units bound by glycosidic bonds that are present in dental tissues mostly in the form of proteoglycans and glycosaminoglycans [1, 6].

Given that the structural building blocks of the tooth are essentially composed of polymeric constituents, it is no surprise that the progress of dentistry and dental biomaterials would seek to approximate the polymeric composition of the natural tooth [7]. Interestingly, however, it was not until the mid 1900s that polymeric materials emerged as an alternative material for dental applications [8].

The origins of dental sciences date back to approximately 500 year before Christ, when reports suggest that Hippocrates and Aristotle studied patterns of tooth eruption, dental extractions techniques and methods for stabilization of loose teeth using metallic wires [8]. Ever since the description of these procedures by antique societies, metals have formed the basis for the majority of dental treatments. Thus, it may be argued that, for a long time, metals formed the basis for clinical dentistry. The ability of polymers to provide excellent aesthetic quality, easy manipulation, tunable physical properties, amongst other advantages, has arguably allowed the greatest transition in dental sciences. In 1949, Hagger developed the first type of polymeric restorative system in an attempt to bond acrylic resin to dentin [9]. This, followed by a wide range of studies on dental polymers, particularly the ones pioneered by Buonocore et al. in 1955, which represented the greatest shift in dental materials development and applications to date. Ever since it was demonstrated that polymeric dental materials had sufficient biocompatibility for direct restorations, the focus of dental materials development shifted from metals to polymers, a trend that has remained virtually untouched since the mid 1900s.

Nowadays, polymers are largely used for restorative applications as a treatment for decayed teeth, as materials for prosthetic applications in the fabrication of partial and complete dentures, in different laboratorial methods for molding and modeling, and more recently for controlled remineralization of teeth and tissue engineering, amongst other applications. In this chapter, we will discuss the applications of polymers in the wide field of clinical dentistry, with particular emphasis in restorative procedures and emerging 'smart' polymeric materials with potential dental applications.

Polymers in Dental Adhesion

Composition and Classification of Dental Adhesives

Adhesion of restorative dental biomaterials to tooth substrates is primarily based on micromechanical interlocking of resin monomers to the components of the hard tissue. In addition to micromechanical retention, chemical bonding can be achieved via functional monomers, which are able to chemically and mechanically bond to the tooth [10, 11]. While commonly classified as generations by industry, the most appropriate way to classify the current adhesive systems is by the dentin surface treatment and application techniques. The application techniques recommended by manufacturers is greatly influenced by the composition of the adhesive polymer [12]. A summary of the current adhesive systems is shown in Table 9.1.

Table 9.1 Contemporary dental adhesive systems and their composition

Clinical steps	Etching	Primer	Resin
Etch-and-rinse (3-steps)	Phosphoric acid (30–35 %)	HEMA, organic solvent (ethanol/acetone/water), proprietary monomers	Hydrophilic and hydrophobic monomers (HEMA, TEGDMA, Bis-GMA, UDMA), initiators
Etch and rinse (2-step)	Phosphoric acid (30–35 %)	Hydrophilic and Hydrophobic monomers (HEMA, TEGDMA, Bis-GMA, UDMA, proprietary monomers), organic solvent (ethanol/acetone/water), fillers, initiators	
Self-etching (2-step)	Functional and hydrophillic acidic monomers (Phenyl-P, 4-MET, 10-MDP, MDPB and HEMA), initiator, solvents and water		Functional, hydrophilic and hydrophobic monomers (Bis-GMA, TEGDMA), initiator
Self etching (1-step)	Functional, hydrophilic acidic and hydrophobic monomers (4 META, Phenyl-P, 10-MDP, HEMA, Bis-GMA, UDMA), initiators, solvents and water		
Universal	Optional Phosphoric acid (30–35 %)	Functional, hydrophilic and hydrophobic monomers(10-MDP, HEMA, Bis-GMA, TEGDMA), proprietary monomers, solvent, initiator	

The basic components of a dental bonding system include a primer, the adhesive resin, an organic solvent and polymerization initiators. Primers contain *hydrophilic* blends of resin monomers/co-monomers. Adhesive resins contain blends of *hydrophobic* monomers/co-monomers. Solvents are added to the systems to enhance resin infiltration into the tissue, whereas photoinitiators are commonly used for convenient operator-controlled photopolymerization of the adhesive. Other ingredients such as fluoride, glutaraldehyde, antimicrobials are also commonly added to the mixture in an attempt to further protect or strengthen the adhesive interface.

The adhesion mechanism is tissue-dependent; in general bonds with greater clinical durability are achieved on enamel surfaces when compared to dentin. The surface treatment, adhesive chemistry, application protocol and different forms of enamel and dentin are also determinant factors in the adhesion process. The main mechanism of bonding to sound enamel is the formation of resin microtags following infiltration of resin monomers into a superficially decalcified microstructured prismatic layer. In dentin, resin tags can also be formed and it is estimated that 60–80 % of the bond strength to dentin is provided by the formation of the hybrid layer, which is the impregnation of the collagen network with the adhesive resin (further details below). The complexity in composition and structure of dentin is a major obstacle for proper interfacial sealing and high bond strength overtime. A proof to the importance of the hybrid layer was poor success rate of earlier dental adhesive systems that did not bond to dentin. Due to the importance of dentin to the extended service-life of a restoration, novel materials have been developed based on high affinity for the dentin structure components. The process of hybrid layer formation is described below.

The Process of Hybrid Layer Formation

In order to properly bond to dentin, resin monomers must interact with the dentin matrix. The term hybrid layer is used to describe the physical interaction between the resin and the demineralized dentin. Adhesion in dentin is mainly obtained by micromechanical inter-locking of cured resins and the exposed dentin collagen network. Earlier adhesive systems provided the foundation for the development of a hybrid layer in dentin. These systems called "etch-and-rinse" remove smear layer—a surface layer composed of organic and inorganic debris resulting from the drilling process—smear plugs and superficially decalcify the dentin with a separate application step of acidic etchant—generally phosphoric acid. Microscopically, a clean surface with the exposed collagen fibrils is apparent and ready for the priming step with hydrophilic-based monomers and subsequent coating with hydrophobic blends of resin monomers. Following resin polymerization, the infiltrated resin will be anchored onto the exposed dentin matrix. This complex process takes place very quickly, usually between 30–90 s.

The primer is constituted of a blend of organic solvents and hydrophilic monomers to enable proper resin infiltration. Following the priming step, a more hydrophobic adhesive layer is applied acting as a barrier for the outward water movement from the dentin tubules, also providing the necessary hydrophobicity to chemically bond the adhesive material with the resin composite, which will make up the bulk of the dental restoration. Because of the presence of water and organic components, the technique is highly sensitive. The surface of dentin must remain hydrated prior to the application of the primer to avoid collapse of the collagen exposed during decalcification. The technique was developed in the early 90s and is called *wet bonding technique*. Overwetting and overdrying the dentin will result in a significant decrease in the bond strength. The later generation of etch-and-rinse system simplified the technique by applying the primer/adhesive at the same time (Table 9.1).

Self-etching systems also have the ability to form hybrid layers however in a limited manner and non-uniform fashion. A thinner hybrid layer is also observed when functional acidic monomers are used to demineralize and simultaneously infiltrate the dentin matrix. The functional monomers in the adhesive blends are ionized in water and etch the dentin surface while penetrating within the collagen framework [12]. The adhesive system is further polymerized in both techniques, resulting in mechanical interlocking with the dentin matrix. Hydrophilic monomers are preferable for penetrating within the dentin matrix after demineralization. However the excess water may result in separation of the hydrophilic and hydrophobic components of the adhesive system, decreasing the mechanical properties of the resin-dentin interface [13]. Good penetration of the adhesive system enveloping the exposed collagen fibrils is important for the success of the hybridization process.

Adhesive Interface Degradation

The hybrid layer is believed to be essential for maintaining the integrity of the resin-dentin bonded interface. The complete replacement of mineral by resin monomers during infiltration is unlikely even with the use of low viscosity hydrophilic monomers and organic solvents [12]. The infiltration of adhesive into demineralized dentin is influenced by the diffusion ability of the resin monomers plus organic solvents within the dentin matrix. Complete enveloping of the dentin matrix is likely not to occur by passive infiltration of the resin monomers due to the size of the molecules and the available spaces within the collagen molecules [1, 14]. The incomplete resin infiltration affects the stability of the interface by establishing pathways for fluid penetration accelerating hydrolytic and enzymatic degradations.

In addition to the hybrid layer, critical components of the adhesive interface are the underlying dentin and the adhesive layer itself (Fig. 9.1). The biomechanical properties of these 3 components are distinct and their integrity overtime also

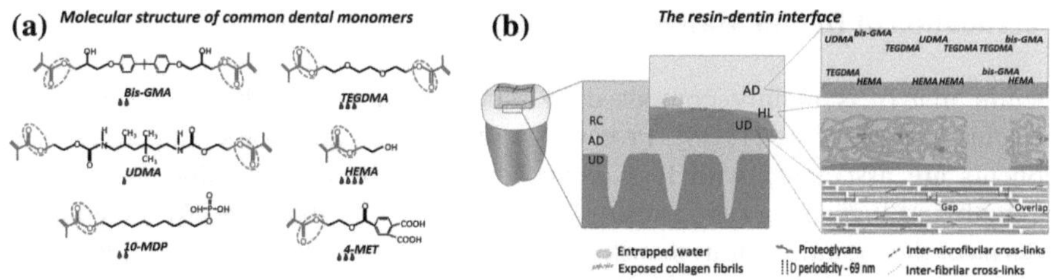

Fig. 9.1 **a** Typical monomer molecules used in dental adhesive systems. **b** Schematic of the resin dentin interface

plays an important role in the service-life of dental restorations. Hydrolytic and enzymatic degradation mechanisms are believed to be major players in the degradation of the interface components. The processes can be accelerated by the chemical, mechanical stresses in the oral environment. Some of the well-established mechanisms of interfacial degradation are described below in detail.

Degradation of Resin at the Interface

The hydrolysis of monomers and breakdown of polymeric chains of methacrylate-based resins are associated with adhesive degradation. After polymerization the adhesive resins absorb water by diffusion through poorly polymerized chains and hydrophilic domains [15–17]. The distance between polymers tends to increase, allowing water to stay entrapped between the polymeric networks, decreasing the mechanical properties of the polymer [16, 18]. The decrease in the modulus of elasticity of the polymer, will allow for polymer chain movement, facilitating the swelling of unreacted monomers [19]. Water can break the ester bonds in methacrylate monomers. In addition to hydrolysis, degradation of 2,2-bis[4-(2-hydroxy-3-methacryloxypropoxy)phenyl]propane (Bis-GMA), by salivary and bacterial esterases has been reported [20, 21]. Hydrophilic monomers are used as priming agents to facilitate the diffusion of resin into the collagen rich layer in dentin. However, hydrophilic monomers such as HEMA (Hydroxyethyl Methacrylate) and diluent monomers with ethylene glycol group (i.e. TEGDMA—triethyleneglycol-dimethacrylate) greatly increase the water sorption of adhesives [22].

The clinical technique can also affect the performance of dental adhesive systems. Significant reduction in the degree of conversion and mechanical properties of adhesive systems was observed when solvents were not properly evaporated [23–26]. The application of simplified-step adhesive systems to an excessively wet dentin surface may lead to phase separation and a hydrophobic-poor and hydrophilic-rich zone may be formed, lowering the stability of the adhesive interface [13]. Acidic monomers remain active when poorly polymerized resulting in continuous etching of the underlying dentin [27].

Degradation of Dentin Matrix at the Interface

Dentin matrix is mainly composed of type I collagen fibrils, non-collagenous proteins and enzymes [1, 28]. Proteolysis of collagen and non-collagenous components are associated with loss of anchorage to the dentin reducing the bond strength and increasing permeability at the resin-dentin interface. At the adhesive interface, the organic dentin matrix can either be left exposed by incomplete resin infiltration or become exposed following degradation of adhesive components. The exposed collagen is vulnerable to hydrolytic and proteolytic degradation. Collagen degradation at the interface has been linked to host-derived enzymes that are commonly latent in fully mineralized dentin [29, 30]. More specifically, the degradation process takes place by activation of host-derived matrix metalloproteinases (MMPs) and cysteine cathepsins [31]. The MMPs are zinc and calcium-dependent proteolytic enzymes capable of degrading the organic network. Collagenolytic (MMP-1, -8 and -13) and gelatinolytic (MMP-2) enzymes, can cleave the collagen triple-helical molecule in ¼ and ¾ fragments. The denatured fragments can be further degraded by gelatinases and other non-specific tissue proteinases.

Proteoglycans (PGs), which represent about 3 % (w/v) of the organic composition of dentin, are organic structures strongly bound to collagen which play important roles on the structure and biomechanics of the matrix. The most prevalent PGs in dentin, decorin and biglycan, contain either one (decorin) or two (byglycan) glycosaminoglycan (GAG) chains attached to a core protein. In mature dentin, negatively charged GAGs provide tissue hydration and organization by interconnecting adjacent fibrils. Selective removal of GAGs and PGs results in decreased mechanical properties of mineralized dentin and also significantly affects the resin-dentin bond strength. Decrease in the resin-dentin bond strength of PGs-depleted dentin matrix has been reported following a re-wetting restorative technique [32]. Resin infiltration is compromised due to the inability of PGs- and GAGs- depleted dentin matrix to re-expand following surface desiccation. Reports have also shown that under hydrated condition, enzymatic removal of PGs may result in better diffusion of monomers into the dentin tubules [33], as PGs control diffusion through the matrix and water displacement. The function of PGs on mature dentin deserves more attention.

Emerging Concepts and Future Prospects for Polymers in Dental Adhesion

It is estimated that resin composite restorations have a service life of 6–7 years, which is far less than half of the service life of dental amalgam. The main reason for replacement of direct adhesive resin composite restorations is secondary caries. Therefore failures at the interface has, to a great extent, inspired development of novel strategies to reduce degradation of the resin-tooth interface. Limitations within the material and intrinsic properties of the dentin have sparked a need to acknowledge the biology nature of the tissue as well as new directions in the resin chemistry that has been used in dental adhesive systems for the past 40 years. Some of the emerging and future concepts are detailed in the two sub-items below.

Material Perspective

Poor degree of conversion of dental resin monomers, elution of un-polymerized monomers and degradation of polymeric chains by enzymatic and hydrolytic challenges, have all been associated with the low stability of the resin at the bonded interface. Novel approaches have focused on improving the adhesion to the dental tissue as well as increasing stability of the resin and resin-dentin interface.

Resin monomers promoting chemical bond to enamel and dentin have been added to many contemporary adhesive systems in an attempt to achieve high bond strength via chemical bonding to the inorganic component of the tissue [34]. Specifically, formation of ionic bonds between 10-methacryloyloxydecyl dihydrogen phosphate monomer (10-MDP) and tissue hydroxyapatite crystals resulting in stable Ca-MDP salts [11]. Other functional monomers are also capable of chemical interaction with the tooth inorganic content. The functional monomers 4-methacryloxyethyl trimellitic acid (4-MET) and 2-methacryloxyethyl phenyl hydrogen phosphate (Phenyl-P) can also interact with hydroxyapatite crystal; however a more stable reaction is observed for Ca-MDP resulting salts [10, 11].

Aiming at establishing a polymeric chain that is less susceptible to degradation, a new class of monomers has been proposed. Silorane-based materials have an oxirane ring-opening mechanism of polymerization which is proposed to reduce polymerization shrinkage. In addition, siloxane molecules are more hydrophobic than methacrylate monomers, which may improve silorane resins` resistance to hydrolysis. However, the mechanical performance of silorane resins are not as predictable as compared to methacrylate resins [35], which may limits its application to areas of non-critical stresses. The substitution of TEGDMA by thiol-ene systems has been studied. Thiol-enes alone may not attain as good mechanical properties as methacrylate resins, but in association, the mechanical properties were equivalent. The methacrylate-thiol-ene resin systems showed increased methacrylate functional group conversion and decreased volumetric shrinkage [36, 37] and are promising alternative dental restorative materials.

Additional improvements on the degree of conversion of the adhesive systems were observed with new and less hydrophobic initiators of polymerization. Camphorquinone and aromatic amines are the most commonly used photoinitiator systems for light-activated dental resins, but they can be excessively hydrophobic making it difficult to activate the more hydrophilic monomers at the adhesive systems. The addition of alternative initiators such as 1-phenyl-1,2-propanedione (PPD), 2,4,6-trimethylbenzoyl-diphenylphosphine oxide (Lucerin-TPO) and bisacylphosphine oxide (BAPO) improve resin polymerization within hydrophilic domains and reduce susceptibility to inactivation by acidic adhesive monomer in self-etching systems. The use of diphenyliodonium hexafluorophosphate (DPIHP) in Bis-GMA and HEMA based experimental adhesives accelerates the resin polymerization and improve the mechanical properties [38].

Biological approaches to reduce degradation of the organic matrix resulted on the investigation of functional monomers to inhibit collagenolytic enzymes. An example is the incorporation of 12-methacryloyloxydodecylpyridinium bromide (MDPB), a polymerizable quaternary ammonium methacrylate [39], into self-etching resin adhesive blends. As for total-etch adhesive systems, an enzyme inhibitory effect can be achieved by adding a quaternary ammonium group, the benzalkonium chloride (BAC), to the etching solution. Studies using experimental materials showed possible incorporating MMP inhibitors in the methacrylate resin composition, aiming to a slow and continuous release of the inhibitors within the adhesive interface.

Tissue Perspective

As a major component of the bonded interface, the dental tissue components have a dramatic effect of the stability of resin-tooth interface. While there is still much to learn about the composition and role of organic components in different forms of dentin and enamel, there is a consensus that the stability of the dentin matrix remains key to the long-term strength and permeability of the interface.

The application of enzyme inhibitors to prevent dentin matrix degradation has been extensively investigated and few materials are already available to allow dental practitioners to rinse the surface with agents such as chlorhexidine (CHX). CHX is a potent antimicrobial agent and it can inhibit MMP-2, -9 and -8 by binding to the enzyme's active sites. Similarly, it interacts with cysteine cathepsins, likely by interacting with the S2 subsites [40, 41]. It has been suggested that low concentrations of CHX (0.05–0.2 %) can inhibit the collagenolytic activity of dentin matrix, however the relative low substantivity of priming solutions may limit the long-term protective effect. Among other synthetic MMP inhibitors are the modified tetracycline. Special attention has been given to Galardin, a hydroxamate-based bisphosphonate, which inhibits MMPs by chelating its zinc active sites [31, 42]. This potential effect against MMP-1, -2, -3, -8 and -9 may reduce the bond strength loss overtime when compared to CHX. Because the inhibitory effect is mainly due to competitive binding of the inhibitory solutions with specific sites, the effectiveness is concentration dependent.

Remineralization of unprotected collagen at the dentin-resin interface has been proposed to preserve the adhesive bond strengths overtime. The biomimetic remineralization strategy is based on the use of polyanionic molecules such as polycarboxylic and polyphosphonic acids, which will be explained with greater detail below. The molecules mimic the mineral nucleation and growth control functions of endogenous non-collagenous proteins bound to collagen. In vitro intra-fibrillar and extra-fibrillar mineralization has been reported at the adhesive interfaces in presence of Portland cement (tricalcium silicate, dicalcium silicate, tricalcium aluminate, and a tetra-calcium aluminoferrite) mineralized using the biomimetic mineralization approach.

Another innovative approach is the biomodification of dentin matrix by multi-functional agents that increase the biomechanical properties and reduce the biodegradation rates of the dentin matrix [43]. Enhanced mechanical properties of biomodified dentin matrices are a result of the presence of non-enzymatic collagen cross-links induced by synthetic and nature-derived agents. These agents are also potent enzyme inhibitors and greatly decrease biodegradation of dentin in presence of host-derived enzymes as well as bacterial collagenase. Plant-derived oligomeric proanthocyanidins (OPACs), in particular, strongly interact with dentin collagen and also non-collagenous components such as PGs and endogenous proteases. Glutaraldehyde is another effective synthetic agent for collagen crosslinking, however due to its toxicity its clinical use is limited. 1-ethyl-3-[3-dimethylaminopropyl] carbodiimide hydrochloride associated with n-hydroxysuccinimide (EDC/NHS) has received much attention as a synthetic option with lower toxicity when compared to glutaraldehyde. Priming dentin with EDC/NHS shows increased long-term stability of the resin-bonded interfaces [44]. Riboflavin [45] has also been studied for this purpose, but the use of UV light may limit its use in clinical setting. Strategies to incorporate most of these agents into the restorative systems are ongoing.

Polymers in Restorative Composites Resins

First introduced over 50 years ago, polymer-based dental materials revolutionized restorative Dentistry primarily due to their outstanding esthetic and adhesive properties. These characteristics have allowed for substantially improved preservation of healthy tooth structures, prevention of postoperative sensitivity, reduction of microleakage, among other advantages compared to dental amalgams.

Over the years, resin based restorative materials have been the focus of a great deal of research, being drastically improved by manufactures, particularly with respect to aesthetic quality and mechanical behavior. Despite great improvements, failure and replacement of dental composite restorations continue to have great impact on clinical outcomes [46]. For instance, restorative composites still present a number of drawbacks, like wear, lack of a consistent degree of conversion, fracture and secondary caries [47, 48].

There have been several attempts to improve clinical performance of composite restorative materials by incorporating novel multifunctional monomers, developing different polymerization strategies or modifying filler components of the formulation. The following sections will explore some of the recent developments in restorative polymer composites.

Composition and Classification of Composite Resins

Composites used in Dentistry were developed in 1962 by combining dimethacrylates (epoxy resin and methacrylic acid) with silanized quartz powder [49]. Modern restorative composites are comprised of synthetic monomers, typically dimethacrylates, reinforcing fillers, typically made from radiopaque glass, quartz or silica, chemicals which promote or modify the polymerization reaction, and silane coupling agents which bond the reinforcing fillers to the polymer matrix [26].

The resin matrix of commercial dental composites has bis-GMA (bisphenol-A-glycidyldimethacrylate) as its predominant base monomer. Due to its high viscosity, bis-GMA is mixed with other dimethacrylates, such as TEGDMA, UDMA or other monomers of lower molecular weight [26, 50] to reduce viscosity. The monomers are heavily reinforced with filler particles, which add dimensional stability, improve wear and strength of the material, also reducing polymerization shrinkage [51].

A number of classification systems have been proposed to describe restorative composites. These materials may be distinguished by their consistency, and classified as flowable, conventional and packable [26]; but the most used classification system is based upon filler particle size. As restorative composites have evolved, the size of filler particles and their size distribution have been changed in an attempt to achieve the best possible mechanical properties while maintaining esthetics.

Initial formulations of dental composites (also known as *macrofill*) had average particle-sizes ranging from 10 to 50 μm. Clinically they were very resistant, but difficult to polish, also retaining poor surface smoothness overtime. *Microfill* composites generally present a wide range of size-distribution of silica particles (40–400 nm). At this size, filler loading represents a challenge for manufacturing composites with higher filler content due to agglomeration of the small particles in the matrix. These characteristics render microfilled composites highly polishable, but generally weak due to their relatively lower filler content and particle size.

One of most recent innovations in composite resins has been the development of *nanofil* composites, containing nanoscale particles ranging from 1 to 100 nm with a more homogenous size distribution. The increased filler content results in a lower amount of resin, which may significantly reduce polymerization shrinkage and improve the physical performance of nanocomposites [52]. Further details on the advantages of nanocomposites are presented in Sect. "Nanocomposites".

The majority of resin composites in clinical use today are categorized in the general term of *hybrid or micro-hybrid composites* [41]. This broad category includes traditional hybrids, midifill, and minifill composites. The "hybrid" denomination implies a resin composite containing submicron inorganic filler particles and fine (over one micron) particles. Traditional hybrid resins consisted of a combination of 10–50 μm filler particles with amorphous spherical silica reinforcing particles of 40 nm. Midifill composites contain average particle sizes slightly greater than 1 μm, but also containing 40 nm-sized fumed silica microfillers. Minifill (also referred as mycrohybrid) materials present refinements in particle size, which generated restorative composites with sub-micron particles averaging from 0.4 to 1 μm.

Most manufacturers have modified the formulation of their mycrohybrids to include more nanoparticles, and have named this category as nanohybrids [26]. The combination of various sizes of filler particles corresponds to an improvement in physical properties as well as acceptable levels of polishability [53].

Emerging Classes of Composite Resins

Anti-caries and Ion-Releasing Polymers

Due to the high frequency of recurrent caries after restorative treatments, much attention has been given to the therapeutic effects manifested by direct restorative materials. Restorative composites have demonstrated to accumulate more biofilm over time, when compared to enamel and other restorative materials, thus favoring the development of recurrent caries around these restorations [54]. Therefore, in an attempt to control or even prevent secondary caries, alternative clinical methods for caries prevention have been proposed including the search for new restorative materials with antibacterial activity.

Great emphasis has been given to the development of fluoride releasing materials, however, the direct antibacterial effect of dental materials is another important property as the inactivation of bacteria is a direct way to eradicate the cause of dental caries. Many attempts for developing dentin-bonding systems and restorative materials presenting antibacterial activity have been performed [55–62].

In the pursuit of developing composites with antibacterial activity, alterations to the resin matrix and filler components have been performed. Alterations of resin matrix constituents have included two relevant methods: firstly, the addition of soluble and immobilized antimicrobial agents in the resin matrix; secondly, the alteration of the filler components by addition of silver. Similarly, the immobilization of an antibacterial agent in a prepolymerized resin filler (PPRF) utilizing an antibacterial monomer has been previously reported [63].

Polymers with Soluble Antimicrobial Agents

The antibacterial effects of the restorative composites are relevant primarily in inhibiting plaque accumulation on the surfaces of the restorative material and tooth structures surrounding the restoration. Soluble antimicrobial agents added to the resin matrix, when exposed to a wet environment, have a tendency to be released from the restorative material, thus preventing plaque accumulation. Commonly, large amounts of these agents are released within a few days, followed by a dramatic decrease in concentration.

Chlorexidine has been the most frequently antibacterial agent incorporated into the resin matrix, and has demonstrated a strong antibacterial activity due to the release of antibacterial agents [64]. However, while a strong effect against bacteria has been obtained, the antibacterial activity drastically decreases over time, since large amounts of the agent are leached out within a few days [65]. Furthermore, it has been reported that the addition of chlorhexidine gluconate at a concentration of as low as 1 % resulted in significant a reduction of tensile and compressive strengths of restorative composite resins strengths [35].

Soluble fluoride agents have also been used to modify the resin matrix and obtain antibacterial properties in resin composites. Fluoride levels leached from composites are mostly much lower compared to levels released from conventional or resin-modified glass-ionomers [66]. Fluoride releasing resin composites might contribute to the decrease in cariogenic composition of dental biofilms if an appropriate amount of fluoride is released in the early stages of biofilm formation [67], yet challenges in developing composites with a sustained fluoride release remain.

Polymers with Immobilized Antimicrobial Agents

The immobilization of antibacterial components in the resin matrix has been another attempt to modify resin components to render restorative materials caries-resistant. This approach is used to obtain antibacterial composites that do not release any antibacterial component. Rather, the immobilized agent acts as a contact inhibitor against bacteria attaching the material surface [32].

To that end, quaternary ammonium dimethacrylate monomers, such as 12-methacryloyloxydodecylpyridinium bromide (MDPB), were copolymerized with resins to yield antibacterial activity. MDPB was developed by combining a quaternary ammonium—which presents a wide spectrum of antibacterial activity—and a methacryloyl group, incorporated into the composite matrix. This agent copolymerizes with other monomers in the composite and thus, the antibacterial component is covalently linked to the polymeric network [32]. The immobilized agent does not leach out of the composite but functions as a contact inhibitor against bacteria attaching to the surface, therefore its effect is not able to reach the tooth structures surrounding the restoration [68]. In summary, the effects of the MDPB-containing composites are not so intensive as the materials that release antibacterial agents. Its effect is mainly bacteriostatic, as the agent cannot penetrate through the cell wall or membrane unlike free antibacterial agents described above [32].

In order to improve the antibacterial activity of these systems, the addition of antibacterial monomers in prepolymerized resin fillers (PPRF) have also been reported. Using this method, the PPRF can be highly cured and washed before they are loaded into the composite, thus ensuring greater immobilization of the antibacterial components than when the antibacterial agent is added to the monomer phase. In an attempt to increase the concentration of MDPB in resin composites, the antibacterial monomer was utilized as a PPRF. The incorporation of MDPB to the composite as a PPRF, for instance, has been shown to allow for an increase of MDPB concentration in the order of 10 times, thus promoting more reliable inhibitory effects on plaque accumulation [69]. An experimental composite prepared by the addition of PPRF-MDPB to a commercially available composite demonstrated to inhibit the progression of artificially induced secondary root caries lesions regardless of adhesive system [70]. The satisfactory results found with MDPB led to the incorporation of quaternary ammonium compounds (QAS) into restorative composites. In recent years, many attempts to incorporate QAS into polymer based restorative materials have been performed, demonstrating good results in antibacterial activity [13, 19, 71, 72]. Therefore, it may be expected that future composites will present relevant antibacterial properties and that this will be a subject of intensive research in future years.

Antimicrobial Fillers

Similar to the modifications described above, alterations to the filler components have been conducted in order to achieve antibacterial composites. Numerous studies have evaluated composites modified by silver-functionalized filler particles. For dental composites, in particular, the use of silver-zeolite, silver-apatite, and silver-supported zirconium phosphate has been reported [46]. Silver-zeolite and silver-apatite show antibacterial effects which are dependent upon the slow release of silver ions, and these effects are expected to last for longer periods of time when compared to materials with embedded antibacterial components. Composites containing silver nanoparticles have demonstrated inhibited biofilm formation and reduction of biofilm viability [73]. However, poor color stability is a common problem for these types of restorative composites.

Low-Shrinkage Composite Resins

Ring-Opening Monomers

One of the main drawbacks in dental composites remains the high polymerization shrinkage of these materials. It is well recognized that the polymerization stresses resulting from polymerization shrinkage of composite restorations can lead to numerous adverse clinical effects, including de-bonding, post-operative sensitivity, marginal discrepancies, among other clinically relevant issues [26]. The extent of shrinkage is generally influenced by the volume of resin, its composition, and the degree of conversion of the cured monomers [41]. Current commercial dental composites have a volumetric shrinkage ranging from 1.6 to 8 vol % [74]. Therefore, the development of non- or minimal-shrinkage dental composites has been the focus of extensive research. Investigators have made several attempts to reduce shrinkage by introducing monomer molecules that present different polymerization strategies to more common linear chain lengthening, such ring-opening monomers like spiro-orthocarbonates [75], epoxy-base resins like the siloranes [76], as well as high-molecular-weight monomers like dimer acid-based dimethacrylates [77], tricyclodecane (TCD) urethane and organically-modified ceramics (ormocers) [78, 79]. Low shrinkage oxiranes, for instance, are cyclic ethers that polymerize through a cationic ring-opening mechanism, in contrast to the free radical polymerization of methacrylates [54, 80]. Oxirane based-resins have shown many advantageous properties, such as improved depth of cure, lower polymerization shrinkage, higher strength, as well as comparable hardness and acceptable glass transition temperature when compared with conventional bis-GMA-based dental composites [81]. However, residual monomers released from oxirane-based composites after polymerization have shown relevant toxicity [82].

With the similar objective of introducing ring-opening monomers into restorative composites, Weinmann et al. [54] described the synthesis of a new monomer system, a 'silorane' which is an epoxy functionalized cyclic siloxane whose name is derived from the combination of its chemical building blocks *silo*xanes and oxi*ranes*. Siloranes were found to be stable and insoluble in biological fluids [24], while showing a much lower mutagenic potential than those of related oxiranes [83]. Silorane's network is generated by the cationic ring-opening polymerization of the cycloaliphatic oxirane moieties. In these systems, polymerization starts with an acidic cation that opens the oxirane ring and generates a new acidic center, a carbocation [16]. After the addition to an oxirane monomer, the epoxy ring is opened to form a chain or, in the case of two- or more multifunctional monomers, a network. The opening of the oxirane rings during the polymerisation process compensates to some degree for the polymerisation shrinkage [61].

The oxirane rings are responsible for the physical properties and the low shrinkage, while the hydrophobic properties of the material are related to the siloxanes [61]. As a consequence, exogenous discolouration and water absorption are reduced. All these reported advantageous characteristics serve to enhance the potential of silorane monomers to be used successfully in dental composite materials. Weinmann et al. [54] observed a low shrinkage rate (<1 %) and seven times more light stability for the silorane in comparison with resin-based methacrylates. The clinical application of siloranes is limited to the posterior teeth because only a few low translucent colours are available. Additionally, due to its hydrophobic properties, a special adhesive system must be used for silorane restorations.

Stress Decreasing Resin (SDR) Technology

Slowing down the polymerization rate is another mechanism that has been utilized to compensate for stresses generated upon polymerization in resin-based composites. These mechanisms increase the material flow capacity, lower stress build-up and thus promote improved interfacial integrity [84]. A recently introduced flowable resin-based composite material, intended to be used as a liner in occlusal and posterior proximal restorations, differs from conventional resin by incorporating a Stress Decreasing Resin (SDR) technology. This material provides an approximate 20 % reduction in volumetric shrinkage and almost an 80 % reduction in polymerization stress compared to a traditional resin system due to the addition of a urethane dimethacrylate structure. This is due in part to the larger size of the SDR resin compared to conventional resin systems (molecular weight of 849 g/mol for SDR resin compared to 513 g/mol for Bis-GMA). The SDR Technology comprises the unique combination of such a large molecular structure with a chemical moiety called a Polymerization Modulator, chemically embedded in the center of the polymerizable resin backbone of the SDR resin monomer [85].

Emerging Classes of Low-Shrinkage Composites

Silsesquioxane (SSQ), an organosilicon compound forming a cage structure, have been studied and present great potential for low-shrinkage nanocomposites. The hardness and modulus of nanocomposites with different percentages of SSQ have been shown to decrease when increased amounts of SSQ monomers were added. Authors have interpreted that the incorporation of SSQ monomers helps to reduce both rigidity and polymerization shrinkage [86]. Therefore, in the correct formulation, SSQ materials have great potential to be used as low-shrinkage composites.

Lee and Rhee [87] developed a bioactive poly(methyl methacrylate)/SiO_2-CaO nanocomposite using either dimethyl-diethoxysilane (DMDES) or tetraethoxysilane (TEOS), which could create 2 and 4 siloxane linkages, respectively, after a sol-gel reaction. According to the authors, this nanocomposite can be applied as filler materials for bone cement as well as dental composite resin, because of its good bioactivity and improved mechanical properties. Chen et al. [88] also developed a low-shrinkage, high-strength nanocomposite by using a 4-epoxycyclohexylmethyl-(3, 4-epoxy) cyclohexane carboxylate (ERL4221) matrix with 55 % of 70- to 100-nm nanosilica fillers through ring-opening polymerization. The nanocomposite was shown to exhibit low polymerization shrinkage strain and a low thermal expansion coefficient comparable with that of the methacrylate-based composites. Other type of resin matrix includes photocurable epoxy-polyols, which were shown to have significant advantages over dimethacrylates, including lower polymer shrinkage, no oxygen inhibition layer, higher strength, and equivalent hardness, as well as acceptable glass transition temperatures [89].

Nanocomposites

Nanotechnology or nanoscience is the field that studies the manipulation of structures on the atomic and molecular scales, and where the dimensions of the resulting supra-atomic and supramolecular structures fall under 100 nm. The National Nanotechnology Initiative defines nanotechnology as the creation of functional materials with characteristic dimensions in the range of 0.1–100 nm. When inorganic phases in an organic/inorganic composite become nanosized, they are called nanocomposites.

The relevance of nanotechnology in Dentistry, as exemplified by the widespread use of nanoparticles in dental composites, is not new [90]. Colloidal silica particles of a diameter of approximately 40 nm have been in use in dental micro-filled and hybrid composites for more than 10 years [91]. Currently, dental nanocomposites are composed of a blend of nanofillers distributed in a dispersed form or as clusters. Nanomers are monodispersed, non-agglomerated, and non-aggregated silica particles of 20 and 75 nm in diameter. Nanocluster fillers are loosely bound agglomerates of nanosized particles that maintain the morphology and properties of individual particles [16].

Nanofillers are usually invisible and offer many advantages to dental composites, such as optical property improvement [92], increase of the overall filler content to as high as 90–95 % of the composite by weight, and reduction of polymerization shrinkage due to a lower amount of the monomeric phase [16].

Nanofillers and nanoclusters enhance the long-term mechanical stability and polishing properties of micro-filled composites [38]. The mechanical stability is achieved in hybrid composites primarily due to larger filler particles in form of "nanoclusters". Wear in composite resins have typically been linked to an increase in surface roughness resulting from removal of resin while filler particle become more exposed to the surface of the restoration, or when filler particles are lost due to abrasion. Contrarily, in nanocomposites, nanoclusters are broken down into individual nanoparticles, and since these particles are smaller than the wavelengths of visible light, roughness is not significantly increased. It has been shown that surface polish of nanocomposites is also preserved for longer periods of time in composites with filler particles of less than 0.4 μm [38].

Although nanocomposites have been marketed as materials presenting superior mechanical performance, in some cases the wear and fatigue properties of composites containing nanoparticles were similar or worse than microfilled composites [4]. Additional studies, nevertheless, report that dental nanocomposites present high translucency, high polish and polish retention similar to those of microfilled composites, while maintaining physical properties and wear resistance equivalent to those of several hybrid composites [5].

Polymers for Denture Base Materials

For a long time, denture base systems relied completely on the use of metallic materials. The first non-metallic denture base material, Vulcanite, was introduced in the 1850s, and served as a denture base system for almost 100 years, when it was then replaced by poly(methyl methacrylate) (PMMA). Although PMMA was first developed in 1931 [93], the first commercially available product was not manufactured until 1935. PMMA for denture base resins is usually marketed as pre-polymerized beads of 35–200 μm in diameter, and cured via emulsion polymerization, whereby the methyl methacrylate (MMA) monomer, supplied as a liquid, is mixed with powder forming a dough upon initiation of curing, which will proceed via addition polymerization; as reinforcements, small proportions of other alkyl methacrylates (ethyl or butyl) may be added to copolymerize with MMA. Other modifications to increase solubility and improve viscosity may be performed by adding small quantities (<5 %) of ethyl acrylate, whereas the most frequently used initiator is benzoyl peroxide (0.5–1.5 %). As the pure MMA is clear, addition of pigments to obtain the various tissue-like shades is also often preformed. Pigments are compounds such as mercuric sulfide, ferric oxide or carbon black. Similarly, opacifiers like zinc or titanium oxides as well as titanium dioxide are typically added to enhance pigmentation and improve aesthetics of denture base materials. Moreover, dyed nylon or acrylic fibers simulating blood vessels underlying the mucosa are commonly added to denture base polymer materials. Monomer liquid also contains a small quantity of cross-linking agent such as ethylene glycoldimethacrylate (EGDMA) [94], which is essential to improve hardness and wear resistance.

In addition to meeting the aesthetic requirements for denture base materials, the simple processing technique and relatively low cost of PMMA have been attributed to its widespread use in dentistry [95]. Oral tissues show good tolerance to PMMA. Also PMMA-based acrylic resins present good color stability, excellent polishing ability, and good marginal adaptation. Yet, the major drawbacks of this group of resins include exothermic polymerization, high polymerization shrinkage, low strength and wear resistance, and potential soft tissue irritation associated with excess free monomer [96].

PMMA was not the only type of polymer to be employed as a denture base material. Other synthetic polymers have also been introduced, including bakelite (phenol-formaldehyde) cellulose nitrate, nylon, epoxy resins, vinyl polymers (polyvinyl chloride and polyvinyl acetate) and polystyrene. Polycarbonates infiltrated with glass filler particles have also been used as denture based materials and, due to their filler content, have shown nine times higher impact properties than PMMA. Yet these materials have the disadvantage of more difficult molding than acrylics, since injection molding is required [97, 98].

Although PMMA satisfies the majority of mechanical, biocompatibility and surface criteria along with reasonable cost and ease of fabrication [99], it still presents relative low impact and flexural strengths, thus leading to high incidence of fractures. Further, the relatively rough surface of PMMA surfaces after fabrication encourage microorganism's adhesion to the denture surfaces adjacent to abutment teeth, with a potential negative impact on oral health and hygiene [100].

Recent improvements to the physical and mechanical properties of the polymeric denture base materials have been obtained by incorporating nanoparticles. For instance, it has been reported that the addition of nanometer ZrO_2 particles improves hardness and flexural strength of denture base PMMA resins [101]. Similarly, embedding carbon nanotubes (CNT), which are well known for having superior mechanical properties, has been attempted as an alternative to reinforce denture base acrylic resins. Two recent studies concluded that a remarkable reduction in polymerization shrinkage [102] and improvement in flexural strength [103] can be obtained. However, the interfacial bonding between carbon nanotubes and the resin matrix has been reported to be weak, as well as a additional factor contributing to crack propagation within the polymer structure. More recently, a new class of glass filler microparticles (ultrafine GM35429) (1.5 μm) modified with 2 % F ion and coated with silane has been incorporated into PMMA for denture base applications. This recent study has shown that the fluoride containing microparticles functioned as a fluoride reservoir with relatively controlled F released over time, while improving mechanical properties and inhibiting microbial adhesion [104].

Polymers for Treatment of Dental Caries

Despite extensive progress in the prevention of tooth decay, caries disease continues to be a major challenge in the dental field [1]. In the US alone, dental treatments are responsible for over $100 billion of the total financial burden associated with the health care system in the country [105]. Therefore, new methods for prevention and treatment of caries in enamel and dentin have long been the focus of great attention in caries research. Although polymers have been used to restore decayed teeth since the late 1940s [8], new strategies have emerged recently, both for preventive treatments and to remineralize decalcified dental structures affected by caries.

Caries Infiltration with Low-Viscosity Polymers

Dental caries starts as small lesions on the surface of dental enamel. These lesions initiate and grow due to the acidic microenvironment that is created in the presence of bacteria colonizing the surface of the tooth. The bacteria-derived acids, combined with enzymes, progress to decalcify the highly organized hydroxyapatite crystallites that constitute about 96 % of enamel, and eventually reach the undelaying dentin [106]. Given the non-homogenous pattern of decalcification and constant variations in pH in the mouth, the appearance of these early enamel lesions is opaque, with loss of luster and whitish or yellowish in color—hence their name "white spot lesions" [107]. Microstructurally, early enamel lesions present a thin surface layer of mineral, while the subsurface lesion is much more porous [108, 109] and acts as diffusion pathways for organic acids and minerals.

Commonly, treatments of enamel white spot lesions have either been preventive (noninvasive), with a combination of fluoride-based remineralization [110] and re-adaptation of the patient's diet, or restorative (invasive), where the lesion is drilled and treated with the polymeric restorative materials and strategies described in sections "Polymers in Dental Adhesion" and "Polymers in restorative composites resins". Recently, monomers that are commonly utilized for adhesive restorative treatments, or combinations thereof, were modified to enable impregnation of white spot lesions with photocrosslinkable materials of low viscosity (Fig. 9.3) [111]. The rational behind this strategy stems from the idea that the infiltrant occludes the lesion porosity and blocks further diffusion pathways for cariogenic acids [111]. Moreover, polymeric resins are much more resistant to acid degradation than enamel apatite is resistant to acidic dissolution, hence further cavitation is prevented after infiltration and photopolymerization (Fig. 9.2).

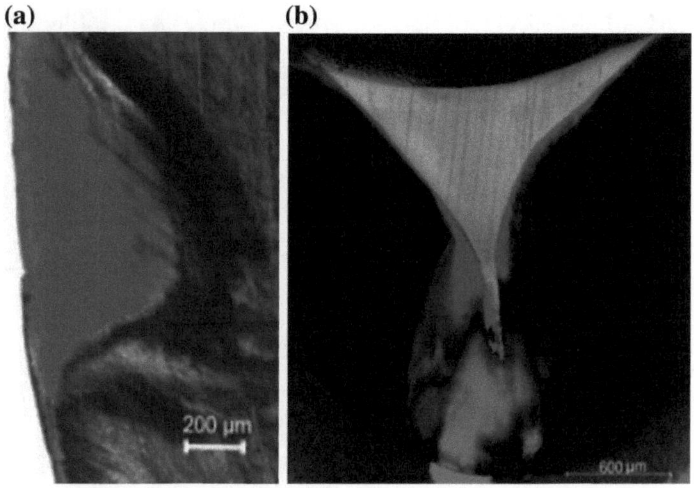

Fig. 9.2 **a** Confocal image of rhodamine-stained enamel proximal lesions treated with resin infiltrant (Icon; DMG). **b** Fissure caries lesions (*green*) infiltrated with resin (*red*) (color figure online). Reproduced with permission from [137] and [138]

Evidently, the ability of polymers to impregnate a porous substrate of intricate microstructural features, such as dental enamel, depends on a series of factors. It has been determined that such interaction may be better described by the Washburn equation [112], which accounts for the penetration of a liquid medium into a porous solid, where the porous solid is assumed to be bundle of open capillaries:

$$d^2 = (\gamma \cos \theta / 2\eta) rt \tag{9.1}$$

$$PC = \frac{\gamma \cos \theta}{2\eta} \tag{9.2}$$

in Eqs. (9.1) and (9.2), d is the distance moved by the liquid, θ the contact angle of the liquid to the substrate, γ the surface tension of the liquid, η is the dynamic viscosity of the liquid, t the penetration time and r is the capillary pore radius [112]. Therefore, from Eq. (9.2), it can be inferred that the penetration coefficient (PC) is heavily influenced by the dynamic viscosity of the liquid, η. Therefore, researchers identified that a combination of monomer molecules of sufficiently low molecular weight would facilitate diffusion into the affected tissues, while a blend of desirable properties after curing would be required for adequate reinforcement of the remainder of the tooth structure [111]. Early formulations of resins allowing for improved infiltration of caries enamel lesions were composed of a mixture of HEMA and ethanol [113–115]. However, mixtures of these components at various ratios showed imperfect hardening after photopolymerization. Formulation leading to the most desirable properties where then developed using blends of TEGDMA, HEMA and 20 % ethanol, which resulted in penetration coefficients of up to 475 cm/s [111].

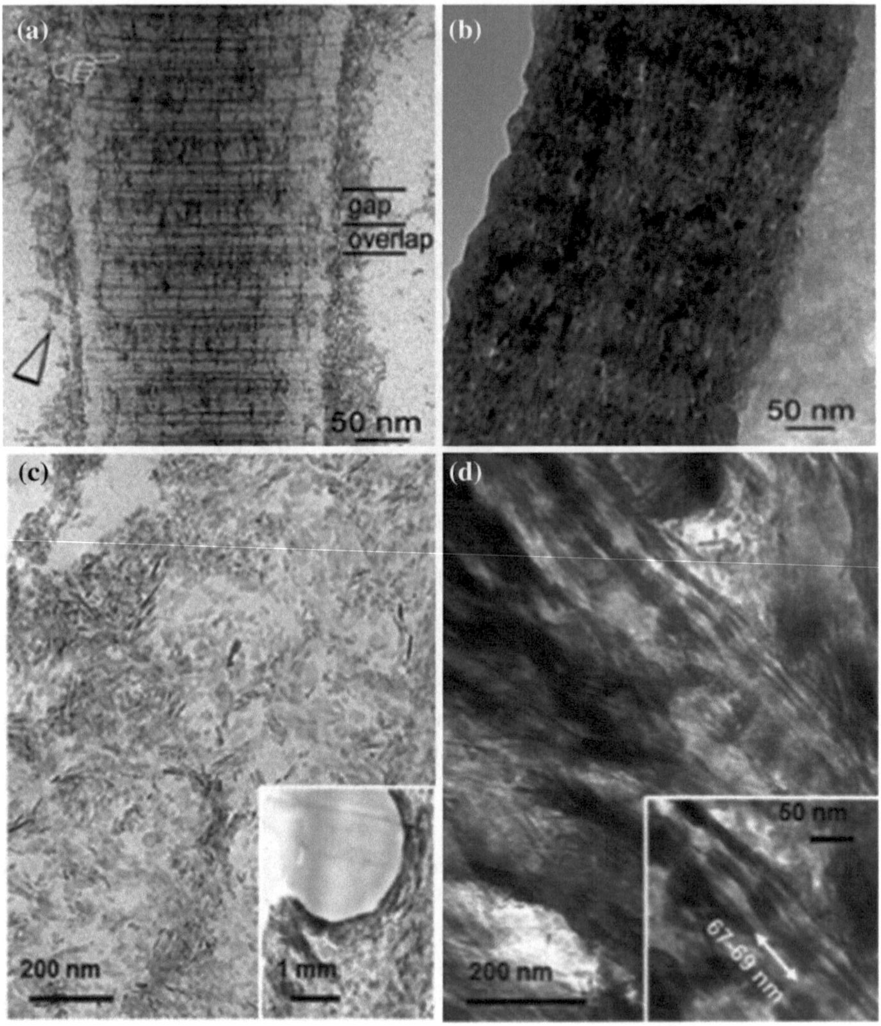

Fig. 9.3 TEM images of reconstituted collagen (**a**) and mineralized collagen using a dual biomimetic analog mineralization protocol (**b**). TEM images of dentin carious lesion (**c**) and lesions after 14 days of PILP-assisted remineralization (**d**). Reproduced with permission from [130] and [132]

Although desirable penetration coefficients could be attained by optimizing the ratios of TEGDMA, HEMA and ethanol, critical challenges associated with this method were not only restricted to minimizing viscosity (and contact angle) of the polymer. Modifying the microstructure of enamel lesions to facilitate impregnation with the resin was also a requirement [116–118]. It has been well known that subsurface lesions in carious enamel are much more porous than the so-called pseudo-intact surface layer, which forms by dissolution and re-precipitation of mineral ions on the enamel surface. According to Eq. (9.1), the capillary pore radius will also have a significant effect on the ability of a viscous fluid to penetrate a porous solid via capillary action. To that end, researchers identified a need to acid-etch the pseudo-intact surface layer of enamel lesions and facilitate diffusion of the viscous fluids of the resins into the body of the lesion [117].

Phosphoric acid has traditionally been used as a conditioner of enamel and dentin for adhesive restorative treatments, as described in section "Polymers in Dental Adhesion". 37 % phosphoric acid has been shown to decalcify enamel and dentin in a desirable pattern, thus facilitating impregnation of adhesive monomers required for placement of composite resin restorations in the tissue matrix. Despite the known efficiency of 37 % phosphoric acid gels in acid-etching enamel and dentin, it has been shown that its effects in increasing the surface porosity of the pseudo intact surface layer of enamel lesions was not sufficient [117]. To overcome this limitation, 15 % hydrochloric acid (generally for 2 min) has been tested and shown to remove about 30 μm of surface enamel, thus allowing for much improved penetration of viscous resins in white spot lesions [116].

Although solid evidence for the efficacy of polymer infiltrants in arresting tooth decay and preventing further demineralization [119–121], a few aspects remain to be answered. Resins composed of mixtures of hydrophobic monomers, as we detailed in section "Polymers in Dental Adhesion", have been extensively demonstrated to undergo hydrolytic degradation in the presence of oral fluids [122]. These conditions have been mostly restricted to dentin, which are not the most common applications of resin infiltrants. Nevertheless, not only these polymers are recommended for infiltration of dentin-affected caries (at early stages), but also marginal degradation due to hydrolyses from oral fluids have been extensively reported for restorative composite resins. It is unclear to which extent resin infiltrated caries will develop similar patterns of degradation over time. Similarly, newer chemistries that enable chemical retention of photolabile resins to hydroxyapatite, such as the 10-MDP molecule currently used in various dental bonding systems, may provide further improvements for the nano- and micro-scale interactions between enamel and polymer resins for infiltration of tooth decay.

Polymers for Assisted Remineralization of Carious Dentin

Although the requirements for caries prevention and diseases development have been well established from many years of research in the field of cariology, our perception of how tooth decay may be remineralized has expanded substantially in the last decade.

One of the primary aspects allowing for such rapid transition has been an improved understanding of the complexity of the mineral-matrix interactions occurring in mineralized tissues, particularly in dentin and bone. Early work has identified that in mineralized tissues, collagen fibrils are reinforced with mineral crystallites that are positioned both intrafibrillarly (inside the fibrils) and extrafibrillarly (outside the fibrils) [123, 124]. This partitioning has been shown to have important implications for remineralization strategies [106]. For instance, it has been shown that the mineral concentration of dentine lacking intrafibrillar mineral (due to dentinogenesis imperfect type II) has little correlation to the tissue's mechanical properties, particularly its elastic modulus [125, 126]. These results led to the hypothesis that, although mineral concentration may be a sufficient endpoint for assessing remineralization of carious enamel, it may not have the same efficiency in evaluating treatment of carious dentin, where the specific interactions between the organic and inorganic components appear to have a greater influence than mineral content alone [106, 125].

Traditionally remineralization of tooth structures have relied on well established concepts of nucleation and crystal growth. Mineral ions interact with the tooth substrate and crystallization occurs at specific thermodynamic conditions that are appropriate for formation of an stable apatite phase in register with the preserved tooth structures. Using these approaches, researchers have been able to demonstrate that in carious dentin, the intrafibrillar mineral that is not fully dissolved upon acidic attack may function as nucleation sites for subsequent deposition of calcium and phosphate within the intrafibrillar compartments of collagen fibrils [127]. This, in turn, has been shown to lead to significant increases in the mechanical properties of partially demineralized dentin.

In nature, however, noncollagenous proteins such as osteopontin, bone sialoprotein, dentin matrix protein 1 (DMP1), dentin sialophosphoprotein (DSPP), and dentin phosphoprotein (DPP), have been associated with the mineralization of the tissue's collagen scaffold [128, 129], thus characterizing a protein-mediated mineralization mechanism that is rather different from the classic remineralization strategies traditionally used in dentistry. It is generally accepted that the carboxylate groups on the polyaspartic acid residues of highly anionic noncollagenous proteins renders these proteins important regulators of biominerlization [130, 131]. Therefore, it has been the focus of much research to develop strategies that enable mimicry of these biological functions using acidic polymers capable of inhibiting apatite nucleation while stabilizing calcium and phosphate ions in an amorphous phase. This conjecture forms the basis for the polymer-assisted mineralization of collagenous tissues that is the focus of contemporary approaches for remineralization of dentin [130]. We point out, as well, that similar polymer-based mineralization strategies have been extensively studied recently to prevent degradation of resin-dentin bonds.

Polymer Induced Liquid Precursor (PILP) System

A recent polymer-assisted biominerlization method that has shown great effectiveness in remineralizing carious dentin is based on a Polymer Induced Liquid Precursor (PILP) methodology (Fig. 9.3) [132, 133]. The PILP process is based on the action of minute amounts of acidic polypeptides which are added to a remineralization solution. The anionic polymer functions be sequestering calcium ions, which then builds up a charge to sequester phosphate or carbonate, thus inducing liquid-liquid phase separation in the crystallizing medium [8, 10, 11] and hence facilitating formation of mineral inside collagen fibrils. Several anionic polymers have been studied as the process-directing agent and tested for their ability to sequester calcium and phosphate ions and form amorphous precursors that could infiltrate the intrafibrillar spaces in demineralized collagen [132–134]. Further studies have also compared poly-L aspartic acid (PASP), poly-L-glutamic acid (PGLU), polyvynilphosphonic acid (PVPA) and polyacrylic acid (PAA). PASP, in particular, represents the original polymeric combination in which a carboxylated group is attached to the amino acid backbone by one methylene group, thus mimicking one of the two most prevalent aminoacids in acidic noncollagenous proteins [131]. PGLU, PAA and PVPA are similar carboxylated molecules that have been tested due to their potential combinatorial effects with PASP in PILP strategies [134]. Results from these studies showed that, among the polymers investigated, PASP and the combination of PASP and PGLU/PASP formed stable mineralization solutions and resulted in effective intrafibrillar mineralization of collagen fibrils. A similar approach was later utilized to remineralize dentin specimens with simulated caries lesions [132].

In the polymer-assisted remineralization, calcium and phosphate ions are sequestered by biomimetic analogs of non-collagenous proteins. Similar to the function of the native proteins, these biomimetic analogs inhibit early crystallization of mineral forming pre-nucleation clusters, which eventually aggregate and form larger amorphous calcium phosphate (ACP) particles, which further stabilize to form apatite crystallites [131].

Dual Biomimetic Analog Strategy

Similar strategies have utilized a dual biomimetic analog strategy to facilitate mineralization of apatite depleted collagen matrices (Fig. 9.3). Contrary to the original PILP method, the dual mineralization strategy utilizes a polyphosphate-containing biomimetic analog which are allowed to bind to the collagen fibrils prior to immersion in a in a poly(anionic) acid-containing mineralization medium [135, 136]. In these systems, polyacrylic acid or polyaspartic acid have originally been used as the phosphoprotein analog for sequestering calcium ions released by a calcium silicate cement, or a supersaturated solutions of calcium and phosphate. Additional biomimetic analogue agents have included polyvinylphosphonic acid, sodium trimetaphosphate or sodium ascorbyl phosphate [130]. The objective of incorporating these analogs is to prevent fluidic amorphous calcium and phosphate particles from agglomerating into larger particles crystalized structures which would prevent the formation of a more stable apatite phase in the intrafibrillar spaces in collagen fibrils. Furthermore, the protein analogues are believed to function as an apatite nucleation inhibitor, preventing auto-transformation of the amorphous phase into apatite prior to their entry into the spaces.

Conclusion

In summary, in this chapter we review emerging concepts of polymeric materials applied to different areas of clinical dentistry. Tooth structures are inherently constituted of natural polymers, such as collagen and noncollagenous proteins. These so-called biopolymers, particularly in dentin, form the substrate onto which dimethacrylate adhesive resins are diffused into to bond restorative composites. Different approaches taking advantage of innovative polymer chemistry and manipulation methods of the natural polymers themselves have been presented as methods to prevent degradation of dentin bonding. Existing and emerging classes of composite resins were also described. Recent noteworthy composites include anti-caries materials with soluble or immobilized antimicrobial agents and antimicrobial fillers. Recent formulations of low-shrinkage composites also represent innovative types of polymers used in restorative dentistry. Ring-opening polymerization methods have been described as well as stress decreasing resins (SDR). Finally, emerging polymers used for denture base materials and prevention/treatment of tooth decay were touched upon. In summary, polymers represent one of major pillars of current restorative dentistry and will continue to evolve with the advent of newer technologies and polymer characterization tools. This review may provide guidance for future developments in the field of polymeric dentistry.

References

1. Bertassoni, L.E., Orgel, J.P., Antipova, O., Swain, M.V.: The dentin organic matrix -limitations of restorative dentistry hidden on the nanometer scale. Acta Biomater. **8**, 2419–2433 (2012)
2. Kumar, G.S.: Orban's oral histology & embryology,13th edn. Elsevier, Amsterdam (2011)
3. Dell, A., Famulok, M., Imperiali, B.: Biopolymers. Chemical and biological approaches for understanding form and function editorial overview. Curr. Opin. Chem. Biol. **4**, 599–601 (2000)
4. Bleicher, F., Couble, M.L., Buchaille, R., Farges, J.C., Magloire, H.: New genes involved in odontoblast differentiation. Adv. Dent. Res. **15**, 30–33 (2001)
5. Mithieux, S.M., Weiss, A.S.: Elastin. Adv. Protein. Chem. **70**, 437–461 (2005)
6. Bertassoni, L.E., Stankoska, K., Swain, M.V.: Insights into the structure and composition of the peritubular dentin organic matrix and the lamina limitans. Micron **43**, 229–236 (2012)
7. Ferracane, J.L.: Current trends in dental composites. Crit. Rev. Oral Biol. Med. **6**, 302–318 (1995)
8. Bertassoni, L.E., Uskokovic, V.: Nanotechnology in dental sciences: moving towards a finer way of doing dentistry. Materials **3**(3), 1674–1691 (2010)
9. Soderholm, K.J.: Dental adhesives… how it all started and later evolved. J. Adhes. Dentistry. **9**(Suppl 2), 227–230 (2007)
10. Van Landuyt, K.L., Yoshida, Y., Hirata, I., Snauwaert, J., De Munck, J., Okazaki, M., et al.: Influence of the chemical structure of functional monomers on their adhesive performance. J. Dent. Res. **87**, 757–761 (2008)
11. Yoshida, Y., Nagakane, K., Fukuda, R., Nakayama, Y., Okazaki, M., Shintani, H., et al.: Comparative study on adhesive performance of functional monomers. J. Dent. Res. **83**, 454–458 (2004)

12. Van Landuyt, K.L., Snauwaert, J., De Munck, J., Peumans, M., Yoshida, Y., Poitevin, A., et al.: Systematic review of the chemical composition of contemporary dental adhesives. Biomaterials **28**, 3757–3785 (2007)
13. Ye, Q., Park, J.G., Topp, E., Wang, Y., Misra, A., Spencer, P.: In vitro performance of nano-heterogeneous dentin adhesive. J. Dent. Res. **87**, 829–833 (2008)
14. Habelitz, S., Balooch, M., Marshall, S.J., Balooch, G., Marshall Jr, G.W.: In situ atomic force microscopy of partially demineralized human dentin collagen fibrils. J. Struct. Biol. **138**, 227–236 (2002)
15. Chiaraputt, S., Mai, S., Huffman, B.P., Kapur, R., Agee, K.A., Yiu, C.K., et al.: Changes in resin-infiltrated dentin stiffness after water storage. J. Dent. Res. **87**, 655–660 (2008)
16. Ito, S., Hashimoto, M., Wadgaonkar, B., Svizero, N., Carvalho, R.M., Yiu, C., et al.: Effects of resin hydrophilicity on water sorption and changes in modulus of elasticity. Biomaterials **26**, 6449–6459 (2005)
17. Malacarne, J., Carvalho, R.M., de Goes, M.F., Svizero, N., Pashley, D.H., Tay, F.R., et al.: Water sorption/solubility of dental adhesive resins. Dent. Mater. **22**, 973–980 (2006)
18. Ferracane, J.L.: Hygroscopic and hydrolytic effects in dental polymer networks. Dent. Mater. **22**, 211–222 (2006)
19. Parthasarathy, R., Misra, A., Park, J., Ye, Q., Spencer, P.: Diffusion coefficients of water and leachables in methacrylate-based crosslinked polymers using absorption experiments. J. Mater. Sci. Mater. Med. **23**, 1157–1172 (2012)
20. Finer, Y., Santerre, J.P.: Salivary esterase activity and its association with the biodegradation of dental composites. J. Dent. Res. **83**, 22–26 (2004)
21. Kostoryz, E.L., Dharmala, K., Ye, Q., Wang, Y., Huber, J., Park, J.G., et al.: Enzymatic biodegradation of HEMA/bisGMA adhesives formulated with different water content. J. Biomed. Mater. Res. B Appl. Biomater. **88**, 394–401 (2009)
22. Park, J., Eslick, J., Ye, Q., Misra, A., Spencer, P.: The influence of chemical structure on the properties in methacrylate-based dentin adhesives. Dent. Mater. **27**, 1086–1093 (2011)
23. Bail, M., Malacarne-Zanon, J., Silva, S.M., Anauate-Netto, A., Nascimento, F.D., Amore, R., et al.: Effect of air-drying on the solvent evaporation, degree of conversion and water sorption/solubility of dental adhesive models. J. Mater. Sci. Mater. Med. **23**, 629–638 (2012)
24. Wang, Y., Spencer, P., Yao, X., Brenda, B.: Effect of solvent content on resin hybridization in wet dentin bonding. J. Biomed. Mater. Res. Part A **82**, 975–983 (2007)
25. Ye, Q., Spencer, P., Wang, Y., Misra, A.: Relationship of solvent to the photopolymerization process, properties, and structure in model dentin adhesives. J. Biomed. Mater. Res. Part A **80**, 342–350 (2007)
26. Yiu, C.K., Pashley, E.L., Hiraishi, N., King, N.M., Goracci, C., Ferrari, M., et al.: Solvent and water retention in dental adhesive blends after evaporation. Biomaterials **26**, 6863–6872 (2005)
27. Wang, Y., Spencer, P.: Continuing etching of an all-in-one adhesive in wet dentin tubules. J. Dent. Res. **84**, 350–354 (2005)
28. Marshall Jr, G.W., Marshall, S.J., Kinney, J.H., Balooch, M.: The dentin substrate: structure and properties related to bonding. J. Dent. **25**, 441–458 (1997)
29. Mazzoni, A., Carrilho, M., Papa, V., Tjaderhane, L., Gobbi, P., Nucci, C., et al.: MMP-2 assay within the hybrid layer created by a two-step etch-and-rinse adhesive: biochemical and immunohistochemical analysis. J. Dent. **39**, 470–477 (2011)
30. Mazzoni, A., Nascimento, F.D., Carrilho, M., Tersariol, I., Papa, V., Tjaderhane, L., et al.: MMP activity in the hybrid layer detected with in situ zymography. J. Dent. Res. **91**, 467–472 (2012)
31. Tjaderhane, L., Nascimento, F.D., Breschi, L., Mazzoni, A., Tersariol, I.L., Geraldeli, S., et al.: Optimizing dentin bond durability: control of collagen degradation by matrix metalloproteinases and cysteine cathepsins. Dent. Mater. **29**, 116–135 (2013)
32. Bedran-Russo, A.K., Pereira, P.N., Duarte, W.R., Okuyama, K., Yamauchi, M.: Removal of dentin matrix proteoglycans by trypsin digestion and its effect on dentin bonding. J. Biomed. Mater. Res. B Appl. Biomater. **85**, 261–266 (2008)

33. Mazzoni, A., Pashley, D.H., Ruggeri Jr, A., Vita, F., Falconi, M., Di Lenarda, R., et al.: Adhesion to chondroitinase ABC treated dentin. J. Biomed. Mater. Res. B Appl. Biomater. **86**, 228–236 (2008)
34. Van Meerbeek, B., Yoshihara, K., Yoshida, Y., Mine, A., De Munck, J., Van Landuyt, K.L.: State of the art of self-etch adhesives. Dent. Mater. **27**, 17–28 (2011)
35. Lien, W., Vandewalle, K.S.: Physical properties of a new silorane-based restorative system. Dent. Mater. **26**, 337–344 (2010)
36. Boulden, J.E., Cramer, N.B., Schreck, K.M., Couch, C.L., Bracho-Troconis, C., Stansbury, J.W., et al.: Thiol-ene-methacrylate composites as dental restorative materials. Dent. Mater. **27**, 267–272 (2011)
37. Cramer, N.B., Couch, C.L., Schreck, K.M., Boulden, J.E., Wydra, R., Stansbury, J.W., et al.: Properties of methacrylate-thiol-ene formulations as dental restorative materials. Dent. Mater. **26**, 799–806 (2010)
38. Guo, X., Wang, Y., Spencer, P., Ye, Q., Yao, X.: Effects of water content and initiator composition on photopolymerization of a model BisGMA/HEMA resin. Dent. Mater. **24**, 824–831 (2008)
39. Tjaderhane, L., Nascimento, F.D., Breschi, L., Mazzoni, A., Tersariol, I.L., Geraldeli, S., et al.: Strategies to prevent hydrolytic degradation of the hybrid layer—a review. Dent. Mater. **29**, 999–1011 (2013)
40. Carrilho, M.R., Carvalho, R.M., de Goes, M.F., di Hipolito, V., Geraldeli, S., Tay, F.R., et al.: Chlorhexidine preserves dentin bond in vitro. J. Dent. Res. **86**, 90–94 (2007)
41. Scaffa, P.M., Vidal, C.M., Barros, N., Gesteira, T.F., Carmona, A.K., Breschi, L., et al.: Chlorhexidine inhibits the activity of dental cysteine cathepsins. J. Dent. Res. **91**, 420–425 (2012)
42. Breschi, L., Martin, P., Mazzoni, A., Nato, F., Carrilho, M., Tjaderhane, L., et al.: Use of a specific MMP-inhibitor (galardin) for preservation of hybrid layer. Dent. Mater. **26**, 571–578 (2010)
43. Bedran-Russo, A.K., Pauli, G.F., Chen, S.N., McAlpine, J., Castellan, C.S., Phansalkar, R.S., et al.: Dentin biomodification: strategies, renewable resources and clinical applications. Dent. Mater. **30**, 62–76 (2014)
44. Bedran-Russo, A.K., Vidal, C.M., Dos Santos, P.H., Castellan, C.S.: Long-term effect of carbodiimide on dentin matrix and resin-dentin bonds. J. Biomed. Mater. Res. B Appl. Biomater. **94**, 250–255 (2010)
45. Chiang, Y.S., Chen, Y.L., Chuang, S.F., Wu, C.M., Wei, P.J., Han, C.F., et al.: Riboflavinultraviolet- A-induced collagen cross-linking treatments in improving dentin bonding. Dent. Mater. **29**, 682–692 (2013)
46. Ferracane, J.L.: Resin composite—state of the art. Dent. Mater. **27**, 29–38 (2011)
47. da Rosa Rodolpho, P.A.: Cenci MS, Donassollo TA, Loguercio AD, Demarco FF. A clinical evaluation of posterior composite restorations: 17-year findings. J. Dent. **34**, 427–435 (2006)
48. Wilder Jr, A.D., May Jr, K.N., Bayne, S.C., Taylor, D.F., Leinfelder, K.F.: Seventeen-year clinical study of ultraviolet-cured posterior composite Class I and II restorations. J. Esthet. Dent. **11**, 135–142 (1999)
49. Bowen, R.L.: Properties of a silica-reinforced polymer for dental restorations. J. Am. Dent. Assoc. **66**, 57–64 (1963)
50. Zimmerli, B., Strub, M., Jeger, F., Stadler, O., Lussi, A.: Composite materials: composition, properties and clinical applications. A literature review. Schweizer Monatsschrift fur Zahnmedizin = Revue mensuelle suisse d'odonto-stomatologie = Rivista mensile svizzera di odontologia e stomatologia/SSO. **120**, 972–986 (2009)
51. Puckett, A.D., Fitchie, J.G., Kirk, P.C., Gamblin, J.: Direct composite restorative materials. Dent. Clin. North Am. **51**(3), 659–675 (2007)
52. Chen, M.H.: Update on dental nanocomposites. J. Dent. Res. **89**, 549–560 (2010)
53. Ferracane, J.L., Berge, H.X., Condon, J.R.: In vitro aging of dental composites in water–effect of degree of conversion, filler volume, and filler/matrix coupling. J. Biomed. Mater. Res. **42**, 465–472 (1998)

54. Beyth, N., Domb, A.J., Weiss, E.I.: An in vitro quantitative antibacterial analysis of amalgam and composite resins. J. Dent. **35**, 201–206 (2007)
55. Beyth, N., Yudovin-Farber, I., Bahir, R., Domb, A.J., Weiss, E.I.: Antibacterial activity of dental composites containing quaternary ammonium polyethylenimine nanoparticles against Streptococcus mutans. Biomaterials **27**, 3995–4002 (2006)
56. Buergers, R., Schneider-Brachert, W., Hahnel, S., Rosentritt, M., Handel, G.: Streptococcal adhesion to novel low-shrink silorane-based restorative. Dent. Mater. **25**, 269–275 (2009)
57. Ehara, A., Torii, M., Imazato, S., Ebisu, S.: Antibacterial activities and release kinetics of a newly developed recoverable controlled agent-release system. J. Dent. Res. **79**, 824–828 (2000)
58. Hiraishi, N., Yiu, C.K., King, N.M., Tay, F.R., Pashley, D.H.: Chlorhexidine release and water sorption characteristics of chlorhexidine-incorporated hydrophobic/hydrophilic resins. Dent. Mater. **24**, 1391–1399 (2008)
59. Syafiuddin, T., Hisamitsu, H., Toko, T., Igarashi, T., Goto, N., Fujishima, A., et al.: In vitro inhibition of caries around a resin composite restoration containing antibacterial filler. Biomaterials **18**, 1051–1057 (1997)
60. Takahashi, Y., Imazato, S., Kaneshiro, A.V., Ebisu, S., Frencken, J.E., Tay, F.R.: Antibacterial effects and physical properties of glass-ionomer cements containing chlorhexidine for the ART approach. Dent. Mater. **22**, 647–652 (2006)
61. Tanagawa, M., Yoshida, K., Matsumoto, S., Yamada, T., Atsuta, M.: Inhibitory effect of antibacterial resin composite against Streptococcus mutans. Caries Res. **33**, 366–371 (1999)
62. Yoshida, K., Tanagawa, M., Matsumoto, S., Yamada, T., Atsuta, M.: Antibacterial activity of resin composites with silver-containing materials. Eur. J. Oral Sci. **107**, 290–296 (1999)
63. Imazato, S.: Antibacterial properties of resin composites and dentin bonding systems. Dent. Mater. **19**, 449–457 (2003)
64. Jedrychowski, J.R., Caputo, A.A., Kerper, S.: Antibacterial and mechanical properties of restorative materials combined with chlorhexidines. J. Oral Rehabil. **10**, 373–381 (1983)
65. Ribeiro, J., Ericson, D.: In vitro antibacterial effect of chlorhexidine added to glassionomer cements. Scand. J. Dent. Res. **99**, 533–540 (1991)
66. Wiegand, A., Buchalla, W., Attin, T.: Review on fluoride-releasing restorative materials–fluoride release and uptake characteristics, antibacterial activity and influence on caries formation. Dent. Mater. **23**, 343–362 (2007)
67. Pandit, S., Kim, G.R., Lee, M.H., Jeon, J.G.: Evaluation of Streptococcus mutans biofilms formed on fluoride releasing and non fluoride releasing resin composites. J. Dent. **39**, 780–787 (2011)
68. Imazato, S., Torii, M., Tsuchitani, Y., McCabe, J.F., Russell, R.R.: Incorporation of bacterial inhibitor into resin composite. J. Dent. Res. **73**, 1437–1443 (1994)
69. Ebi, N., Imazato, S., Noiri, Y., Ebisu, S.: Inhibitory effects of resin composite containing bactericide-immobilized filler on plaque accumulation. Dent. Mater. **17**, 485–491 (2001)
70. Thome, T., Mayer, M.P., Imazato, S., Geraldo-Martins, V.R., Marques, M.M.: In vitro analysis of inhibitory effects of the antibacterial monomer MDPB-containing restorations on the progression of secondary root caries. J. Dent. **37**, 705–711 (2009)
71. Cheng, L., Weir, M.D., Limkangwalmongkol, P., Hack, G.D., Xu, H.H., Chen, Q., et al.: Tetracalcium phosphate composite containing quaternary ammonium dimethacrylate with antibacterial properties. J. Biomed. Mater. Res. B Appl. Biomater. **100**, 726–734 (2012)
72. Cheng, L., Weir, M.D., Zhang, K., Wu, E.J., Xu, S.M., Zhou, X., et al.: Dental plaque microcosm biofilm behavior on calcium phosphate nanocomposite with quaternary ammonium. Dent. Mater. **28**, 853–862 (2012)
73. Cheng, L., Weir, M.D., Xu, H.H., Antonucci, J.M., Kraigsley, A.M., Lin, N.J., et al.: Antibacterial amorphous calcium phosphate nanocomposites with a quaternary ammonium dimethacrylate and silver nanoparticles. Dent. Mater. **28**, 561–572 (2012)
74. Rawls, H.R., Upshaw, J.E.: Restorative resins. In: Anusavice, K.J. (ed.) Phillip's science of dental materials, 11th edn, pp. 399–441. WB Saunders, Philadelphia (2003)
75. Eick, J.D., Robinson, S.J., Byerley, T.J., Chappelow, C.C.: Adhesives and nonshrinking dental resins of the future. Quintessence Int. **24**, 632–640 (1993)

76. Weinmann, W., Thalacker, C., Guggenberger, R.: Siloranes in dental composites. Dent. Mater. **21**, 68–74 (2005)
77. Trujillo-Lemon, M., Ge, J., Lu, H., Tanaka, J., Stansbury, J.: Dimethacrylate derivates of dimer acid. J. Polymer. Sci. **44**, 3921–3929 (2006)
78. Wolter H, Storch W, Ott H. New inorganic/organic copolymers (ormocerâ®s) for dental applications. In: MRS Online Proceedings Library. **346**, 143 (1994)
79. Moszner, N., Gianasmidis, A., Klapdohr, S., Fischer, U.K., Rheinberger, V.: Sol-gel materials 2. Light-curing dental composites based on ormocers of cross-linking alkoxysilane methacrylates and further nano-components. Dent. Mater. **24**, 851–856 (2008)
80. Aleixo, A.R., Guiraldo, R.D., Fugolin, A.P., Berger, S.B., Consani, R.L., Correr, A.B., et al.: Evaluation of contraction stress, conversion degree, and cross-link density in lowshrinkage composites. Photomed Laser Surg. **32**, 267–273 (2014)
81. Eick, J.D., Kostoryz, E.L., Rozzi, S.M., Jacobs, D.W., Oxman, J.D., Chappelow, C.C., et al.: Invitro biocompatibility of oxirane/polyol dental composites with promising physical properties. Dent. Mater. **18**, 413–421 (2002)
82. Bettencourt, A.F., Neves, C.B., de Almeida, M.S., Pinheiro, L.M., Oliveira, S.A., Lopes, L.P., et al.: Biodegradation of acrylic based resins: A review. Dent. Mater. **26**, e171–e180 (2010)
83. Schweikl, H., Schmalz, G., Weinmann, W.: The induction of gene mutations and micronuclei by oxiranes and siloranes in mammalian cells in vitro. J. Dent. Res. **83**, 17–21 (2004)
84. Ilie, N., Hickel, R.: Investigations on mechanical behaviour of dental composites. Clin Oral Investig. **13**, 427–438 (2009)
85. Jin, X., Bertrand, S., Hammesfahr, P.: New radically polymerizable resins with remarkably low curing stress. J. Dent. Res. **88**, 1651 (2009)
86. Soh, M.S., Yap, A.U., Sellinger, A.: Physicomechanical evaluation of low-shrinkage dental nanocomposites based on silsesquioxane cores. Eur. J. Oral Sci. **115**, 230–238 (2007)
87. Lee, K.H., Rhee, S.H.: The mechanical properties and bioactivity of poly(methyl methacrylate)/SiO(2)-CaO nanocomposite. Biomaterials **30**, 3444–3449 (2009)
88. Chen, M.H., Chen, C.R., Hsu, S.H., Sun, S.P., Su, W.F.: Low shrinkage light curable nanocomposite for dental restorative material. Dent. Mater. **22**, 138–145 (2006)
89. Tilbrook, D.A., Clarke, R.L., Howle, N.E., Braden, M.: Photocurable epoxy-polyol matrices for use in dental composites I. Biomaterials **21**, 1743–1753 (2000)
90. Uskoković, V., Bertassoni, L.E.: Nanotechnology in dental sciences: moving towards a finer way of doing dentistry. Materials **3**, 1674–1691 (2010)
91. Jandt, K.D., Sigusch, B.W.: Future perspectives of resin-based dental materials. Dent. Mater. **25**, 1001–1006 (2009)
92. Mitra, S.B., Wu, D., Holmes, B.N.: An application of nanotechnology in advanced dental materials. J. Am. Dent. Assoc. **134**, 1382–1390 (2003)
93. Rueggeberg, F.A.: From vulcanite to vinyl, a history of resins in restorative dentistry. J. Prosthetic. Dentistry **87**, 364–379 (2002)
94. Jagger, D., Harrison, A., Jandt, K.: The reinforcement of dentures. J. Oral Rehabil. **26**, 185–194 (1999)
95. Cunningham, J.: Bond strength of denture teeth to acrylic bases. J. Dentistry **21**, 274–280 (1993)
96. Jo, L.J., Shenoy, K.K., Shetty, S.: Flexural strength and hardness of resins for interim fixed partial dentures. Indian J. Dent. Res. **22**, 71 (2011)
97. Irini, S.D.: Polymeric materials in dentistry 1st edn. Nova Science, Hauppauge (2010)
98. Khindria, S., Mittal, S., Sukhija, U.: Evolution of denture base materials. J. Indian Prosthodontic Soc. **9**(2), 64–69 (2009)
99. McCord, J.F.: Contemporary techniques for denture fabrication. J. Prosthodontics. **18**, 106–111 (2009)
100. Raj, P.A., Dentino, A.R.: New phosphated poly (methyl methacrylate) polymers for the prevention of denture-induced microbial infection: an in vitro study. Clin. Cosmet. Investig. Dentistry **3**, 25 (2011)

101. Zhang, X., Zhang, X., Zhu, B., Qian, C.: [Effect of nano ZrO2 on flexural strength and surface hardness of polymethylmethacrylate]. Shanghai kou qiang yi xue=. Shanghai. J. Stomatology. **20**, 358–363 (2011)
102. Turagam, N., Prasad Mudrakola, D.: Effect of micro-additions of carbon nanotubes to polymethylmethacrylate on reduction in polymerization shrinkage. J. Prosthodontics. **22**, 105–111 (2013)
103. Wang, R., Tao, J., Yu, B., Dai, L.: Characterization of multiwalled carbon nanotube—polymethyl methacrylate composite resins as denture base materials. J. Prosthetic. Dentistry. **111**(4), 318–326 (2013)
104. Albakri, I.S.M., Naoum, S., Martin, E., ALomari, W., Ellakwa, A.: Fluoride release, recharge and flexural properties of polymethylmethacrylate containing fluoridated glass fillers. Aus. Dent. J **59**(2), 208–214 (2014)
105. Services UDoHaH. NHEA—National health expenditure projections 2009–2019. Washington, DC (2006)
106. Bertassoni, L.E., Habelitz, S., Kinney, J.H., Marshall, S.J., Marshall Jr, G.W.: Biomechanical perspective on the remineralization of dentin. Caries Res. **43**, 70–77 (2009)
107. Cochrane, N.J., Cai, F., Huq, N.L., Burrow, M.F., Reynolds, E.C.: New approaches to enhanced remineralization of tooth enamel. J. Dent. Res. **89**, 1187–1197 (2010)
108. Huang, T.T., He, L.H., Darendeliler, M.A., Swain, M.V.: Correlation of mineral density and elastic modulus of natural enamel white spot lesions using X-ray microtomography and nanoindentation. Acta Biomater. **6**, 4553–4559 (2010)
109. Huang, T.T., Jones, A.S., He, L.H., Darendeliler, M.A., Swain, M.V.: Characterisation of enamel white spot lesions using X-ray micro-tomography. J. Dent. **35**, 737–743 (2007)
110. Ten Cate, J.M., Featherstone, J.D.: Mechanistic aspects of the interactions between fluoride and dental enamel. Crit. Rev. Oral. Bio. Med. **2**, 283–296 (1991)
111. Paris, S., Meyer-Lueckel, H., Colfen, H., Kielbassa, A.M.: Penetration coefficients of commercially available and experimental composites intended to infiltrate enamel carious lesions. Dent. Mater. **23**, 742–748 (2007)
112. Fan, P.L., Seluk, L.W., O'Brien, W.J.: Penetrativity of sealants: I. J. Dent. Res. **54**, 262–264 (1975)
113. Davila, J.M., Buonocore, M.G., Greeley, C.B., Provenza, D.V.: Adhesive penetration in human artificial and natural white spots. J. Dent. Res. **54**, 999–1008 (1975)
114. Robinson, C., Brookes, S.J., Kirkham, J., Wood, S.R., Shore, R.C.: In vitro studies of the penetration of adhesive resins into artificial caries-like lesions. Caries Res. **35**, 136–141 (2001)
115. Gray, G.B., Shellis, P.: Infiltration of resin into white spot caries-like lesions of enamel: an in vitro study. Eur. J. Prosthodontics. Restorative. Dentistry. **10**, 27–32 (2002)
116. Meyer-Lueckel, H., Paris, S.: Improved resin infiltration of natural caries lesions. J. Dent. Res. **87**, 1112–1116 (2008)
117. Meyer-Lueckel, H., Paris, S., Kielbassa, A.M.: Surface layer erosion of natural caries lesions with phosphoric and hydrochloric acid gels in preparation for resin infiltration. Caries Res. **41**, 223–230 (2007)
118. Meyer-Lueckel, H., Paris, S., Mueller, J., Colfen, H., Kielbassa, A.M.: Influence of the application time on the penetration of different dental adhesives and a fissure sealant into artificial subsurface lesions in bovine enamel. Dent. Mater. **22**, 22–28 (2006)
119. Paris, S., Hopfenmuller, W., Meyer-Lueckel, H.: Resin infiltration of caries lesions: an efficacy randomized trial. J. Dent. Res. **89**, 823–826 (2010)
120. Paris, S., Meyer-Lueckel, H.: Infiltrants inhibit progression of natural caries lesions in vitro. J. Dent. Res. **89**, 1276–1280 (2010)
121. Paris, S., Meyer-Lueckel, H., Kielbassa, A.M.: Resin infiltration of natural caries lesions. J. Dent. Res. **86**, 662–666 (2007)
122. Tay, F.R., Hashimoto, M., Pashley, D.H., Peters, M.C., Lai, S.C., Yiu, C.K., et al.: Aging affects two modes of nanoleakage expression in bonded dentin. J. Dent. Res. **82**, 537–541 (2003)

123. Lees, S., Page, E.A.: A study of some properties of mineralized turkey leg tendon. Connect. Tissue Res. **28**, 263–287 (1992)
124. Arsenault, A.L.: Image analysis of collagen-associated mineral distribution in cryogenically prepared turkey leg tendons. Calcif. Tissue Int. **48**, 56–62 (1991)
125. Kinney, J.H., Habelitz, S., Marshall, S.J., Marshall, G.W.: The importance of intrafibrillar mineralization of collagen on the mechanical properties of dentin. J. Dent. Res. **82**, 957–961 (2003)
126. Kinney, J.H., Pople, J.A., Driessen, C.H., Breunig, T.M., Marshall, G.W., Marshall, S.J.: Intrafibrillar mineral may be absent in dentinogenesis imperfecta type II (DI-II). J. Dent. Res. **80**, 1555–1559 (2001)
127. Bertassoni, L.E., Habelitz, S., Marshall, S.J., Marshall, G.W.: Mechanical recovery of dentin following remineralization in vitro–an indentation study. J. Biomech. **44**, 176–181 (2011)
128. Veis, A.: Mineral-matrix interactions in bone and dentin. J. Bone. Mineral. Res. **8**(Suppl 2), S493–S497 (1993)
129. Boskey, A.L.: Biomineralization: conflicts, challenges, and opportunities. J. Cell. Biochem. Suppl. **30–31**, 83–91 (1998)
130. Niu, L.N., Zhang, W., Pashley, D.H., Breschi, L., Mao, J., Chen, J.H., et al.: Biomimetic remineralization of dentin. Dent. Mater. **30**, 77–96 (2014)
131. Gower, L.B.: Biomimetic model systems for investigating the amorphous precursor pathway and its role in biomineralization. Chem. Rev. **108**, 4551–4627 (2008)
132. Burwell, A.K., Thula-Mata, T., Gower, L.B., Habelitz, S., Kurylo, M., Ho, S.P., et al.: Functional remineralization of dentin lesions using polymer-induced liquid-precursor process. PLoS ONE **7**, e38852 (2012)
133. Thula-Mata, T., Burwell, A., Gower, L.B., Habeliz, S., Marshall, G.W. : Remineralization of artificial dentin lesions via the Polymer-Induced Liquid-Precursor (PILP) Process. In: Materials Research Society symposia proceedings Materials Research Society, vol. 1355, p. 1114 (2011)
134. Thula, T.T., Svedlund, F., Rodriguez, D.E., Podschun, J., Pendi, L., Gower, L.B.: Mimicking the nanostructure of bone: comparison of polymeric process-directing agents. Polymers **3**, 10–35 (2011)
135. Tay, F.R., Pashley, D.H.: Guided tissue remineralisation of partially demineralised human dentine. Biomaterials **29**, 1127–1137 (2008)
136. Kim, Y.K., Gu, L.S., Bryan, T.E., Kim, J.R., Chen, L., Liu, Y., et al.: Mineralisation of reconstituted collagen using polyvinylphosphonic acid/polyacrylic acid templating matrix-protein analogues in the presence of calcium, phosphate and hydroxyl ions. Biomaterials **31**, 6618–6627 (2010)
137. Paris, S., Bitter, K., Renz, H., Hopfenmuller, W., Meyer-Lueckel, H.: Validation of two dual fluorescence techniques for confocal microscopic visualization of resin penetration into enamel caries lesions. Microsc. Res. Tech. **72**(7), 489–494 (2009)
138. Paris, S., Lausch, J., Selje, T., Dö rfer, C.E., Meyer-Lueckel, H.: Comparison of sealant and infiltrant penetration into pit and fissure caries lesions in vitro. J. Dent. **42**, 432–438 (2014)

Chapter 10
Polymers in Oncology

Manuela Curcio, Ortensia Ilaria Parisi and Francesco Puoci

Abstract Over the past decade nanoparticulate polymers has been established both in pharmaceutical and in clinical research. These kinds of systems are expected to stay in the blood for long time and accumulate in pathological sites with affected and leaky vasculature, such as tumors or inflammatory areas, via the enhanced permeability and retention (EPR) effect, facilitating targeted delivery of specific drugs and genes into poorly accessible areas. Moreover, minimally invasive cancer biomarkers are greatly required for routine clinical practice, for example to deliver hydrophobic imaging agents. Finally, in the last years nano-scaled polymeric systems able to combine both therapy and imaging were designed and developed in a new research field that is called theranostics (or theragnostics). This chapter summarizes the different kinds of polymeric systems used to synthesize therapeutic, diagnostic and theranostic agents in cancer treatment with particular attention to nanoparticulate systems.

Keywords Nanomaterials · Cancer therapy · Diagnostics · Theranostics · Polymer-based materials

M. Curcio (✉) · O.I. Parisi · F. Puoci
Department of Pharmacy, Health and Nutritional Sciences,
University of Calabria, 87036 Rende, CS, Italy
e-mail: manuela.curcio@unical.it

O.I. Parisi
Department of Informatics, Modeling, Electronics and Systems Engineering,
University of Calabria, 87036 Rende, CS, Italy

F. Puoci (ed.), *Advanced Polymers in Medicine*, DOI 10.1007/978-3-319-12478-0_10

Abbreviations

CMV	Cytomegalovirus
DDS	Drug delivery systems
DOTA	1,4,7,10-tetraazacyclododecane-1,4,7,10- tetrakisacetic acid
DOX	Doxorubicin
EGFR	Epidermal growth factor receptor
EPR	Enhanced permeability and retention
FA	Folic acid
GOx	Glucose oxidase
HPMA	N-(2-hydroxypropyl)methacrylamide
LCST	Lower critical solution temperature
LHRH	Luteinizing hormone-releasing hormone
MMA	Methyl methacrylate
MMP	Matrix metalloproteinase
MR	Magnetic resonance
MRI	Magnetic resonance imaging
NBA	O-nitrobenzyl acrylate
NIPAAM	N-isopropylacrylamide
NIR	Near-infrared
NIRF	Near-infrared fluorescence
NIS	Sodium iodide symporter
OEGMA	Oligo(ethylene glycol) monomethyl ether methacrylate
P(AA/MAA)	Poly(acrylic/methacrylic acid)
Pc	Phthalocyanines
PCL	Poly(ε-caprolactone)
PcSi-(OH)(mob)	Monosubstituted phthalocyanine
PDT	Photodynamic therapy
PEG	Poly(ethylene glycol)
PEG-A	Poly(ethyleneglycol)monoacrylate
PEGMEM	Peg methyl ether methacrylate
PEG-PPS-PEG	Peg-β-poly(propylene sulfide)-β–peg
PEGPTMBPEC	Peg-β-poly(2,4,6-trimethoxybenzylidenepentaerythritol carbonate)
PLA	Polylactic acid
PNIPAAM	Poly(N-isopropylacrylamide)
PPI G4	Generation 4 polypropylenimine
PPS	Poly(propylene sulfide)
Ps	Polymersome
PTX	Paclitaxel
QDs	Quantum dots
RF	Radio-frequency
SPIONs	Superparamagnetic iron oxide nanoparticles
TNPs	Theranostic nanoparticles
VP	N-vinyl-2-pyrrolidone

Introduction

Nanomedicine is the term indicating the medical application of nanotechnology. It aims to solve the problems, related to diseases, at the nanoscale where most of the biological molecules exist and operate [1].

The use of nanotechnology has revealed a tremendous potential when applied to cancer treatment, prevention, monitoring and diagnosis [2, 3]. Properly engineered nanosized material can target a tumor, sense pathophysiological defects in tumors, deliver therapeutic drugs, genes, or imaging agents, respond to external triggers to release the agent, and monitor the therapeutic response. Moreover, since these nanoparticles are 100- to 10,000-fold smaller than cancer cells, they can easily pass through cell barriers. Nanoparticulate systems also allow a selective drug targeting to solid tumors, in virtue of the EPR effect (Fig. 10.1).

This occurs because of the abnormalities of tumor vasculature, namely hypervascularization, aberrant vascular architecture, extensive production of vascular permeability factors and lack of lymphatic drainage [4], which stimulate the extravasation of nanoparticles and the accumulation of drugs in the tumor interstitium, improving their therapeutic efficacy and reducing harmful non-specific side effects [5]. In addition, nanosized materials administered intravenously (i.v.) escape renal clearance due to their large size.

When loaded with imaging agents, these kinds of systems offers opportunities to exploit optical imaging or MRI in cancer imaging, and guided hyperthermia therapy.

In literature, several examples of nanoparticulate systems with a variety of composition for cancer treatment are reported, including liposomes, polymeric nanoparticles, gold nanoparticles, paramagnetic nanoparticles, and so on. Among others, polymeric materials offer unique advantages such as the easy preparation,

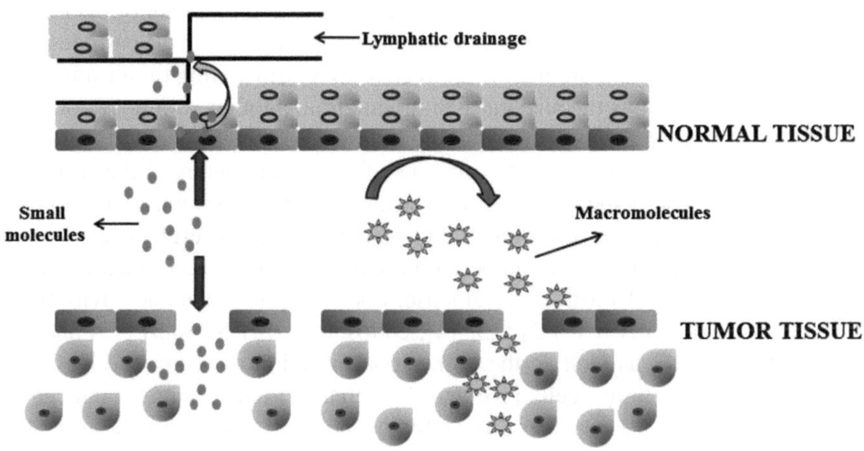

Fig. 10.1 Representation of EPR effect

mechanical strength, versatility and the possibility to easily modulate their physico-chemical properties.

This chapter is focused on the recent advances in the design and synthesis of polymeric nanosized materials in cancer therapy, diagnosis and theranostics.

Nano-sized Polymers in Therapeutic

The combination of controlled release technology and targeted drug delivery may provide a more efficient and less harmful solution to overcome the limitations found in conventional chemotherapy. Recent interest has been focused on developing nanoscale delivery vehicles based on synthetic or natural polymers capable of controlling the release of chemotherapeutic agents directly inside cancer cells [6–8]. Depending from the chemical-physical properties, these systems can release encapsulated drugs through surface or bulk erosion, diffusion, or swelling followed by diffusion, in a time- or condition-dependent manner. Moreover, the release may be constant over a long period, or it may be triggered by the environment or other external events [9]. In general, controlled-release polymer systems can provide drug levels in the optimum range over a longer period of time than other drug delivery methods, thus increasing the efficacy of the drug and maximizing patient compliance.

Generally, the exploited processes to deliver drug-encapsulated in nanoparticles to cancerous tissues are passive and active targeting. As described above, the first approach uses the unique properties of the tumor microenvironment, such as the leaky tumor vasculature, which is highly permeable to macromolecules and the dysfunctional lymphatic drainage system, which results in enhanced fluid retention in the tumor interstitial space [10]. As before explained, the tumor-specific deposition, also known as the EPR effect, occurs as the nanoparticles extravasate out of tumor microvasculature, leading to an accumulation of drugs in the tumor interstitium. The extent of nanoparticles extravasation depends on the size of open inter-endothelial gap junctions and trans-endothelial channels. In general, particles with diameters less than 200 nm are the most effective for extravasating tumor microvasculature [11, 12]. Besides the size particle modulation, another strategy to obtain a passive drug targeting consists in designing engineered materials able to program the drug delivery in response to the variations of some parameters of the surrounding environment. The responsiveness or smartness of these systems refers to their ability to receive, transmit a stimulus, and respond with a useful effect. Typical stimuli are the variations of pH, temperature, redox potential, light, magnetic field, and concentrations of electrolytes or glucose. For example, the acidic environment of cancerous tissues (pH 6.5–7.2) [13, 14], endosomes (pH 5.0–6.5) [15] and lysosomes (pH 4.5–5.0), as well as the higher concentration of redox species in the intracellular space of tumor cells [16] and the enhanced temperature in cancer tissue, can be exploited in anticancer drug delivery and intracellular drug delivery.

The responses of the so-called "smart" drug delivery vehicles can be dissolution/precipitation, swelling/collapsing, hydrophilic/hydrophobic transition, bond cleavage, degradation, drug release, and so on. The second strategy to specifically deliver the drug in tumor site is active targeting. Active tumor targeting is typically achieved by conjugating a targeting molecule, that can recognize and bind to specific ligands that are unique to cancer cells, on the particle surface. In the following sections, the main classes of polymeric nanosized materials to be used in targeted cancer therapy are described.

Dendrimers

Dentritic polymers, or dendrimers, are synthetic, highly branched, spherical, monodispersed macromolecules with an average diameter of 1.5–14.5 nm [17, 18]. The typical dendrimer structure consists of an initiator core, highly branched layers composed of repeating units, and multiple active terminal groups. They can be synthesized with either divergent methods (outward from the core) or convergent methods (inward towards the core). Tomalia was the first to synthesize the 3D (polyamidoamine) dendrimers using divergent methods [19]. These dendrimers contain tertiary amines that allow the binding of a number of molecules. In the convergent approach, established by Frechet [20], the dendrimer results from the generation of monomers added to a main core. Dendrimers have emerged as an important class of drug complexing/encapsulating systems and in literature several examples of the employment of these materials as drug delivery vehicles have been reported, although one limitation lies in the effort of controlling the rate of drug release. The encapsulated, complexed, drugs tend to be released rapidly (before reaching the target site) and in the dendrimer-drug conjugates, it is the chemical linkage that controls the drug release. However, dendrimers offer several advantages as drug carriers targeting cancer. One major advantage is their surface functionality providing the selective coupling of imaging agents, targeting ligands and/or other components to increase tumor specificity [1]. In a work of 2002, Henrik et al. [21] proposed biodegradable polyester dendrimers based on 2,2-bis(hydroxymethyl)-propanoic acid monomers for intracellular release of DOX after hydrolysis of the hydrazone linkage. Moreover, DOX was conjugated to a biodegradable dendrimer with optimized blood circulation time through the careful design of size and molecular architecture Specifically, the DOX-dendrimer controlled drug-loading through multiple attachment sites, solubility through PEGylation, and drug release through the use of pH-sensitive hydrazone dendrimer linkages. In culture, DOX dendrimers were N10 times less toxic than free DOX toward colon carcinoma cells. Upon intravenous administration to tumor bearing mice, tumor uptake of DOX-dendrimers was nine-fold higher than intravenous free DOX and caused complete tumor regression and 100 % survival of the mice after 60 days [22].

The promising properties of polyester dendrimers as a drug delivery system has led to further studies based on tunable architectures and molecular weights to optimize tumor accumulation [23, 24].

Nanogels

Nanogels are nanosized hydrogel particles formed by physical or chemical cross-linked polymer networks. The main characteristic of these systems consists in their ability to retain considerable amount of water, but also the biocompatibility, the stability in aqueous media and the versatility in release drugs in a controlled manner are common properties of this class of materials. Nanogels made from synthetic polymers offer well-defined morphologies that can be customized to gel networks with biocompatible and degradable properties. Bisht et al. [25] synthesized polymeric nanoparticle encapsulated formulation of curcumin—nanocurcumin—utilizing the micellar aggregates of cross-linked and random copolymers of NIPAAM, with VP and PEG-A. Further, the mechanism of action of nanocurcumin on pancreatic cancer cells mirrors that of free curcumin, including induction of apoptosis, blockade of nuclear factor kappa B activation, and downregulation of pro-inflammatory cytokines (i.e. IL-6, IL-8 and TNF-α). Nanocurcumin provides an opportunity to expand the clinical repertoire of this efficacious agent by enabling soluble dispersion.

Nanogel networks formed of stimuli responsive units extensively regulate the drug release profile and have found large application in delivery of anticancer drugs. Nanogels generated with polymer chains containing ionizable repeating groups are suitable for pH-dependant release [26]. The construction of nanogel networks with P(AA/MAA) units and PNIPAAM chains underlies a rapid increase in the hydrophilicity LCST of the copolymer at all the pH ranges, particularly pH < 5 [27]. Polyampholytic or zwitterionic polymeric gel particles have also received priority owing to their interior structural features. These features enable a response under all pH conditions owing to their effectiveness at a wide range of isoelectric points [28]. MMA diethyl acrylate-diethy phthalate nanogels stabilized by PEGMEM resulted in varied sizes under different pH conditions, with size following an order of pH $9 > 2 > 5$ [29].

Polymeric Micelles

Polymeric micelles result from the auto assembly of di-block amphiphilic copolymers and are composed of two separated functional segments: inner core and outer shell [30]. The outer shell controls the in vivo pharmacokinetic behavior, while the inner core is responsible for drug loading capacity, stability and drug release behavior. The suitable PM size, too large for extravasation from normal vessel walls and renal excretion, and too small for extravasation from tumor blood vessels, combined with the pathophysiological characteristics of solid tumor tissues, hypervascularity, incomplete vascular architecture, secretion of vascular permeability factors and absence of effective lymphatic drainage leads to EPR effect in solid tumors [4, 31] and warrants the passive targeting of these systems.

Biocompatible, targeted sterically stabilized micelles have been used as nanocarriers for camptothecin, a topoisomerase I inhibitor used in cancer therapy.

Moreover, stealth micelle formulations have stabilizing PEG coronas to minimize opsonization of the micelles and maximize serum half-life. Currently, SP1049C, NK911, and Genexol-PM have been approved for clinical use [32]. SP1049C is formulated as DOX-encapsulated pluronic micelles. NK911 is DOX-encapsulated micelles from a copolymer of PEG-DOX-conjugated poly(aspartic acid), and Genexol-PM is a paclitaxel-encapsulated PEG-PLA micelle formulation. Polymer micelles have several advantages over other drug delivery systems, including increased drug solubility, prolonged circulation half-life, selective accumulation at tumor sites, and lower toxicity.

Polymersomes

Ps are vesicular systems made from synthetic amphiphilic block copolymers [33, 34] that are organized to form hollow spheres containing an aqueous solution in the core surrounded by a bi-layer membrane. The bi-layer membrane is composed of hydrated hydrophilic coronas both at the inside and outside of the hydrophobic middle part of the membrane separating and protecting the fluidic core from the outside medium. Compared to polymeric micelles, the main advantages of these systems is the possibility to load hydrophilic, hydrophobic or amphiphilic compounds, exploiting the aqueous core or the membrane bilayers. The aqueous core can be utilized for the encapsulation of therapeutic molecules such as drugs, enzymes, other proteins and peptides, and DNA and RNA fragments [35–37]. On the other hand, the membrane can be considered as a reservoir system for both hydrophobic [38, 39], and amphiphilic (i.e. octadecyl rhodamine B [40, 41]) molecules similar to cell membranes, which incorporate cholesterol and membrane proteins.

These properties make polymersomes very attractive materials for various applications in drug delivery, biomedical imaging and diagnostics [42].

In principle, drug release from Ps is governed by the diffusion of the drug through the membrane [43], but many examples of smart Ps, in which the physical-chemical properties of the starting block copolymers are modulated to respond to external stimuli (i.e. pH, temperature, redox conditions, light, magnetic field, ionic strength and concentration of glucose), are reported in literature and proposed in cancer therapy.

Ps based on PEGPTMBPEC were reported by Chen et al. and in vitro studies demonstrated that the release of paclitaxel as well as DOX from these Ps was faster at mildly acidic conditions than at physiological pH due to the faster degradation of PTMBPEC at mildly acidic conditions [39].

The occurrence of oxidation-reduction (redox) reactions in the body has also been reported as a means to control spatial drug release in the body [44, 45]. Oxidative conditions exist in extracellular fluids and inflamed or tumor tissues, while intracellular compartments are known to be reductive [46, 47]. Hubbell and co-workers developed oxidation responsive Ps based on PEG-PPS-PEG [48]. The hydrophobic PPS was oxidized and transformed within 2 h into hydrophilic poly(sulfoxides) and poly(sulfones) upon exposure to hydrogen peroxide in the (GOx)/glucose/oxygen system, leading to destabilization of the vesicular structure. Reduction-sensitive disulfide block copolymer, PEG-SS-PPS was used to prepare Ps that can protect therapeutics in the extracellular environment but releasing their contents within the early endosome when the Ps are taken up by cells [49].

Polymeric Nanoparticles in Diagnostic

The conventional imaging agents currently used in clinics for diagnosis suffer from disadvantages including the non-specificity, in vivo instability and toxicity. For example, imaging molecules such as the fluorophores compounds, including blue, green, or red fluorescence dyes with visible range (400–600 nm), have significant limitations such as tissue auto-fluorescence and light absorbing components [hemoglobin, deoxyhemoglobin (max. abs. 560 nm), and water] [50].

Consequently, delivery of low concentrations of contrast agents to region of interest affects image quality. In addition, they have limited chemical modification sites without significantly changing their biological activities. Due to their enormous versatility, nanoparticulate systems offer multifunctional capabilities to encapsulate and transport high concentrations of imaging probes selectively to diseased site inside the body.

Polymer-based imaging probes have a large surface areas (easy modification with a wide range of imaging moieties), improved plasma half-lives and stability, less toxicity, and improved targeting.

They help the detection process of tumor cells by concentrating and protecting the marker from degradation, in order obtain a more sensitive analysis.

Currently, the modalities available for imaging of nanoparticles include optical imaging, MRI, nuclear imaging, computed tomography, and ultrasound [51].

Optical imaging, which includes fluorescence and bioluminescence detection, and radionucleotide-based imaging are both very sensitive but typically have a resolution greater than several millimeters. This can be limiting, especially in small animal models in which higher resolution is more informative. Optical imaging is also restricted to a depth of only several centimeters, and quantification of the signal can be problematical due to significant tissue absorption of the signal. By contrast, MRI and computer tomography are much less sensitive but demonstrate a resolution less than 1 mm. MRI can image deep tissues and has the added advantage of not exposing patients to radiation. However, data acquisition is slow compared with other approaches [52].

For each of these imaging modalities, novel nanoparticles have been developed that can enhance tissue contrast or can identify specific biological changes.

Streptavidin-coated fluorescent polystyrene nanospheres [Fluospheres® (green fluores cence) and TransFluospheres® (red fluorescence)] were used in single color flow cytometry to detect the EGFR on A431 cells (human epidermoid carcinoma cells) [53]. The results showed that the fluorescent nanospheres provided a sensitivity 25-fold that of the conjugate streptavidin–fluorescein. The encapsulation of fluorescent markers resulted in objects that were brighter and more concentrated than when simple conjugates of single dyes were used. The same fluorescent nanoparticles were used in combination with R-Phycoerythrin (R-PE, reagent for flow cytometry) in multicolor flow cytometry, enabling the concomitant detection of the CD3 and CD4 receptors on JURKAT cells (human acute T-cell leukemia cells) [53].

Another approach consists in functionalizing nanoparticles with target-specific biomolecules for controlling the navigation under in vivo conditions.

Weissleder and colleagues [54] developed a method to image tumor-associated lysosomal protease activity in a xenograft mouse model in vivo using autoquenched NIRF probes. NIRF probes were bound to a long circulating graft copolymer consisting of poly-L-lysine and methoxypolyethylene glycol succinate. Following intravenous injection, the NIRF probe carrier accumulated in solid tumors due to its long circulation time and leakage through tumor neovasculature.

Moreover, multimodal polymeric micelles have been developed for the visualization of cancer cells, known to overexpress a specific receptor, by both optical and nuclear techniques [55]. To achieve active targeting, specific peptide sequences were conjugated to nanoparticles, increasing the specificity of tumor imaging [56].

Moreover, Yang et al. [57] developed PEG-coated micelles with embedded near-infrared fluorescent dye for dual optical and nuclear imaging applications, showing a prolonged blood residence and effective accumulation inside solid tumors in mice. In another work, polymeric NPs containing the fluorogenic probe Cy5.5 and the dark quencher BHQ-312, linked together by a peptide sequence specific for a MMP for in vivo tumor imaging were developed by Lee and coworkers [58]. MMPs are a family of zinc-dependent proteins involved in inflammatory diseases and cancer progression. When these NPs are exposed to the specific MMP, fluorescence emission of Cy5.5 occurs, due to the enzymatic cleavage of the peptide bond between Cy5.5 and the quencher. The specificity of tumor imaging is usually enhanced by the conjugation of NPs with specific antibodies. Other moieties used in specific targeting include folic acid [59–61], peptides [62, 63] and cell ligands [64].

Engineered Polymers in Theranostic

Conventional cancer chemotherapy presents relevant limitations associated with the non-selectivity of cytotoxic drugs, their narrow therapeutic indices and limited cellular penetration. Furthermore, during the anticancer treatment, the real-time evaluation of the therapeutic efficacy is of considerable importance in the aim to evaluate patient response.

A possible interdisciplinary approach to overcome these drawbacks is the development of innovative therapeutic strategies involving the use of tumor-targeted nanodevices able to promote specific drug accumulation at the pathological site, but also able to act as diagnostic molecular imaging agents. In this context lies *Theranostics* also called theragnostics, which is an innovative and emerging treatment strategy that combines disease diagnosis with therapy and describes any material for this kind of applications. Theranostic approaches can involve the coupling of imaging with several types of therapy leading to imaging-guided drug delivery, but also image-guided gene delivery, photodynamic therapy, hyperthermia and radiation therapy [65]. *Theranostic agents* are characterized by the presence of both diagnostic and therapeutic functions within a single system that enables both diagnosis and targeted therapy at the same time, but also the monitoring of the therapeutic response to the treatment increasing the drug efficacy and safety.

In the last decades, the development of theranostic nanoparticles has received considerable attention due to their ability to be selectively delivered to tumors by passive or active targeting [66]. These TNPs, indeed, are designed for both cancer imaging (diagnosis) and treatment (i.e. chemotherapy or gene therapy).

A specific type of TNPs is the "activation" theranostic nanoparticles which are monitored for their kinetics in tumors. When imaging shows maximum nanoparticle accumulation in the tumor site, a physical source is applied in order to allow the burst release of the anticancer agent which is delivered rapidly and locally [1].

Different types of materials are used in the aim to prepare theranostic agents and, among them, imaging ones include photoluminescent mostly fuorescent groups, quantum dots [67], magnetic compounds and contrast agents for magnetic resonance imaging [68], while common therapeutic approaches are drug delivery [69], gene delivery [70], photodynamic therapy [71], hyperthermia and radiation therapy [71].

In this context, the present book chapter aims to focus the attention on *polymer-based materials for theranostics*.

A drug delivery system is defined as a device that enables the introduction of a therapeutic agent in the body and improves its efficacy and safety, with a reduction of the side effects, by controlling the rate, the time and the place of release. Polymeric nanoparticles are widely employed as effective DDS due to their ease of processing and the possibility to control their chemical and physical properties via molecular synthesis. Furthermore, the ability of nano-sized particles to preferentially accumulate in tumor tissues provides a platform for improved tumor diagnostics [50]. Therefore, by combining targeted delivery with advanced imaging technologies, it is possible to develop new polymer-based systems able to diagnose and treat cancer at the same time.

A polymer-based material for theranostics should consist of four main components (Fig. 10.2) [66]:

- the *polymeric component*, which offers stability, biocompatibility, solubility and biodegradability;
- the *imaging component*, such as quantum dots, magnetic nanoparticles or contrast agent;
- the *therapeutic component*, that carries a drug, a gene or provokes therapy for example a photosensitiser that is used for photodynamic therapy;
- the specific *targeting agent*, usually an antibody or peptide.

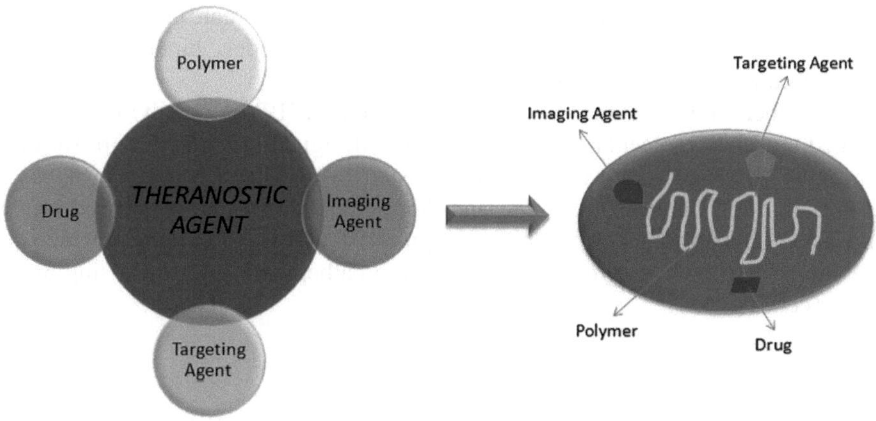

Fig. 10.2 Schematic representation of a theranostic agent and its main components

Image-guided drug delivery allows to monitor the biodistribution of the drug at real time and at the target site, quantify the drug release and evaluate the drug efficacy [69] while in image-guided gene therapy the incorporation of an imaging agent or labelled polymer or gene on the polyplex offers the ability to monitor the complex through the transfection/gene delivery procedure.

Polymer-Drug Conjugates

Polymer-drug conjugates offer several advantages such as increased circulations times, decreased toxicity, passive tumor targeting and incorporation of different functionalities including active targeting moieties or contrast agents [72–74].

N-(2-hydroxypropyl)methacrylamide is widely employed to prepare polymer-drug conjugates due to its non-toxicity, non-immunogenicity and stability in systemic circulation [75, 76] and several contrast agents have been associated with HPMA copolymer conjugates for in vitro and in vivo molecular imaging. Two different approaches are employed in order to functionalize HPMA copolymers with diagnostic and therapeutic moieties including copolymerization and chemical conjugation. The first one may be the preferred conjugation method due to the flexibility to conjugate single or multimodal diagnostic agents and chemotherapeutic drugs, while the other one allows the direct conjugation of the contrast agents and therapeutics to the copolymer.

Paramagnetically labeled HPMA copolymer conjugates were synthesized by free radical copolymerization of HPMA with monomers containing a chelating ligand, followed by complexation with $Gd(OAc)_3$ [77], in the aim to study a non-invasive method of using contrast enhanced MRI to visualize the real-time pharmacokinetics, biodistribution and tumor accumulation of copolymer conjugates in tumor-bearing mice. Contrast enhanced MRI resulted in a real-time, three-dimensional visualization of blood circulation, pharmacokinetics, biodistribution and tumor accumulation of the conjugates.

In another study, polymeric nanocarriers based on HPMA copolymer and conjugated with low molecular weight drugs were designed in order to improve their efficacy [78]. The diagnostic system consisted of self-quenched Cy5 (SQ-Cy5) as near-infrared fluorescence probe and the therapeutic system was based on the anticancer agent paclitaxel. HPMA copolymer-PTX/SQ-Cy5 systems enable site-specific release upon enzymatic degradation in cathepsin B-overexpressing breast cancer cells.

Dendrimers

Among polymeric architectures, dendrimers are a unique class of repeatedly branched polymeric macromolecules characterized by three main parts including a core, an inner shell and an outer shell. They are versatile polymeric particles which can be designed for variable functionality for each of these parts and to feature controlled properties such as solubility and thermal stability. Due to the presence of many chain-ends and, therefore, improved reactivity properties compared to traditional linear polymers [79], dendrimers could undergo several chemical modifications for particular applications including imaging modalities. Furthermore, their surface functionalities provide the selective coupling of imaging agents, targeting ligands and/or other components to increase tumour specificity [1]. This kind of materials has been widely studied both in cancer therapy and diagnosis for example for photodynamic therapy (activation therapies) [80] and hyperthermia therapies using gold nanoparticles [81].

Gadolinium has been complexed with dendrimers and it was observed that this complex enhanced conventional MR images in a dendrimer molecular weight dependent way and substantially better, compared with conventional diethylenetriaminepentaacetic acid Gd (III) chelates [82].

Phthalocyanines have promising potential as near-infrared theranostic agents for fluorescence image-guided drug delivery and treatment of tumors by photodynamic therapy. However, clinical application of phthalocyanines is limited by their poor water solubility and insufficient selectivity for cancer cells. In the aim to overcome these drawbacks, a dendrimer-based theranostic platform for tumor-targeted delivery of phthalocyanines was developed by the modification of the Pc molecule with a hydrophobic linker which enhances physical encapsulation of the hydrophobic drug into a generation 4 polypropylenimine dendrimer (Fig. 10.3) [83].

The surface of the resulting Pc–PPIG4 complexes was modified with poly(ethylene glycol) and luteinizing hormone-releasing hormone peptide in order to improve biocompatibility and tumor-targeted delivery, respectively. The performed imaging experiments showed that the LHRH targeted nanocarrier was capable of an efficient internalization into cancer cells. Furthermore, the prepared formulation exhibited

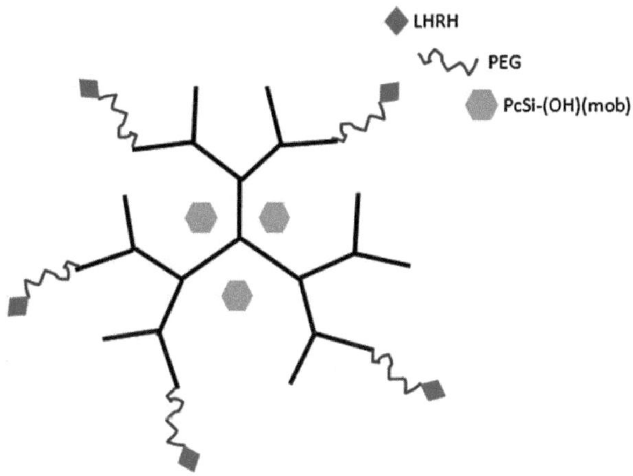

Fig. 10.3 Schematic representation of theranostic agent based on phthalocyanine-loaded dendrimer

low dark cytotoxicity (IC50 = 28 μg/mL) while light irradiation of the cancer cells transfected with the prepared theranostic agents resulted in significant PDT effects (IC50 = 0.9 μg/mL). The obtained results demonstrated the potential application of the developed dendrimer-based nanocarrier as an efficient NIR theranostic agent.

The main limitations of adenovirus-mediated gene therapy are high prevalence of neutralizing antibodies, widespread expression of the coxsackie-adenovirus receptor and adenovirus sequestration by the liver. Grünwald et al. [84] used the sodium iodide symporter as a theranostic gene in the aim to investigate whether coating of adenovirus with synthetic dendrimers could be useful to develop adenoviral vectors for combination of systemic oncolytic virotherapy and NIS-mediated radiotherapy. For this purpose, replication-deficient (Ad5-CMV/NIS) and replication-selective (Ad5-E1/AFP-E3/NIS) adenovirus serotype 5 carrying the hNIS gene were coated with poly(amidoamine) dendrimers generation 5. The obtained results showed efficient liver detargeting and tumor retargeting of adenoviral vectors after coating with synthetic dendrimers representing a promising strategy for systemic NIS gene therapy. Furthermore, NIS could work as a theranostic gene allowing the noninvasive imaging of NIS expression by ^{123}I scintigraphy.

Hydrogels

Thermoresponsive hydrogels are characterized by the ability to transition between hydrophilic and hydrophobic states as a function of temperature. By coupling the temperature sensitivity with the ability to quickly respond to an external magnetic field, it is possible to develop novel hydrogels to be employed as platform systems for long-term MR theragnosis.

A long-term theranostic hydrogel system for solid tumors was prepared via simple physical mixing, which consisted of three main parts including the thermosensitive/biodegradable poly(organophosphazene) hydrogel, PEGylated cobalt ferrite nanoparticles and the anticancer drug paclitaxel [85]. It was observed that the theranostic hydrogel gradually degraded over 28 days, PTX was released out from the polymeric matrix over the same period in vitro and the in vivo efficacy of long-term MR theragnosis was estimated successfully over 3 weeks by using high field (4.7 T) animal MRI and solid tumor-bearing mice. Based on these results, the synthesized hydrogel system showed adequate properties to be used as biodegradable platform for long-term MR theragnosis.

Another study reports on the development of spherically shaped thermoresponsive magnetic hydrogels (~200 nm) based on poly(N-isopropylacrylamide) encapsulation of Fe_3O_4 magnetic nanostructures for theranostic application [86]. The synthesized system demonstrated multimodal imaging and remote RF-triggered drug release leading to cell death for cancer simultaneous therapy and diagnostic application.

A stable injectable magnetic nanoparticle incorporated hydrogel system was prepared as an alternative for the long-term drug release and diagnosis to the cancer patients [87]. The injectable hydrogel system consisted of aminated guar gum, DOX and iron oxide-zinc sulphide core-shell nanoparticles as biodegradable polymer and gelling agent, anticancer drug and imaging agent, respectively. The in vitro drug releasing tendency of DOX is seen up to 21st day of incubation demonstrating the sustained delivery over long period. Furthermore, studies reveal that the core-shell nanoparticles can be released slowly from the hydrogel to provide the healing and diagnosis of the solid tumor. Based on these results, the prepared thermoresponsive injectable hydrogel system has promising applications such as sustained drug release, hyperthermia and theranostic for the solid tumor treatment.

Polymeric Micelles

Currently, polymeric micelles are widely accepted as drug and imaging agent delivery systems due to their ease of formation, stability, ability to encapsulate hydrophobic molecules and therapeutic success in preclinical and clinical studies [88].

Theranostic phospholipid based polymeric micelles were synthesized for the encapsulation of the anticancer drug DOX and CdSe quantum dots together (Fig. 10.4) [89].

DOX and QDs were co-encapsulated into the hydrophobic core of the micelles, the release kinetics was carried out in order to confirm the sustained release of the DOX and the therapeutic efficacy of the obtained micellar formulation was tested in vitro using HeLa cell line. In the aim to evaluate the cellular uptake behavior of the micelles, in vitro imaging studies were also performed. The results indicated the sustained release of the drug and the potential of these micellar systems as efficient optical fluorescence imaging and controlled drug delivery systems.

In another work, Li et al. [90] prepared UV irradiation-responsive amphiphilic diblock copolymer micelles exhibiting light-triggered hydrophobic-hydrophilic

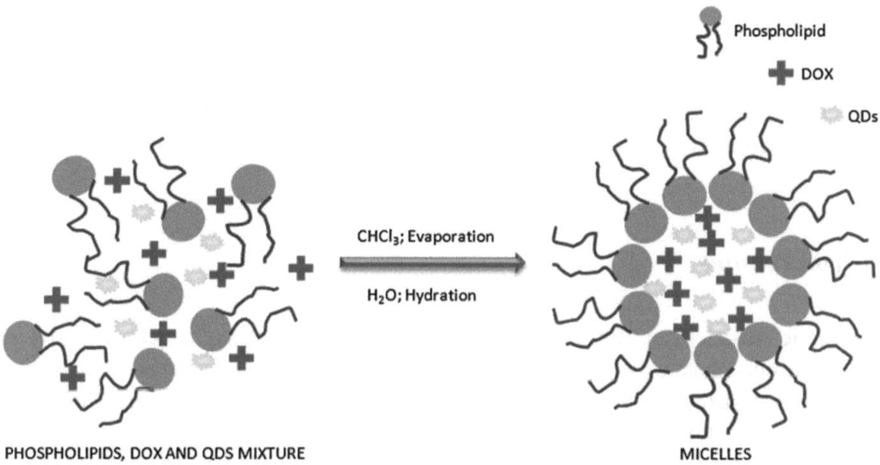

Fig. 10.4 Schematic representation of the synthetic strategy of the phospholipid micelles encapsulating DOX and QDs

transition within micellar cores and the concomitant enhancement of magnetic resonance imaging contrast performance and of the release rate of encapsulated hydrophobic drugs. POEGMA-b-P(NIPAAM-co-NBA-co-Gd) diblock copolymer covalently labeled with Gd^{3+} complex (Gd) in the light-responsive block was synthesized at first, then the obtained amphiphilic diblock copolymer spontaneously self-assembled in aqueous solution into micellar nanoparticles which can physically encapsulate DOX as a model chemotherapeutic drug. Upon UV irradiation, the photocleavage of hydrophobic NBA moieties led to a hydrophobic-hydrophilic transition within micellar cores, triggering micelle microstructural changes and core swelling. During this process, the microenvironment surrounding Gd^{3+} complexes was subjected to a transition from being hydrophobic to hydrophilic, leading to the enhancement of MR imaging contrast performance and of the drug release rate. The reported approach of light-triggered co-enhancement of MR imaging contrast performance and drug release profiles represents an innovative strategy for the preparation of smart polymeric theranostic nanocarriers.

In another study, two types of amphiphilic diblock copolymers, PCL-*b*-P(OEGMA-FA) and PCL-*b*-P(OEGMA-Gd) were synthesized via the combination of atom transfer radical polymerization, ring-opening polymerization and "click" post-functionalization in the aim to prepare mixed diblock copolymer micelles able to act as an integrated multifunctional platform for the cancer cell-targeted delivery of chemotherapeutic drugs and magnetic resonance imaging contrast enhancement [91]. Mixed micelles co-assembled from PCL-*b*-P(OEGMA-FA) and PCL-*b*-P(OEGMA-Gd) possess hydrophobic PCL cores for loading chemotherapeutic drugs and hydrophilic POEGMA outer coronas functionalized with folic acid and DOTA-Gd moieties for synergistic functions of targeted delivery and MR imaging contrast enhancement. An anticancer drug, such as paclitaxel, was physically encapsulated into mixed polymeric micelles in order to perform in vitro drug release measurements. The obtained results indicated that the synthesized mixed micellar nanocarriers were characterized by synergistically integrated functions of cancer-targeted drug delivery, controlled release and MR imaging contrast enhancement confirming their potential application as a novel theranostic platforms.

Polymersomes

Polymeric vesicles, or polymersomes, are versatile vehicles characterized by the ability to encapsulate both hydrophobic and hydrophilic molecules and co-deliver therapeutic and diagnostic agents at the same time. These vesicular structures offer improved control over the membrane thickness and stability and are able to efficiently load drugs and imaging agents via covalent or non-covalent forces, incorporate targeting strategies, prolong systemic circulation and increase tumor accumulation.

Chiang et al. [92] developed a novel and stable tumor-targeting polymersome carrier system for improved cancer theranosis. The DOX-loaded magnetic polymersomes were prepared by the self-assembly of lipid-containing copolymer, poly(acrylic acid-co-distearin acrylate) in aqueous solution containing citric acid-coated superparamagnetic iron oxide nanoparticles and followed by DOX loading via electrostatic attraction. In order to further functionalize these artificial vesicles, chitosan and poly(γ-glutamic acid-co-γ-glutamyl oxysuccinimide)-g-poly(ethyleneglycol)-folate were deposited in sequence onto the outer surfaces of SPION/DOX-loaded polymersomes to form the layered polyelectrolyte gels via electrostatic interactions and in situ covalent crosslinking. When these theranostic polymersomes were effectively internalized by HeLa cells, they exhibited several interesting characteristics including: highly stable colloidal structure against large volume dilution and protein adsorption, rapid drug release in the intracellular acidic endosomes/lysosomes and/or under high frequency magnetic fields, superior anticancer efficacy by the combined active tumor-targeting via FA receptor-mediated endocytosis and magneto-thermo-chemotherapy and enhanced MRI sensitivity. The combined effects of both pH and magnetic hyperthermia-triggered drug release and thermo-therapy has led to a higher cytotoxicity than the treatment by DOX alone. The obtained results confirmed the potential application of this kind of systems as an advanced cancer theranostic nanodevice.

In another study, the development of polymersomes based on poly(trimethylene carbonate)-block-poly(L-glutamic acid) copolymer and able to encapsulate up to 6 % (w/w) of DOX together with 30 % (w/w) of superparamagnetic iron oxide nanoparticles was reported [93]. The prepared vesicular structures, containing SPIONs and DOX and fluorescently labeled with fluorescein isothiocyanate showed an increase of drug release when the sample was exposed to the high frequency alternating magnetic field.

Kokkoli et al. [94] reported on the use of peptide-functionalized polymersomes composed of poly(1,2-butadiene)-b-poly(ethylene oxide) for siRNA delivery.

The prepared polymeric vesicles were, indeed, functionalized with peptide targeting ligands in the aim to enhance cellular uptake and confer an active targeting modality to the vesicles. The resulted polyplex was followed in vitro by monitoring the encapsulated carboxyfluorescein and the obtained results confirmed that the prepared polymersomes represent a promising first generation model system for targeted delivery of siRNA.

Conclusions

Nanomedicine is the term indicating the medical application of nanotechnology which is the engineering of functional systems at the molecular scale.

Nowadays, nanosized materials are attracting considerable attention and significant research interest due to their potential applications in fields including cancer treatment, prevention, monitoring and diagnosis.

The present book chapter aims to focus the attention on polymer-based materials which represent a reliable and inexpensive substrate to synthesize therapeutic and diagnostic agents in cancer treatment. Furthermore, polymeric materials offer more functionalities where specific targeting moieties and therapeutic and imaging components can be attached for simultaneous targeted therapy and imaging providing innovative theranostic agents characterized by great potential in monitoring and treatment of cancer.

References

1. Wang, M., Thanou, M.: Targeting nanoparticles to cancer. Pharmacol. Res. **62**, 90–99 (2010)
2. Ferrari, M.: Cancer nanotechnology: opportunities and challenges. Nat. Rev. Cancer **5**, 161–171 (2005)
3. Srinivas, P.R., Barker, P., Srivastava, S.: Nanotechnology in early detection of cancer. Lab. Investig. **82**, 657–662 (2002)
4. Maeda, H., Wu, J., Sawa, T., Matsumura, Y., Hor, K.: Tumor vascular permeability and the EPR effect in macromolecular therapeutics: a review. J. Controlled Release **65**, 271–284 (2000)
5. Greish, K.: Enhanced permeability and retention (EPR) effect for anticancer nanomedicine drug targeting. Methods Mol. Biol. **624**, 25–37 (2010)
6. Dong, Y.C., Feng, S.S.: Nanoparticles of montmorillonite (mmt)/poly (d,l-lactide-co-glycolide) (plga) for oral delivery of anticancer drugs. Biomaterials **26**, 6068–6076 (2005)
7. Chawla, J.S., Amiji, M.M.: Biodegradable poly (ε-caprolactone) nanoparticles for tumor-targeted delivery of tamoxifen. Int. J. Pharm. **249**, 127–138 (2002)
8. Farokhzad, O.C., Langer, R.: Nanomedicine: developing smarter therapeutic and diagnostic modalities. Adv. Drug Delivery Rev. **58**, 1456–1459 (2006)
9. Langer, R., Tirrell, D.A.: Designing materials for biology and medicine. Nature **428**, 487 (2004)
10. Matsumura, Y., Maeda, H.: A new concept for macromolecular therapeutics in cancer chemotherapy: mechanism of tumoritropic accumulation of proteins and the antitumor agent SMANCS. Cancer Res. **46**, 6387–6392 (1986)

11. Kong, G., Braun, R.D., Dewhirst, M.W.: Hyperthermia enables tumor-specific nanoparticle delivery: effect of particle size. Cancer Res. **60**, 4440–4445 (2000)
12. Yuan, F., Leunig, M., Huang, S.K., Berk, D.A., Papahadjopoulos, D., Jain, R.K.: Microvascular permeability and interstitial penetration of sterically stabilized (stealth) liposomes in a human tumor xenograft. Cancer Res. **54**, 3352–3356 (1994)
13. Engin, K., Leeper, D.B., Cater, J.R., Thistlethwaite, A.J., Tupchong, L., Mcfarlane, J.D.: Extracellular pH distribution in human tumours. Int. J. Hyperthermia **11**, 211–216 (1995)
14. Thistlethwaite, A.J., Leeper, D.B., Moylan, D.J., Nerlinger, R.E.: pH distribution in human tumors. Int. J. Radiat. Oncol. Biol. Phys. **11**, 1647–1652 (1985)
15. Sun, H.H., Andresen, T.L., Benjaminsen, R.V., Almdal, K.: Polymeric nanosensors for measuring the full dynamic ph range of endosomes and lysosomes in mammalian cells. J. Biomed. Nanotechnol. **5**, 676–682 (2009)
16. Schafer, F.Q., Buettner, G.R.: Redox state of the cell as viewed through the glutathione disulfide/glutathione couple. Free Radic. Biol. Med. **30**, 1191–1212 (2001)
17. Andresen, T.L., Jensen, S.S., Jørgensen, K.: Advanced strategies in liposomal cancer therapy: problems and prospects of active and human specific drug release. Prog. Lipid Res. **44**, 68–97 (2005)
18. Patri, A.K., Majoros, I.J., Baker, J.R.: Dendritic polymer macromolecular carriers for drug delivery. Curr. Opin. Chem. Biol. **6**, 466–471 (2002)
19. Tomalia, D.A., Uppuluri, S., Swanson, D.R., Brothers, H.M., Piehler, L.T., Li, J., Meier, D.J., Hagnauer, G.L., Balogh, L.: Dendritic macromolecules: a fourth major class of polymer architecture—new properties driven by architecture. Mater. Res. Soc. Symp. P **543**, 289–298 (1999)
20. Hawker, C.J., Frechet, J.M.J.: Preparation of polymers with controlled molecular architecture. a new convergent approach to dendritic macromolecules. J. Am. Chem. Soc. **112**, 7638–7647 (1990)
21. Ihre, H.R., Padilla De Jesús, O.L., Szoka, F.C., Fréchet, J.M.: Polyester dentritic systems for drug delivery applications: design, synthesis and characterization. Bioconjugate Chem. **13**, 443–452 (2002)
22. Lee, C.C., Gillies, E.R., Fox, M.E., Guillaudeu, S.J., Fréchet, J.M., Dy, E.E., Szoka, F.C.: A single dose of doxorubicin-functionalized bow-tie dendrimer cures mice bearing C-26 colon carcinomas. Proc. Natl. Acad. Sci. U.S.A. **103**, 16649–16654 (2006)
23. Gillies, E.R., Dy, E., Fréchet, J.M.J., Szoka, F.C.: Biological evaluation of polyester dendrimers: poly(ethylene oxide) "bow-tie" hybrids with tunable molecular weight and architecture. Mol. Pharm. **2**, 129–138 (2005)
24. Gillies, E.R., Fréchet, J.M.J.: Designing macromolecules for therapeutic applications polyester dendrimer-poly(ethylene oxide) "bow-tie" hybrids with tunable molecular weight and architecture. J. Am. Chem. Soc. **124**, 14137–14146 (2002)
25. Bisht, S., Feldmann, G., Soni, S., Ravi, R., Karikar, C., Maitra, A., Maitra, A.: Polymeric nanoparticle-encapsulated curcumin ("nanocurcumin"): a novel strategy for human cancer therapy. J. Nanobiotech. **5**, 3 (2007)
26. Siegel, R.A.: Hydrophobic weak polyelectrolyte gels: studies of swelling equilibria and kinetics. Adv. Polym. Sci. **109**, 233–267 (1993)
27. Das, M., Mardyani, S., Chan, W.C.W., Kumacheva, E.: Biofunctionalized pH-responsive microgel for cancer cell targeting. Adv. Mater. **18**, 80–83 (2006)
28. Kihara, N., Adachi, Y., Nakao, K., Fukutomi, T.: Reaction of methyl thioglycolate with chloromethylstyrene microgel: preparation of core–shell-type microgel by chemical modification. J. Appl. Polym. Sci. **69**, 1863–1873 (1998)
29. Beng, H.T., Palaniswamy, R., Kam, C.T.: Poly(L-lysine-g-ethylene glycol)/oligo(lactic acid)-b-pluronic F127-b-oligo(lactic acid) nanogels. Macromol. Rapid Commun. **27**, 522–528 (2006)
30. Gong, J., Chen, M., Zheng, Y., Wang, S., Wang, Y.: Polymeric micelles drug delivery system in oncology. J. Controlled Release **159**, 312–323 (2012)
31. Torchilin, V.: Tumor delivery of macromolecular drugs based on the EPR effect. Adv. Drug Deliv. Rev. **63**, 131–135 (2011)

32. Sutton, D., Nasongkla, N., Blanco, E., Gao, J.: Functionalized micellar systems for cancer targeted drug delivery. Pharm. Res. **24**, 1029–1046 (2007)
33. Du, J.Z., O'Reilly, R.K.: Advances and challenges insmart and functional polymer vesicles. Soft Matter **5**, 3544–3561 (2009)
34. Meng, F., Zhong, Z.: Polymersomes spanning from nano- to microscales: advanced vehicles for controlled drug delivery and robust vesicles for virus and cell mimicking. J. Phys. Chem. Lett. **2**, 1533–1539 (2011)
35. Pangburn, T.O., Petersen, M.A., Waybrant, B., Adil, M.M., Kokkoli, E.: Peptide- and aptamer-functionalized nanovectors for targeted delivery of therapeutics. J. Biomech. Eng. Trans. ASME **131**, 1–20 (2009)
36. Kim, K.T., Meeuwissen, S.A., Nolte, R.J.M., van Hest, J.C.M.: Smart nanocontainers and nanoreactors. Nanoscale **2**, 844–858 (2010)
37. Liu, G., Ma, S., Li, S., Cheng, R., Meng, Liu H., Zhong, Z.: The highly efficient delivery of exogenous proteins into cells mediated by biodegradable chimaeric polymersome. Biomaterials **31**, 7575–7585 (2010)
38. Ahmed, F., Pakunlu, R.I., Brannan, A., Bates, F., Minko, T., Discher, D.E.: Biodegradable polymersomes loaded with both paclitaxel and doxorubicin permeate and shrink tumors, inducing apoptosis in proportion to accumulated drug. J. Control Release **116**, 150–158 (2006)
39. Chen, W., Meng, F.H., Cheng, R., Zhong, Z.Y.: pH-sensitive degradable polymersomes for triggered release of anticancer drugs: a comparative study with micelles. J. Controlled Release **142**, 40–46 (2010)
40. Battaglia, G., Ryan, A.J.: Bilayers and interdigitation in block copolymer vesicles. J. Am. Chem. Soc. **127**, 8757–8764 (2005)
41. Lomas, H., Massignani, M., Abdullah, K.A., Canton, I., Lo Presti, C., MacNeil, S., Du, J.Z., Blanazs, A., Madsen, J., Armes, S.P., Lewis, A.L., Battaglia, G.: Non-cytotoxic polymer vesicles for rapid and efficient intracellular delivery. Faraday Discuss. **139**, 143–159 (2010)
42. Massignani, M., Lomas, H., Battaglia, G.: Polymersomes: a synthetic biological approach to encapsulation and delivery. Mod. Tech. Nano. Microreact. React. **229**, 115–154 (2010)
43. Saylor, D.M., Kim, C.S., Patwardhan, D.V., Warren, J.A.: Diffuse-interface theory for structure formation and release behavior in controlled drug release systems. Acta Biomater. **3**, 851–864 (2007)
44. Bodor, N.: Redox drug delivery systems for targeting drugs to the brain. Ann. N. Y. Acad. Sci. **507**, 289–306 (1987)
45. Corti, A., Duarte, T.L., Paolicchi, A., Dominici, S., Jones, G.D.D., Dilda, P., Hogg, P.J., Pompella, A.: Gamma-glutamyltransferase of cancer cells at the crossroads of redox regulation, tumor progression, drug resistance and drug targeting. Anticancer Res. **28**, 3451–3452 (2008)
46. Tew, K.D., Ali-Osman, F.: Redox pathways in cancer drug discovery. Curr. Opin. Pharmacol. **7**, 353–354 (2007)
47. Grundl, T.: A review of the current understanding of redox capacity in natural, disequilibrium systems. Chemosphere **28**, 613–626 (1994)
48. Napoli, A., Boerakker, M.J., Tirelli, N., Nolte, R.J.M., Sommerdijk, N.A.J.M., Hubbell, J.A.: Glucose-oxidase based self-destructing polymeric vesicles. Langmuir **20**, 3487–3491 (2004)
49. Cerritelli, S., Velluto, D., Hubbell, J.A.: PEG-SS-PPS: reduction-sensitive disulfide block copolymer vesicles for intracellular drug delivery. Biomacromolecules **8**, 1966–1972 (2007)
50. Park, K., Lee, S., Kang, E., Kim, K., Choi, K., Kwon, I.: New generation of multifunctional nanoparticles for cancer imaging and therapy. Adv. Funct. Mater. **19**, 1553–1566 (2009)
51. Sato, N., Kobayashi, H., Hiraga, A., Saga, T., Togashi, K., Konishi, J., Brechbiel, M.W.: Pharmacokinetics and enhancement patterns of macromolecular MR contrast agents with various sizes of polyamidoamine dendrimer cores. Magn. Reson. Med. **46**, 1169–1173 (2001)
52. Minchin, R.F., Martin, D.J.: Minireview: nanoparticles for molecular imaging-an overview. Endocrinology **151**, 474–481 (2010)
53. Bhalgat, M.K., Haugland, R.P., Pollack, J.S., Swan, S., Haugland, R.P.: Green- and red-fluorescent nanospheres for the detection of cell surface receptors by flow cytometry. J. Immunol. Methods **219**, 57–68 (1998)

54. Weissleder, R., Tung, C.H., Mahmood, U., Bogdanov Jr, A.: In vivo imaging of tumors with protease-activated near-infrared fluorescent probes. Nat. Biotechnol. **17**, 375–378 (1999)
55. Canfarotta, F., Whitcombe, M.J., Piletsky, S.A.: Polymeric nanoparticles for optical sensing. Biotechnol. Adv. **31**, 1585–1599 (2013)
56. Mulder, W.J.M., Castermans, K., Van Beijnum, J.R., Oude Egbrink, M.G.A., Chin, P.T.K., Fayad, Z.A.: Molecular imaging of tumor angiogenesis using αvβ3-integrin targeted multimodal quantum dots. Angiogenesis **12**, 17–24 (2009)
57. Yang, Z., Zheng, S., Harrison, W.J., Harder, J., Wen, X., Gelovani, J.G., et al.: Long-circulating near-infrared fluorescence core-cross-linked polymeric micelles: synthesis, characterization, and dual nuclear/optical imaging. Biomacromolecules **8**, 3422–3428 (2007)
58. Lee, S., Ryu, J.H., Park, K., Lee, A., Lee, S.Y., Youn, I.C., et al.: Polymeric nanoparticle-based activatable near-infrared nanosensor for protease determination in vivo. Nano. Lett. **9**, 4412–4416 (2009)
59. Hong, G., Yuan, R., Liang, B., Shen, J., Yang, X., Shuai, X.: Folate-functionalized polymeric micelle as hepatic carcinoma-targeted, MRI-ultrasensitive delivery system of antitumor drugs. Biomed. Microdevices **10**, 693–700 (2008)
60. Suen, W.L.L., Chau, Y.: Specific uptake of folate-decorated triamcinolone-encapsulating nanoparticles by retinal pigment epitheliumcells enhances and prolongs antiangiogenic activity. J Control Release **167**, 21–28 (2013)
61. Yoo, M.K., Park, I.K., Lim, H.T., Lee, S.J., Jiang, H.L., Kim, Y.K., Choi, Y.J., Cho, M.H., Cho, C.S.: Folate-PEG-superparamagnetic iron oxide nanoparticles for lung cancer imaging. Acta Biomater. **8**, 3005–3013 (2008)
62. Rowe, M.D., Tham, D.H., Kraft, S.L., Boyes, S.G.: Polymer-modified gadolinium metal–organic framework nanoparticles used as multifunctional nanomedicines for the targeted imaging and treatment of cancer. Biomacromolecules **10**, 983–993 (2009)
63. Zhang, L., Xue, H., Gao, C., Carr, L., Wang, J., Chu, B., Jiang, S.: Imaging and cell targeting characteristics of magnetic nanoparticles modified by a functionalizable zwitterionic polymer with adhesive 3,4-dihydroxyphenyl-l-alanine linkages. Biomaterials **31**, 6582–6588 (2010)
64. Chen, G., Chen, W., Wu, Z., Yuan, R., Li, H., Gao, J., Shuai, X.: MRI-visible polymeric vector bearing CD3 single chain antibody for gene delivery to T cells for immunosuppression. Biomaterials **30**, 1962–1970 (2009)
65. Krasia-Christoforou, T., Georgiou, T.K.: Polymeric theranostics: using polymer-based systems for simultaneous imaging and therapy. J. Mater. Chem. B **1**, 3002–3025 (2013)
66. Bhojani, M.S., Van Dort, M., Rehemtulla, A., Ross, B.D.: Targeted imaging and therapy of brain cancer using theragnostic nanoparticles. Mol. Pharm. **7**, 1921–1929 (2010)
67. Ho, Y.P., Leong, K.W.: Quantum dot-based theranostics. Nanoscale **2**, 60–68 (2010)
68. Shubayev, V.I., Pisanic, T.R., Jin, S.: Magnetic nanoparticles for theragnostics. Adv. Drug Deliv. Rev. **61**, 467–477 (2009)
69. Lammers, T., Kiessling, F., Hennink, W.E., Storm, G.: Nanotheranostics and image-guided drug delivery: current concepts and future directions. Mol Pharmaceutics **7**, 1899–1912 (2010)
70. Payne, C.K.: Imaging gene delivery with fluorescence microscopy. Nanomedicine **2**, 847–860 (2007)
71. Juzenas, P., Chen, W., Sun, Y.P., Coelho, M.A.N., Generalov, R., Generalova, N., Christensen, I.L.: Quantum dots and nanoparticles for photodynamic and radiation therapy of cancer. Adv. Drug. Deliv. Rev. **60**, 1600–1614 (2008)
72. Lammers, T.: Improving the efficacy of combined modality anticancer therapy using HPMA copolymer-based nanomedicine formulations. Adv. Drug Deliv. Rev. **62**, 203–230 (2010)
73. Pike, D.B., Ghandehari, H.: HPMA copolymer-cyclic RGD conjugates for tumor targeting. Adv. Drug Deliv. Rev. **62**, 67–183 (2010)
74. Pola, R., Studenovsky, M., Pechar, M., Ulbrich, K., Hovorka, O., Vetvicka, D., Rihova, B.: HPMA-copolymer conjugates targeted to tumor endothelium using synthetic oligopeptides. J. Drug Target **17**, 763–776 (2009)
75. Lammers, T., Ulbrich, K.: HPMA copolymers: 30 years of advances. Adv. Drug Deliv. Rev. **62**, 119–121 (2010)

76. Kopecek, J., Kopeckova, P.: HPMA copolymers: origins, early developments, present, and future. Adv. Drug Deliv. Rev. **62**, 122–149 (2010)
77. Wang, Y., Ye, F., Jeong, E.K., Sun, Y., Parker, D.L., Lu, Z.R.: Noninvasive visualization of pharmacokinetics, biodistribution and tumor targeting of poly[n-(2-hydroxypropyl) methacrylamide] in mice using contrast enhanced mri. Pharm. Res. **24**, 1208–1216 (2007)
78. Ferber, S., Baabur-Cohen, H., Blau, R., Epshtein, Y., Kisin-Finfer, E., Redy, O., Shabat, D., Satchi-Fainaro, R.: Polymeric nanotheranostics for real-time non-invasive optical imaging of breast cancer progression and drug release. Cancer Lett. Article (2014 in press)
79. Frechet, J.M.J.: Functional polymers and dendrimers: reactivity, molecular architecture, and interfacial energy. Science **263**, 1710–1715 (1994)
80. Wolinsky, J.B., Grinstaff, M.W.: Therapeutic and diagnostic applications of dendrimers for cancer treatment. Adv. Drug Deliv. Rev. **60**, 1037–1055 (2008)
81. Shi, X.G., Wang, S.H., Meshinchi, S., Van Antwerp, M.E., Bi, X., Lee, I., Baker, J.R.: Dendrimer-entrapped gold nanoparticles as a platform for cancer-cell targeting and Imaging. Small **3**, 1245–1252 (2007)
82. Wiener, E.C., Brechbiel, M.W., Brothers, H., Magin, R.L., Gansow, O.A., Tomalia, D.A., Lauterbur, P.C.: Dendrimer-based metal chelates: a new class of magnetic resonance imaging contrast agents. Magn. Reson. Med. **31**, 1–8 (1994)
83. Taratula, O., Schumann, C., Naleway, M.A., Pang, A.J., Chon, K.J., Taratula, O.: A multifunctional theranostic platform based on phthalocyanine-loaded dendrimer for image-guided drug delivery and photodynamic therapy. Mol. Pharmaceutics **10**, 3946–3958 (2013)
84. Grünwald, G.K., Vetter, A., Klutz, K., Willhauck, M.J., Schwenk, N., Senekowitsch-Schmidtke, R., Schwaiger, M., Zach, C., Wagner, E., Göke, B., Holm, P.S., Ogris, M., Spitzweg, C.: Systemic image-guided liver cancer radiovirotherapy using dendrimer-coated adenovirus encoding the sodium iodide symporter as theranostic gene. J. Nucl. Med. **54**, 1450–1457 (2013)
85. Kim, J.I., Lee, B.S., Chun, C., Cho, J.K., Kim, S.Y., Song, S.C.: Long-term theranostic hydrogel system for solid tumors. Biomaterials **33**, 2251–2259 (2012)
86. Jaiswal, M.K.I., De, M., Chou, S.S., Vasavada, S., Bleher, R., Prasad, P.V., Bahadur, D., Dravid, V.P.: Thermoresponsive magnetic hydrogels as theranostic nanoconstructs. ACS Appl. Mater. Interfaces **6**, 6237–6247 (2014)
87. Murali, R., Vidhya, P., Thanikaivelan, P.: Thermoresponsive magnetic nanoparticle – Aminated guar gumhydrogel system for sustained release of doxorubicin hydrochloride. Carbohydr. Polym. **110**, 440–445 (2014)
88. Janib, S.M., Moses, A.S., MacKay, J.A.: Imaging and drug delivery using theranostic nanoparticles. Adv. Drug Deliv. Rev. **62**, 1052–1063 (2010)
89. Kumar, R., Kulkarni, A., Nagesha, D.K., Sridhar, S.: In vitro evaluation of theranostic polymeric micelles for imaging and drug delivery in cancer. Theranostics **2**, 714–722 (2012)
90. Li, Y.I., Qian, Y., Liu, T., Zhang, G., Liu, S.: Light-triggered concomitant enhancement of magnetic resonance imaging contrast performance and drug release rate of functionalized amphiphilic diblock copolymer micelles. Biomacromolecules **13**, 3877–3886 (2012)
91. Liu, T., Qian, Y., Hu, X., Ge, Z., Liu, S.: Mixed polymeric micelles as multifunctional scaffold for combined magnetic resonance imaging contrast enhancement and targeted chemotherapeutic drug delivery. J. Mater. Chem. **22**, 5020–5030 (2012)
92. Chiang, W.H., Huang, W.C., Chang, C.W., Shen, M.Y., Shih, Z.F., Huang, Y.F., Lin, S.C., Chiu, H.C.: Functionalized polymersomes with outlayered polyelectrolyte gels for potential tumor-targeted delivery of multimodal therapies and MR imaging. J. Controlled Release **168**, 280–288 (2013)
93. Oliveira, H., Pérez-Andrés, E., Thevenot, J., Sandre, O., Berra, E., Lecommandoux, S.: Magnetic field triggered drug release from polymersomes for cancer therapeutics. J. Controlled Release **169**, 165–170 (2013)
94. Pangburn, T.O., Georgiou, K., Bates, F.S., Kokkoli, E.: Targeted polymersome delivery of sirna induces cell death of breast cancer cells dependent upon orai3 protein expression. Langmuir **28**, 12816–12830 (2012)

[illegible] HPMA copolymers, origins, early developments, present and future. Adv Drug Deliv Rev 62:122–149 (2010)
[illegible]

Chapter 11
Polymers in Drug Delivery: Fundamentals

Luis Díaz-Gómez, Angel Concheiro and Carmen Alvarez-Lorenzo

Abstract Drug delivery has experienced an outstanding advance in the last few decades. Two key elements have contributed in a large extent to such a progress: the better knowledge of the physio/pathological environments through which the drugs have to pass through to reach their targets, and the development of novel excipients that actively participate in the accomplishment of the aimed delivery. In this context polymers occupy an outstanding position due to the versatility of the synthesis routes and the possibility of tuning their features and performances to fulfill the needs of every particular application. Polymers can finely regulate the site and the rate at which the drug is released from the formulation, improve drug solubility, contribute to the stability in the physiological environment, and help the drug to overcome cellular barriers, facilitating the contact with the therapeutic diana. This Chapter reviews the role of polymers on the evolution of drug delivery systems and the current performances they are expected to play in improving the efficiency and safety of the treatments with both old and novel active pharmaceutical ingredients (APIs). An analysis of how polymers themselves are contributing to optimize classical methods of preparing drugs dosage forms and to envision advanced drug nanocarriers is also included. Whenever possible, the information was organized trying to offer structure-property-functionality relationships, with examples of commercially available materials.

Keyword Polymer excipients · Drug dosage forms · Polysaccharides · Polyesters · Coating · Drug solubilization · Drug permeability · Gene delivery

L. Díaz-Gómez · A. Concheiro · C. Alvarez-Lorenzo (✉)
Dept Farmacia Y Tecnología Farmacéutica, Facultad de Farmacia,
Universidad de Santiago de Compostela, 15782 Santiago de Compostela, Spain
e-mail: carmen.alvarez.lorenzo@usc.es

F. Puoci (ed.), *Advanced Polymers in Medicine*, DOI 10.1007/978-3-319-12478-0_11

Abbreviations

ABC	ATP binding cassette
API	Active pharmaceutical ingredient
ATP	Adenosine triphosphate
BCRP	Breast cancer resistant protein
CAP	Cellulose acetate phthalate
EMA	European Medicines Agency
FDA	US Food and Drug Administration
HLB	Hydrophilic-lipophilic balance
HPC	Hydroxypropylcellulose
HPMC	Hydroxypropyl methylcellulose
MCC	Microcrystalline cellulose
MRP	Multidrug resistant proteins
P-gp	P-glycoprotein
PAA	Poly(acrylic acid)
PAMAM	Polyamidoamine
PCL	Poly-ε-caprolactone
PEI	Polyethyleneimine
PEO	Poly(ethylene oxide)
PGA	Poly(glycolic acid)
PLA	Poly(lactic acid)
PLGA	Polylactic-co-glycolic acid
PPO	Poly(propylene oxide)
PVP	Polyvinylpyrrolidone
ROS	Reactive oxygen species
SMCC	Silicified microcrystalline cellulose
T_g	Glass transition temperature

Evolution of Drug Dosage Forms

Since ancient times humans have dedicated strong efforts to identify remedies that could ameliorate wounds and diseases and to implement suitable ways to administer those remedies in an efficient way. Dosage forms appeared as a tool to facilitate the administration of drugs that could not be directly applied or ingested, for example due to the small amount required for the effect or its unpleasant taste. Ebers papyrus (16th century BC) and other antique documents describe hundreds of recipes based in natural remedies that required, for example, the previous boiling in water to extract the active substances and to enable the intake, or the mixing with components (mostly fats) for a prolonged permanence on the application site (cataplasms or ointments) or an easier swallow (solid preparations). Thus, together with the remedy containing the active components, some other materials named *excipients* (derived from the Latin verb *excipere*, which literally means to mix) had to be incorporated to the medicines in order to make easier their administration and to maintain their stability for a while. The initial role of excipients was that of acting as vehicles, and as such the most used ones were milk, honey and wine. Despite the efforts spent for many centuries in having adequate medicines, relevant advances in composition and preparation did not occur until the scientific method was introduced in the age of Enlightenment [1].

Evolution of knowledge in chemistry, physiology and pharmacology together with the industrial revolution in the 19th century made it possible the design and manufacture of more complex dosage forms, which are still used nowadays such as tablets or capsules, for isolated or newly synthesized active pharmaceutical ingredients (APIs) [2]. Industrial revolution was a milestone for the wide access of the population to medicines, and prompted the search of excipients able to face up to the growing challenges of the new manufacturing procedures [3]. Advances in pharmacokinetics and born of biopharmacy in the mid 20th century, made pharmacists and clinicians to realize about the importance of preparing dosage forms that not only contain the adequate amount of active substance, but that also can release it at the adequate rate when the medicine enters into contact with the physiological fluids. For systemic treatments, the amount and the rate at which unaltered drugs reaches blood stream (*bioavailability*) was set as a main criterion of quality of a medicine. As a consequence, the requirement of drug dissolution test for solid dosage forms was established for first time in 1970 [4].

Current pharmacological treatments aim to adapt drug administration to the therapeutic needs of the patient so that, using the lowest possible dose, the disease process can be cured or its symptoms alleviated. Local, systemic and targeted release dosage forms are the main approaches to afford this aim (Fig. 11.1). Acute processes require that once the medicine is administered either locally or systemically, the drug is immediately transferred from the dosage form to the body. Conversely, the treatment of a chronic condition demands a prolonged supply of drug in order to maintain effective therapeutic drug levels for a sufficiently long period of time. Targeting is particularly useful when the disease requires the use of drugs that are very unstable in the biological medium and thus should be protected from degradation before reaching the site of action, drugs that are highly toxic for the non-target tissues and may cause untoward effects if systemically distributed (e.g. antitumor agents), or drugs that should reach cellular structures that are not easily accessible from the general circulation (e.g. cell nucleus in gene therapy). Thus, depending on the particular therapeutic aim and the administration route, drug dosage forms have to fulfill a wide variety of highly demanding performances.

When the medicine is administered through a non-parenteral route, the drug has to be transferred from the dosage form to the neighbor biological environment. Dissolved drug molecules can either accumulate in the tissue in contact with the dosage form (Fig. 11.1a; e.g., skin, ophthalmic or bronchial application) for local treatment, or can pass through the membranes and enter into the bloodstream (Fig. 11.1b), from where the drug will be distributed throughout the body, reaching the site of action (systemic effect) and the elimination organs.

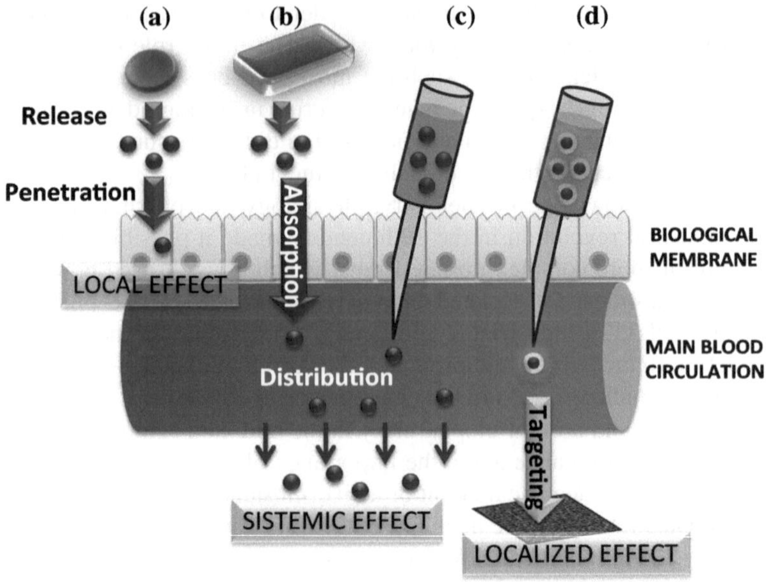

Fig. 11.1 Medicines can be designed: (i) to exert a local effect on the application site by means of drug release and penetration in surrounding cells (**a**), (ii) to exert a systemic effect by releasing the drug in a place suitable for drug absorption (**b**) and/or biodistribution (**c**), (iii) or to target the drug to profound specific tissues or cells via direct transport of the drug (inside nanocarriers) through the blood stream towards the target (**d**). In either case, the drug has to be released from the dosage form to get access to the pharmacological target and exert the therapeutic effect, but the release occurs in different sites and at different rates

Intravenous solutions allow direct incorporation of the drug to the blood stream (Fig. 11.1c). Parenteral route offers also the possibility of administering colloidal (nanometric) carriers with the drug encapsulated for specific delivery to specific tissues or cells (targeting) (Fig. 11.1d).

Except for target delivery systems, drug release and passage through biological membranes are steps that occur sequentially. As a consequence, the slower process determines the overall rate of transfer of drug from the dosage form to the blood circulation; that is, the slower process is the limiting step for drug absorption. If both drug absorption and clearance are rapid, repeated administrations at short time intervals may be required to maintain effective plasma levels. The possibility of modulating the rate of absorption of a drug by applying technological means able to adjust the release from the dosage form is the basis of the *modified release dosage forms*. This group comprises prolonged (sustained)-release, delayed-release and pulsate-release forms (Table 11.1).

Prolonged release dosage forms, also known as rate-programmed release systems, pursue simplification of dosing regimens, by spacing the intervals between successive administrations of doses, and attenuation of peaks in drug levels [5]. The second generation of controlled release systems, called activation-modulated

Table 11.1 Classification of drug dosage forms according to drug release profile as stated in the USP 37–NF 32 (2014)

Dosage form	Drug release pattern	Performance
Conventional	Immediate release	Release depends on the physico-chemical properties of the drug
Modified release	Prolonged	Release occurs at slower rate than from conventional dosage form
	Delayed	Release does not occur until a certain lag time or a certain stimulus triggers it
	Pulsate	Sequential release pulses of one or more therapeutic substances

ones, appeared to regulate not only the rate, but also the site at which drug release should occur. The first devices were developed for site-specific release of orally administered medicines, but rapidly adapted to other routes. In these systems, drug release is activated by physical (swelling), chemical (e.g., pH) or biochemical (e.g., enzymatic degradation) stimuli. Common examples of oral delayed-release formulations are the enteric systems for release in the intestine of irritant or labile drugs, and the time-retard systems for fitting of drug release to circadian rhythm of pathological processes. Some pulsate-release formulations have been developed for sequential release of one or various therapeutic substances by combining particles that degrade at different rates after activation; parenteral administration of pulsate-release systems has been successfully applied for vaccination. Most modified-drug release devices commercialized belong to the two first generations. The third generation of controlled release systems pursues the feedback-regulation of drug release, by testing the patient condition, especially illness evolution. These new systems present the singularity of integrating components that play an active role in the therapeutic treatment [6].

Polymer Excipients

As introduced above, the roles that a given dosage form is expected to play are very varied, but can be gathered into three large groups: (i) facile drug dosing and patient acceptability; (ii) enhanced safety of the treatment and reproducibility of the therapeutic response; and (iii) improved drug efficacy (Table 11.2). The dosage form has to provide the adequate physical properties to facilitate the administration, but also have to correct/modulate physicochemical and biopharmaceutical properties of the drug, such as solubility or permeability, which are critical for the effectiveness of treatment. Poor aqueous solubility is a common problem among new chemical entities, because the current drug discovery methods favor the selection of highly hydrophobic molecules. In other cases, hydrophilicity and large molecular weight hinder the pass through biological membranes. Current diversity of requirements regarding spatio-temporal regulation of drug release also make

Table 11.2 Main functions of the drug dosage forms

Category	Performance
Facile drug dosing and patient acceptability	Adequate physical format for administration
	Simple and rational dosing
	Correction of unpleasant organoleptic properties
Enhanced safety of the treatment and reproducibility of the therapeutic response	Improved physical and chemical stability of the drug
	Protection against microbial contamination
	Minimization of toxicity and untoward effects
Improved drug efficacy	Modulation of drug solubility, release rate and permeability
	Enhanced bioavailability
	Modulation of drug biodistribution
	Easy adherence to the treatment

design and development of drug dosage forms a highly challenging task. To ensure the quality of medicines, the dosage form has to contribute to the chemical and physical stability of the drug, both in the course of the manufacturing process and during storage.

The diversity of roles that dosage forms are called to play is only possible thanks to strong efforts in the finding/synthesis of suitable excipients able to face up to the increasing complexity of production processes and increasingly stringent quality requirements. The United States Pharmacopeia (USP37/NF32, 2014) classifies the excipients in more than 40 functional categories according to their most common application in the formulation of pharmaceuticals. Such large list of functions can be reorganized in main four categories:

- Processability, i.e., they facilitate the manufacture of the dosage form;
- Stabilization, to overcome problems related to the stability of the drug or the dosage form;
- Correction of organoleptic properties; and
- Modulation of drug bioavailability (altering solubility, permeability or drug release rate) or the access (targeting) to specific tissues or cell structures.

As material science progresses, novel and everyday more sophisticated materials are being evaluated as excipients for drug dosage forms. It should be noticed that, among other materials, polymers occupy a relevant position as versatile excipients able to perform one or more functions simultaneously. Multifunctional excipients are particularly attractive because they simplify development and manufacturing processes and reduce costs. Currently, natural, semi-synthetic and synthetic polymers are common excipients (Fig. 11.2). Natural polymers, mainly polysaccharides and protein derivatives, have been largely used for many years to cover the demands of classical dosage forms (tablets, capsules, gels) and are still widely used today because the good biocompatibility of most of them, biodegradability in the body or in the environment, and obtaining from renewable sources.

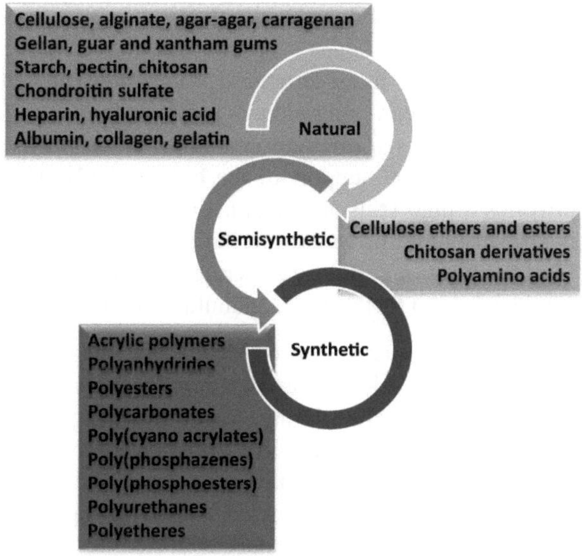

Fig. 11.2 Examples of natural, semi-synthetic and synthetic polymers used to prepare drug dosage forms

Improvements in the extraction and characterization methods make natural polymers reliable materials for quality standards. Moreover, some natural polymers perform as multifunctional or can be easily derivatized to modulate their solubility and biodegradability patterns or to endow them with responsiveness to certain stimuli. Synthetic polymers have the advantage of being prepared on demand to fit to specific requirements, setting a priori their functional groups and molecular weight. Outstanding examples of biodegradable and non-biodegradable polymers are poly(L,D-lactic-co-glycolic acid) (PLGA) and polyethylene glycol (PEG), respectively.

In the next sections, examples of polymer excipients suitable for specific functionalities are analyzed.

Polymers as Manufacture Aids and Sustained Release Formulations Components

Processing requirements are notably different depending on the physical state of the dosage form. Manufacture of dosage forms requires excipients that are able to overcome deficiencies of the drug regarding processing and contribute to rapid and reproducible production of manageable medicines. Hydrophilic polymers may also contribute to slow down drug release by increasing the viscosity of liquid formulations or by forming gel matrix networks when solid formulations become wet. In contrast, hydrophobic polymers can help regulate drug release by means of hydrolytic or enzymatic degradation mechanisms.

Cellulose and Cellulose Derivatives

Cellulose is the main structural component of cell walls in higher plants and consists in linear, unbranched polysaccharide of β-1,4-linked D-glucose units. Cellulose chains form long crystalline microfibrils aligned with each other's to provide structural support to the cell wall [7]. The strong structure of cellulose provides a high resistance against enzymatic reactions that degrade the chains. It is also insoluble in water and indigestible by the human gastrointestinal system. Modifications of cellulose structure leads to materials widely used in the pharmaceutical field to facilitate the manufacture of drugs:

- Microcrystalline cellulose (MCC). It is obtained by treatment of cellulose with hydrochloric acid to partially depolymerise the structure. After purification by filtration and spray-drying, a free-flowing powder of small aggregates of cellulose fibers is obtained [8]. Polymer compactability can be modified by varying the degrees of polymerization and of crystallinity. It is commonly used as diluent in wet granulation and as filler in capsules. The most known commercial brands are Avicel® and Emcocel®.
- Silicified MCC. Commercialized as Prosolv SMCC®, it is produced by co-processing MCC (98 %) with colloidal silicon dioxide (2 %) and commonly used as filler binder and glidant [9]. This excipient has better properties for direct compaction, such as flowability and packaging properties. In addition, silicified MCC has higher bulk density than does regular MCC and maintains compactation properties after wetting and drying.
- Cellulose ethers. Derivatives more hydrophilic than cellulose and thus that can easily disperse in water are obtained via substitution of one or more hydroxyl groups of the D-glucose units with alkyl, hydroxyalkyl and carboxyalkyl molecules. Applications of cellulose derivatives depend on the degree of substitution because it determines the strength of the interaction with water. Non-ionic cellulose ethers, such as hydroxypropylcellulose (HPC) and hydroxypropyl methylcellulose (HPMC) are commonly used in tableting as binders and film-coating components. Gelling features of medium-high substituted cellulose ethers make them suitable to create gel barriers when tablets enter into contact with physiological fluids, which can sustain drug release. They are also suitable as thickener agents for the formulation of solutions and suspensions. Low substituted non-ionic cellulose ethers behave as disintegrants of tablets and pellets [10]. Co-processed excipients containing MCC, HPMC and crospovidone show excellent flowability, compressibility and mixing ability, and therefore notably improve manufacturability of solid dosage forms.

Starch

Starch is a storage carbohydrate consisting of glucose monomers organized as amylose and amylopectin chains. Starches are used in solid oral formulations as diluents, binders and disintegrants. Deficient flow properties of natural starches can be overcome by substitution with acetate groups, prepared by partial reaction of the hydroxyl groups of starch with acetic acid anhydride in an acetyl esterification reaction [8, 11]. Alternatively, flow properties can be improved via chemical and/or mechanical processing to break all or part of the starch granules (namely, the bonds between amylose and amylopectin molecules) in a process named pregelatinization. Partial pregelatinization renders the starch flowable, directly compressible, and suitable for preparing oral capsules. Both partial and fully pregelatinized can be used in wet granulation processes. Combination of pregelatinized starch with amylose and amylopectine leads to multifunctional excipients that are effective as binders, disintegrants, flow aids and lubricants [12]. Most known commercial brands are Starch 1500®, Sepistab ST200® and C*PharmGel®.

Natural Anionic Polysaccharides

Anionic polysaccharides extracted from seaweeds (alginate, agar, carrageenans; Fig. 11.3) and plant cell walls (pectin) and exudates (gum arabic) are largely used as thickening and gelling agents. Alginate is a linear polysaccharide composed of β(1-4)-D-mannosyluronic acid (M) and α(1-4)-L-gulosyluronic acid (G) blocks. The ratio and the distribution of the M and G blocks (Fig. 11.3) notably affect to the sensitiveness of alginate to pH and calcium ions because the different relative position of the carboxylic acid group in each block [13]. Alginate also offers a wide range of possibilities of derivatization to improve its performance [14]. Alginic acid and its sodium, calcium, ammonium and potassium salts have been shown suitable for oral and topical dosage forms, acting as diluent and disintegrant in solid forms and as thickener, emulsifier and taste-masking agent in liquid and semisolid. Alginic acid is particularly suitable for preparing microcapsules, pellets and microspheres that are easily cross-linked in the presence of calcium ions [15].

Carrageenans or carrageenins are hydrocolloids extracted from some red seaweeds. They mainly consists of linear β-D-galactose and 3,6-anhydro-α-D-galactose copolymers with a variable density in sulfated groups, which leads to three different families: kappa (κ, 1 sulfate group per dimer) which has a helical tertiary structure and strong gelling capability; iota (ι, 2 sulfate groups per dimer); and lambda (λ, 3 sulfate groups per dimer) which does not form gels (Fig. 11.3). Only κ-carrageenan hydrogels exhibit pH- and temperature-sensitiveness [16]. At low concentration, carrageenans are added to emulsions to increase the physical stability. They are also used as pelletizer agents for extrusion-spheronization, binder agents in tableting, and as components of hard and soft capsule shells.

Agar or agar-agar is obtained from the cell walls of some species of red algae or seaweeds and is widely employed as emulsifying and suspending agent, thickener, and tablet binder. Agar is a heterogeneous mixture of two unbranched polysaccharides: agaropectin and agarose, which share the same galactose-based backbone (Fig. 11.3). Agaropectin is heavily modified with acidic side-groups, such as sulphate and pyruvate, while agarose has neutral charge and possesses longer chains [17]. Thus, depending on the composition, agar are designed as neutral agarose, pyruvated agarose (with little sulfation) and sulfated galactan.

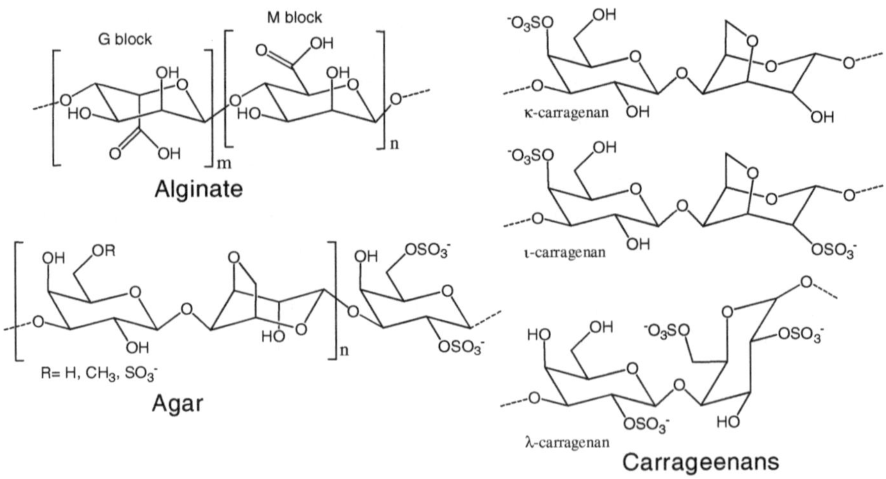

Fig. 11.3 Structure of some anionic polysaccharides used as pharmaceutical excipients

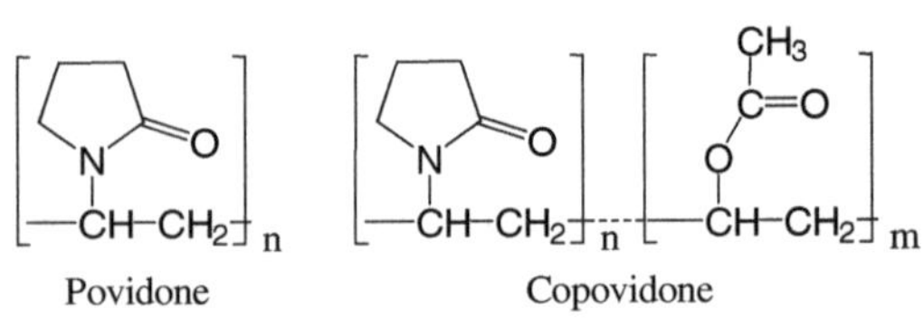

Fig. 11.4 Repeating units of povidone and copovidone

Polyvinylpyrrolidone

Polyvinylpyrrolidone (PVP), also known as povidone and commercialized as Kollidon® (Fig. 11.4), is a synthetic linear polymer widely used in pharmaceutical industry. It is highly soluble in water, but also in some organic solvents such as butanol. The thickening ability of PVP depends on its molecular weight, and several grades can be distinguished which are identified with a K-value (average molecular weight estimated from relative viscosity values). PVP is also used as adhesive and binding agent in tablets, and as taste masker in oral solutions and chewing tablets. Chemically and physically cross-linked insoluble PVP (crospovidone) has good flow properties and strong swelling capability, performing as disintegrant of tablets. Water-soluble copolymers of N-vinylpyrrolidone and vinylacetate (copovidone; Fig. 11.4) are used as binders and as film-forming agents of tablets, pellets and granules. Compared to PVP grades, copovidone has lower hygroscopicity, better dry binding properties, and higher plasticity [18].

Acrylic Acid-Based Polymers

High molecular weight, crosslinked, acrylic acid-based polymers are known as Carbopol® and Noveon®. Carbopol® homopolymers consists of acrylic acid crosslinked with allyl sucrose or allylpentaerythritol. There exist also Carbopol® copolymers (with C10-C30 alkyl acrylate) and interpolymers (which contain a block copolymer of polyethylene glycol and a long chain alkyl acid ester). Noveon® polycarbophil is a polymer of acrylic acid crosslinked with divinyl glycol [19].

These polymers have microgel structure and behave as thickening agents in lotions, creams and gels, oral suspensions, and in transdermal gel reservoirs. They are also useful to communicate controlled release properties to solid dosage forms. In contact with the aqueous media, acrylic acid-based polymers form gel matrices that hinder drug diffusion more efficiently than other polymers. It should be noticed that due to the presence of carboxylic acid groups, acrylic acid-based polymers undergo relevant conformational changes as a function of pH and ionic strength. At pH above the pKa (5.5–6.5), the ionized polymer chains expand and can easily entangle with neighbor chains forming highly structured, viscoelastic gels.

Polyesters

Polyesters are biocompatible and biodegradable polymers including poly(lactic acid) (PLA), poly(glycolic acid) (PGA), poly(lactic-co-glycolic acid) (PLGA), and poly-ε-caprolactone (PCL). These biocompatible polymers are widely used to encapsulate drugs in micro/nanoparticles and in macroscopic implants [20, 21]. Poly(α-hydroxy) esters are not biodegraded by enzymes in the body, but undergo hydrolytic degradation via surface or bulk degradation pathways. Surface degradation occurs when the rate of hydrolytic chain scission and the production of oligomers and monomers which diffuse into the surroundings is faster than the rate of water intrusion into the polymer bulk. As a consequence, the formulation erodes over time without affecting the molecular weight of the polymer bulk. Bulk degradation occurs when water penetrates the entire polymer structure, causing hydrolysis throughout the entire polymer matrix and thus overall reduction in molecular weight. In the case of PLGA, if the generated carboxyl-containing species do not diffuse out the matrix, they can act as internal autocatalyzer that accelerates the bulk degradation compared to the surface. Due to these biodegradation patterns, PLGA formulations exhibit bi/triphasic release profiles: initial burst of drug close to the surface, slow release of the entrapped drug until the molecular weight of the polymer becomes lower than a critical threshold, and rapid release when most polymer has degraded [22]. PCL is less used mainly because it bioerodes at slower rate than other aliphatic polyesters, but has the advantage of degrading in neutral species and not in acid byproducts [23].

Polymers for Coating

Coating of solid dosage forms allows facing up to a variety of formulation demands: taste masking, improvement of appearance, easy swallowing, prolonged stability and spatiotemporal control of drug release [24, 25].

Shellac is an excellent film-forming natural polyester resin secreted by insects. It consists in a complex mixture of aliphatic and alicyclic acids, which serves as moisture barrier of tablets and pellets due to its low permeability to water and oxygen [26, 27]. Shellac films protect drugs from degradation in the gastric environment. However, its use is limited by stability problems.

Cellulose ethers also exhibit good filmogenic features. Low-viscosity grades are suitable for aqueous film-coating, while higher-viscosity grades are used with organic solvents. HPMC films are gastrosoluble. Oppositely, ester derivatives of HPMC such as hypromellose acetate succinate or hypromellose phthalate can provide enteric films that resist prolonged contact with the strongly acidic medium, but dissolve in the mildly acidic or neutral intestinal environment. Cellulose esters, particularly acetate and acetate phthalate (CAP), are commonly applied to solid-dosage forms either by coating from organic or aqueous solvent systems, or by direct compression. CAP has the advantage of being compatible with most plasticizers [28].

Pectin, amylose, dextran and inulin provide coatings that degrade by enzymes of colonic flora. These polysaccharides are commonly combined with cellulose ethers or esters or synthetic polymers to obtain biphasic release profiles or colon-specific release [29–31]. Drugs conjugated to dextran (linear polymer backbone of α-D-glucopyranose units) show enhanced stability in the upper part of the gastro-intestinal tract, but they can be absorbed in the colon [32].

There is a large list of methacrylate copolymers that can provide specific performances as film-coating materials (Table 11.3) [33, 34]. Protective coatings seal the formulation, masking unpleasant odor and taste. Gastroresistant films aim to provide protection of the drug against gastric fluid and of gastric mucosa from aggressive drugs. Films insoluble at any pH, but permeable can provide sustained-release along the entire gastrointestinal tract [8, 34]. Similarly, polyvinyl acetate films are insoluble in dilute acid and alkali media and thus act as diffusion barriers over a long period of time.

Polymers That Enhance Drug Solubility or Dissolution Rate

A large majority of active substances are poorly soluble in water, which limits the feasibility of dissolution of the therapeutic dose. Moreover, certain treatments require that the drug is rapidly bioavailable when administered in oral solid dosage forms. Among other technological strategies, the use of polymers as solubilising and release-rate enhancer excipients has received a strong attention [35].

Table 11.3 Synthetic polymers commonly used as film-forming agents for coating of solid dosage forms. Data taken from references [8, 34]

Function	Composition	Features	Trade names
Protective	Cationic copolymer based on dimethylaminoethyl methacrylate, butyl methacrylate, and methyl methacrylate	Soluble pH < 5, permeable pH > 5	Eudragit® E 100, E 12.5, E PO
	Polyethylene glycol with side chains of polyvinyl alcohol	Water-soluble	Kollicoat® IR
Enteric	Poly(methacrylic acid-co-ethyl acrylate) 1:1; poly(methacrylic acid-co-methyl methacrylate) 1:2; poly(methyl acrylate-co-methyl methacrylate-co-methacrylic acid) 7:3:1	Soluble pH > 5.5–7.0	Eudragit® L 30 D-55, L 100-55, L 100, L 12.5, S 100, S 12.5, FS 30 D. Acryl-EZE® 93A, MP Kollicoat® MAE
Sustained-release	Poly(ethyl acrylate-co-methyl methacrylate-co-trimethylammonioethyl methacrylate chloride) 1:2:0.2 and 1:2:0.1; poly(ethyl acrylate-co-methyl methacrylate) 2:1	Insoluble, low or high permeability	Eudragit® RL 100, RL PO, RL 30D, RL 12.5, RS 100, RS PO, RS 30D, RS 12.5, NE 30D, NE 40 D, NM 30D
			Kollicoat® EMM
	Polyvinylacetate		Kollicoat® SR

Self-Assembly Polymers

Amphiphilic polymers, mainly block copolymers, may self-assembly in aqueous medium rendering structures similar to micelles of conventional surfactants (polymeric micelles) or vesicles that resemble liposomes (polymersomes). The hydrophobic regions of the polymer chains form the core, while the hydrophilic blocks extend towards the aqueous phase as a shell. The resultant polymeric micelles can host drugs of diverse polarity in the core or in the core-shell interface, enhancing the apparent solubility of the drug up to several orders of magnitude [36]. A variety of amphiphilic polymers have been synthetized. Common examples of hydrophilic blocks are poly(ethylene oxide) (PEO), poly(N-vinyl pyrrolidone), poly(N-isopropylacrylamide) or poly(acrylic acid) (PAA). Suitable hydrophobic blocks may be PLA, PCL, poly(propylene oxide) (PPO), poly(trimethylene carbonate), polyethers, polypeptides, and poly(β-aminoester)s [37–39].

Commercially available grades of sequential PEO-PPO-PEO or reverse PPO-PEO-PPO triblock copolymers of Pluronic® family (also known as poloxamers) are already components of topical, oral and parenteral formulations approved by US Food and Drug Administration (FDA) and European Medicines Agency (EMA) [37, 40]. Related X-shape copolymers with a central ethylenediamine group and four branches of PEO-PPO are commercialized as Tetronic® (poloxamine) [41]. These block copolymers are available in a number of varieties differing in length of hydrophilic PEO and hydrophobic PPO blocks and hydrophilic-lipophilic balance (HLB), which in turn enables the preparation of micelles with cores displaying a variety of sizes and hydrophobic environment [37, 40]. The choice of the core-forming segment is a critical issue for a variety of properties of polymeric micelles such as stability, drug-loading capacity, and drug-release profile. In general, polymeric micelles exhibit better thermodynamic (lower critical micellar concentration) and kinetic (less prone to rapid disassembly) stability than conventional micelles. The main advantage is that once diluted in the physiological fluids, drug-loaded polymeric micelles maintain their stability for minutes to hours even the polymer concentration in the medium is well below the critical micellar concentration. This feature endows polymeric micelles with ability to circulate for a prolonged time in the blood stream if the surface is endowed with stealth features. Although Pluronics are non-degradable biomaterials, molecules around 10–15 KDa are filtered by kidney and eliminate in the urine [42]. Pluronic formulations have been widely investigated demonstrating their usefulness to enhance solubilization of poorly-water soluble drugs and also prolonging their release profile in oral, rectal, topical, ophthalmic, nasal and injectable preparations.

An amphiphilic copolymer composed of PEG, polyvinylcaprolactam and polyvinylacetate side chains (Soluplus®; Fig. 11.5) has also shown excellent solubilising properties for class II drugs, particularly crystalline drugs [43–45]. This copolymer as well as some other block copolymers cited above can be also incorporated to solid dosage forms and create self-micellizable systems that accelerate drug release.

Polymers for Solid Dispersions

Solid dispersions provide drug particles of reduced size, promote wetting, avoid agglomeration, and change the crystalline state of the drug, which in turn lead to an increase in drug dissolution rate and even solubility [46]. Common techniques to prepare solid dispersions require (i) dissolution of the drug and the polymer in a common solvent followed by spray-drying or freeze-drying; or (ii) mixing in solid state followed by cogrinding or melt extrusion [47, 48]. Suitable polymers are those that can be dissolved in a variety of organic media if the solution approach is going to be applied, or that exhibit low temperature of melting (if crystalline) or low glass transition temperature, T_g (if amorphous) for methods that require melting [48, 49]. In the solid dispersion, molecular interactions between drug and polymer or formation of eutectic products notably favor drug dissolution process [50, 51].

Poloxamer, PVP, copovidone and PEG are suitable solubilizing agents for solid dispersions. Soluplus® enable hot-melt extrusion to be carried out at low temperature without the addition of other excipients such as plasticizers [52]. Some hyperbranched polymers (e.g. Hybrane®, Fig. 11.5) of reduced T_g are also suitable for

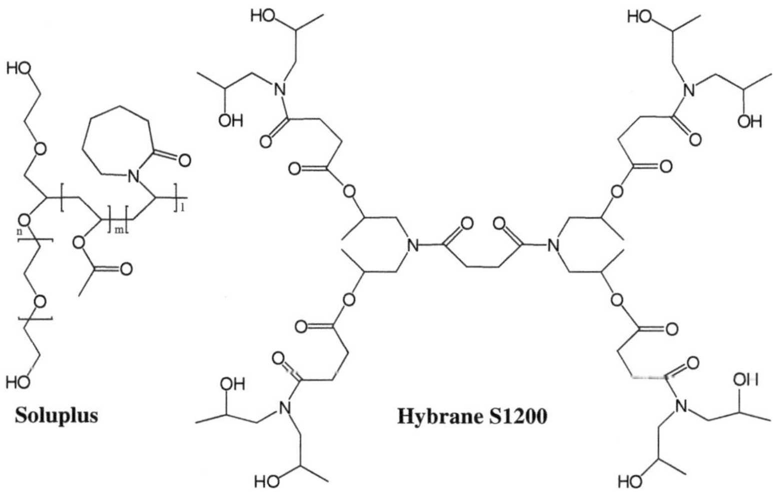

Fig. 11.5 Structure of Soluplus® and Hybrane® S1200 amphiphilic polymers

this technique and their pharmaceutical potential is under research [53]. Compared to other techniques, the advantage of hot-melt extrusion is that it can work in a continuous mode without the use solvents. Requirements for biocompatible polymers used in hot-melt extrusion are thermoplastic behavior, T_g in the 50–180 °C, low hygroscopicity, and ability to solubilize hydrophobic drugs. For this later requirement, polymers bearing hydrogen bond acceptor or donor groups or amide moieties are particularly adequate.

Polymers That Enhance Drug Permeability

Non-parenteral administration requires that the drug molecules can pass through the lipid bilayer of cell membranes close to the administration site (for local effect) or through the entire physiological membranes that act as a barrier for the access to the blood stream. Once in the blood, the drug molecules themselves or incorporated in suitable nanocarriers should extravase towards the target tissues. Several structures and physicochemical phenomena oppose to drug permeation: the gap between cells is very small; drug molecules have to partition between aqueous phase and oily phase of the bilayer membrane; efflux pumps expel molecules from inside cells to the outer cellular medium; or cytochromes at the membrane can degrade the passing through molecules [54]. Cell penetration in the target site has also to overcome similar problems.

Polymers may enhance drug permeability if they can (i) open the intercellular spaces, (ii) increase the fluidity of the lipid membrane, (iii) inhibit or evade efflux pumps, (iv) inhibit or evade enzymatic activity, and/or (v) facilitate the access to the cell by an alternative mechanism.

Chitosan is a semisynthetic polyssacharide obtained via deacetylation or enzymatic degradation of chitin. Its backbone consists of β-1,4-linked D-glucosamines with a variable degree of N-acetylation (40–98 %) and molecular weight (50–2,000 kDa) [55]. Chitosan favors the transport of drugs across membranes due to its bioadhesion properties and the transient opening of the tight junctions [56, 57]. Limited solubility of chitosan at physiological pH can be overcome with the use of derivatives. The N-substitution of some primary amine of chitosan with carboxyl groups can yield monocarboxymethyl chitosan which exhibits zwitterionic character [58]. N-trimethyl chitosan obtained by partial quaternization of chitosan is water-soluble in a range of pH between 1 and 9, and has been shown efficient for buccal penetration of high molecular weight molecules and for gene delivery [59, 60]. Other cationic polymers like poly-L-lysine, poly-L-arginine and polyethyleneimine (PEI) are also able to induce reversible opening of tight junctions.

Mucoadhesive polymers, such as derivatives of PAA and thiol-functionalized polymers, enable a strong attachment to cysteine groups of glycoproteins from mucus layer, resulting in an increased residence time and enhanced permeability [61, 62]. Functionalization with thiol groups notably increases the mucoadhesion strength of chitosan, PAA derivatives, alginate or carboxymethyl cellulose [63–65].

A variety of polymers have been shown able to inhibit efflux pumps and thus to notably increase drug accumulation inside cells [66]. Efflux pump proteins are active membrane transporters (encoded by the ATP Binding Cassette, ABC, gene family) involved in the expelling of a broad range of structurally diverse compounds out of healthy cells, protecting them from adverse xenobiotics [67]. Efflux pumps affect the absorption, distribution, metabolism and elimination of endogenous substances and also of drugs, ultimately decreasing their bioavailability. P-glycoprotein (P-gp), one of the most studied mammalian ABC proteins, is ubiquitous distributed throughout the body, with the highest levels found in the epithelial cell surfaces, mainly at the apical membranes of the intestines, liver and kidney, and the blood-brain barrier [68]. Other important drug-related efflux pumps are the multidrug resistant proteins (MRP) 1 and 2 as well as the breast cancer resistant protein (BCRP), which overexpressed in tumor cells and lead to low concentrations of anticancer agents, being responsible for multidrug resistance and, consequently, for the chemotherapy failure [69]. Efflux pumps are polyspecific because the drug-binding site is a large and flexible region which contains multiple hydrophilic electron donor/acceptor groups, charged groups and aromatic aminoacids providing a number of subsites where drugs can bind [70].

The development of compounds able to selectively block or to inhibit the ATP-dependent transport function of these proteins is a very important issue for the improvement of the drug therapy, mainly in the fields of oral delivery, brain targeting and cancer therapy [71]. Oral bioavailability of drugs substrate of efflux pumps can be improved by co-administration of efflux pump inhibitors. In the case of cancer treatment, modulators of drug efflux pumps are not expected to kill multidrug resistant cells, but to restore the cytotoxic effect of coadministered anticancer agents. The modulators or inhibitors of efflux pumps can be categorized into two groups: (i) small molecule inhibitors, and (ii) polymeric inhibitors. The polymers have the advantage of being pharmacologically inactive avoiding the toxicity problems related to the active small inhibitors. Natural polysaccharides, such as dextran, anionic gums, or sodium alginates have been proved to inhibit efflux pumps at concentration above 0.05 % [72]. Synthetic polymers based on PEO block copolymers [73] and dendritic [74] and thiolated [75] polymers are effective even at lower concentration. Moreover, hydrophilic polymeric inhibitors are not absorbed from the gastrointestinal tract and thus act locally without causing systemic adverse effects.

In general terms, drug-polymers formulations can overcome multidrug resistance phenomena following two different approaches: (i) circumventing efflux pump transport or (ii) inhibiting efflux transporter proteins [72]. Polymeric micelles and polymer-drug conjugates take advantage of the first approach since the micelles or the conjugates can be uptaken via endocytosis, escaping from membrane diffusion affected by efflux pumps. Differently, unimers of block copolymers, e.g. Pluronics, enhance in vivo intracellular drug accumulation due to the inhibition of P-gp, MRP1 and MRP2 pumps [76, 77]. Pluronic® P85 (4,600 Da) is so far one of the most potent inhibitor of efflux pumps. The unimers rapidly bind cell membrane, penetrate into the cells and co-localizes with the mitochondria. This leads to inhibition of the respiratory chain, decreases oxygen consumption and causes ATP depletion. The inhibition of the ATPase and depletion of ATP and the fluidization of the membrane hinders the activity of the efflux pumps, enabling a more efficient entry of drugs into the cells. In the multidrug resistant cancer cells, the production of reactive oxygen species (ROS) and the release of cytochrome C, due to the impairment of mitochondrial respiration, enhances drug-induced apoptosis and prevents the activation of the anti-apoptotic cellular defense [78].

Polymers for Gene Delivery

Gene material cannot easily enter into cells and is extremely unstable in the extracellular medium. Therefore, systemic administration of gene material requires nanocarriers that can deliver it in the appropriate cells. Most polymers intended as non-viral gene vectors are cationically charged in order to form complexes with DNA which is anionic at physiological pH. The resultant colloidal polyplexes should exhibit removable stealth surface to enable the transport through biological barriers without preventing the entrance into the target cells. The polycation should also perform as endosomolytic component to facilitate the escape of DNA from endosomes in order to avoid degradation, traverse the cytoplasm intact and enter into the nucleus [79].

Although very efficient regarding DNA complexation, highly charged cationic polymers, such as PEI, poly(L-lysine) and polyamidoamine dendrimers (PAMAM), exhibit toxicity problems. Thus, combination of cationic moieties with hydrophilic non-ionic components (e.g. grafted with Pluronic, carbohydrates or cyclodextrins) or even anionic groups (e.g. glycolic acid, polyacrylic acid) is under investigation [80].

Acknowledgments This work was supported by MICINN (SAF2011-22771), Xunta de Galicia (CN 2012/045), and FEDER. L. Diaz-Gomez acknowledges MICINN for a FPI fellowship (BES-2012-051889).

References

1. Allen, L.V., Popovich, N.G., Ansel, H.C.: Ansel's Pharmaceutical Dosage Forms and Drug Delivery Systems. Lippincott Williams & Wilkins, Baltimore (2011). Chapter 1
2. Krówczynski, L.: The development of pharmaceutical technology (chronological tabulated facts). Pharmazie **40**, 346 (1985)
3. Alvarez-Lorenzo, C., Concheiro, A.: From drug dosage forms to intelligent drug-delivery systems: a change of paradigm. In: Alvarez-Lorenzo, C., Concheiro, A. (eds.) Smart materials for drug delivery, vol. 1, p. 1. Royal Society of Chemistry Publishing, Cambridge (2013)
4. Dokoumetzidis, A., Macheras, P.: A century of dissolution research: from Noyes and Whitney to the biopharmaceutics classification system. Int. J. Pharm. **321**, 1 (2006)
5. Hoffman, A.S.: The origins and evolution of "controlled" drug delivery systems. J. Control. Release **18**, 153 (2008)
6. Alvarez-Lorenzo, C., Concheiro, A.: Smart drug delivery systems: from fundamentals to the clinic. Chem. Comm. **50**, 7743 (2014)
7. Hon, D.N.S.: Cellulose and its derivatives: structures, reactions and medical uses. In: Dumitriu, S. (ed.) Polysaccharides in Medicinal Applications, p. 87. Marcel Dekker, New York (1996)
8. Rowe, R.C., Sheskey, P.J., Cook, W.G., Fenton, M.E.: Handbook of Pharmaceutical Excipients. Pharmaceutical Press, London (2012)
9. Zhang, Y., Law, Y., Xhakrabarti, S.: Physical properties and compact analysis of commonly used direct compression binders. AAPS PharmSciTech **4**, 489 (2003)
10. Alvarez-Lorenzo, C., Gomez-Amoza, J.L., Martinez-Pachecho, R., Souto, C., Concheiro, A.: Evaluation of low-substituted hydroxypropylcellulose as filler-binders for direct compression. Int. J. Pharm. **197**, 107 (2000)
11. Chen, L., Li, X., Li, L., Guo, S.: Acetylated starch-based biodegradable materials with potential biomedical applications as drug delivery systems. Curr. Appl. Phys. **7**(s1), 90 (2007)
12. Rashid, I., Al Omari, M.M.H., Badwan, A.A.: From native to multifunctional starch-based excipients designed for direct compression formulation. Starch **65**, 552 (2013)
13. Lee, Y.K., Mooney, D.J.: Alginate: properties and biomedical applications. Prog. Polym. Sci. **37**, 106 (2012)
14. Pawar, S.N., Edgar, K.J.: Alginate derivatization: a review of chemistry, properties and applications. Biomaterials **33**, 3279 (2012)
15. Tonnesen, H.H., Karlsen, J.: Alginate in drug delivery systems. Drug. Dev. Ind. Pharm. **28**, 621 (2002)
16. Coviello, T., Matricardi, P., Marianecci, C., Alhaique, F.: Polysaccharide hydrogels for modified release formulations. J. Control. Rel. **119**, 5 (2007)
17. Freile-Pelegrín, Y., Murano, E.: Agars from three species of Gracilaria (Rhodophyta) from Yucatán Peninsula. Bioresour. Technol. **96**, 295 (2005)
18. Bühler, V.: Kollidon®, polyvinylpyrrolidone excipients for the pharmaceutical industry, 9th edn. BASF, Ludwigshafen (2008)

19. Lubrizol.: Pharmaceutical Bulletin 1. http://www.lubrizol.com/Life-Science/Documents/Pharmaceutical/Bulletins/Bulletin-01—Polymers-for-Pharmaceutical-Applications.pdf (2011). Accessed on June 2014
20. Danhier, F., Ansorena, E., Silva, J.M., Coco, R., Le Breton, A., Preat, V.: PLGA-based nanoparticles: an overview of biomedical applications. J. Control. Release. **161**, 505 (2012)
21. Tahara, K., Sakai, T., Yamamoto, H., Takeuchi, H., Kawashima, Y.: Establishing chitosan coated PLGA nanosphere platform loaded with wide variety of nucleic acid by complexation with cationic compound for gene delivery. Int. J. Pharm. **354**, 210 (2008)
22. Makadia, H.K., Siegel, S.J.: Poly lactic-co-glycolic acid (PLGA) as biodegradable controlled drug delivery carrier. Polymers **3**, 1377 (2011)
23. Woodruff, M.A., Hutmacher, D.W.: The return of a forgotten polymer—Polycaprolactone in the 21st century. Progr. Polym. Sci. **35**, 1217 (2010)
24. Joshi, S., Petereit, H.U.: Film coatings for taste masking and moisture protection. Int. J. Pharm. **457**, 395 (2013)
25. Maroni, A., Zema, L., Loreti, G., Palugan, L., Gazzaniga, A.: Film coatings for oral pulsatile release. Int. J. Pharm. **457**, 362 (2013)
26. Farag, Y., Leopold, C.S.: Development of shellac-coated sustained release pellet formulations. Eur. J. Pharm. Sci. **42**, 400 (2011)
27. Pearnchob, N., Siepmann, J., Bodmeier, R.: Pharmaceutical application of shellac: moisture-protective and taste-masking coatings and extended-release matrix tablets. Drug. Dev. Ind. Pharm. **29**, 925 (2003)
28. Felton, L.A., Porter, S.C.: An update on pharmaceutical film coating for drug delivery. Expert. Opin. Drug Del. **10**, 421 (2013)
29. Wong, T.W., Colombo, G., Sonvico, F.: Pectin matrix as oral drug delivery vehicle for colon cancer treatment. AAPS. Pharm. Sci. Tech. **12**, 201 (2011)
30. Siew, L.F., Basit, A.W., Newton, J.M.: The properties of amylose–ethylcellulose films cast from organic-based solvents as potential coatings for colonic drug delivery. Eur. J. Pharm. Sci. **11**, 133 (2000)
31. Vervoort, L., Kinget, R.: In vitro degradation by colonic bacteria of inulin HP incorporated in Eudragit films. Int. J. Pharm. **129**, 185 (1996)
32. Brøndsted, H., Andersen, C., Hovgaard, L.: Crosslinked dextran—a new capsule material for colon targeting of drugs. J. Control. Release. **53**, 7 (1998)
33. Nollenberger, K., Albers, J.: Poly(meth)acrylate-based coatings. Int. J. Pharm. **457**, 461 (2013)
34. Bühler, V.: Kollicoat grades. BASF, Ludwigshafen (2007)
35. Fahr, A., Liu, X.: Drug delivery strategies for poorly water-soluble drugs. Expert. Opin. Drug. Del. **4**, 403 (2007)
36. Lu, Y., Park, K.: Polymeric micelles and alternative nanonized delivery vehicles for poorly soluble drugs. Int. J. Pharm. **453**, 198 (2013)
37. Chiappetta, D.A., Sosnik, A.: Poly(ethylene oxide)-poly(propylene oxide) block copolymer micelles as drug delivery agents: improved hydrosolubility, stability and bioavailability of drugs. Eur. J. Pharm. Biopharm. **66**, 303 (2007)
38. Rangel-Yagui, C.O., Pessoa, A., Tavares, L.C.: Micellar solubilization of drugs. J. Pharm. Pharm. Sci. **8**, 147 (2005)
39. Kwon, G.S.: Polymeric micelles for delivery of poorly water-soluble compounds. Crit. Rev. Ther. Drug Carrier Syst. **20**, 357 (2003)
40. Kabanov, K.V., Batrakova, E.V., Alakhov, V.Y.: Pluronic block copolymers as novel polymer therapeutics for drug and gene delivery. J. Control. Release. **82**, 189 (2002)
41. Alvarez-Lorenzo, C., Rey-Rico, A., Sosnik, A., Taboada, P., Concheiro, A.: Poloxamine-based nanomaterials for drug delivery. Front. Biosci. (Elite edition) **2**, 424 (2010)
42. Dumortier, G., Groissord, J.L., Agnely, F., Chaumeil, J.C.: A review of poloxamer 407 pharmaceutical and pharmacological characteristics. Pharm. Res. **211**, 2709 (2006)

43. Linn, M., Collnot, E.M., Djuric, D., Hempel, K., Fabian, E., Kolter, K., Lehr, C.M.: Soluplus® as an effective absorption enhancer of poorly soluble drugs in vitro and in vivo. Eur. J. Pharm. Sci. **45**, 336 (2012)
44. Cespi, M., Casettari, L., Palmieri, G.F., Perinelli, D.R., Bonacucina, G.: Rheological characterization of polyvinyl caprolactam–polyvinyl acetate–polyethylene glycol graft copolymer (Soluplus®) water dispersions. Colloid. Polym. Sci. **292**, 235 (2014)
45. Shamma, R.N., Basha, M.: Soluplus®: A novel polymeric solubilizer for optimization of Carvedilol solid dispersions: formulation design and effect of method of preparation. Powder Technol. **237**, 406 (2013)
46. Vo, C.L.N., Park, C., Lee, B.J.: Current trends and future perspectives of solid dispersions containing poorly water-soluble drugs. Eur. J. Pharm. Biopharm. **85**, 799 (2013)
47. Serajuddin, A.T.M.: Solid dispersion of poorly water-soluble drugs: Early promises, subsequent problems, and recent breakthroughs. J. Pharm. Sci. **88**, 1058 (1999)
48. Kumar, S., Gupta, S.K.: Pharmaceutical solid dispersion technology: a strategy to improve dissolution of poorly water-soluble drugs. Recent. Pat. Drug. Deliv. Formul. **7**, 111 (2013)
49. Wilson, M., Williams, M.A., Jones, D.S., Andrews, G.P.: Hot-melt extrusion technology and pharmaceutical application. Ther. Deliv. **3**, 787 (2012)
50. Leuner, C., Dressman, J.: Improving drug solubility for oral delivery using solid dispersions. Eur. J. Pharm. Biopharm. **50**, 47 (2000)
51. Janssens, S., van den Mooter, G.: Review: physical chemistry of solid dispersions. J. Pharm. Pharmacol. **61**, 1571 (2009)
52. Hardung, H., Djuric, D., Shaukat, A.: Combining HME & solubilization: Soluplus®-the solid solution. Drug. Deliv. Tech. **10**, 3 (2010)
53. Ravina-Eirin, E., Gomez-Amoza, L., Martinez-Pacheco, R.: Utility of the hyperbranched polymer hybrane S1200 for production of instant-release particles by hot melt extrusion. Drug. Dev. Ind. Pharm. **39**, 1107 (2013)
54. Deli, M.A.: Potential use of tight junction modulators to reversibly open membranous barriers and improve drug delivery. Biochim. Biophys. Acta **1788**, 892 (2009)
55. Illum, L.: Chitosan and its use as a pharmaceutical excipient. Pharm. Res. **15**, 1326 (1998)
56. Smith, J., Wood, E., Dornish, M.: Effect of chitosan on epithelial cell tight junctions. Pharm. Res. **21**, 43 (2004)
57. Di Colo, G., Zambito, Y., Zaino, C.: Polymeric enhancers of mucosal epithelia permeability: synthesis, transepitheliar penetration-enhancing properties, mechanism of action, safety issues. J. Pharm. Sci. **97**, 1652 (2008)
58. Thanou, M., Nihot, M.T., Jansen, M., Verhoef, J.C., Junginger, H.E.: Mono-N-carboxymethyl chitosan (MCC), a polyampholytic chitosan derivative, enhances the intestinal absorption of low molecular weight heparin across intestinal epithelia in vitro and in vivo. J. Pharm. Sci. **90**, 38 (2001)
59. Sandri, G., Rossi, S., Bonferoni, M.C., Ferrari, F., Zambito, Y., Di Colo, G., Caramella, C.: Buccal penetration enhancement properties of N-trimethyl chitosan: influence of quaternization degree on absorption of a high molecular weight molecule. Int. J. Pharm. **297**, 146 (2005)
60. Mourya, V., Inamdar, B.: Trimethyl chitosan and its applications in drug delivery. J. Mater. Sci. Mater. Med. **20**, 1057 (2009)
61. Andrews, G.P., Laverty, T.P., Jones, D.S.: Mucoadhesive polymeric platforms for controlled drug delivery. Eur. J. Pharm. Biopharm. **71**, 505 (2009)
62. Clausen, A.E., Bernkop-Schnurch, A.: In vitro evaluation of the permeation-enhancing effect of thiolated polycarbophil. J. Pharm. Sciences. **89**, 1253 (2000)
63. Iqbal, J., Shahnaz, G., Perera, G., Hintzen, F., Sarti, F., Berkop-Schnurch, A.: Thiolated chitosan: development and in vivo evaluation of an oral delivery system for leuprolide. Eur. J. Pharm. Biopharm. **80**, 85 (2012)
64. Bernkop-Schnurch, A., Kast, C.E., Richter, M.F.: Improvement in the mucoadhesive properties of alginate by the covalent attachment of cysteine. J. Control. Release. **28**, 277 (2001)

65. Trapani, A., Palazzo, C., Contino, M., Perrone, M.G., Cioffi, N., Ditaranto, N., Colabufo, N.A., Conese, M., Trapani, G., Puglisi, G.: Mucoadhesive properties and interaction with P-glycoprotein (P-gp) of thiolated-chitosans and -glycol chitosans and corresponding parent polymers: a comparative study. Biomacromol **15**, 882 (2014)
66. Bernkop-Schnürch, A., Grabovac, V.: Polymeric efflux pump inhibitors in oral drug delivery. Am. J. Drug. Del. **4**, 263 (2006)
67. Eckford, P.D.W., Sharom, F.J.: ABC efflux pump-based resistance to chemotherapy drugs. Chem. Rev. **109**, 2989 (2009)
68. Leveque, D., Jehl, F.: P-glycoprotein and pharmacokinetics. Anticancer. Res. **15**, 331 (1995)
69. Yokoyama, M.: Polymeric micelles as a new drug carrier system and their required considerations for clinical trials. Expert. Opin. Drug. Del. **7**, 145 (2010)
70. Loo, T.W., Clarke, D.M.: Recent progress in understanding the mechanism of P-glycoprotein-mediated drug efflux. J. Membrane. Biol. **206**, 173 (2005)
71. Varma, M.V., Perumal, O.P., Panchagnula, R.: Functional role of P-glycoprotein in limiting peroral drug absorption:optimizing drug delivery. Curr. Opin. Chem. Biol. **10**, 367 (2006)
72. Werle, M.: Natural and synthetic polymers as inhibitors of drug efflux pumps. Pharm. Res. **25**, 500 (2008)
73. Kabanov, A.V., Batrakova, E.V., Alakhov, V.Y.: Pluronic block copolymers for overcoming drug resistance in cancer. Adv. Drug Deliv. Rev. **54**, 759 (2002)
74. D'Emanuele, A., Jevprasesphant, R., Penny, J., Attwood, D.: The use of a dendrimer-propranolol prodrug to bypass efflux transporters and enhance oral bioavailability. J. Control. Release. **95**, 447 (2004)
75. Föger, F., Hoyer, H., Kafedjiiski, K., Thaurer, M., Bernkop-Schnürch, A.: In vivo comparison of various polymeric and low molecular mass inhibitors of intestinal P-glycoprotein. Biomaterials **27**, 5855 (2006)
76. Kabanov, A.V., Alkhov, VYu.: Pluronic® block copolymers in drug delivery: from micellar nanocontainers to biological response modifiers. Critical. Rev. Therap. Drug. Carrier. Syst. **19**, 1 (2002)
77. Cambón, A., Rey-Rico, A., Barbosa, S., Soltero, J.F.A., Yeates, S.G., Brea, J., Loza, M.I., Alvarez-Lorenzo, C., Concheiro, A., Taboada, P., Mosquera, V.: Poly(styrene oxide)-poly(ethylene oxide) block copolymers: From "classical" chemotherapeutic nanocarriers to active cell-response inducers. J. Control. Release. **167**, 68 (2013)
78. Alakhova, D.Y., Rapoport, N.Y., Batrakova, E.V., Timoshin, A.A., Li, S., Nicholls, D., Alakhov, V.Y., Kabanov, A.V.: Differential metabolic responses to pluronic in MDR and non-MDR cells: a novel pathway for chemosensitization of drug resistant cancers. J. Control. Release. **142**, 89 (2010)
79. Kan, P.L., Schätzlein, A.G., Uchegbu, I.F.: Polymers used for the delivery of genes in gene therapy. In: Uchegbu, I.F., Schätzlein, A.G. (eds.) Polymers in Drug Delivery, p. 183. CRC/Taylor and Francis, Boca Raton (2006)
80. Yue, Y., Wu, C.: Progress and perspectives in developing polymeric vectors for in vitro gene delivery. Biomater. Sci. **1**, 152 (2013)

Chapter 12
Drug Delivery Systems: Smart Polymeric Materials

Roberta Cassano and Sonia Trombino

Abstract Over the last two decades the smart polymeric materials have involved the interest of the scientific community because they can be used in the design and formulation of dosage forms that respond, with a considerable variation of their properties, to changes in their environment. As result, these materials control the drug release into specific physiological compartments. Concerning on the environmental stimuli these include pH, temperature, light, chemicals, etc. The smart polymeric materials stimuli-responsive can be synthetics or naturals and have been used in the biotechnological, medicinal and engineering fields. The present chapter is aimed to focus the importance of this category of drug delivery systems and, in particular, it provides a summarizing overview of the range of smart polymeric materials and the drug delivery systems that exploit them.

Keywords Smart polymers · Stimuli · pH · Light · Electric field · Magnetic field · Ultrasound · Temperature · Ion · Enzyme · Glucose · Hydrogels · Nanotubes · Films · Membranes · Nanoparticles · Microparticles · Micelles · Biosensor

Abbreviations

AA	Acrylic acid
AEMA	2-acetoacetoxyethylmethacrylate
BMA	Butyl methacrylate

R. Cassano (✉) · S. Trombino
Department of Pharmacy and Health and Nutrition Sciences, University of Calabria, Arcavacata di Rende, 87036 Cosenza, Italy
e-mail: roberta.cassano@unical.it

S. Trombino
e-mail: sonia.trombino@unical.it

F. Puoci (ed.), *Advanced Polymers in Medicine*, DOI 10.1007/978-3-319-12478-0_12

CST	Critical solution temperature
DDS	Drug delivery systems
DEAAm	*N,N*-diethylacrylamide
DHP	Disulfide-crosslinked heparin-Pluronic
DMAEMA	2-(dimethylamino)ethyl methacrylate
DNQ	2-diazo-1,2-napthoquinone
DSC	Differential scanning calorimetry
EVAc	Ethylene-vinyl acetate copolymer
5-FU	5-fluoruracil
GSH	Glutathione
HA	Hyaluronic acid
IPN	Interpenetrating polymer network
IPMCs	Ionic polymeric-metal composites
LC	Liquid crystal
LCST	Lower critical solution temperature
LMWGs	Low-molecular-weight hydrogelators
MBAAm	*N,N′*-methylenebisacrylamide
ME	Merocyanine
MEMS	Micro-electro-mechanical-systems
MNPs	Magnetic nanoparticles
MSCs	Mesenchymal stem cells
NIPAAm	*N*-isopropylacrylamide
PAA	Poly(acrylamide)
PAAc	Poly(acrylicacid)
PAAm-g-XG	Poly(acrylamide-grafted-xanthan gum)
PbAEs	Poly(b-amino esters)
PCL-PEG-PCL	Poly(ε-caprolactone)-block-poly(ethyleneglycol)-block-poly(ε-caprolactone)
PDAAEMA	Poly(*N,N*-diakylamino ethylmethacrylates)
PEG	Poly(ethylene glycol)
PEG–PPS–PEG	((Poly(ethylene glycol))–(poly(propylene sulfide))–PEG)
PEI	Poly(ethylene imine)
PEO–PPO–PEO	Poly(ethylene oxide)-poly(propylene oxide)-poly(ethylene oxide)
PL	Poly(lysine)
PLGA	Poly(lactic/glycolic acid)
PLLA-PEG-PLLA	Poly(*L*-lactic acid)-poly(ethylene glycol)-poly(*L*-lactic acid)
PMAA	Polymethacrylic acid
pMWNTs	Pristine multi-walled carbon nanotubes
PNIPAAm	Poly(*N*-isopropylacrylamide)
PNVC	Poly(*N*-vinylcaprolactam)
PSS	Sulphonated-polystyrene
PT	Polythiophene
PVA	Polyvinyl acetate
PVDF	Poly(vinylidene fluoride)

RCM	Rate controlling membranes
UCST	Upper critical solution temperature
SP-*hb*-PG	Spiropyran-initiated hyperbranched polyglycerol
SPION	Superparamagnetic iron oxide
SR	Stimuli-responsive
ULS	Ultrasound

Introduction

Stimuli-Responsive (SR) materials, also called "smart materials" have been attracting great interest within scientific community in the last few decades [1–4]. They possess unique properties that have made this class of materials very promising for several applications in the field of nanoscience. In particular, the smart materials undergo changes in response to small external variations in environmental conditions or to physical or biochemical stimuli. In addition, there are dual SR materials that simultaneously respond to more than one stimulus [5–7]. For instance, temperature-sensitive polymers may also respond to pH changes [8–11].

Many efforts have been carried out to find new solutions for developing SR materials for the reason that a smart response to external or internal stimuli allows a better localization of the system in the desired biological compartment and a controlled release of the loaded drug at the site interested from the pathological event. The polymers have proved interesting for the development of stimuli-responsive materials due to their chemistry that permits to modulate the properties by inserting sensible chemical moieties, a responsive compound. In this case, the polymer serves only as a carrier for that compound. On the other hand, SR systems containing polymers can be also designed with a responsive polymers. These systems strictly path the normal physiological process of the disease state where the amount of drug released is precious according to the physiological need [12]. Biopolymers such as proteins, carbohydrates and nucleic acid are all basic components of living organic systems that are responsible for the cells construction and process [13, 14]. These natural polymers have led to the development of numerous synthetic polymers that have been designed to simulate these biopolymers. In particular, a great range of polymeric materials has been synthesized to response to different stimuli such temperature, light, solvent, ionic strength, electric, magnetic, mechanical, pH, enzymes and receptors (Fig. 12.1) [15]. These polymers might recognize one or more of the listed stimuli as a signal, judge the magnitude of this signal, and then change their chain conformation in direct response [16].

The responses are manifested as variations in the shape, surface, solubility, degree of intermolecular association and others [17]. Particularly, the subsequent polymer structure and property alterations lead to the overall characteristic switching. The extraordinariness of these polymers lies not only in the fast structural macroscopic changes but also these transitions being reversible. Therefore, the polymer is capable of returning to its initial state as soon as the trigger is removed

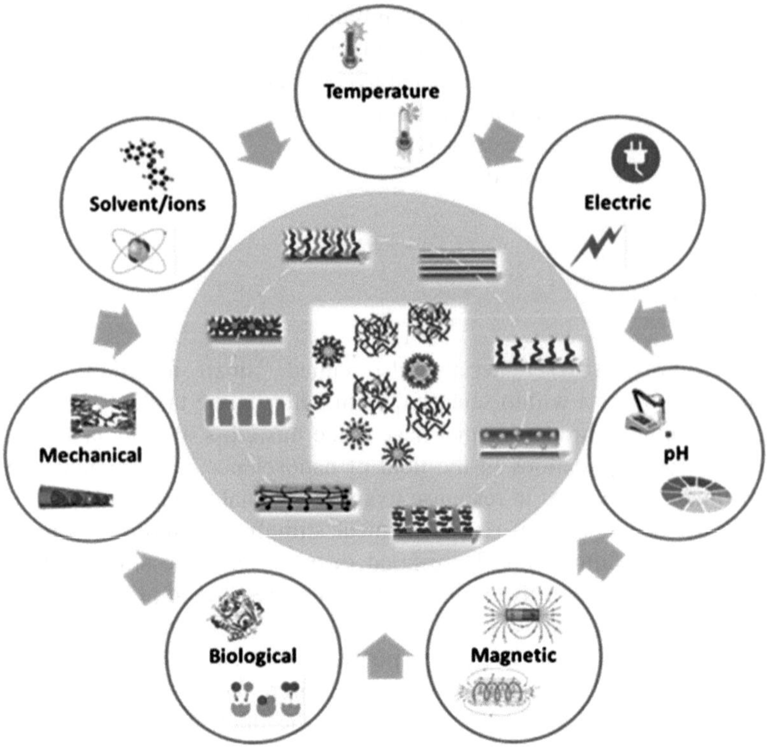

Fig. 12.1 Stimuli of SR polymers

[13, 14]. There is a great deal of literature available about the different types of SR polymers. These materials have been utilized in the form of cross-linked hydrogels, reversible hydrogels, micelles, modified interfaces and conjugated solutions.

The main aim of this review is to highlight the various smart polymeric materials and the drug delivery systems (DDS) that exploit them. These are useful to realize biomimetic devices [18], intelligent medical instruments and auxiliaries [19, 20], electrochemical devices [21], artificial muscles [22], heat shrinkable materials for electronics packaging [23], microelectromechanical systems [24] and actuators and sensors [25].

Stimuli-Responsive Polymers

The stimuli that commonly drive the changes within SR polymers are represented in Fig. 12.1 [5–7]. These ones, commonly classified as physical, chemical, or biological, are also classified as both external or internal stimuli. The polymeric SR materials are too known as self-regulated devices, where the release rate is controlled by a mechanism of feedback that is produced within the body to control the structural changes in the polymer network and exhibit the desired drug release, without any external mediation [26, 27]. On the other hand, externally controlled SR polymers depend on the applied stimuli that are produced with the support of different stimuli-generating strategies, which results in pulsed drug delivery which may be defined as the rapid and transient release of a certain amount of drug within a short time period immediately after a predetermined off-release period [15, 26, 27].

Physically Dependent Stimuli

A very effective way of achieving site-specific drug targeting is by employing externally regulated polymeric drug delivery systems that are responsive to stimuli such as temperature, electric field, light, ultrasound, magnetic fields and mechanical deformation that typically modify the polymeric chain dynamics. Temperature is the most common stimulus for SR polymers.

Temperature-Responsive Polymers

Temperature-sensitive or thermo-responsive hydrogels and polymers have attracted great attention in different fields because some diseases manifest a temperature modification [28, 29]. In particular, they are characterized by a critical solution temperature (CST) around which the hydrophobic and hydrophilic interactions between the polymeric chains and the aqueous media brusquely change within a small temperature range bringing to the disruption of intra- and intermolecular interactions and resulting in chain collapse or expansion. Typically, these polymer solutions possess a temperature above which one polymer phase exists, namely upper critical solution temperature (UCST), and below which a phase separation occurs with the formation of an hydrogel [30]. On the other hand, polymer solutions that appear as monophasic below a specific temperature and biphasic above it generally possess a so-called lower critical solution temperature (LCST). The LCST is a fascinating phenomenon found for various water soluble polymers which tend to phase-separate from solution upon heating. The most investigated temperature-responsive polymer featuring a LCST in water is the poly(N-isopropylacrylamide) (PNIPAAm). The LCST of PNIPAAm was of ~32 °C, proximate to the human body temperature. By altering the temperature of PNIPAAm solution in water, its solubility behavior can be reversibly changed from hydrophilic-soluble to hydrophobic-insoluble and thus can be induced externally (Fig. 12.2). Then, above the LCST, the polymer become increasingly insoluble leading to gel formation.

The phenomenon of transition from a solution to a gel is commonly referred to as sol-gel transition. The sol–gel transition of thermosensitive hydrogels can be

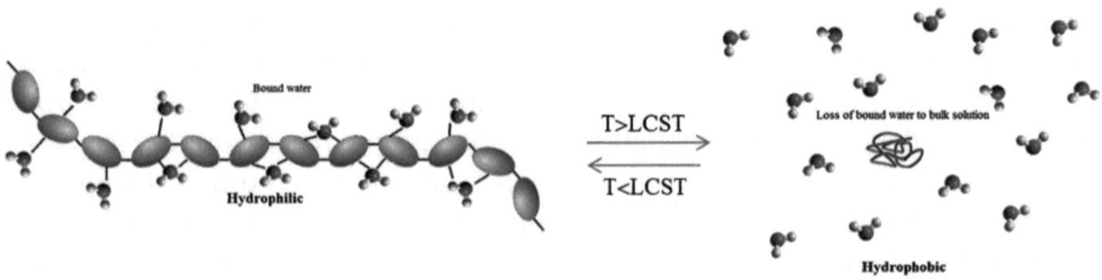

Fig. 12.2 Thermoresponsive polymers: reversible switch from a hydrophilic swollen state to a hydrophobic collapsed state

experimentally verified by a number of techniques such as spectroscopy [31–33], differential scanning calorimetry (DSC) [31, 32] and rheology [33].

Other *N*-substituted polyacrylamides [34, 35], and further classes of polymers such as poly(oligoethyleneoxide-(meth)acrylate)s [36], poly(2-oxazoline)s [37], poly(*N*-vinylalkylamides), e.g. poly(*N*-vinylcaprolactam) (PNVC) [38], copolymers such as poly(*L*-lactic acid)-poly(ethylene glycol)-poly(L-lactic acid) (PLLA-PEG-PLLA) triblock copolymers [39], poly(ethylene oxide)-poly(propylene oxide)-poly(ethylene oxide) (PEO–PPO–PEO) copolymers [40] and many natural polymers [41], e.g. polysaccharides and proteins, utilize temperature change as the trigger that determines their gelling behavior without any additional external factor. Researchers have used them alone or in combination to fabricate thermally responsive hydrogels with desired properties. Hydrogels based on these polymers have been interesting for biomedical uses as they can swell in situ under physiological conditions and provide the advantage of convenient administration.

Temperature-Responsive Polymers Applications

The major advantage of thermosensitive polymeric systems is the avoidance of toxic organic solvents, the ability to transport both hydrophilic and lipophilic drugs, reduced systemic side effects, site-specific drug delivery, and sustained release properties.

Hydrogels responsive to temperature are being used to obtain an on–off drug release profile in response to a gradual change of temperature [42–44]. In particular, hydrogels PNIPAAm-BMA based loading indomethacin were analyzed for their on-off release profile. The on state was reached at low temperatures and off state at high temperatures. This behavior is due to the formation of scarcer permeable gel surface layer when the temperature was rapidly changed. This layer acts as barrier whose formation was regulated through the length of the methacrylate alkyl side-chain [45]. Thermo-responsive polymers were used also to overcome the limited therapeutic activity and insolubility of antitumoral drugs due to their toxicity and to the limited accessibility of tumors. The literature reports on the development of different systems (prodrugs, liposomes, micro- and nano-particles), such as anti-cancer drugs carriers, whose therapeutic efficacy is rather limited [46, 47]. Instead, soluble polymeric drug carriers have proved capable to increase drug tumor permeability [48] but, these carriers fail to intrinsically target a specific physiological compartment.

Thermo-responsive polymeric micelles can be used to target adriamycin at the tumoral site. In particular, block copolymers containing hydrophobic polymers, such as poly(butyl methacrylate) (PBMA) and end-functionalized PNIPAAm [49–51], forming a micellar structure in aqueous solution below the transition temperature of PNIPAAm, act as an inert material in the hydrated form. Upon 32 °C, the polymeric chains became hydrophobic due to their dehydration and aggregation and precipitation occur. The cores of micelles then acted as a reservoir for the hydrophobic drug adriamycin.

However, use of PNIPAAm is limited due to cytotoxicity attributed to the presence of quaternary ammonium in its structure, its non-biodegradability and its ability to activate platelets upon contact with body fluids. Many efforts have been made to decrease the initial burst drug release related to thermosensitive systems due to slow in vivo sol–gel transition. Literature data suggest that significant progress in release characteristics can be achieved by optimizing the chain-length ratio between hydrophilic and hydrophobic segments. A novel triblock polymeric system poly(ε-caprolactone)-block-poly(ethylene glycol)-block-poly(ε-caprolactone) (PCL-PEG-PCL) showed a noticeable decrease in initial burst release by coupling to a peptide. Moreover, in vitro drug release studies showed a wide-ranging sustained-release profile for over 1 month [52] (Fig. 12.3).

With the aim to develop a drug delivery system with thermal stimuli responsing, Nozawa et al. have been investigated liquid crystal (LC)-entrapped membranes, polymer alloyed membranes and LC-adsorbed membranes for the transport and release of indomethacin. Polymer alloyed membranes were obtained by polymerizing acrylic monomers in presence of LC and LC-adsorbed membrane were obtained by adsorbing LC into porous hydrophobic polymer membrane. Permeation experiments showed that below and above the gel-liquid crystal phase transition temperature of the LC, the extent of thermo-sensitivity for LC-adsorbed

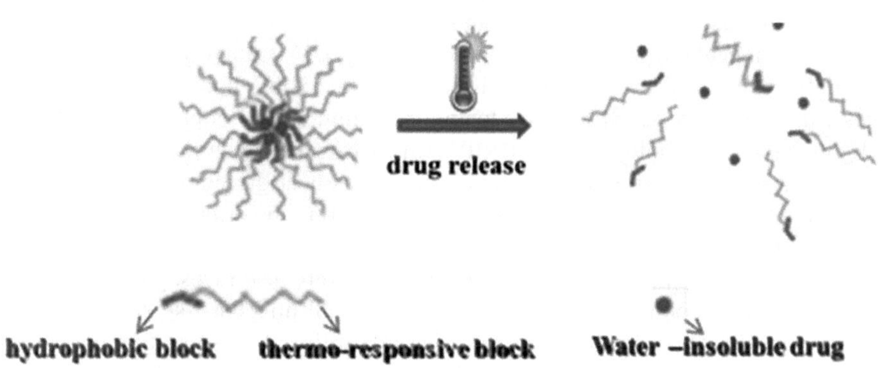

Fig. 12.3 Drug release from a polymeric system

membranes was greater than that for the alloyed membrane. The permeability ratio was found to be about 120 with the LC-adsorbed membrane. The obtained results indicated that the LC-adsorbed membrane was an useful candidate as a thermo-responsive system for DDS [53].

Photo-Responsive Polymers

Photo-sensitive polymers have received increasingly attention in recent years because light can be applied straightaway and under specific conditions with high accuracy. The light is both negligibly absorbed by both cells and tissue and greatly consequently by the polymers. This makes light-responsive polymers highly advantageous for applications in wide fields including drug release, biomaterials, and artificial tissues [54–60]. Photo-responsive polymers contain light-sensitive chromophore moieties. Without external stimuli, these polymers can maintain their structures but, upon light absorption, these moieties can be broken from the polymer chain that can be degraded into smaller molecular fragments. Generally, light-sensitive polymers, UV or visible light sensitive, are classified into two main categories that are the side-chain-type polymer containing the chromophores as lateral groups of the chain backbone and the main-chain-type structure possessing single or multiple photosensitive species covalently- or non-covalently connected to the backbone. Chromophores groups are azobenzene [11, 61], spiropyran [62, 63] and nitrobenzyl [64, 65] and a variety of azobenzene or spiropyran-containing photo-responsive polymers such as poly(acrylamide) (PAA) [41, 66] and PNIPAAm [43, 44].

Photo-Responsive Polymer for the Drug Controlled Delivery

UV-sensitive hydrogels could be synthesized by introduction of bis(4-dimethyl-amino) phenylmethyl leucocyanide, a leuco derivative molecule, into the polymeric matrix in which ionization of the leuco derivative with UV radiation result in discontinuous swelling caused by an increase in osmotic pressure within the gel due to the appearance of cyanide ions formed by UV irradiation [67]. When the UV light is removed the hydrogels shrink. Instead, visible light–responsive materials can be prepared [68] by introducing trisodium salt of copper chlorophyllin, a light-sensitive chromophore, to PNIPAAm hydrogels. When the light is applied the chromophore absorbs it which is dissipated as heat giving an increase of the hydrogel temperature that alters its swelling promoting the drug release.

Polymeric vesicles obtained from the self-assembly of a photocleavable amphiphilic block copolymer, as a light-triggered DDS, were also investigated. The vesicles disintegrate upon UV irradiation, yielding small micellar-like structures, and simultaneously releasing their payload. The versatility of these system was tested both for low molecular weight molecules, proteins, enzymes and DNA. By varying the UV intensity, the loaded drug was released in a controlled manner [69].

Recently, spiropyran-initiated hyperbranched polyglycerol (SP-*hb*-PG) micelles were reported [70]. These carriers responded to UV/visible light and could dissociate due to conversion of the hydrophobic chromophore SP to zwitterionic and hydrophilic merocyanine (ME). In addition, chromophores such as coumarin, *o*-nitrobenzyl, stilbene, dithienylethene and 2-diazo-1,2-napthoquinone (DNQ) have been employed in light-responsive micelles, which can respond either to UV/visible or NIR irradiation to undergo structural or phase changes and trigger the drug release from micelles [71–74].

Ichimura and coworkers reported about photo-responsive polymer membranes based on poly(vinyl alcohol) derivatives having AZB side chains with different lengths, filled with liquid crystal (LC), and investigated the photo-response of LC alignment. They found that liquid crystal alignment changes were possible if the AZB unit was linked to poly(vinyl alcohol) backbone by a sufficient long spacer. The response times could be reduced by using high intensity sources [75]. Moreover, when visible light illuminates the surface of the membrane, the azobenzene moieties straighten out and the liquid crystals fall into line, which allows drug to easily flow through the holes. But when ultraviolet light illuminates the surface, the dye molecules bend into a new shape and the liquid crystals scatter into random orientations, clogging the tunnel and blocking drug from penetrating (Fig. 12.4).

Electro-Responsive Polymers

Increasing research and development efforts have been dedicated to the field of electro-responsive polymers (ERPs) due to their advantages of precise control via the magnitude of the current, the duration of an electrical pulse or the interval between pulses [76, 77]. ERPs are promising candidate materials for the design of drug delivery technologies, especially in conditions where an "on-off"

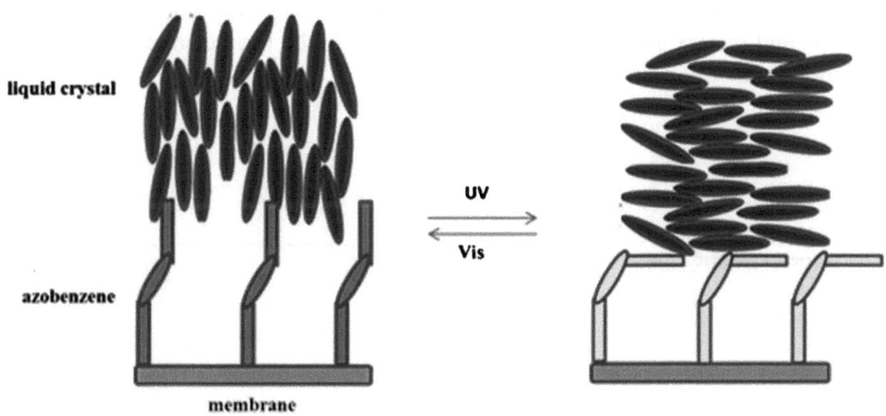

Fig. 12.4 Photo-controlled alignment in liquid crystals

drug release mechanism is required. Typical ERPs are naturally occurring polymers such as chitosan, alginate and hyalouronic acid are commonly employed to prepare electro-responsive materials. Major synthetic polymers that have been used include polythiophene (PT) or sulphonated-polystyrene (PSS), polyaniline, polypyrrole, ethylene vinyl acetate, and polyethylene.

In some cases, combinations of natural and synthetic polymers have been used. Most polymers that exhibit electro-sensitive behavior are polyelectrolytes and they undergo deformation under an electric field due to anisotropic swelling or de-swelling as the charged ions move towards the cathode or anode (Fig. 12.5). Greatest stress is felt by the region surrounding the anode and smaller stress near the vicinity of the cathode. This stress gradient contributes to the anisotropic gel deformation under an electric field [78, 79].

Neutral polymers that exhibit electro-sensitive behaviour require the presence of a polarizable component with the ability to respond to the electric field. A rapid bending of gel in silicon oil was observed in the case of lightly cross-linked poly(dimethylsiloxane)-containing electrosensitive colloidal SiO_2 particles.

These polymers can show swelling, shrinking or bending in response to an external field [80, 81] and they may be blended into responsive hydrogels in conjunction with the desired drug to obtain a patient-controlled drug release system useful for neurotransmitters and vaccine delivery. The "on-off" drug release mechanism can be achieved through the environmental-responsive nature of the interpenetrating hydrogel-EAP complex via (i) charged ions initiated diffusion of drug molecules due to an increase in osmotic pressure in the polymer; (ii) conformational changes that occur during redox switching of EAPs; or (iii) electro-erosion. For example, when an electrochemical stimulus is applied to multilayer polyacrylamide films, the combined effects of H ions migrating to the region of the cathode and the electrostatic attraction between the anode surface and the negatively charged acrylic acid groups lead to shrinking of the film on the anode side [78, 82].

The hydrogel-EAP composites include other implications such as, application towards biosensors, DNA hybridizations, micro-surgical tools and miniature bioreactors and may be utilized to their full potential in the form of injectable devices as nanorobots or nano-biosensors.

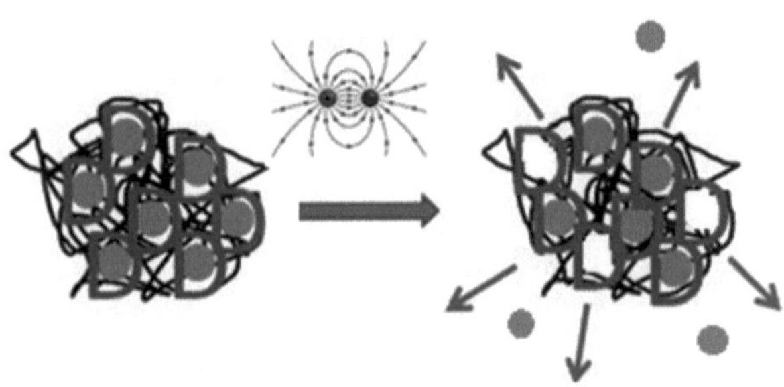

Fig. 12.5 De-swelling of the polymeric drug delivery device due to electric field

Electro-Responsive Polymeric Drug Delivery Systems

ERPs poly(2-acrylamido-2-methyl-propane sulphonic acid-co-n-butylmethacrylate) based were used to delivery edrophonium hydrochloride and hydro-cortisone in a pulsatile manner [83]. The control of drug release was achieved by varying the intensity of electric stimulation in distilled deionized water. For a positively charged drug, the release pattern depends on ion exchange between hydrogen ion produced by electrolysis of water and positively charged solute.

Liu and coworkers have been also designed and successfully realized a novel micro-electro-mechanical-systems (MEMS) based polymer drug delivery microsystem. The device consists of an array of metallic contacts, able to create an uniform electric field. In particular, a hydrogel polymer matrix loaded with hematoxylin dye, as model of hydrophilic drug, has been studied. The delivery microsystem operated at normal body temperature (37 °C) under an applied voltage of 20 V. The release rate and dose were accurately controlled. The polymer responds to the electrical stimulus by shrinking and releases the hematoxylin dye into solution. The release of hematoxylin in the media was monitored using ultraviolet-visible spectrophotometry.

Different drugs can be encapsulated within the hydrogel polymer matrix. The de-swelling of the polymer upon exposure to the applied electric field allows the encapsulated drug to be released from the matrix. The control of the applied voltage can be used to achieve pulsatile drug delivery. Alternatively, small volumes of drug may be continuously delivered to maintain the optimal therapeutic dose for the patient [84].

An electro-responsive drug delivery system was also developed using poly(acrylamide-grafted-xanthan gum) (PAAm-g-XG) hydrogel for transdermal delivery of ketoprofen [85]. When a swollen PAAm-g-XG hydrogel was placed between a pair of electrodes, a de-swelling of the hydrogel was observed in the vicinity of electrodes carrying the electric stimulus. Ketoprofen-loaded PAAm-g-XG hydrogel was also crosslinked with poly(vinyl alcohol) to prepare films as rate controlling membranes (RCM). The in vitro drug permeation study from the formulations was performed through excised rat abdominal skin. The drug permeation across the skin was significantly improved in the presence of electric stimulus as compared to passive diffusion and was found to be dependent upon the applied electric current strength and crosslink density of RCM. A pulsated pattern of drug release was observed as the electric stimulus was switched *on* and *off*. These PAAm-g-XG hydrogel could be useful as transdermal drug delivery systems actuated by an electric signal to provide on-demand release of drugs.

Pristine multi-walled carbon nanotubes (pMWNTs) were incorporated into a polymethacrylic acid (PMAA)-based hydrogel matrix by in situ radical polymerisation [86]. The effect of pMWNTs and cross-linker concentration on the electrical and mechanical properties of the hydrogel was carefully studied. The incorporation of pMWNTs into the polymeric network improved the electrical properties of the hydrogel. Moreover, the drug release from the gels was significantly enhanced at high pMWNT concentrations. But, the presence of pMWNTs within the hydrogel matrix affected the hydrogel mechanical properties by decreasing the pore size and, consequently, the swelling/de-swelling of the gels. The damage on the gel surfaces after electrical stimulation and the loss of the pulsatile release profile at high cross-linker concentrations, suggested that the mechanism of drug release involved a compacting effect and intensified the stress on the polymeric network as a result of the electrical properties of pMWNTs.

Ultrasonically Responsive Polymers

An innovative approach of exploiting ultrasound in drug delivery consists on the application of the ultrasonic waves directly at the polymers or the hydrogel matrix [87]. For the ultrasonically responsive polymers the release mechanism is driven by the cavitation. In particular, the ultrasound (ULS) energy generates both high and low pressure waves, resulting in an alternative growth and shrinkage of gas-filled microbubbles. These high-low pressure waves regulate the intermittent opening of the pores of the polymer, thus inducing the delivery of the respective drugs.

The most widely employed polymers for the ULS-responsive uses could be biodegradable or non-biodegradable. The biodegradables ones include polyglycolides, polylactides, bis(p-carboxyphen-oxy)alkane anhydride with sebacic acid. Instead, the non-biodegradables materials are ethylene-vinyl acetate copolymers or the poly(lactide-co-glycolide) microspheres, PHEMA hydrogels, the PEO-b-PPO-b-PEO micelles and the poly(HEMA-co-DMAEMA) hydrogels. The releasing agents are *p*-nitroaniline, *p*-amino-hippurate, bovine serum albumin and insulin. When exposed to ultrasound, these bioerodible polymers respond rapidly and reversibly. It is believed that the ultrasound also causes an increase in temperature in the delivery system, which allows the diffusion [88, 89]. ULS-responsive polymers are advantageous because they are non-invasive and capable of penetrating deep into the interior of the body and thus drug delivery can be focused and carefully controlled through a number of parameters including frequency, power density, duty cycles and time of application [90, 91]. Biologically the ultrasound action is related to the generation of thermal energy, perturbation of cell membranes, and enhanced permeability of blood capillaries [92].

Application of Ultrasound in Drug Delivery

Ultrasound responsive drug delivery systems have great potential for applications requiring stimulated release in vivo with a high degree of control over spatial and temporal location. Numerous carriers for ultrasonically enhanced drug delivery have been explored including polymeric ultrasound contrast agents with targeting potential, modified lipospheres and nano-/micro-bubble-enhanced chemotherapy (Fig. 12.6) [93–97]. Miyazaki and coworkers used ULS-responsive matrix ethylene-vinyl acetate copolymer (EVAc) based to achieve a 27-fold increase in the release of 5-fluoruracile. The ultrasound strength increase results in a proportional

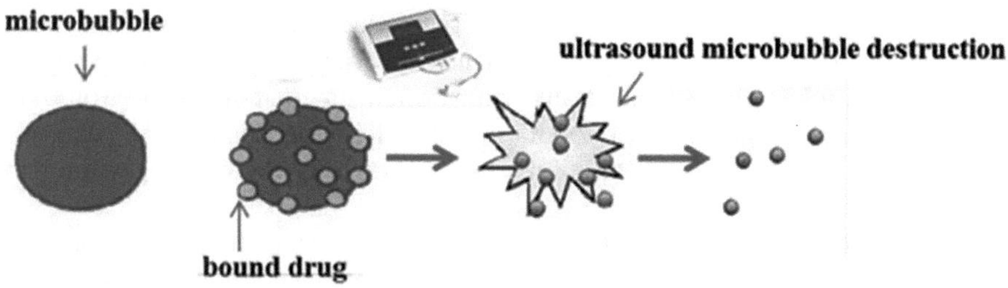

Fig. 12.6 Action of ultrasound targeted microbubble destruction. Microbubbles are attached with drugs or genes

increase in the amount of 5-FU release [98]. EVAc systems were also tested as delivery device of insulin. It was found that exposure of insulin-loaded matrices to ULS significantly reduced the blood glucose levels on the rats [99].

Kwok et al. have reported on the development of ULS-sensitive barrier membranes able to give a pulsatile drug release. A co-polymer of 2-hydroxyl methacrylate (HEMA) and PEG dimethacrylate was loaded with particulate insulin and PEG, after which the surface of the polymer was coated with methylene chains. Upon exposure to ultrasound the methylene chains became disordered, permitting the insulin to diffuse out of the matrix [100, 101].

In addition, Suzuki et al. [102] achieved tumor-specific ultrasound-enhanced gene transfer with novel liposomal bubbles, which entrapped an ultrasound imaging gas. Extraordinarily, the bubble liposomes healthy transferred genes, only at the site of ultrasound exposure, into tumor cells and solid tumor tissue [103–106].

Magnetically-Responsive Polymers

The use of an oscillating magnetic field to modulate the rates of drug delivery from a polymeric matrix was one kind of method to achieve externally controlled drug delivery systems [107]. When planning a magnetic-responsive delivery system characteristics such as the magnetic properties of the carrier particles, field strength and geometry, drug/gene binding capacity and physiological parameters like the depth to target, the rate of blood flow, vascular supply and body weight need to be considered [108]. Magnetic targeting is based on the attraction of magnetic polymer carrier to an external magnetic field source that effectively traps it in the field at the target site and pulls it toward the magnet [109–113]. In order to maintain the magnetic loaded carrier at a specific location, the externally applied field must have a relatively strong gradient. When the drug is released from the magnetic matrix this is no longer responsive to the applied field.

Several carriers for magnetically enhanced drug delivery have been studied including nanoparticles with a magnetic core and a polymer shell and liposomes which have a magnetic core and an artificial liposomal shell are reported [114–119]. These materials may also be embedded in hydrogels which can carry drugs that are released upon heating [110, 120]. To produce highly efficient magnetic-responsive materials, the "doping" of polymer materials with magnetic nanoparticles (MNPs), made of inorganic matter (most often superparamagnetic iron oxide (SPION) Fe_3O_4 or g-Fe_2O_3, or "soft" metallic iron, but also "hard" magnetic materials e.g. Co, Ni, FeN, FePt, FePd…), appeared to be the more appealing and efficient solution.

Many hydrophilic polymers were proposed to host magnetic nanoparticles, in particular thermosensitive gels like poly(*N*-isopropylacrylamide) (PNIPAAm). However, PNIPAAm and other polymers exhibiting a LCST are generally less polar than polyvinyl acetate (PVA) and can be inefficient for trapping the MNPs due to the absence of hydrogen bonds and to a mesh size of typically 10–20 nm, i.e. larger than the size of superparamagnetic iron oxide MNPs (5–10 nm) [121]. To overcome this problems, strategies reported in the Fig. 12.7 concerning on a statistical copolymer network with a chelating comonomer such as 2-acetoacetoxyethylmethacrylate (AEMA) [122], a semi-interpenetrated network with alginate chains wrapping the MNPs [123] or a composite network of PNIPAAm and poly(ethylene glycol) (PEG) using PEG400–dimethacrylate as crosslinker of NIPAAm [124] were proposed.

Magnetic Field Responsive DDS

By merging magnetic and polymer materials one can obtain composites with exceptional magnetic responsive features. In this context, magnetic responsive micro- and nano-particles have been explored as possible drug carriers for site-specific drug targeting [125, 126]. Cytotoxic anti-cancer drugs were attached to these carriers and injected into the subject both via intravenous or intra-arterial injection. External magnetic fields generated by rare earth permanent magnets were then used to direct and concentrate the drug at the tumor site [127]. Subcutaneous implants of EVAc-insulin, capable of decreasing glucose levels in diabetic rats for 105 days, were also designed [128, 129]. Additionally, Hsieh et al. embedded magnetic steel beads in an EVAc copolymer matrix that was loaded with bovine serum albumin as a model of drug. They demonstrated increased rates of drug release in

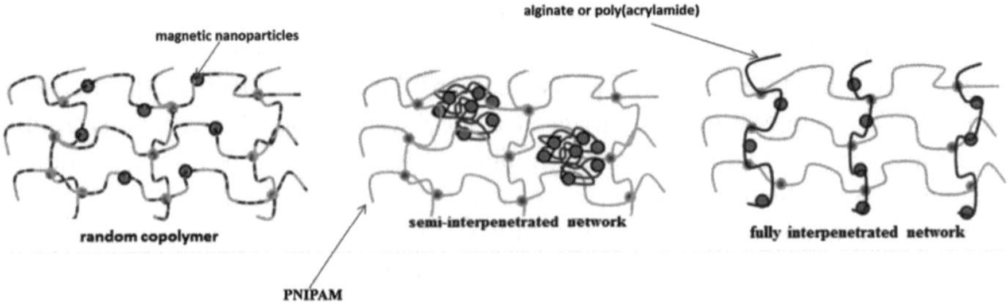

Fig. 12.7 Strategies proposed to trap magnetic nanoparticles inside a hydrogel network

the presence of an oscillating magnetic field [117, 130]. During the exposure to the magnetic field, the beads oscillate within the matrix, on the other hand creating compressive and tensile forces. This consecutively acts as a pump to push an increased amount of the drug out of the polymer matrix. In vivo studies were later conducted demonstrating the effectiveness of an optimized version of this system, consisting of EVAc-protein matrices containing magnetic beads, loaded with insulin. In particular, was demonstrated that glucose levels can be repeatedly decreased on demand by applying an oscillating magnetic field [131–134].

Chemically Dependent Stimuli

Stimuli that occur internally are classified as chemical or biological. The pH as well as the ionic strength, redox and solvent are defined chemically-dependent stimuli.

pH-Responsive Polymers

pH sensitive polymers are materials which respond to the changes in the pH of the surrounding medium by varying their dimensions. Such materials increase its size (swell) or collapse depending on the pH of their environment (Fig. 12.8). This behavior is due to the presence of certain functional groups in the polymer chain such as acidic or basic groups that can either accept or release a proton in response to changes in environmental pH.

The pH is an important environmental parameter for biomedical applications, because pH changes occur in several specific or pathological sites.

The changes along the gastrointestinal tract from acidic in the stomach ($pH = 2$) to basic in the intestine ($pH = 5–8$) has to be considered for oral delivery of any kind of drug. Certain cancers as well inflamed or wound tissue exhibit a pH different from 7.4 as it is in circulation. For example chronic 7.4 and 5.4 and cancer tissue is also reported to be acidic extracellularly [135–137].

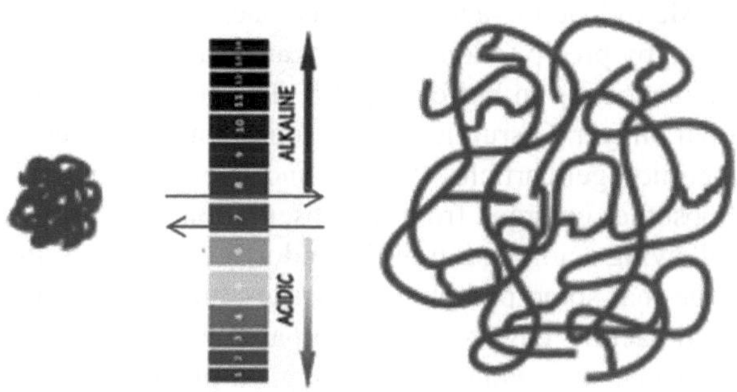

Fig. 12.8 Swelling-de-swelling transition of a pH responsive hydrogel

Consequently, this parameter can be exploited for a direct response at a certain tissue or in a cellular compartment. As mentioned above, pH responsive polymers consist of polymers with a large number of ionisable groups known as polyelectrolytes. Polyelectrolytes are classified into two types: weak polyacids and weak polybases. Weak polyacids accept protons at low pH and release protons at neutral and high pH [138]. Poly(acrylicacid)(PAAc) and poly(methacrylicacid) (PMAA) are commonly used pH-responsive polyacids [139, 140]. As the environmental pH changes, the pendant acidic group undergoes ionization at specific pH called as pKa. This rapid change in the charge of the attached group causes alteration in the molecular structure of the polymeric chain. This transition to expanded state is mediated by the osmotic pressure exerted by various stimuli responsible for controlling drug release from smart polymeric delivery systems [26–143]. pH responsive polymers typically include also chitosan [144], albumin [145], gelatin [146], poly(acrylic acid) (PAAc)/chitosan IPN [147], poly(methacrylic acid-g-ethylene glycol) [P(MAA-g-EG)] [148, 149], poly(ethylene imine) (PEI) [150], poly(*N*,*N*-diakylamino ethylmethacrylates) (PDAAEMA), and poly(lysine) (PL) [151, 152].

pH-Stimuli Sensitive Polymer DDS

Oral pH sensitive drug delivery systems are gaining importance because they are able to deliver the drug at specific part of the gastrointestine. Antibiotics, especially macrolide ones like erythromycin, enzymes and proteins are rapidly degraded by gastric juices. Others, such as acidic drugs like NSAID's (e.g., diclofenac, valproic acid, or acetylsalicylic acid) cause a local irritation of the stomach mucosa.

Recently, it has been reported that aqueous dispersions or suspensions can be produced, in which the drug is present in enteric-coated form. The enteric-coated time *clock system* consists of a tablet core covered with a mixture of hydrophobic material and surfactant, which is applied as an aqueous dispersion [153]. The drug release from the core of the time clock system occurs after a pre-determined lag time.

Many polyanionic materials, such as PAAc, are pH sensitive and the degree of swelling of such polymers can be modulated by changing the pH. The use of these systems, too in conjunction with temperature-sensitive lipids, offers potential to target drugs to areas of inflammation or to achieve site-specific, pulsatile drug delivery [154].

Methylene-bis-acrylamide/methacrylic acid anionic microgels were also prepared by precipitation polymerization and loaded with doxorubicin and condensed by incubating in buffer at pH 5. The condensed particles were then coated with a lipid bilayer. Disruption of the lipid bilayer by electroporation was shown to cause the microgel particles to swell and release their drug. The concept of pH-sensitive liposomes emerged from the observation that certain enveloped viruses infect cells following acidification of the endosomal lumen to infect cells and from the knowledge that some pathological tissues (tumors inflamed and infected tissue) have a more acidic environment compared to normal tissues. Although, pH-sensitive liposomes are stable at physiological pH, they destabilize under acidic conditions, leading to the release of their aqueous contents [155]. The liposomes are internalized by endocytosis after binding to cell surface receptors. In addition, pH-sensitive hydrogels have been used in making biosensors and permeation switches [156]. The pH-sensitive hydrogels for these applications are usually loaded with enzymes that change the pH of the local microenvironment inside the hydrogels. One of the common enzymes used in pH-sensitive hydrogels is glucose oxidase which transforms glucose to gluconic acid. The formation of gluconic acid lowers the local pH, thus affecting the swelling of pH-sensitive hydrogels.

Soleimani and Sadeghi have reported on a super-absorbent hydrogel, starch-g-poly(sodium acrylate-co-2-hydroxy ethyl methacrylate) (starch-g—poly(NaAA-co-HEMA)) based, showing a maximum water absorbency in solutions with pH = 8. This hydrogel exhibited high sensitivity to pH, so that, several swelling changes of it or drug releasing percent were observed in lieu of pH variations in a wide range. Furthermore, the reversible swelling–deswelling behavior in solutions with acidic and basic pH, makes the hydrogels suitable candidates for controlled releasing systems [157].

Ion-Responsive Polymers and Their Applications

Ionic polymers were increasingly attractive for many applications in biotechnology and medicine such as drug delivery. They are also called polyelectrolytes, ionic gels, or ionic hydrogels. They dissociate, in a solution, into polyions and a larger number of oppositely charged counter ions. Interactions between polyions and counter ions cause phase transition, change in diffusivity and change in order of magnitude in equilibrium swelling. Typical examples of pH-sensitive polymers are PAAc, PMAA, poly(ethylene imine), and poly(N,N-dimethyl aminoethyl methacrylamide) [108–110, 158, 159].

Shahinpoor and Kim presented the fundamental properties and characteristics of ionic polymeric-metal composites (IPMCs) as biomimetic sensors, actuators and artificial muscle. The IPMC is composed of a perfluorinated ionic polymer layer, whose surfaces are coated by a conductive medium such as platinum. A strip of perfluorinated ionic membrane bends toward the anode under influence of an electric potential. The water containing counter ions moves toward anode creating a motion of the actuator [160]. Ion-exchange resins are frequently used for taste-masking, counterion-responsive drug release and sustained drug release. Polymers responding to ions in the saliva and gastrointestinal fluids are also used for controlled drug release in oral drug formulations.

Redox-Sensitive Polymers as DDS

Polymers containing labile groups present an advantageous opportunity to develop redox-responsive biodegradable systems. Disulfide linkages have been broadly applied in reduction-responsive polymeric drug delivery systems [117]. In fact, they are unstable in a reducing environment, being cleaved in favour of corresponding thiol groups [115, 116]. Polyanhydrides [111, 112], poly(lactic/glycolic acid) (PLGA) [113], and poly(b-amino esters) (PbAEs) [114], linking acid labile moieties, also induce redox responsiveness. PbAEs are useful to prepare efficient carriers for cytotoxic agents. On the other hand, poly(NiPAAm-co-Ru(bpy)3) finds application in the development of artificial muscles. Nguyen et al. reported on a polymeric nanogel useful to enhance the stability, redox responsiveness, and the efficacy for intracellular protein delivery. The thiolated heparin-Pluronic conjugate was self-assembled and oxidized to form a disulfide-crosslinked nanogel network under a diluted aqueous condition. The disulfide-crosslinked heparin-Pluronic (DHP) nanogels with encapsulated RNase A were characterized by in vitro release and cytotoxicity tests depending on the existence of glutathione (GSH). The DHP nanogels exhibited reduced hydrodynamic size, higher encapsulation degree, and augmentable release responding to the GSH concentration. The cytotoxicity data confirmed that DHP nanogels were more effective for the intracellular delivery of RNase A compared to non-crosslinked nanogel [161].

Moreover, novel redox-responsive polycationic hydrogels of *N,N*-diethylacrylamide (DEAAm) and 2-(dimethylamino)ethyl methacrylate (DMAEMA) were successfully synthesized by cross-linking reactions via quaternary ammonium compounds with a disulfide. The ability of the polymer network to enclose and release substances by reductive cleavage or oxidative formation of disulfide bonds was shown exemplarily using different dyes. The redox-responsive character was proven by oscillatory rheological measurements and different material properties of polycationic polymer discs were also investigated. Because of its polycationic structure, this polymeric system could be a promising compound for complexation of DNA-like substances. Its ability for selective release in reductive environments, like tumor tissues, could possibly be used in medical applications or in chemotherapy [162].

Biologically Responsive Polymers

Biologically dependent stimuli characteristically include analytes and biomacromolecules such as receptors, enzymes, glutathione, glucose, and metabolites that are over-produced in inflammation.

Glucose Responsive Polymers as Drug Carriers

Glucose sensitive materials are generated through the conjugation of glucose oxidase (GOx) to a smart pH-sensitive polymer. These systems are potentially useful for the insulin delivery [6, 119]. The incorporation of GOx may provide controlled access to the substrate and release of the product via disruption of the barrier function of the membrane. GOx oxidizes glucose to gluconic acid, which causes a pH change in the environment [4] and, subsequently, drastic changes in the polymer conformation. Hubbell et al. described glucose oxidase (GOx) encapsulated within PEG–PPS–PEG ((poly(ethylene glycol))–(poly(propylene sulfide))–PEG) polymersome [163]. This enzyme-loaded polymersome is permeable to glucose resulting in intravesicular formation of H_2O_2 upon generation of gluconic acid. Peroxide generation causes polymersome destabilization and particle destruction. This type of enzyme-amplified approach to particle degradation may have utility in drug delivery and the detection of biological analytes.

One of the most popular applications of glucose-sensitive polymers is the fabrication of insulin delivery systems for the treatment of diabetic patients. Delivering insulin is different from delivering other drugs, since insulin has to be delivered in an exact amount at the exact time of need. Many devices have been developed for this purpose and all of them have a glucose sensor built into the system. In a glucose-rich environment, such as the bloodstream after a meal, the oxidation of glucose to gluconic acid catalysed by glucose oxidase (GluOx) can lower the pH to approximately 5.8. This enzyme is probably the most widely used in glucose sensing, and makes possible to apply different types of pH-sensitive hydrogels for modulated insulin delivery [164].

Enzyme-Responsive Polymers

Among a range of external stimuli that have been utilized for the design of novel responsive polymers, enzymes have recently result to be a promising triggering subject. Enzyme-catalyzed reactions are highly selective and efficient toward specific substrates under mild conditions. They are involved in all biological and metabolic processes, serving as the main protagonists in the chemistry of living organisms at a molecular level. The integration of enzyme-catalyzed reactions with responsive polymers can additional increase the design of DDS characterized by high specificity and selectivity. In most enzyme-responsive polymer systems, enzymes are used to destroy the polymer or its assemblages. In addition, two other different types of systems, namely, enzyme-triggered self-assembly and aggregation of synthetic polymers and enzyme-triggered sol-to-gel and gel-to-sol transitions, are known (Fig. 12.9).

The major advantage of enzyme responsive polymers is that they do not require an external trigger. For instance, polymer systems based on alginate/chitosan or DEXS/chitosan microcapsules are responsive to chitosanase [126]. On the other hand, azo-aromatic bonds are sensitive to azo-reductase [127]. These enzymes, naturally produced by bacteria principally located in the colon, are capable of degrading polysaccharides like pectin, chitosan, amylase/amylopectin, cyclodextrin and dextrin [120, 125, 165].

Enzyme-Sensitive Polymers as DDS

Enzyme-sensitive polymers have been exploited frequently and they have become one of the most important branches of drug delivery systems. Zhang et al.

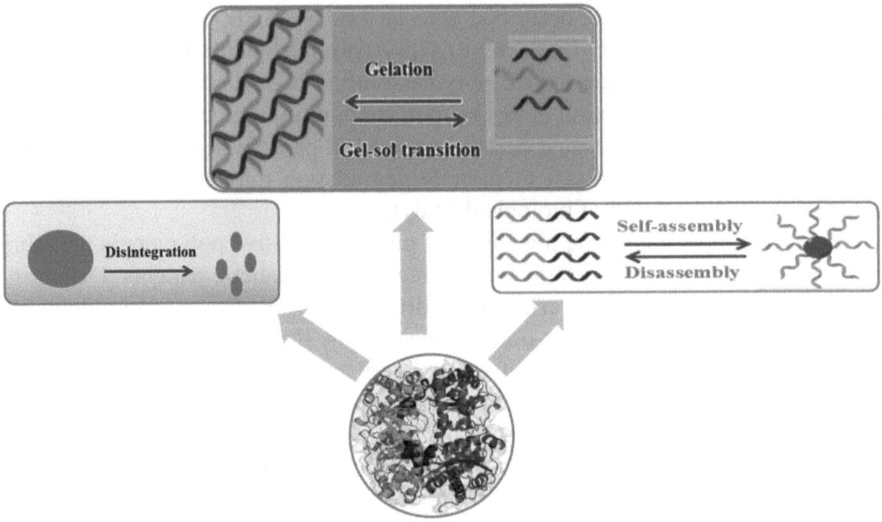

Fig. 12.9 Scheme of three main types of enzyme-responsive polymeric materials

prepared and synthesized mPEGylated peptide dendrimer–drug conjugate as a promising candidate of drug delivery system via a two-step click reaction with excellent characteristics and functionalities. A tetra-peptide sequence GFLG, which was cleavable in the presence of cathepsin B overexpressed in the tumor cells, was employed as linker to connect the anticancer drug DOX to mPEGylated peptide dendrimer. Due to the controlled release of drug and the particular nanoscale size, mPEGylated dendrimer–GFLG–DOX conjugate was found to have obviously improved in vivo antitumor efficacy over commercial DOX formulation at an equal dose, as well as low side effects, which were measured by changes in body weight and histological analysis. Overall, the structural design of mPEGylated peptide dendrimer–DOX conjugate-based nanoparticle in this study may provide useful strategy for design and preparation of peptide dendrimer as a safe and effective drug delivery system [166]. The use of enzyme catalysis as a tool to disassemble self-assembled hydrogels to control the release encapsulated drug provides a further opportunity to design a wide range of enzyme-specific low-molecular-weight hydrogelators (LMWGs). Vemula and coworkers reported a novel approach for controlled delivery of multiple drugs by an enzyme triggered hydrogel degradation mechanism. In particular, they described the synthesis of LMWGs (amphiphiles) from well-known drug acetaminophen (which is known as Tylenolreg), and their ability to self-assemble into nanoscale structures in aqueous solutions to form hydrogels that subsequently encapsulate a second drug such as curcumin which is a known chemopreventive hydrophobic drug. Upon enzyme triggered degradation, hydrogels showed single and double drug delivery at physiological conditions in vitro. After treating with prodrug amphiphiles, mesenchymal stem cells (MSCs) retain their stem cell properties such as maintaining their adhesive and proliferation capacities with high viability. This new platform approach will have prospective effect on hydrogel based drug delivery research through developing drug delivery vehicles from a wide range of prodrug-based gelators [167].

Inflammation-Responsive Smart Polymers

The inflammation is one of the manifestations of immune response and the chief immune components involved are the cells of the polymorphonuclear leukocytes (PML) [168]. These include the neutrophils, eosinophils and basophils. Apart from these, T-cell and B-cell lymphocytes and macrophages are also involved in the amplification of these signals. One of the hallmarks of inflammatory response is the generation of free radicals. Thus design of a system with bonds that will lyse due to the action of free radicals (for example, OH^-, the hydroxyl radical) will enable release of drugs at the site of inflammation. Polyglycerolpolyglycidylether cross-linked with hyaluronic acid was used as the polymer matrix. The hyaluronic cross-links were degraded rapidly in the presence of hydroxyl radicals resulting in release of the drug. This system enables rapid release of drug at the site of inflammation [169].

Polymers with Dual Stimuli-Responsiveness

It is possible to obtain polymeric structures sensitive simultaneously to more than one stimulus. Particularly interesting are the dual temperature- and pH-responsive smart polymers that are attracting increasing attention recently for their advantages in biotechnological and biomedical applications. In this respect, Leung and coworkers have prepared smart core-shell microgels based on PNIPAAm, N,N′-methylenebisacrylamide (MBAAm) and chitosan or PEI in the absence of surfactants. The materials exhibited a well-defined core-shell structure consisting of temperature-sensitive cores, based on PNIPAAm, and pH-sensitive shells, made of cationic water-soluble polymers [170]. Moreover, Kuckling et al. prepared copolymers of NIPAAm with acrylamide derivatives bearing carboxylic groups attached to spacers with different chain length and studied the influence of both temperature and pH on their properties [171]. pH/temperature dual stimuli-responsive microcapsules have been prepared by incorporating carboxyl groups into PNIPAAm hydrogel shells by random copolymerization of NIPAAm and acrylic acid (AA) to endow the microcapsules with temperature responsiveness as well as pH responsiveness [172, 173]. The reversible change in hydrogen bonding between the two components NIPAAm and AA and water, and the ionization of carboxylate groups under different environmental condition resulted in the dual-stimuli response. Chitosan based PNIPAAm films having both thermal and pH sensitivity were prepared by combination of chitosan with PNIPAAm and PEG [174].

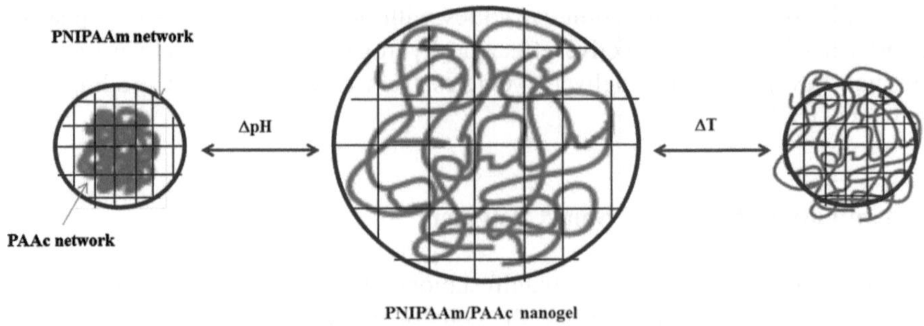

Fig. 12.10 Schematic representation of dual-sensitive nanogels

The resulting film had an LCST at around 32 °C, due to the presence of PNIPAAm, and showed pH responsiveness due to the amino groups of chitosan component. Poly(vinylidene fluoride) (PVDF) hydrophobic films grafted with PAA demonstrated convective permeability that changed significantly with the pH and/or the salt concentration of the surrounding fluids [175].

Nanogels with pH and temperature dual stimuli-responsive properties characterized by interpenetrating polymer network (IPN) structure, based on PNIPAAm and PAAc, were also synthesized by in situ polymerization of acrylic acid and N,N-methylenebisacrylamide (Fig. 12.10). These IPN nanogels have the advantage of less mutual interference between the temperature-responsive and pH-responsive components, which is beneficial for their applications in controlled drug release and sensors [176].

References

1. Galaev, I.Y., Mattiasson, B.: Smart polymers and what they could do in biotechnology and medicine. Trends Biotechnol. **17**, 335–340 (1999)
2. Hoffman, A.S., Stayton, P.S., Bulmus, V., Chen, G., Chen, J., Cheung, C., Chilkoti, A., Ding, Z., Dong, L., Fong, R., Lackey, C.A., Long, C.J., Miura, M., Morris, J.E., Murthy, N., Nabeshima, Y., Park, T.G., Press, O.W., Shimoboji, T., Shoemaker, S., Yang, H.J., Monji, N., Nowinski, R.C., Cole, C.A., Priest, J.H., Harris, J.M., Nakamae, K., Nishino, T., Miyata, T.: Founder's award, society for biomaterials. Sixth world biomaterials congress 2000, Kamuela, HI, May 15–20, 2000. Really smart bioconjugates of smart polymers and receptor proteins. J. Biomed. Mater. Res. **52**, 577–586 (2000)
3. Kikuchi, A., Okano, T.: Intelligent thermoresponsive polymeric stationary phases for aqueous chromatography of biological compounds. Prog. Polym. Sci. **27**, 1165–1193 (2002)
4. Qiu, Y., Park, K.: Environment-sensitive hydrogels for drug delivery. Adv. Drug Deliv. Rev. **53**, 321–339 (2001)
5. Jeong, B., Gutowska, A.: Lessons from nature: stimuli-responsive polymers and their biomedical applications. Trends Biotechnol. **20**, 305–311 (2002)
6. Gil, E.S., Hudson, S.M.: Stimuli-responsive polymers and their bioconjugates. Prog. Polym. Sci. **29**, 1173–1222 (2004)

7. Delcea, M., Möhwald, H., Skirtach, A.G.: Stimuli-responsive LbL capsules and nanoshells for drug delivery. Adv. Drug Deliv. Rev. **63**, 730–747 (2011)
8. Pinkrah, V.T., Snowden, M.J., Mitchell, J.C., Seidel, J., Chowdhry, B.Z., Fern, G.R.: Physicochemical properties of poly(N-isopropylacrylamide-co-4-vinylpyridine) cationic polyelectrolyte colloidal microgels. Langmuir **19**, 585–590 (2003)
9. Peng, T., Cheng, Y.L.: PNIPAAm and PMAA co-grafted porous PE membranes: living radical co-grafting mechanism and multi-stimuli responsive permeability. Polymer **41**, 2091–2100 (2001)
10. Bignotti, F., Penco, M., Sartore, L., Peroni, I., Mendichi, R., Casolaro, M., D'Amore, A.: Synthesis, characterisation and solution behaviour of thermo- and pH-responsive polymers bearing L-leucine residues in the side chains. Polymer **41**, 8247–8256 (2000)
11. Gan, L.H., Gan, Y.Y., Deen, G.R.: Poly(N-acryloyl-N'-propylpiperazine): a new stimuli-responsive polymer. Macromolecules **33**, 7893–7897 (2000)
12. Kost, J., Langer, R.: Responsive polymeric delivery systems. Adv. Drug Deliv. Rev. **46**, 125–148 (2001)
13. Galaev, I.Y., Mattiasson, B.: Smart polymers and what they could do in biotechnology and medicine. Trends Biotechnol. **17**, 335–340 (1999)
14. Kumar, A., Srivastava, A., Galaev, I.Y., Mattiasson, B.: Smart polymers: physical forms and bioengineering applications. Prog. Polym. Sci. **32**, 1205–1237 (2007)
15. Liechty, W.B., Kryscio, D.R., Slaughter, B.V., Peppas, N.A.: Polymers for drug delivery systems. Annu. Rev. Chem. Biomol. Eng. **1**, 149–173 (2010)
16. Okano, T.: Biorelated Polymers and Gels-Controlled Release and Applications in Biomedical Engineering. Academic Press, San Diago (1998)
17. Roy, D., Cambre, J.N., Sumerlin, B.S.: Future perspectives and recent advances in stimuli responsive materials. Prog. Polym. Sci. **35**, 278–301 (2010)
18. Xie, T., Xiao, X.: Self-peeling reversible dry adhesive. Chem. Mater. **20**, 2866–2868 (2008)
19. Lendlein, A., Langer, R.: Biodegradable, elastic shapememory polymers for potential biomedical applications. Science **96**, 1673–1676 (2002)
20. Zhu, Y., Hu, J., Yeung, K.: Effect of soft segment crystallization and hard segment physical crosslink on shape memory function in antibacterial segmented polyurethane ionomers. Acta Biomater. **5**, 3346–3357 (2009)
21. Scrosati, B.: Application of Electroactive Polymers. Chapman and Hall, London (1993)
22. Bar-Cohen, Y.: Proceedings of the 42nd AIAA Structures, Structural Dynamics, and Materials Conference (SDM), Gossamer Spacecraft Forum (GSF), Seattle (2001)
23. Charlesby, A.: Atomic Radiation and Polymers. Pergamon, New York (1960)
24. Gall, K., Dunn, M.L., Liu, Y., Finch, D., Lake, M., Munshi, N.A.: Shape memory polymer nanocomposites. Acta Mater. **50**, 5115–5126 (2002)
25. Bar-Cohen, Y., Zhang, Q.: Electroactive polymer actuators and sensors. MRS Bull. **33**, 173–181 (2008)
26. Gupta, P., Vermani, K., Garg, S.: Hydrogels: from controlled release to pH-responsive drug delivery. Drug Discov. Today **7**, 569–579 (2002)
27. Kikuchi, A., Okano, T.: Pulsatile drug release control using hydrogels. Adv. Drug Deliv. Rev. **54**, 53–77 (2002)
28. Nakayama, M., Okano, T., Miyazaki, T., Kohori, F., Sakai, K., Yokoyama, M.: Molecular design of biodegradable polymeric micelles for temperature-responsive drug release. J. Control Release **115**, 46–56 (2006)
29. Bromberg, L.E., Ron, E.S.: Temperature-responsive gels and thermogelling polymer matrices for protein and peptide delivery. Adv. Drug Deliv. Rev. **31**, 197–221 (1998)
30. Peppas, N.A., Bures, P., Leobandung, W., Ichikawa, H.: Hydrogels in pharmaceutical formulations. Eur. J. Pharm. Biopharm. **50**, 27–46 (2000)
31. Li, L., Shan, H., Yue, C.Y., Lam, Y.C., Tam, K.C., Hu, X.: Thermally induced association and dissociation of methyl cellulose in aqueous solutions. Langmuir **18**, 7291–7298 (2002)
32. Liu, Y.Y., Shao, Y.H., Lü, J.: Preparation properties and controlled release behaviors of pH-induced thermosensitive amphiphilic gels. Biomaterials **27**, 4016–4024 (2006)

33. Yin, X., Hoffman, A.S., Stayton, P.S.: Poly(N-isopropylacrylamide-co-propylacrylic acid) copolymers that respond sharply to temperature and pH. Biomacromolecules **7**, 1381–1385 (2006)
34. Kabanov, A.V., Batrakova, E.V., Alakhov, V.Y.: Pluronic block copolymers as novel polymer therapeutics for drug and gene delivery. J. Control Release **82**, 189–212 (2002)
35. Joly-Duhamel, C., Hellio, D., Djabourov, M.: All gelatin networks: 1. Biodiversity and physical chemistry. Langmuir **18**, 7208–7217 (2002)
36. Lutz, J.F.: Polymerization of oligo(ethylene glycol) (meth)acrylates: toward new generations of smart biocompatible materials. J. Polym. Sci. A Polym. Chem. **46**, 3459–3470 (2008)
37. Hoogenboom, R.: Poly(2-oxazoline)s: a polymer class with numerous potential applications. Angew. Chem. Int. Ed. **48**, 7978–7994 (2009)
38. Jeong, B., Kim, S.W., Bae, Y.H.: Thermosensitive sol-gel reversible hydrogels. Adv. Drug Deliv. Rev. **54**, 37–51 (2002)
39. Ruel-Gariepy, E., Leroux, J.C.: In situ forming hydrogels-review of temperature-sensitive systems. Eur. J. Pharm. Biopharm. **58**, 409–426 (2004)
40. Takahashi, M., Shimazaki, M., Yamamoto, J.: Thermoreversible gelation and phase separation in aqueous methyl cellulose solutions. J. Polym. Sci. B **39**, 91–100 (2001)
41. Klouda, L., Mikos, A.G.: Thermoresponsive hydrogels in biomedical applications. Eur. J. Pharm. Biopharm. **68**, 34–45 (2008)
42. Bae, Y.H., Okano, T., Kim, S.W.: "On-off" thermocontrol of solute transport. II. Solute release from thermosensitive hydrogels. Pharm. Res. **8**, 531–537 (1991)
43. Bae, Y.H., Okano, T., Kim, S.W.: On-off thermocontrol of solute transport. II solute release from thermosensitive hydrogels. Pharm. Res. **8**, 624–628 (1991)
44. Okano, T., Bae, Y.H., Jacobs, H., Kim, S.W.: Thermally on-off switching polymers for drug permeation and release. J. Controlled Release **11**, 255–265 (1990)
45. Okuyama, Y., Yoshida, R., Sakai, K., Okano, T., Sakurai, Y.: Swelling controlled zero-order and sigmoidal drug release from thermoresponsive poly(N-isopropylacrylamide-co-butyl methacrylate) hydrogel. J. Biomater. Sci. Polym. **4**, 545–556 (1993)
46. Jones, M., Leroux, J.: Polymeric micelles: a new generation of colloidal drug carriers. Eur. J. Pharm. Biopharm. **48**, 101–111 (1999)
47. Allen, T.M.: Liposomal drug formulations, rationale for development and what we can. Expect for the future. Drugs **56**, 747–756 (1998)
48. Matsumura, Y., Maeda, H.: A new concept for macromolecular therapeutics in cancer chemotherapy: mechanism of tumoritropic accumulation of proteins and the antitumor agent smancs. Cancer Res. **46**, 6387–6392 (1986)
49. Chung, J.E., Yokoyama, M., Yamato, M., Aoyagi, T., Sakurai, Y., Okano, T.: Thermoresponsive drug delivery from polymeric micelles constructed using block copolymers of poly(N-isopropylacrylamide) and poly(butylmethacrylate). J. Controlled Release **62**, 115–127 (1999)
50. Chung, E., Yokoyama, M., Okano, T.: Inner core segment design for drug delivery control of thermo- responsive polymeric micelles. J. Controlled Release **65**, 93–103 (2000)
51. Kohori, F., Sakai, K., Aoyagi, T., Yokoyama, M., Yamato, M., Sakurai, Y., Okano, T.: Control of adriamycin cytotoxic activity using thermally. Colloids Surf. B **16**, 195–205 (1999)
52. Honey, P.J., Rijo, J., Anju, A., Anoop, K.R.: Smart polymers for the controlled delivery of drugs—a concise overview. Acta Pharm. Sinica B **4**, 120–127 (2014)
53. Nozawa, I., Suzuki, Y., Sato, S., Sugibayashi, K., Morimoto, Y.: Preparation of thermoresponsive polymer membranes. I. J. Biomed. Mat. Res. **25**, 243–254 (1991)
54. Yan, B., Boyer, J.C., Habault, D., Branda, N.R., Zhao, Y.: Near infrared light triggered release of biomacromolecules from hydrogels loaded with upconversion nanoparticles. J. Am. Chem. Soc. **134**, 16558–16561 (2012)
55. Fomina, N., McFearin, C.L., Sermsakdi, M., Morachis, J.M., Alrnutairi, A.: Low power, biologically benign NIR light triggers polymer disassembly. Macromolecules **44**, 8590–8597 (2011)

56. Habault, D., Zhang, H.J., Zhao, Y.: Light-triggered self-healing and shape-memory polymers. Chem. Soc. Rev. **42**, 7244–7256 (2013)
57. Yan, Y., Yue, L., Li, H.L., Maher, E., Li, Y.G., Wang, Y.Z., Wu, L.X., Yarn, V.W.W.: Photo-responsive self-assembly of an azobenzene-ended surfactant-encapsulated polyoxometalate complex for modulating catalytic reactions. Small **8**, 3105–3110 (2012)
58. Schumers, J.M., Fustin, C.A., Gohy, J.F.: Light-responsive block copolymers. Macromol. Rapid Commun. **31**, 1588–1607 (2010)
59. Gilot, J., Abbel, R., Lakhwani, G., Meijer, E.W., Schenning, A.P.H.J., Meskers, S.C.J.: Polymer photovoltaic cells sensitive to the circular polarization of light. Adv. Mater. **22**, E131–E134 (2010)
60. Narayan, K.S., Kumar, N.: Light responsive polymer field-effect transistor. Appl. Phys. Lett. **79**, 1891–1893 (2001)
61. Gan, L.H., Roshan, G., Loh, X.J., Gan, Y.Y.: New stimuli responsive copolymers of N-acryloyl-N′-alkyl piperazine and methyl methacrylate and their hydrogels. Polymer **42**, 65–69 (2001)
62. Aoyagi, T., Ebara, M., Sakai, K., Sakurai, Y., Okano, T.: Novel bifunctional polymer with reactivity and temperature sensitivity. J. Biomater. Sci. Polym. **11**, 101–110 (2000)
63. Aoki, T., Muramatsu, M., Nishina, A., Sanui, K., Ogata, N.: Thermosensitivities of optically active hydrogels constructed with N-(L)-(1-hydroxymethyl)propylmethacrylamide. Macromol. Biosci. **4**, 943–949 (2004)
64. Bae, Y.H., Okano, T., Kim, S.W.: Insulin permeation through thermosensitive hydrogels. J. Controlled Release **9**, 271–279 (1989)
65. Hirokawa, Y., Tanaka, T.: Volume phase transition in a nonionic gel. J. Chem. Phys. **81**, 6379–6380 (1984)
66. Bae, Y.H., Okano, T., Kim, S.W.: A new thermo-sensitive hydrogel: Interpenetrating polymer networks from N-acryloylpyrrolidine and poly(oxyethylene). Makromol. Chem. Rapid Commun. **9**, 185–189 (1988)
67. Mamada, A., Tanaka, T., Kungwachakun, D., Irie, M.: Photoinduced phase transition of gels. Macromolecules **23**, 1517–1519 (1990)
68. Suzuki, A., Tanaka, T.: Phase transition in polymer gels induced by visible light. Nature **346**, 345–347 (1990)
69. Cabane, E., Malinova, V., Menon, S., Palivan, C.G., Meier, W.: Photoresponsive polymersomes as smart, triggerable nanocarriers. Soft Matter **7**, 9167–9176 (2011)
70. Son, S., Shin, E., Kim, B.S.: Light-responsive micelles of spiropyran initiated hyperbranched polyglycerol for smart drug delivery. Biomacromolecules **15**, 628–634 (2014)
71. Chen, Z., He, Y., Wang, Y., Wang, X.: Amphiphilic diblock copolymer with dithienylethene pendants: synthesis and photo-modulated self-assembly. Macromol. Rapid Commun. **32**, 977–982 (2011)
72. Jin, Q., Mitschang, F., Agarwal, S.: Biocompatible drug delivery system for photo-triggered controlled release of 5-fluorouracil. Biomacromolecules **12**, 3684–3691 (2011)
73. Menon, S., Thekkayil, R., Varghes, S., Das, S.: Photoresponsive soft materials: synthesis and photophysical studies of a stilbene-based diblock copolymer synthesis and photophysical studies of a stilbene-based diblock copolymer. J. Polym. Sci. A Polym. Chem. **49**, 5063–5073 (2011)
74. Liu, G.Y., Chen, C.J., Li, D.D., Wang, S.S., Ji, J.: Near-infrared light-sensitive micelles for enhanced intracellular drug delivery. J. Mater. Chem. **22**, 16865–16871 (2012)
75. Seki, T., Fukuda, R., Tamakia, T., Ichimura, K.: Alignment photoregulation of liquid crystals on precisely area controlled azobenzene langmuir-blodgett monolayers. Thin Solid Films **243**, 675–678 (1994)
76. Anal, A.K.: Stimuli-induced pulsatile or triggered release delivery systems for bioactive compounds. Recent Pat. Endocr. Metab. Immune Drug Discov. **1**, 83–90 (2007)
77. Mendes, P.M.: Stimuli-responsive surfaces for bio-applications. Chem. Soc. Rev. **37**, 2512–2529 (2008)

78. Gong, J.P., Nitta, T., Osada, Y.: Electrokinetic modeling of the contractile phenomena of polyelectrolyte gels-one dimensional capillary model. J. Phys. Chem. **98**, 9583–9587 (1994)
79. Kwon, I.C., Bae, Y.H., Okano, T., Kim, S.W.: Drug release from electric current sensitive polymers. J. Controlled Release **17**, 149–153 (1991)
80. Jones, D.P., Carlson, J.L., Samiec, P.S., Sternberg Jr, P., Mody Jr, V.C., Reed, R.L., Brown, L.A.S.: Glutathione measurement in human plasma. Clin. Chim. Acta **275**, 175–184 (1998)
81. Koo, A.N., Lee, H.J., Kim, S.E., Chang, J.H., Park, C., Kim, C., Park, J.H., Lee, S.C.: Disulfide-cross-linked PEG-poly(amino acid)s copolymer micelles for glutathione-mediated intracellular drug delivery. Chem. Commun. **44**, 6570–6572 (2008)
82. Tanaka, T., Nishio, I., Sun, S.-T., Ueno-Nishio, S.: Collapse of gels in an electric. Field. Sci. **218**, 467–469 (1982)
83. Zhao, X., Kim, J., Cezar, C.A., Huebsch, N., Lee, K., Bouhadir, K., Mooney, D.J.: Active scaffolds for on-demand drug and cell delivery. Proc. Natl. Acad. Sci. U.S.A. **108**, 67–72 (2011)
84. Liu, Y., Servant, A., Guy, O.J., Al-Jamal, K.T., Williams, P.R., Hawkins, K.M., Kostarelos, K.: Liposomes: from a clinically established drug delivery system to a nanoparticle platform for theranostic nanomedicine. Proc. Eng. **25**, 984–987 (2011)
85. Kulkarni, R.V., Sa, B.: Electroresponsive polyacrylamide-grafted-xanthan hydrogels for drug delivery. J. Bioact. Compat. Polym. **24**, 368–384 (2009)
86. Servant, A., Bussy, C., Al-Jamal, K., Kostarelos, K.: Design, engineering and structural integrity of electro-responsive carbon nanotube-poly(methyl) methacrylate hydrogels for pulsatile drug release. J. Mater. Chem. B **1**, 4593–4600 (2013)
87. Haba, Y., Harada, A., Takagishi, T., Kono, K.: Rendering poly(amidoamine) or poly(propylenimine) dendrimers temperature sensitive. J. Am. Chem. Soc. **126**, 12760–12761 (2004)
88. Burakowska, E., Zimmerman, S.C., Haag, R.: Photoresponsive crosslinked hyperbranched polyglycerols as smart nanocarriers for guest binding and controlled release. Small **5**, 2199–2204 (2009)
89. Chen, W., Tomalia, D.A., Thomas, J.L.: Unusual pH-dependent polarity changes in PAMAM dendrimers: evidence for pH-responsive conformational changes. Macromolecules **33**, 9169–9172 (2000)
90. Liu, Y., Bryantsev, V.S., Diallo, M.S., Goddard III, W.A.: PAMAM dendrimers undergo pH responsive conformational changes without swelling. J. Am. Chem. Soc. **131**, 2798–2799 (2009)
91. Yang, K., Weng, L., Cheng, Y., Zhang, H., Zhang, J., Wu, Q., Xu, T.: Host-guest chemistry of dendrimer-drug complexes. 6. Fully acetylated dendrimers as biocompatible drug vehicles using dexamethasone 21-phosphate as a model drug. J. Phys. Chem. B **115**, 2185–2195 (2011)
92. Kohman, R.E., Zimmerman, S.C.: Degradable dendrimers divergently synthesized via click chemistry. Chem. Commun. **45**, 794–796 (2009)
93. Cho, S.Y., Allcock, H.R.: Dendrimers derived from polyphosphazene poly(propyleneimine) systems: encapsulation and triggered release of hydrophobic guest molecules. Macromolecules **40**, 3115–3121 (2007)
94. Kostiainen, M.A., Rosilo, H.: Low-molecular-weight dendrons for DNA binding and release by reduction-triggered degradation of multivalent interactions. Chem. Eur. J. **15**, 5656–5660 (2009)
95. Ong, W., McCarley, R.L.: Chemically and electrochemically mediated release of dendrimer end groups. Macromolecules **39**, 7295–7301 (2006)
96. Azagarsamy, M.A., Sokkalingam, P., Thayumanavan, S.: Enzyme triggered disassembly of dendrimer-based amphiphilic nanocontainers. J. Am. Chem. Soc. **131**, 14184–14185 (2009)
97. Azagarsamy, M.A., Yesilyurt, V., Thayumanavan, S.: Disassembly of dendritic micellar containers due to protein binding. J. Am. Chem. Soc. **132**, 4550–4551 (2010)
98. Miyazaki, S., Hou, W.M., Takada, M.: Controlled drug release by ultrasound irradiation. Chem. Pharm. Bull. **33**, 428–431 (1985)
99. Miyazaki, S., Yokouchi, C., Takada, M.: External control of drug release: controlled release of insulin from a hydrophilic polymer implants by ultrasound irradiation in diabetic rats. J. Pharm. Pharmacol. **40**, 716–717 (1988)

100. Kwok, C.S., Mourad, P.D., Crum, L.A., Ratner, B.D.: Surface modification of polymers with self-assembled molecular structure: multitechnique surface characterization. Biomacromolecules **1**, 139–148 (2000)
101. Kwok, C.S., Mourad, P.D., Crum, L.A., Ratner, B.D.: Self-assembled molecular structures as ultrasonically-responsive barrier membranes for pulsatile drug delivery. J. Biomed. Mater. Res. **57**, 151–164 (2001)
102. Kotharangannagari, V.K., Sánchez-Ferrer, A., Ruokolainen, J., Mezzenga, R.: Photoresponsive reversible aggregation and dissolution of rod-coil polypeptide diblock copolymers. Macromolecules **44**, 4569–4573 (2011)
103. Koyama, T., Hatano, K., Matsuoka, K., Esumi, Y., Terunuma, D.: Synthesis and characterization of photo-responsive carbosilane dendrimers. Molecules **14**, 2226–2234 (2009)
104. Chan, Y., Wong, T., Byrne, F., Kavallaris, M., Bulmus, V.: Acid-labile core cross-linked micelles for pH-triggered release of antitumor drugs. Biomacromolecules **9**, 1826–1836 (2008)
105. Katayama, Y., Sonoda, T., Maeda, M.: A polymer micelle responding to the protein kinase A signal. Macromolecules **34**, 8569–8573 (2001)
106. Gonzalez, D.C., Savariar, E.N., Thayumanavan, S.: Fluorescence patterns from supramolecular polymer assembly and disassembly for sensing metallo- and nonmetalloproteins. J. Am. Chem. Soc. **131**, 7708–7716 (2009)
107. Hsieh, D.S.T., Langer, R., Folkman, J.: Magnetic modulation of release of macromolecules from polymers. Proc. Natl. Acad. Sci. U.S.A. **78**, 1863–1867 (1981)
108. Salamone, J.C., Rodriguez, E.L., Lin, K.C., Quach, L., Watterson, A.C., Ahmed, I.: Aqueous salt absorption by ampholytic polysaccharides. Polymer **26**, 1234–1238 (1985)
109. Morrison, M.E., Dorfman, R.C., Clendening, W.D., Kiserow, D.J., Rossky, P.J., Webber, S.E.: Quenching kinetics of anthracene covalently bound to a polyelectrolyte. 1. Effects of ionic strength. J. Phys. Chem. **98**, 5534–5540 (1994)
110. Szczubiałka, K., Jankowska, M., Nowakowska, M.: Smart polymeric nanospheres as new materials for possible biomedical applications. J. Mater. Sci. Mater. Med. **14**, 699–703 (2003)
111. Leong, K.W., Brott, B.C., Langer, R.: Bioerodible polyanhydrides as drug carrier matrices I: characterization, degradation and release characteristics. J. Biomed. Mater. Res. **19**, 941–955 (1985)
112. Mathiowitz, E., Jacob, J.S., Jong, Y.S., Carino, G.P., Chickering, D.E., Chaturvedi, P., Santos, C.A., Vijayaraghavan, K., Montgomery, S., Bassett, M., Morrell, C.: Biologically erodable microspheres as potential oral drug delivery systems. Nature **386**, 410–414 (1997)
113. Cohen, S., Yoshioka, T., Lucarelli, M., Hwang, L.H., Langer, R.: Controlled delivery systems for proteins basedon poly(lactic/glycolic acid) microspheres. Pharm. Res. **8**, 713–720 (1991)
114. Shenoy, D., Little, S., Langer, R., Amiji, M.: Poly(ethylene oxide)-modiWed poly(beta-amino ester) nanoparticles as a pH-sensitive system for tumor-targeted delivery of hydrophobic drugs: part 3. Therapeutic efficacy and safety studies in ovarian cancer xenograft model. Pharm. Res. **22**, 2107–2114 (2005)
115. Cerritelli, S., Velluto, D., Hubbell, J.A.: PEG-SS-PPS: reduction-sensitive disulfide block copolymer vesicles for intracellular drug delivery. Biomacromolecules **8**, 1966–1972 (2007)
116. Oh, J.K., Siegwart, D.J., Lee, H.-I., Sherwood, G., Peteanu, L., Hollinger, J.O., Kataoka, K., Matyjaszewski, K.: Biodegradable nanogels prepared by atom transfer radical polymerization as potential drug delivery carriers: synthesis, biodegradation, in vitro release, and bioconjugation. J. Am. Chem. Soc. **129**, 5939–5945 (2007)
117. Matsumoto, S., Christie, R.J., Nishiyama, N., Miyata, K., Ishii, A., Oba, M., Koyama, H., Yamasaki, Y., Kataoka, K.: Environment-responsive block copolymer micelles with a disulfide cross-linked core for enhanced siRNA delivery. Biomacromolecules **10**, 119–127 (2008)
118. Yoshida, R., Yamaguchi, T., Kokufuta, E.: Self-oscillation of polymer gels coupled with the Belousov–Zhabotinsky reaction. J. Artif. Organs. **2**, 135–140 (1999)

119. Chaterji, S., Kwon, I.K., Park, K.: Smart polymeric gels. Prog. Polym. Sci. **32**, 1083–1122 (2007)
120. Chambin, O., Dupuis, G., Champion, D., Voilley, A., Pourcelot, Y.: Colon-specific drug delivery: influence of solution reticulation properties upon pectin beads performance. Int. J. Pharm. **321**, 86–93 (2006)
121. Galicia, J.A., Cousin, F., Dubois, E., Sandre, O., Cabuil, V., Perzynski, R.: Static and dynamic structural probing of swollen Polyacrylamide ferrogels. Soft Matter **5**, 2614–2624 (2009)
122. Papaphilippou, P.C., Pourgouris, A., Marinica, O., Taculescu, A., Athanasopoulos, G.I., Vekas, L., Krasia-Christoforou, T.: Fabrication and characterization of superparamagnetic and thermoresponsive hydrogels based on oleic-acid-coated Fe_3O_4 nanoparticles, hexa(ethylene glycol) methyl ether methacrylate and 2-(acetoacetoxy)ethyl methacrylate. J. Magn. Magn. Mater. **323**, 557–563 (2011)
123. Li, Z., Shen, J., Ma, H., Lu, X., Shi, M., Li, N., Ye, M.: Poly(acrylamide/laponite) nanocomposite hydrogels: swelling and cationic dye adsorption properties. Polym. Bull. **68**, 1153–1169 (2012)
124. Satarkar, N.S., Zach Hilt, J.: Magnetic hydrogel nanocomposites forremote controlled pulsatile drug release. Acta Biomater. **4**, 11–16 (2007)
125. Vandamme, T.F., Lenourry, A., Charrueau, C., Chaumeil, J.C.: The use of polysaccharides to target drugs to the colon. Carbohydr. Polym. **48**, 219–231 (2002)
126. Itoh, Y., Matsusaki, M., Kida, T., Akashi, M.: Enzyme-responsive release of encapsulated proteins from biodegradable hollow capsules. Biomacromolecules **7**, 2715–2718 (2006)
127. Akala, E.O., Kopečková, P., Kopeček, J.: Enzyme-responsive release of encapsulated proteins from biodegradable hollow capsules. Biomaterials **19**, 1037–1047 (1998)
128. Miyata, K., Kakizawa, Y., Nishiyama, N., Harada, A., Yamasaki, Y., Koyama, H., Kataoka, K.: Block catiomer polyplexes with regulated densities of charge. J. Am. Chem. Soc. **126**, 2355–2361 (2004)
129. Boas, U., Heegaard, P.M.H.: Dendrimers in drug research. Chem. Soc. Rev. **33**, 43–63 (2004)
130. Zrinyi, M.: Intelligent polymer gels controlled by magnetic fields. Colloid Polym. Sci. **278**, 98–103 (2000)
131. Cheng, Y., Xu, Z., Ma, M., Xu, T.: Pharmaceutical applications of dendrimers: promising nanocarriers for drug discovery. J. Pharm. Sci. **97**, 123–143 (2007)
132. Patri, A.K., Majoros, I.J., Baker Jr, J.R.: Dendritic polymer macromolecular carriers for drug delivery. Curr. Opin. Chem. Biol. **6**, 466–471 (2002)
133. Zhou, J., Wang, L., Ma, J., Wang, J., Yu, H., Xiao, A.: Temperature and pH-responsive star amphiphilic block copolymer prepared by a combining strategy of ring-opening polymerization and reversible addition–fragmentation transfer polymerization. Eur Polym J **46**, 1288–1298 (2010)
134. Yang, Z., Zhang, W., Zou, J., Shi, W.: Synthesis and thermally responsive characteristics of dendritic poly(ether-amide) grafting with PNIPAAm and PEG. Polymer **48**, 931–938 (2007)
135. Dissemond, J., Witthoff, M., Brauns, T.C., Haberer, D., Goos, M.: Untersuchungen zum pH-Wert des Milieus chronischer Wunden im Rahmen einer modernen Wundtherapie. Hautarzt **54**, 959–965 (2003)
136. Rofstad, E.K., Mathiesen, B., Kindem, K., Galappathi, K.: Acidic extracellular. pH promotes experimental metastasis of human melanoma cells in athymic nude mice. Cancer Res. **66**, 6699–6707 (2006)
137. Vaupel, P., Kallinowski, F., Okunieff, P.: Blood flow, oxygen and nutrient supply, and metabolic microenvironment of human tumors: a review. Cancer Res. **49**, 6449–6465 (1989)
138. Chan, A., Orme, R.P., Fricker, R.A., Roach, P.: Remote and local control of stimuli responsive materials for therapeutic applications. Adv. Drug Deliv. Rev. **65**, 497–514 (2013)
139. Foss, A.C., Goto, T., Morishita, M., Peppas, N.A.: Development of acrylic-based copolymers for oral insulin delivery. Eur. J. Pharm. Biopharm. **57**, 163–169 (2004)
140. Peng, C.L., Yang, L.Y., Luo, T.Y., Lai, P.S., Yang, S.J., Lin, W.J., Shieh, M.J.: Development of pH sensitive 2-(diisopropylamino)ethyl methacrylate based nanoparticles for photodynamic therapy. Nanotechnology **21**, 155013 (2010)

141. Park, S.Y., Bae, Y.H.: Novel pH-sensitive polymers containing sulfonamide groups. Macromol. Rapid Commun. **20**, 269–273 (1999)
142. Lee, Y.M., Shim, J.K.: Preparation of pH/temperature responsive polymer membrane by plasma polymerization and its riboflavin permeation. Polymer **38**, 1227–1232 (1997)
143. Soppimath, K.S., Kulkarni, A.R., Aminabhavi, T.M.: Chemically modified Polyacrylamide-g-Guar Gum- based crosslinked anionic microgels as pH-sensitive drug delivery systems: preparation and characterization. J. Controlled Release **75**, 331–345 (2001)
144. Abdelaal, M.Y., Abdel-Razik, E.A., Abdel-Bary, E.M., El-Sherbiny, I.M.: Study on chitosan-poly(vinyl alcohol) interpolymeric pH-responsive hydrogel films for controlled drug delivery. J. Appl. Polym. Sci. **103**, 2864–2874 (2007)
145. Park, H.-Y., Song, I.-H., Kim, J.-H., Kim, W.-S.: Preparation of thermally denatured albumin gel and its pH-sensitive swelling. Int. J. Pharm. **175**, 231–236 (1998)
146. Kurisawa, M., Yui, N.: Gelatin/dextran intelligent hydrogels for drug delivery: dual-stimuli-responsive degradation in relation to miscibility in interpenetrating polymer networks. Macromol. Chem. Phys. **199**, 1547–1554 (1998)
147. Lee, J.W., Kim, S.Y., Kim, S.S., Lee, Y.M., Lee, K.H., Kim, S.J.: Synthesis and characteristics of interpenetrating polymer network hydrogel composed of chitosan and poly(acrylic acid). J. Appl. Polym. Sci. **73**, 113–120 (1999)
148. Nakamura, K., Murray, R.J., Joseph, J.I., Peppas, N.A., Morishita, M., Lowman, A.M.: Oral insulin delivery using P(MAA-g-EG)hydrogels: effects of network morphology on insulin delivery characteristics. J. Controlled Release **95**, 589–599 (2004)
149. Zhang, J., Peppas, N.A.: Synthesis and characterization of pH- and temperature-sensitive poly(methacrylic acid)/poly(N-isopropylacrylamide) interpenetrating polymeric network. Macromolecules **33**, 102–107 (1999)
150. Sideratou, Z., Tsiourvas, D., Paleos, C.M.: Quaternized poly(propylene imine) dendrimers as novel pH-sensitive controlled-release systems. Langmuir **16**, 1766–1769 (2000)
151. Burke, S.E., Barrett, C.J.: pH-responsive properties of multilayered poly(Llysine)/hyaluronic acid surfaces. Biomacromolecules **4**, 1773–1783 (2003)
152. Toncheva, V., Wolfert, M.A., Dash, P.R., Oupicky, D., Ulbrich, K., Seymour, L.W.: Novel vectors for gene delivery formed by self-assembly of DNA with poly(L-lysine) grafted with hydrophilic polymers. Biochim. Biophys. Acta **1380**, 354–368 (1998)
153. Wilding, R.S.S., Davis, F., Pozzi, P., Furlani, A.: Enteric coated timed release systems for colonic targeting. Int. J. Pharm. **111**, 99–102 (1994)
154. Hongkee, S., Chien, Y.H., Park, H., Hwang, S.J., Park, K., Lloyd, A.W.: In: Drug delivery and targeting in new generation technologies. Taylor and Francis, New York (2001)
155. Ellens, H., Bentz, J., Szoka, F.C.: pH-induced destabilization of phosphatidylethanolamine-containing liposomes: role of bilayer contact. Biochemistry **23**, 1532–1538 (1984)
156. Hoffman, A.S.: Intelligent polymers, controlled drug delivery: challenge and strategies. American Chemical Society, Washington, DC (1997)
157. Soleimani, F., Sadeghi, M.: Synthesis of pH-sensitive hydrogel based on Starch-Polyacrylate Superabsorbent. J Biomat Nanobiotech **3**, 310–314 (2012)
158. Corpart, J.M., Candau, F.: Aqueous solution properties of ampholytic copolymers prepared in microemulsions. Macromolecules **26**, 1333–1343 (1993)
159. Kathmann, E.E.L., White, L.A., McCormick, C.L.: Electrolyte- and pH-responsive zwitterionic copolymers of 4-[(2acrylamido-2-methylpropyl)-dimethylammonio]butanoate with 3-[(2-acrylamido-2methyl-propyl)dimethylammonio]propanesulfonate. Macromolecules **30**, 5297–5304 (1997)
160. Shahinpoor, M., Kim, K.J.: Ionic polymer-metal composites: I fundamentals. Smart Mater Struct. J. **10**, 819–833 (2001)
161. Nguyen, D.H., Choi, J.H., Joung, Y.K., Park, K.D.: Disulfide-crosslinked heparin-pluronic nanogels as a redox-sensitive nanocarrier for intracellular protein delivery. J. Bioact. Compat. Polym. **26**, 287–300 (2011)
162. Dollendorf, C., Hetzer, M., Ritter, H.: Polymeric redox-responsive delivery systems bearing ammonium salts cross-linked via disulfides. Beilstein J. Org. Chem. **9**, 1652–1662 (2013)

163. Napoli, A., Boerakker, M.J., Tirelli, N., Nolte, R.J.M., Sommerdijk, N.A.J.M., Hubbell, J.A.: Glucose-oxidase based self-destructing polymeric vesicles. Langmuir **20**, 3487–3491 (2004)
164. Podual, K., Doyle, I.I.I., Peppas, N.A.: Preparation and dynamic response of cationic copolymer hydrogels containing glucose oxidase. Polymer **41**, 3975–3983 (2000)
165. Sinha, V.R., Kumria, R.: Polysaccharides in colon-specific drug delivery. Int. J. Pharm. **224**, 19–38 (2001)
166. Zhang, C., Pan, D., Luo, K., Li, N., Guo, C., Zheng, X., Gu, Z.: Dendrimer–doxorubicin conjugate as enzyme-sensitive and polymeric nanoscale drug delivery vehicle for ovarian cancer therapy. Polym. Chem. (2014). doi:10.1039/C4PY00601A
167. Vemula, P.K., Cruikshank, G.A., John, G., Karp, J.M.: Enzyme responsive acetaminophen hydrogels. Massachussett Institute of Technology Open Access Article (2014)
168. Rao, N.A.: Role of oxygen free radicals in retinal damage associated with experimental uveitis. Trans. Am. Ophthalmol. Soc. **88**, 797–850 (1990)
169. Nobuhiko, Y., Jun, N., Teruo, O., Yasuhisa, S.: Regulated release of drug microspheres from inflammation responsive degradable matrices of crosslinked hyaluronic acid. J. Controlled Release **25**, 133–143 (1993)
170. Leung, M.F., Zhu, J., Li, P., Harris, F.W.: Novel synthesis and properties of smart core-shell microgels. Macromol. Symp. **226**, 177–185 (2005)
171. Kuckling, D., Adler, H.-J.P., Arndt, K.F., Ling, L., Habicher, W.D.: Temperature and pH-dependent solubility of novel poly(N-isopropylacrylamide)-copolymers. Macromol. Chem. Phys. **201**, 273–280 (2000)
172. Gao, H.F., Yang, W.L., Min, K., Zha, L.S., Wang, C.C., Fu, S.K.: Thermosensitive poly(N-isopropylacrylamide)nanocapsules with controlled permeability. Polymer **46**, 1087–1093 (2005)
173. Gu, J.X., Xia, F., Wu, Y., Qu, X.Z., Yang, Z.Z., Jiang, L.: Programmable delivery of hydrophilic drug using dually responsive hydrogel cages. J. Controlled Release **117**, 396 (2007)
174. Sun, H., Liu, S., Ge, B., Xing, L., Chen, H.: Cellulose nitrate membrane formation via phase separation induced by penetration of nonsolvent from vapor phase. J. Membr. Sci. **295**, 2–10 (2007)
175. Kontturi, K., Mafé, S., Manzanares, J.A., Svarfvar, B.L., Viinikka, P.: Modeling of the salt and pH effects on the permeability of grafted porous membranes. Macromolecules **29**, 5740–5746 (1996)
176. Liu, X., Guoa, H., Zhaa, L.: Study of pH/ temperature dual stimuli-responsive nanogels with interpenetrating polymer network structure. Polym. Inter. **61**, 1144–1150 (2012)

Chapter 13
Polymers in Nephrology

Jörg Vienken and Oliver Gottschalk

Abstract The use of polymers in nephrology represents a success story. Their selection, chemical modification and application in medical devices applied to hemodialysis (HD) and peritoneal dialysis (PD) allows for the successful treatment of more than 2.5 million dialysis patients worldwide in 2013 (HD: 2,250,000; PD: 272,000). Properties of polymer families applied for the production of membranes, tubing, PD-bags and filter housing material refer to performance, sterilization and blood compatibility. For all polymers, including those for housings and tubing, the amount of leachables has currently received increasing interest. It can be explained by the notion that treatment durations increase and the number of elderly patients with an impaired immune system is on the rise. New developments and selection of new polymers should target unspecific adsorption characteristics and interactive systems.

Keywords Membrane polymers · Leachables · Biocompatibility · Biostability

Abbreviations

ACE	Angiotensin converting enzyme
ACEi	ACE-inhibitor
BPA	Bis Phenol A
CA	Cellulose acetate
CDA	Cellulose-di-acetate
CTA	Cellulose-tri-acetate
C3a, C5a	Activated complement factors 3 and 5 in its desarginine variation
DEHP	Di-ethyl-hexyl phthalate (also DOP)
DINCH	Di-isononyl-cyclohexane

J. Vienken (✉) · O. Gottschalk
Nephro-Solutions AG, Harvesterhuder Weg 49, 20149 Hamburg, Germany
e-mail: vienken.usingen@gmail.com

F. Puoci (ed.), *Advanced Polymers in Medicine*, DOI 10.1007/978-3-319-12478-0_13

EVOH	Ethyl-vinyl alcohol copolymer (also EVAL)
HD	Hemodialysis
IgE	Immunoglobulin E
ETO	Ethylene oxide
LDL	Low density lipoprotein
MDA	4,4′-Methylene-di-aniline
PAN	Polyacrylonitrile
PAES	Poly(aryl)ethersulfone
PD	Peritoneal dialysis
PEPA	Polyester polymer alloy
PES	Polyethersulfone
PC	Polycarbonate
PMMA	Polymethylmethacrylate
PSu	Polysulfone
PP	Polypropylene
PUR	Polyurethane
PVP	Polyvinylpyrrolidone
SC	Sieving coefficient
TOTM	Tri-octyl trimellitate
VEGF	Vascular endothelial growth factor

Introduction

The treatment of patients suffering from end stage kidney disease by hemodialysis (HD) or peritoneal dialysis (PD) represents a success story in medical application of polymers. At the beginning of the twentieth century, John Abel in the United States [1] and Georg Haas in Germany [2, 3] started their research on blood purification techniques and treated animals and humans with kidney failure. It can be assumed that they might have had a dream at that time: their inventions would be generally accepted by the medical community and become a routine therapy. This dream shed light on the situation of dialysis at that time, when the famous German clinician Franz Volhard (1872–1950) has stated in the late 1920s "Dialysis is useless and even dangerous!" As a consequence of this opinion, Georg Haas abandoned his research on the artificial kidney shortly afterwards. This dream, however, has come true about 100 years later. In 2014, more than 2.5 million patients owe their life to hemodialysis or peritoneal dialysis. Dialysis has thus, developed from an experimental to a routine therapy whilst simultaneously patient survival considerably improved. Some figures may illustrate this notion. A recent survey specified the situation of dialysis patients in Japan [4] and reported that in 2011 more than 80,000 patients underwent dialysis for longer than 10 years and an impressive high number of more than 11,000 patients were successfully exposed to hemodialysis for even more than 25 years. The longest survivor in Japan currently dialyzes longer than 43 years [4] with an exposure to foreign polymer material during that time.

Table 13.1 Classical membrane polymers abandoned by manufacturers in the past

Polymer name	Manufacturer	Reason
Cuprophan®, Hemophan®	Membrana GmbH	Loss of market share, alleged lack of biocompatibility
Polycarbonate (PC)	Gambro	Only as flat sheet membrane available
Cellulose acetate (CA)	Cordis Dow	Loss of market share, manufacturing company dis-appeared from market

The number of dialysis patients and consequently the need for more filters, bags, and tubing will further increase in upcoming years, as the number of dialysis patients worldwide will increase by 6 % annually. It will reach the figure of 4 million patients in the year 2020.

These figures illustrate three facts:

(a) Long term survival on dialysis is possible due to a better understanding of physiological mechanisms and improved medical therapies.
(b) The current average annual cost of treatment, guestimated to be about 50,000 US-$ in 2009 [5], is no obstacle for increasing patients numbers. Disposable medical devices, such as filters and tubing that are manufactured on the basis of an economy of scale, as well as improved logistics for the provision of these goods, may contribute to this effect.
(c) The need for improving the quality/purity of medical devices becomes increasingly important due to the extended exposure of long term dialysis patients to polymers and medical devices. "Leachables" from polymers might become one of the key-words of the next decades.

Medical devices for dialysis therapy have been optimized and adapted to medical needs in recent years. Polymers have been carefully investigated and qualified for optimized blood compatibility and selected for their suitability under specific manufacturing and cost conditions. As a consequence, some polymers did not survive this careful screening process in the past (Table 13.1).

Membrane Polymers in the Market Place

The fate of the famous Cuprophan® dialysis membrane may serve as an example. Dialysis membranes, made from regenerated cellulose (e.g., Cuprophan®), used to be the golden standard for dialysis membranes for about four decades. Its manufacturers profited from a worldwide market share of more than 70 % in the 1970s. It could be shown, that the production capacity for Cuprophan® dialysis membranes paralleled the development of patient numbers in the 1970s. However in 2006 and about 35 years later, its main producer (Membrana GmbH, Germany) decided to cease the production of dialyzers with this membrane polymer. It can be argued that its alleged lack of blood compatibility and the availability of alternate biocompatible polymers provoked this development. A famous publication challenged this membrane polymer already in 1985 and thus, anticipated this situation by asking: "Cellulose membranes, time for a change?" [6].

Since then, only cellulosic dialysis membranes, made from derivatives of cellulose acetate, CDA and CTA, are commercially available. As a consequence, many scientific publications in which properties and outcomes of Cuprophan® application are compared are invalid today even if they are in favor of other membrane polymers. However, they are of importance and should not be neglected as they may serve for advising scientists on how to select polymers for developing new biomaterials.

For instance, the knowledge gained in these publications about adequate testing of membrane polymers, the effects of polymer composition to related clinical sequelae, etc., can be successfully used for the selection and the characterization of new polymers.

Polymers for New Therapies and the System's Approach?

Unfortunately and despite many improvements in polymer behavior and performance, dialysis as a membrane-based procedure for blood purification is still an incomplete renal replacement therapy, as the mortality and morbidity of the affected patients remain high compared to the healthy population. To date, the following questions have not yet been answered satisfactorily:

1. "Is it possible to improve patient mortality by either improved devices with optimized polymers, or by modified and more efficient treatment modes?"
2. "Is it possible to improve patient survival through the introduction of completely new concepts, such as wearable artificial kidneys (WAKs) or through regenerative therapies?"

First successful attempts into this direction have been made with the introduction of convective therapies such as high-flux dialysis or hemodiafiltration (HDF). Increased pore sizes achieved with high-flux membranes allow for the removal of families of molecules and the possible high ultrafiltration rates improve removal by convective transport. The concept of a dialysis dose, based on the amount of a substitution fluid, called high-volume hemodiafiltration, turned out to be successful further [7, 8]. The ESHOL study published in 2013 [8] has proven a 30 % reduction of mortality in HD-patients given that this cohort has been treated by HDF with a substitution volume of more than 20 L. In a parallel arm of this clinical trial, patients were treated by normal high-flux dialysis. Obviously, treatment modes, such as high volume HDF combined with the application of high-flux membranes, has led to this advantage. As a consequence, polymers have to be suitable for this treatment mode and allow for an adequate ultrafiltration (water permeability), hydrophilicity and porosity in case of membranes.

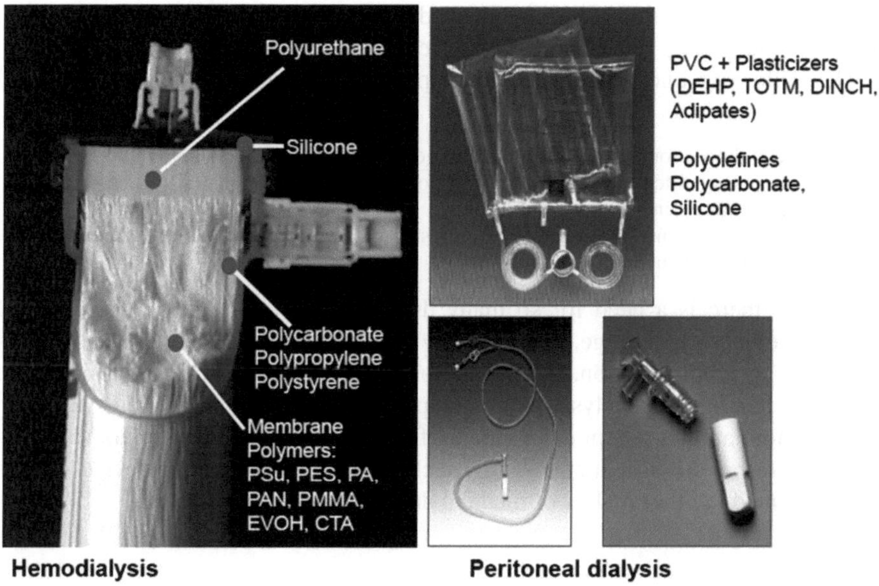

Fig. 13.1 Polymers used for medical devices for dialysis and peritoneal dialysis. Polyurethane (PUR) is applied as potting material for capillary membranes, silicone rings guarantee a leakage-free system, polycarbonate and polypropylene are used for casings, and a series of polymers are incorporated as membrane materials (*PSu*-polysulfone, *PES*-polyether-sulfone, *PA*-polyamide, *PAN*-polyacrylonitrile, *PMMA*-polymethylmethacrylate, *CTA*-cellulose-tri-acetate). *PVC*-polyvinylchloride as a biomaterial for tubing needs plasticizers for its flexibility, such as *DEHP/DOP*-di-ethyl-hexylphthalate/di-octyl-phthalate, *TOTM*-tri-octyl trimellitate, *DINCH*-di-isononyl-cyclohexane

Finally, it's important to note, that a "systems approach" is obligatory when comparing different polymers in medical application. The exclusive study of the properties and characteristics of individual polymers in nephrology is not sufficient. In fact, one should consider a series of mutual interactions, e.g., between different polymers in a single device, their behavior within the device during different therapies, polymer interactions with the actual medication and other bystander conditions, such as long term stability [9]. Figure 13.1 depicts the variety of polymers used for medical devices in dialysis, such as dialyzers and tubing.

This paper will discuss properties, requirements for use and characteristics related to possible clinical outcomes of polymers that are used in dialysis therapy.

Polymers for Dialyzers and Dialysis Membranes

For some people, it's unbelievable and may sound like a surprise: 900 different types of dialyzers are commercially available worldwide in 2014. They differ in geometric design, membrane polymer and surface area, capillary geometry and undulation and can further be distinguished by their sterilization technique, steam, ethylene oxide gas, γ-rays, ß-rays, and E-beam.

The following questions may come up and bother clinic administrators and nephrologists:

Is there a real need for so many different types of polymers and filters?

Are so many filters desired by the nephrological community based on the specific healthcare requirements of dialysis therapies?

Is this market situation artificial and only stimulated by the international competition of dialyzer manufacturers?

Obviously, there is a need for so many different dialysis filters. The cohorts of dialysis patients vary in age, gender, body weight, blood volume, comorbid conditions, drug administration, predisposition to allergies and other physiological bystander conditions. Dialysis as a therapy for chronically ill patients tends to become more and more a practical model for personalized dialysis treatment regimen with respect to all patients. Thus, such a diversity of medical devices that is unprecedented in other realms of medical device technology, is needed.

Polymers for Dialyzer Housing

Recent years have seen a mayor change in the geometry of dialyzer housing and the corresponding membranes. For many years, Kiil dialyzers have been the work-horse of dialysis therapy. Here, the patient's blood was circulated in a parallel flow mode through four cellophane channels made up of eight cellophane membranes. On the outside of the cellophane sheets dialysis fluid circulated at reduced hydrostatic pressure in the grooves of plastic boards [10]. The dimensions of the plastic boards were 970 × 340 × 20 mm and made of an epoxy resin compound. In fact, this size and the long lasting preparation time limited its use to a small number of patients. Improvements have been made with the introduction of the parallel plate dialyzers from Gambro/Hospal, fabricated with a polycarbonate housing and containing either a flat sheet Cuprophan or a PAN-membrane. Flat sheet dialyzers never dominated the market, because the mayor breakthrough came with the development of capillary-membrane dialyzers in 1968 [11]. Richard Steward, the first author on the first publication on capillary membranes spun his capillary membranes from saponified cellulose acetate polymers [11]. The concept of this device facilitated practical dialysis therapy and enabled manufacturers to produce filters in large quantities. There is certainly no doubt that the development of capillary dialyzers was the reason for the expansion of patient numbers worldwide. Figure 13.2 depicts the scheme of a modern capillary dialyzer.

Standard dialyzer housings are made from polycarbonate. Its transparency and easy handling for labelling and sterilization is highly welcome by physicians and manufacturers. During the last decade, new developments have led to the

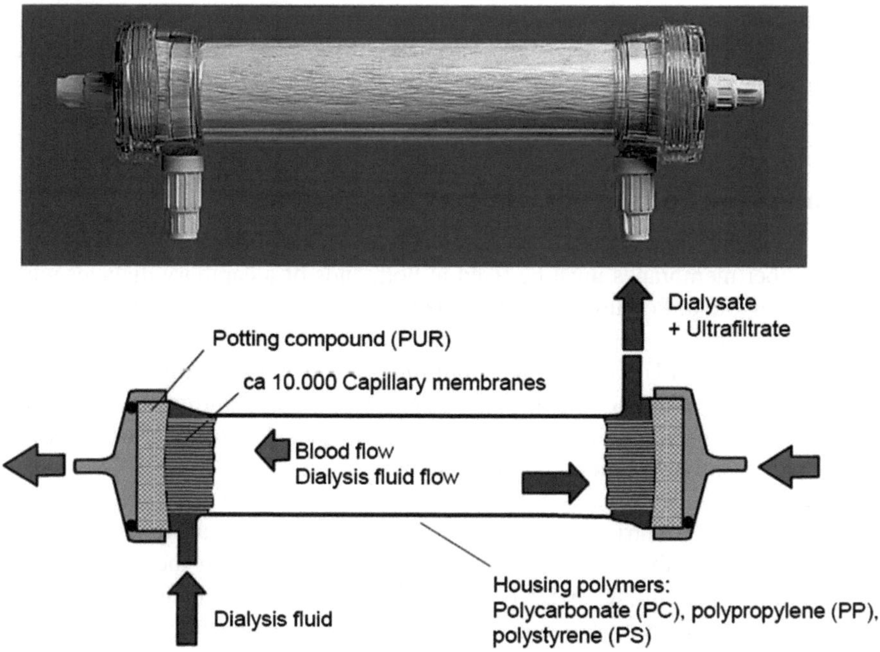

Fig. 13.2 The standardly used "artificial kidney" is a dialyzer that contains more than 10,000 capillary membranes. Blood is guided through these hollow fibers whereas the dialysis fluid is perfused in an opposite direction. Due to size, reproducibility and perfection of engineering features this type of dialyzer now dominates the dialysis market, mostly as a single-use device, since many years. The annual production capacity for hollow fibers in 2013 made from different polymers is about 450,000,000 km. This figure is equivalent to three-times the distance between the Earth and the sun

introduction of housings made from two other polymers. Polypropylene (PP) was introduced for its polysulfone Fx-class by Fresenius Medical Care [12], and for the Sureflux-dialyzers provided by Nipro Medical Corporation, Japan. Polystyrene as housing material is available for PMMA dialyzers by Toray Industries, Japan.

Dialyzer cages made of polypropylene (PP) are not transparent, they appear opaque. However, they offer advantages that are appreciated by both, manufacturers and physicians. Medical grade PP is available at a cheaper price than medical grade polycarbonate which adds to lower manufacturing cost. In contrast to polycarbonate, PP does not release bis-phenol A (BPA). BPA is termed an exogenous hormone or endocrine disruptor because it interferes with the estrogen receptor at cell surfaces similar to the plasticizer di-ethyl-hexyl phthalate (DEHP). As a consequence of this interaction, BPA is made responsible for some adverse clinical effects, such as diabetes mellitus type II [13], impact on gene transcription [14], modulation of VEGF secretion [15]. Reports on dialysis patients describe its high protein-binding and thus explain its presence in the blood of dialysis patients in high amounts [16].

Compared to polycarbonate, however, handling of polypropylene in terms of labelling and sterilization needs special knowhow. It's use as housing for medical devices is thus limited to engineering plastics experts.

Polymers for Potting of Capillary Membranes

Hollow fiber membranes must be fixed at both ends of a capillary dialyzer with a potting compound. Polyurethane has turned out to be the most suitable biomaterial for this purpose.

Polyurethanes (PUR or PU) are traditionally and most commonly formed by reacting a di- or poly-isocyanate with a polyol in a polyaddition reaction. While most polyurethanes are thermo-setting polymers that do not melt when heated, thermoplastic polyurethanes are also available.

Unfortunately, isocyanates are the most frequent cause of occupational asthma in industrialized countries. Exposure to isocyanates may result in the formation of specific IgE antibodies [17, 18]. There are also reports in the literature, that 4,4′-Methylene-di-aniline (MDA) can be released from aromatic polyurethanes after gamma-irradiation or steam sterilization [17, 19] suggesting the advantage of aliphatic polyurethanes in contrast to its aromatic derivatives.

Finally, polyurethane polymers used as potting material in dialyzers are known for effectively binding and adsorbing the sterilization gas ethylene oxide (ETO). Due to the very slow release kinetics of ETO, a dialysis patient may be continuously exposed to the gas and IgE-antibodies against an albumin-ETO conjugate are found in dialysis patients and severe allergic reactions could be observed in hypersensitive patients [18]. A rigorous rinsing of the dialyzer prior to its clinical use allowed for avoiding this "first-use syndrome". Dialyzer manufacturers meanwhile have improved the quality of dialyzers by reducing the PUR potting mass to its minimum necessary amount.

Polymers for Dialysis Membranes

The selection of the polymer material for the production of dialysis membranes has significant implications on the quality of hemodialysis therapy. Only a limited number of polymers are suitable for the spinning and extrusion process involved in the manufacture of capillary membranes. The selection was originally based on experiences from textile fiber production. Further, biochemical and physical properties that may result from the membrane formation process, determine the selection of a polymer. The ideal polymer family should allow the production of biocompatible dialysis membranes and possess a stable physical stability. The latter guarantees an easy production process and sterilization without problems.

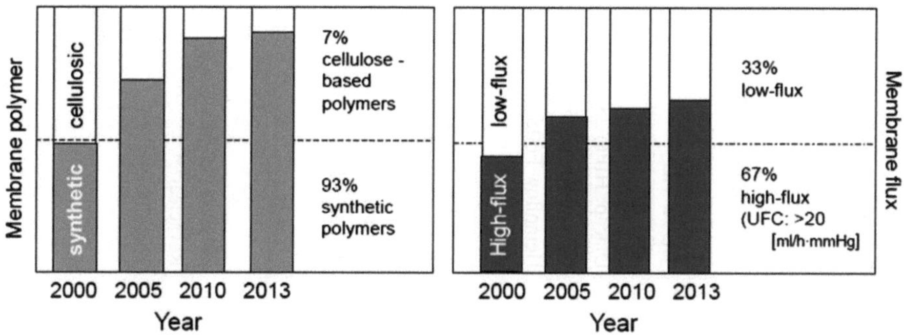

Fig. 13.3 Worldwide changes of dialysis membrane properties observed between the years 2000 and 2013. Cellulose-based membranes have lost their importance and market share continuously. They are replaced by synthetic polymers as membrane materials. In addition "flux" has become an issue either. High-flux membranes, characterized by their ultrafiltration coefficient to be UFC => 20 [ml/h·mmHg] are now used in more than two thirds of all dialysis centers

The majority of patients with kidney disease are currently treated with dialyzers containing synthetic membranes with high-flux properties [20]. Figure 13.3 depicts changes in market shares for membrane flux and polymer type from the year 2000 to 2013 [21]. The figure shows that membrane polymers have evolved as part of a routine therapy, essentially in line with clinical observations and constantly changing clinical requirements [20].

Eighteen different membrane polymers can be attributed to four synthetic and to one cellulosic membrane family. They will be described shortly in the following and characterized by features that outline their specific individual advantages or disadvantages. Table 13.2 depicts an actualized list of polymers used for dialysis membranes and the appropriate manufacturers of dialyzers. Their characteristics will be discussed below.

Membrane Families, Their Main Features and Specific Properties?

Polymers for the manufacturing of dialysis membranes can be grouped as families and are described in the following.

Group 1, Polysulfone-family Members: Polysulfone (PSu, Fresenius Medical Care, Germany), Polyethersulfone (PES, Membrana, Nipro Medical Corporation, Japan), Polyester polymer alloy (PEPA, Nikkiso, Japan), Blends from Polyamide/Polysulfone (PA/PSu, Gambro, Sweden), as well as blends made of PES/PVP. Recent research on membranes with antioxidant features have led to the production of a polysulfone membrane with immobilized Vitamin E (PSu/Vit E, ASAHI, Japan).

Membranes from polysulfone dominate the dialysis market since many years. Today, 93 % of all synthetic membranes stem from the parent polyarylethersulfone

Table 13.2 Dialysis membranes listed according to their polymers and dialyzer manufacturers

Type of polymer (polymer groups)	Membrane manufacturer (in alphabetic sequence, *exclusive membrane producer)	Dialyser manufacturer (if different from membrane manufacturer)	Dialyser types (examples)
Synthetic dialysis membranes (polymer groups)			
Polysulfone (PSu) membranes			
Asahi Polysulfone (APS™)	Asahi Kasei Medical Co., Ltd., Tokyo, Japan		APS-650 Leoceed-16 N
REXBRANE™			REXEED™-13A
VitabranE™			ViE-A, ViE
α Polysulfon	BBraun Melsungen AG, Melsungen, Germany		Diacap®HI PS 12
α Polysulfon+			Diacap®HIFlo 23
Amembris			Xevonta Hi 12
Fresenius Polysulfone®	Fresenius Medical Care AG,		Hemoflow F60S
Helixone®			$FX_{classix}60$
Helixone®plus	Bad Homburg, Germany		$FX_{Cordiax}60$
Fibron Polysulfone	Fibron AG*, Teterow, Germany	Allmed Medical GmbH, Pulsnitz, Germany	Polypure® 16H
		Haidylena, Giza, Egypt	Platinum H3
Minntech Polysulfone	MEDIVATORS Inc. (previously Minntech), Minneapolis, USA		Renaflo® II
Toraysulfone®	Toray Medical Co., Ltd., Chiba, Japan		TS-1.3S
Poly(aryl)ethersulfone (PAES) membranes			
Polyamix™	Gambro Dialysatoren GmbH, Hechingen		Polyflux®140H
Poracton™			Revaclear™
HCO—membrane	Germany		Theralite™

(continued)

Table 13.2 (continued)

Type of polymer (polymer groups)	Membrane manufacturer (in alphabetic sequence, *exclusive membrane producer)	Dialyser manufacturer (if different from membrane manufacturer)	Dialyser types (examples)
DIAPES®	Membrana GmbH*, Wuppertal, Germany	Allmed Medical GmbH, Pulsnitz, Germany	Ruby 160
		Bellco S.r.l., Mirandola, Italy	BLS 812G
		Haidylena, Giza, Egypt	HPH 160 S
		Medica S.p.A., Medolla, Italy	L3
		Meditechlab, Thiais, France	MF 7
		Nipro Corp., Osaka, Japan	SureLyzer® PES-150DH
Purema®	Membrana GmbH*, Wuppertal, Germany	Allmed Medical GmbH, Pulsnitz, Germany	Biorema 16H
		Bain Medical Equipment Co., Ltd, Guangzhou, China	DORA B-16H
		Baxter International Inc., Deerfield, USA	Xenium 130LF
		Bellco S.r.l., Mirandola, Italy	Phylter™15G
		Etropal JSC, Etropole, Bulgaria	PH 160
		Haidylena, Giza, Egypt	Biopure 160 HF
		Medica S.p.A., Medolla, Italy	Smartflux HFP 150
		Meditechlab, Thiais, France	MP 60
		MTP Medical Technologies Gesellschaft mbH, Pirna, Germany	VitaPES® 150 HF
		Nephros Inc., River Edge, USA	Olpur™
		Nipro Corp., Osaka, Japan	PureFlux®-130H,
		NxStage GmbH & Co. KG, Göttingen, Germany	Filter in System One®-Cassette

(continued)

Table 13.2 (continued)

Type of polymer (polymer groups)	Membrane manufacturer (in alphabetic sequence, *exclusive membrane producer)	Dialyser manufacturer (if different from membrane manufacturer)	Dialyser types (examples)
Polyester-Polymer Alloy (PEPA®)	Nikkiso Co., Ltd., Tokyo, Japan		FLX-15GW
Polynephron™	Nipro Corp., Osaka, Japan	Nipro Corp., Osaka, Japan	ELISIO™-13H
		Baxter International Inc., Deerfield, USA	Xenium XPH130
Polyacrylonitrile (PAN) membranes			
AN69, AN69®ST	Gambro Hospal	Gambro Hospal/Baxter Healthcare	Nephral®ST
HeprAN™	Meyzieu, France		Evodial®1.3
Other synthetic dialysis membranes			
Ethylene vinyl alcohol copolymer (EVAL™, EVOH)	Asahi Kasei Medical Co., Ltd., Tokyo, Japan		KF-201-1.3C
Polymethylmethacrylate (PMMA)	Toray Medical Co., Ltd., Chiba, Japan		Filtryzer® BG-1.3U
Cellulose-tri-acetate (CTA) membranes			
Cellulose-tri-acetate (CTA)	Nipro Corp., Osaka, Japan	Nipro Corp., Osaka, Japan	SUREFLUX™-13L
		Baxter International Inc., Deerfield, USA	TRICEA 150G

*Companies providing membranes or membrane bundles but no complete dialysers to the market

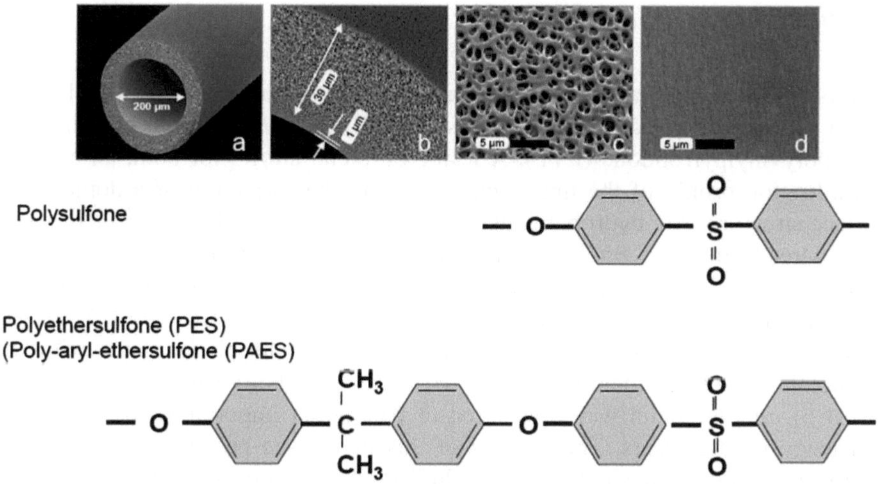

Fig. 13.4 Chemical structure and characteristics of polysulfone (PSu) polymers used for dialysis membranes. Its specific chemical characteristics are shown in the *panel above*. PSu- membrane dimensions are depicted in the *centered panel*: **a** capillary cross section, inner diameter 200 μm, **b** cross section of the membrane wall; the membrane is only 1 μm thick and backed by a rather open support structure of 39 μm that maintains mechanical stability, **c** view on the outer membrane surface area, showing its high porosity, **d** view on the rather smooth inner membrane surface area where pore sizes are between 1 and 3 nm. The *lower panel* shows the detailed molecular structure of polysulfone (PSu) and polyethersulfone (PES)

family of which 71 % are from polysulfone (PSu) and 22 % from polyethersulfone (PES). Polysulfone belongs to a family of thermoplastic polymers which are known for their thermal and chemical stability. They contain the subunits "aryl-SO_2-aryl" and "benzyl-SO_2-benzyl" (Fig. 13.4) of which the polysulfone group provides the name of the polymer.

What Is the Difference Between Polysulfone (PSu) and Polyarylethersulfone (PES/PAES)?

Polysulfone, polyethersulfone and polyarylethersulfon are used as synonyms by many scientists due to their great similarity in performance and chemical stability. Generally spoken, polysulfones (PSu) are a group of polymers that contain sulfone- and alkyl- or aryl- (e.g., arylether-) groups. According to the chemical nomenclature, only those polymers belong to the polysulfone family, that contain an additional isopropylidene group. Polymers without the isopropy-lidene group are called polyarylethersulfones (PAES) or in short polyethersulfones (PES) (Fig. 13.4).

Modification of PSu Membranes

The polysulfone polymer, as such, is a hydrophobic polymer and must be rendered hydrophilic at least in part. This is generally achieved through blending PSu with polyvinylpyrrolidone (PVP). A PSu/PVP blend allows for both, an efficient ultrafiltration profile of the final membrane, and the formation of a domain-like surface structure with hydrophilic and lipophilic spots at the blood contacting surface. Already in 1983, Streicher and Schneider reported on their clinical experiments in dialysis with the first PSu membrane in its high-flux version. To their surprise, they were able to observe a high sieving coefficient (SC = 0.7) and an efficient removal of ß$_2$-microglobulin and compared its performance with the glomerular basement membrane [22]. This was long before the removal capacity of ß$_2$-microglobulin was considered of paramount importance for membrane efficiency in later years. The success of this membrane polymer can be further attributed to appropriate and efficient solute and fluid removal capabilities and to a pronounced intrinsic blood compatibility [23].

It is possible to affect blood compatibility and biocompatibility of so called non-physiological interfaces by chemical modifications of the polymer contact zone. The contact zone between blood and the membrane polymer represents such a non-physiological interface [24]. Blood compatibility of artificial surfaces is primarily determined by protein adsorption and protein adsorption depends on surface properties of the membrane. A general scheme of how surface reactivities are influenced by the chemical composition of a membrane is depicted in Fig. 13.5.

As a consequence, none of the surfaces with single-characteristics properties satisfies biocompatibility sufficiently. Domain-like surface structures are essential

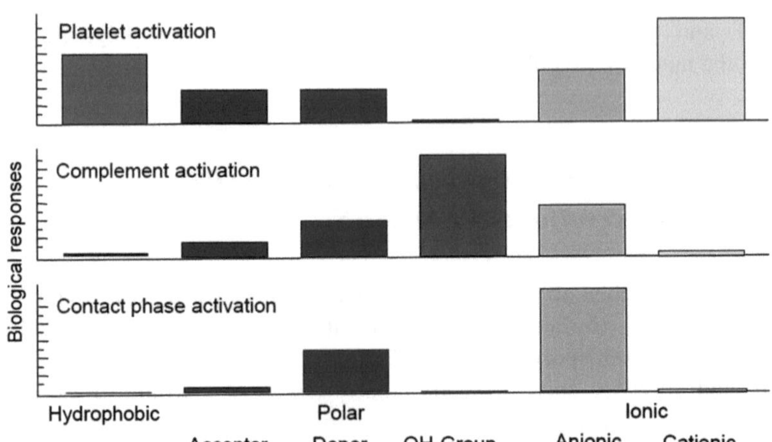

Fig. 13.5 Overall biological response as a function of surface properties. Inert surfaces for the anticoagulation system are hydrophobic, cationic charged and OH-group bearing. Inert systems for complement are also hydrophobic and cationic (modified from [24])

in order to achieve optimized blood compatibility (see above). Poylsulfone/polyvinylpyrrolidone blends (PSu/PVP) offer such domain-like structures with the well-known biocompatibility features.

PSu Membranes and Endotoxin Binding Capacity

A further major advantage of PSu-membranes relates to their adsorptive capacity for bacterial endo-toxins. Dialysis therapies with high-flux membranes expose the patients to large volumes of dialysis fluid, e.g., during high-volume hemodiafiltration [7, 8]. Should these fluids be contaminated with endotoxins that derive from the outer cell wall of Gram-negative bacteria during cell growth or lysis, there is a risk of these substances entering the patient's bloodstream [25, 26]. Endotoxins activate a number of physiological pathways, triggering the generation of potent pro-inflammatory substances, such as cytokines (IL-1, IL-6, TNF, etc.) and growth factors (e.g., VEGF) [26]. Subsequent inflammation, the underlying mechanism for most related disease states including chronic kidney failure, is widely recognized to be a major risk factor for cardiovascular disease-related mortality in dialysis patients.

Depending on their chemical constitution and microstructures, polysulfone membranes are able to prevent entry of endotoxins into the patient's blood stream [27–29, Fig. 13.6]. However, polysulfone and polysulfone membranes are not all alike.

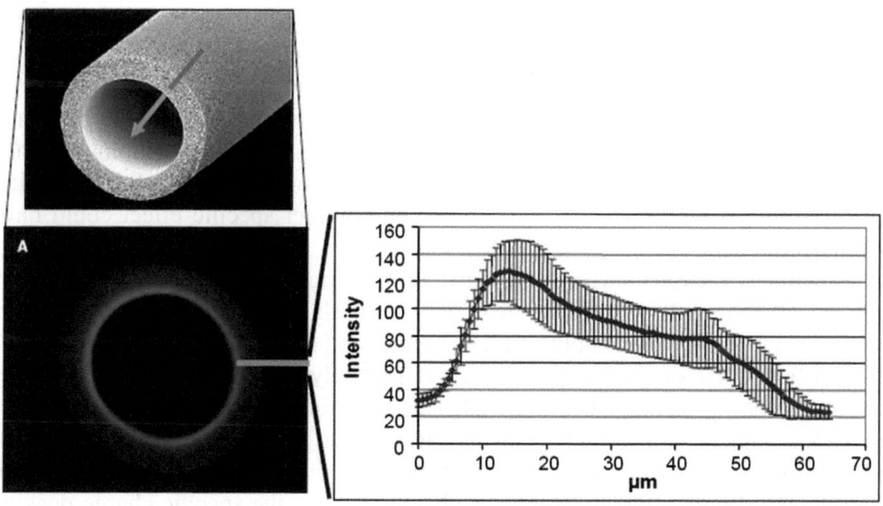

Fig. 13.6 Endotoxin adsorption at the inner layer of a membrane made of a polysulfone/poyl vinylpyrrolidone blend. This adsorption capacity prevents endotoxins possibly originating from contaminated dialysis fluid to enter the patient's blood stream

Weber and coworkers were able to show in an in vitro model, that endotoxin adsorption depends both, on chemical composition and the manufacturing process of the membrane [30]. In fact, hydrophobic parts of the lipopolysaccharide molecule (LPS, endotoxin) are considered to interact with hydrophobic entities within the polysulfone structure thereby facilitating their removal [29] (Tables 13.3 and 13.4).

As a summary, it is possible to improve both, blood compatibility and the adsorption of dialysate contaminants, such as endotoxins, through a chemical modification of the membrane poly-mer, as realized in some polysulfone dialysis membranes.

Group 2, Polyacrylonitrile family Members: PAN (ASAHI Kasei Medical, Japan), AN69, AN69ST, AN69-Heparin (Gambro/Hospal/Baxter Healthcare, Sweden, France, USA).

Already in 1972, Rhône Poulenc introduced the first synthetic highly permeable dialysis membrane to the market. This membrane was made from a copolymer, the hydrophobic polyacrylo-nitrile (PAN) and the hydrophilic Na-Methallyl-sulfonate and was called AN69 [31]. Later, a PAN membrane, fabricated exclusively with the PAN-polymer was also offered by ASAHI Kasei Medical in Japan.

This membrane will be discussed in more detail because related data may serve for the characterization of other negatively charged polymers in medical application.

The chemical structure of the PAN (AN69) copolymer membrane is depicted in Fig. 13.7.

Due to its microstructure and its high electronegativity based on the methallylsulfonate compound, the copolymer AN69 shows a high adsorptive capacity and similar to other negatively charged membranes, both, at its surface and within its wall. This holds true for those positively charged proteins, like the polyamines spermidin, cadaverin or putrescin that originate from the ornithine metabolism, for complement fragments C3a, C5a and Complement factor D [32–34]. Consequently, low complement activation is observed during hemodialysis with AN69. Further, the specific adsorption features of this membrane polymer may affect the therapeutic availability of proteins or drugs, such as recombinant erythropoietin (rh-EPO) [35–37]. With a subcutaneous administration of rh-EPO during dialysis with AN69, however, this membrane-polymer specific effect could have been overcome [37].

Negatively charged surfaces are cited as favoring the activation of the contact phase system [38, 39]. However, there are results showing negatively charged surfaces, that do not promote contact phase activation [40, 41] as the involved adsorption of factor XII and factor XIIa are not remarkably different from a wide variety of other blood proteins. Obviously, other determining factors play a role, such as preceding platelet activation [41] or the specific charge density of negative charges at the surface of the membrane. Contact phase activation may be avoided, given that the density of negative charges is above or below the specific charge density. Clinical observations, however, have shown that negatively charged membranes of a defined charge density activate the kallikrein-kinin system and that this reaction vwas amplified by a simultaneous administration of the pharmaceutical drug

Table 13.3 Outline of properties and structures of some representatives of polysulfone membranes

Membrane producer	Type	Permeabilities	Sterilization	Wall structure Inner diameter of capillary
Asahi Kasei Medical	Asahi Polysulfone (APS™)	High-flux	Gamma rays	Asymmetric wall thickness: 40 μm Inner diameter: 200 μm
	REXBRANE™	High-flux	Gamma rays	Asymmetric wall thickness: 45 μm Inner diameter: 185 μm
		Low-flux	E-beam	
	VitabranE™	High-flux	Gamma rays	Asymmetric wall thickness: 45 μm Inner diameter: 200 μm wall thickness: 45 μm Inner diameter: 185 μm
	ViE			
	ViE-A			
BBraun Avitum	α Polysulfon	High-flux, low-flux	Gamma rays	Asymmetric wall thickness: 40 μm Inner diameter: 200 μm
	α Polysulfon	High-flux	Gamma rays	Asymmetric wall thickness: 40 μm Inner diameter: 200 μm
	Amembris	High-flux, low-flux	Gamma rays	Asymmetric wall thickness: 40 μm Inner diameter: 200 μm
Fresenius Medical Care	Fresenius Polysulfone®	High-flux, low-flux	Inline-steam,	Asymmetric wall thickness: 40 μm Inner diameter: 200 μm
			E-Beam, ETO	
	Helixone®	High-flux, low-flux, mid-flux	Inline-steam	Asymmetric wall thickness: 35 μm Inner diameter: 185 μm
	Helixone®plus	High-flux	Inline-steam	Asymmetric
Toray Medical	Toraysulfone®	High-flux	Gamma rays	Asymmetric wall thickness: 40 μm Inner diameter: 200 μm

Table 13.4 Outlines properties and structures of some representatives of polyethersulfone membranes

Membrane producer	Type	Permeabilities	Sterilization	Wall structure Inner diameter of capillary
Gambro Hospal	Polyamix™	High-flux	Steam	Three layer structure Wall thickness: 50 μm Inner diameter: 200 μm
Baxter Healthcare	(PAES/PVP/PA)	Low-flux		
	Poracton™	High-flux	Steam	
Membrana GmbH	DIAPES® Bellco, Nipro MTP/Serumwerk Bernburg	High-flux Mid-flux (HP), Low-flux	ETO, heat, steam, Gamma rays, E-beam	Asymmetric wall thickness: 30 μm Inner diameter: 200 μm
	Purema® Baxter, Bellco Nipro, MTP/Serumwerk Bernburg	High-flux Low-flux	ETO, heat, steam, Gamma rays E-beam	Asymmetric wall thickness: 30 μm Inner diameter: 200 μm
Nikkiso	Polyester-Polymer Alloy (PEPA®)	High-flux	Gamma rays	Three layer structure: Skin-porous layer-skin
Nipro	Polynephron™	High-flux	Gamma rays	Asymmetric wall thickness: 40 μm Inner diameter: 200 μm

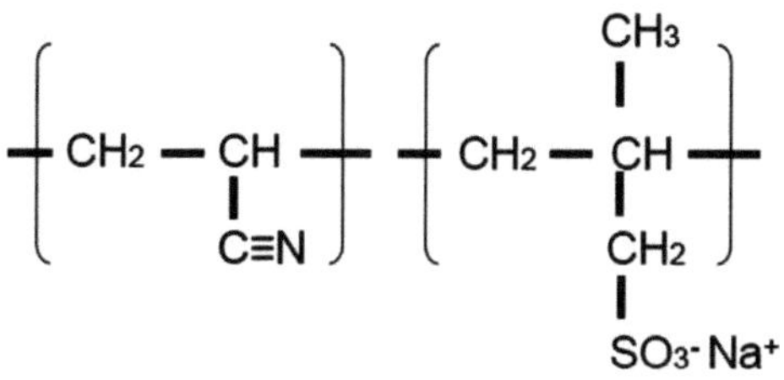

Fig. 13.7 Chemical structure of the AN69–PAN membrane. This membrane is a copolymer made from polyacrylonitrile and [Na^{+} methallylsulfonate^{-}]

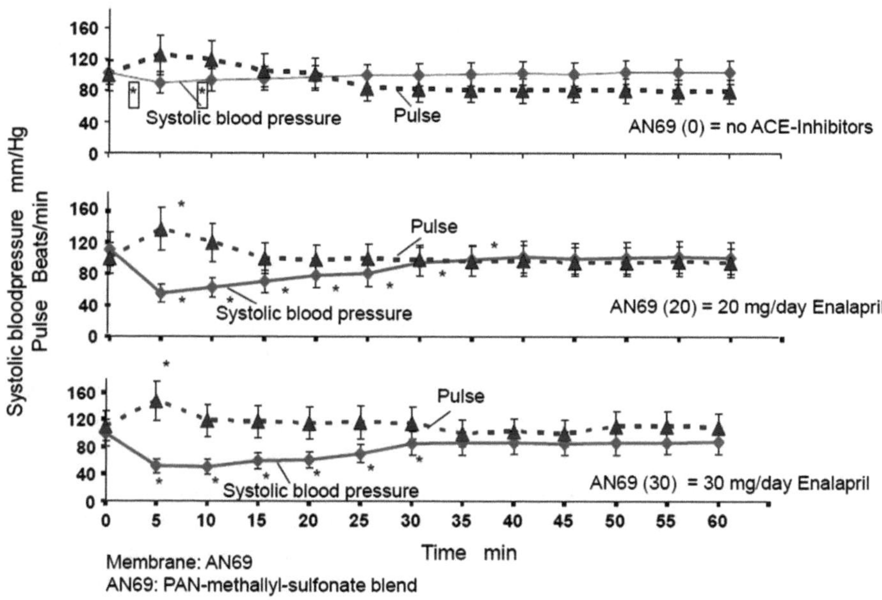

Fig. 13.8 Sheep model on hemodialysis: given that a negatively charged dialysis membrane, such as AN69, is used together with ACE-inhibitors (Enalapril), a dose dependent blood pressure drop is observed (modified from [46])

ACE-inhibitor [42–45]. Clinical and biochemical observations showed that by this means, the vasodilator bradykinin is activated. A severe blood pressure drop followed in those hemodialysis patients who had been treated with such a membrane. Clinical consequences in terms of blood pressure drop and duration were dependent on ACEi dose (Fig. 13.8, [46]). The effect is currently mentioned in leaflets that accompany medicinal drugs and alert for contraindications. They could, however prevented by changing the pH of the buffer solution (Fig. 13.9, [47, 48]). This observation should be kept in mind, when other negatively charged polymers are used in clinical application, such as, for instance, for adsorber particles made from dextran sulfate or acrylic acid.

Blood-compartment	Rinsing solution	pH	Bradykinin generation fmol/ml (mean)
Citrated plasma	Phosphate	5.0	97.867
(pH: 7.1)	Phosphate	7.0	21.633
	NaHCO (1.4%)	8.0	207
	NaCl Control	6.0	36.975
Heparinized plasma	Phosphate	5.0	12.568
(pH: 7.4)	Phosphate	7.0	672
	$NaHCO_3$ (1.4%)	8.0	90
n = 6	NaCl - Control	6.0	168

Recirculation of plasma through PAN - AN69 - minidialysers

Fig. 13.9 The formation of bradykinin after blood contact with negatively charged surfaces can be prevented by varying the blood pH through applying different buffers. Bicarbonate buffer fits best for both, citrated and heparinized plasma. Of course, these adaptations require to be performed locally in the extracorporeal blood circuit (adapted from [48])

Similar observations have also been reported for negatively charged white blood cell removal filters [49], for LDL adsorber particles made of dextran sulfate [50]. Fatal consequences on the basis of this mechanism have been reported for the heparin contaminant "over sulfated chondroitin sulfate" [51].

A modification of the AN69 membrane achieved by coating the membrane with a polyethyleneimine layer has led to the development of the AN69-ST membrane [52]. This coating neutralized the electronegativity (zeta potential) of the original polyacrylonitrile AN69 membranes and showed reduced generation of kinins. A comparison of AN69 and AN69-ST membranes in an ex vivo model of plasma showed that plasma dialysis with AN69 membranes led to significant bradykinin and des-Arg(9)-bradykinin release, which was potentiated by the administration of ACE-inhibitors (ACEi). This kinin formation was dramatically decreased by AN69-ST membranes, even in the presence of an ACEi, and kinin recovery in the dialysates was also significantly lower with these membranes [52].

A further most recent modification of the polyacrylonitrile membrane allowed for the immobilization of heparin in order to be able to perform hemodialysis treatment with reduced amounts of the anticoagulant. The introduction of positive charges offers binding sites for the negatively charged heparin molecule. Early observations on this effect stem from the clinical use of the positively charged cellulosic membrane "Hemophan" and the positively charged AN69ST membrane [53, 54]. Recent developments have led to the production of the cationic HeprAN-membrane in 2008, that has been grafted with heparin on its bulk polymer and been successfully used in clinical trials [31, 55].

Group 3, Polymethylmethacrylate family Member: polymethylmethacrylate (PMMA, Toray Industries, Japan) with of a series of different PMMA modifications (Table 13.5).

Table 13.5 PMMA membrane and manufacturer

Membrane producer	Type	Permeabilities	Sterilization	Wall structure Internal diameter of capillary
Toray Industries	PMMA	Low flux	Gamma rays	Homogeneous
Japan		High flux	Wet	Internal diameter: 200 μm Wall thickness 20/30 μm Spacer yarns around fiber

In 1977, Tory Industries introduced their dialysis membranes fabricated from polymethylmethacrylate (PMMA). They were the first to be sterilized by gamma rays [56], because the PMMA polymer shows disadvantages when sterilized with ETO. The desorption kinetics for this sterilizing gas, e.g., the reduction to 1/10 of its initial residual value, amounts up to 3 years. Dialysis membranes from PMMA exhibit specific adsorptive features at their surface. The middle molecule ß2-microglobulin is effectively adsorbed in its wall structure as well as serum free light chains [57]. Observations about improvement of anemia in dialysis are also reported [58] and a recent report documents on improvements in the skin disease "*prurigo nodularis*" [59, 60], when patients received a dialysis with PMMA membranes. The authors comment on this finding as follows: "The therapeutic effect might be due to a better removal of unknown uremic toxins using a highly permeable membrane with adsorption capacity" [59]. Some PMMA membranes exhibit negative charges at their blood-contacting surface. Consequently, reports on anaphylactoid reactions related to contact phase activation can be found in the literature [61] and discussions circled around the same arguments as described above for the AN69 membrane.

Group 4, Ethylene vinyl alcohol copolymer family Member: Ethylene vinyl alcohol copolymer (EVAL, EVOH, Kawasumi/Kuraray Laboratories, Japan) with of a series of different EVAL/EVOH modifications (Table 13.6).

The ethylene vinyl alcohol copolymer (EVAL/EVOH) is a hydrophilic and uncharged synthetic polymer blend [62]. The polymer used to fabricate EVOH membranes is a random copolymer of ethylene and vinylalcohol. Due to its original hydrophilicity, no hydrophilizing agents, such as polyvinylpyrrolidone (PVP), are needed. EVOH membranes have a smooth surface and retain structural water. As a consequence, they adsorb few plasma proteins and membrane fouling during

Table 13.6 EVAL/EVOH membrane and manufacturer

Membrane producer	Type	Permeabilities	Sterilization	Wall structure Internal diameter of capillary
Kawasumi	EVAL	Middle flux	Gamma rays	Homogenous
Laboratories Inc, Japan	EVOH		wet	Inner diameter: 175 μm Wall thickness: 60 μm Inner diameter: 175 μm Wall thickness: 25 μm

Table 13.7 CDA and CTA membrane and manufacturer

Membrane producer	Type	Permeabilities	Sterilization	Wall structure Internal diameter of capillary
Nipro, Japan	Cellulose-di-acetate	Low flux	Gamma rays	Homogenous Inner diameter: 200 μm Wall thickness: 15 μm
	Cellulose-di-acetate	High flux		
ASAHI Kasei Medical, Japan	Vit-E coated cellulose	Low flux	Gamma rays	Homogeneous Inner diameter: 200 μm Wall thickness: 25 μm
	Exebrane (Terumo)			

treatment is reduced. Reports on its biocompatibility show that the membrane offers specific advantages when its impact on cell-cell interactions is assessed. Cell aggregates formed with erythrocytes, neutrophils and platelets and their dynamic interactions came out positive when compared with other membrane polymers [63]. As one of the consequences, reduced neutrophil activation can be related to a reduced oxidative stress [64]. EVAL membranes exhibit less but larger pores than its counterparts and thus, offer a good permeability for larger uremic retention products whilst having a moderate UF-coefficient.

Group 5, Classical cellulose family Members: cellulose-di-acetate (CDA), cellulose-tri-acetate (CTA), (Nipro Medical), cellulose modified with Vitamin E (ASAHI Medical) (Table 13.7).

Cellulosic membranes have dominated the market for many years. The discussion about the alleged lack of blood compatibility has finally provoked the end of their production of regenerated unmodified cellulose membranes (Cuprophan®) in 2006.

When it became clear, that the OH-groups of cellulose are involved in complement activation through forming ester bonds with the C3b molecule, chemical modifications of cellulose have been performed already in 1983 [65]. At that time, a cellulose acetate modification provided better results in terms of leukocyte activation than the classical Cuprophan membrane. It appeared that blocking the OH-groups by esterification with acetic acid yields better results [65]. Replacing the hydroxyl group by acetyl groups further renders the membrane partly hydrophobic and leads to a reduced protein adsorption. Today, only membranes made of cellulose-di-acetate (CDA) and cellulose-tri-acetate (CTA) are available. When analyzing the protein adsorption capacity of CTA membranes with the help of proteomics, it could be shown that CTA bound more proteins (239 spots) than the polysulfone Helixone membrane (179 spots). This is in contrast to many early reports that cellulose acetate membranes exhibit only a low binding capacity for peptides/proteins [66].

There are also reports in the literature that attribute allergic reactions to the therapy with cellulose acetate membranes. The clinical finding of hearing loss, red-eye-syndrome, etc., after a treatment with cellulose-di-acetate membranes was attributed to polymer degradation due to saponification of cellulose acetate. This might have happened during gamma irradiation for sterilization [67]. Current CTA membranes are submitted to optimized gamma sterilization processes through reducing the presence of oxygen during the sterilization procedure [68].

Polymer Developments for Future Membrane Applications

Currently used polymers in nephrology have to satisfy many needs. These requirements differ according to both, technical production and clinical application. Polymers for dialysis membranes should be suitable for a reproducible membrane manufacturing, allow an easy sterilization and show long term stability, at least along the time line of the expiry date of the final product. As an example for blood compatibility, steam sterilization for dialyzers represents now the most widely technique for dialyzers (Fig. 13.10).

Polymers applied for products in nephrology should therefore be able to resist the necessary temperature and pressure conditions, i.e. 121 °C and 1 bar.

Clinical parameters related to polymers applied in dialyzers refer to blood compatibility and biostability. Membrane polymers should have adsorptive capacity for specific uremic retention products, even when these are unknown yet [59]. Adsorption of endotoxins [27–30] and of anaphyla-toxins, such as C3a and C5a [34] have considerably contributed to the safety and biocompatibility of dialysis treatments.

Extractables and leachables, that are released from polymers, have turned to become an issue, since more and more dialysis patients undergo this therapy for

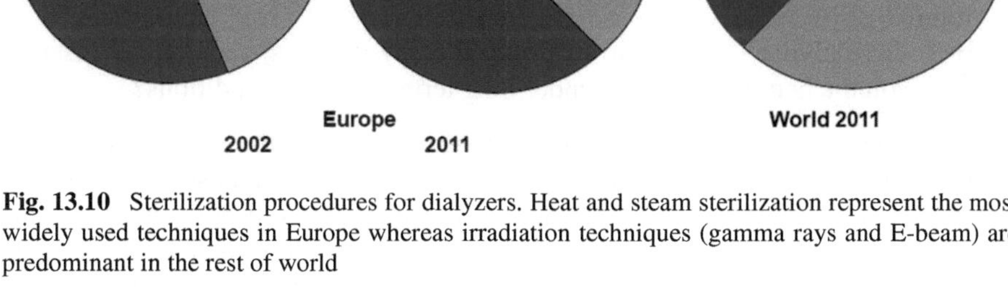

Fig. 13.10 Sterilization procedures for dialyzers. Heat and steam sterilization represent the most widely used techniques in Europe whereas irradiation techniques (gamma rays and E-beam) are predominant in the rest of world

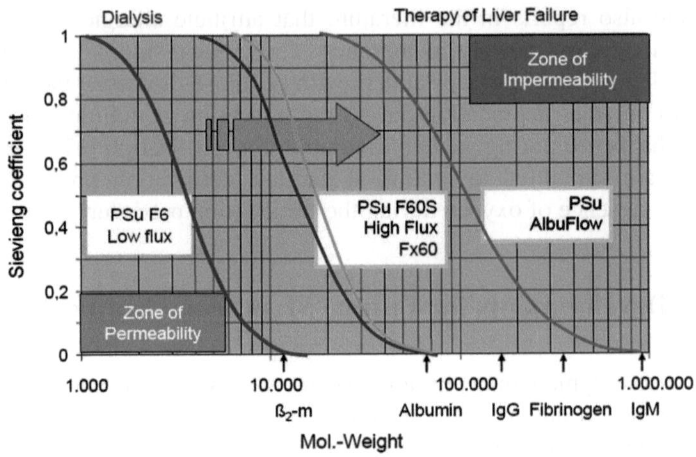

Fig. 13.11 Sieving coefficient curve for dialyzers as a tool for optimizing blood purification techniques. Shifting the curve to larger molecular weights with more open membranes allows for performing therapies, such as haemodiafiltration and liver failure therapies

longer periods of time [4] and thus, leachables that are not cleared by the failing kidney, might accumulate in the patient with deleterious consequences. This also holds true for polymers applied to dialyzer housing and tubing. Much effort has already been invested in order to improve this situation by selecting the optimal polymer or abandoning mal-performing types.

Chemical modification techniques of polymers primarily aim at altering the surface and bulk properties of the final product in order to enhance its performance in the biological environment. Currently applied polymers, e.g. for dialysis membranes, have reached a satisfactory level. They offer a high degree of both, performance adaptability and blood compatibility after an appropriate chemical modification. As an example, the sieving coefficient curve of dialysis membranes can be shifted towards larger molecular weights and thus be adapted to medical needs (Fig. 13.11).

Two questions may still arise:

1. Which requirements determine the selection of polymers in nephrology in the future?
2. How can polymers contribute to future therapy changes, such as for instance high volume hemodiafiltration under long term exposure conditions?

Current dialysis techniques are still and mostly based on the removal of matter or the removal of uremic retention solutes. Transport mechanisms for removal are diffusion and convection. Only apheresis techniques use both, filtration and adsorption processes. What about adding adsorption as a third removal mechanism also to dialysis? Ronco and Tetta have recently addressed this similar question and proposed to add adsorption features to the current therapies [69, 70].

Adsorption onto the membrane does contribute to the removal of noxious compounds, such as interleukin-1 and interleukin-6 (IL-1, IL-6), tumor necrosis factor (TNF), peptides and ß2-microglobulin [71]. As a result of the restricted surface area of dialyzers, however, adsorption capacity will rapidly be saturated. Acceptable rates of net removal by adsorption can only be achieved if the surface area is drastically increased by specifically designed devices [75, 76] or blood purification systems combining filtration and adsorption mechanisms in two devices, either arranged in parallel or in series.

Further complications may arise in that uremic toxicity depends on individual patient characteristics [72] and an increased capacity of the albumin molecule to bind toxins in the uremic state [73, 74], that leads to the accumulation of protein-bound uremic toxins. Consequently, either protein-permeable membranes will play a major role in the future or adsorber systems should be implemented in addition.

Results are already available as some polymers used for dialysis membranes exhibit intrinsic and specific adsorptive features for endotoxins [27–30], complement proteins or even unknown peptides [59].

However, the need for specific adsorptive features of polymers may still be questionable. Which argument supports this notion? Already in 1978, Henne and coworkers received a patent for their invention on a combination of tubular cellulosic membranes with carbon adsorber particles for the unspecific removal

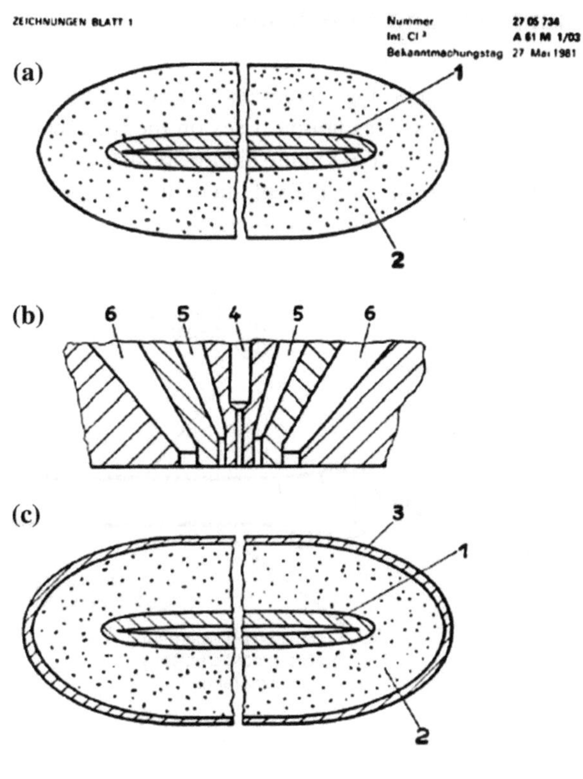

Fig. 13.12 In an early invention form 1978 adsorption and filtration are combined. One of two concentrically arranged tubular membranes is prefilled with carbon adsorber particles

of uremic retention products (Fig. 13.12, [75]). A similar approach is currently pursued at Twente University in the Netherlands, where scientists successfully inserted adsorber particles into the wall of capillary membranes and improved its membrane performance in in vitro experiments [76]. Of course, current carbon adsorber beads are cheap and thus easily available, however adsorption is still unspecific. Improvements could be realized by using charged beads or beads that bear immobilized antibodies for a specific removal. This proposal, however, should be seen under the premise that a culprit molecule for kidney failure has not yet been identified. Exemptions are water, potassium and phosphate.

The picture also shows the spinning orifices for the two membranes in the center (Adapted from [71]).

Proteome analyses of the ultrafiltrate of low- and high-flux membranes, moreover, have shown that around 1,000 different peptides can be found here [77]. In light of these observations, it may be reasonable to suggest that the removal of groups of different molecules might be more advantageous than focusing on single toxins. That approach would favor either or both, the use of non-specifically acting adsorber beads or the application of highly efficient filtration techniques, such as high-volume hemodiafiltration [8]. Polymer development for future therapies must be seen under these conditions and first results can already be reported [78, 79].

Summary and Conclusion

Polymers in nephrology represent a success story among all polymer applications for medical devices. This notion bases on the fact, that currently more than 2.5 million patients suffering from kidney failure are successfully treated in 2013 [21]. The quality and performance of the polymers that are part of the necessary medical devices can be attributed to this success. However, several factors have still to be considered.

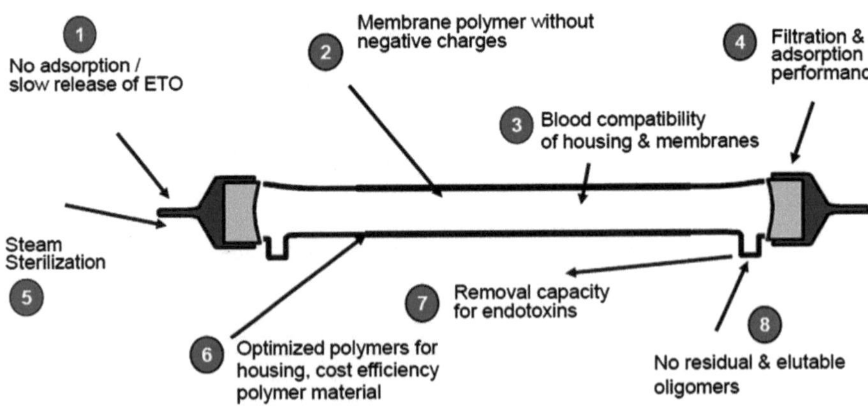

Fig. 13.13 Requirements for polymers to be used in blood purification therapies

A polymer will always remain one part of the extracorporeal system. Polymers may interfere with administered drugs, sterilization techniques or the specific pathological situation of an individual patient, e.g. his or her hypersensitivity, blood composition (uremia, diabetes) or even the individual circadien rhythm that affects physiological parameters. Figure 13.13 depicts a summary of properties for polymers that are and will be selected for future therapies.

References

1. Abel, J., Rowntree, L., Turner, B.: On the removal of diffusible substances from the circulating blood of living animals by means of dialysis. J. Pharmacol. Exp. Ther. **5**, 275–283 (1913)
2. Haas, G.: Dialysieren des strömenden Bluts am Lebenden. Klin Wochenschr **2**, 1888 (1923)
3. Haas, G.: Die Methodik der Blutauswaschung (Dialysis in vivo). In: Abderhalden, E (ed.) Handbuch der biologischen Arbeitsmethoden, Abt V, pp. 717–754. Urban-Schwarzenberg, Berlin/Wien (1935)
4. Nakai, S., Watanabe, Y., Masakane, I., Wada, A., Shoji, T., Hasegawa, T., Nakamoto, H., Yamagata, K., Kazama, K., Fujii, N., Itami, N., Shinoda, T., Shigematsu, T., Marubayashi, S., Morita, O., Hashimoto, S., Suzuki, K., Kimata, N., Hanafusa, N., Wakai, K., Hamano, T., Ogata, S., Tsuchida, K., Taniguchi, M., Nishi, H., Iseki, K., Tsubakihara, Y.: Overview of regular dialysis treatment in Japan (as of 31 December 2011). Ther. Apher. Dial. **17**, 567–611 (2013)
5. Knauf, F., Aronson, P.: ESRD as a window into America's cost crisis in health care. J. Am. Soc. Nephrol. **20**, 2093–2097 (2009)
6. Henderson, L., Chenoweth, D.: Cellulose membranes–time for a change? Contrib. Nephrol. **44**, 112–126 (1985)
7. Canaud, B., Bragg-Gresham, J., Marshall, M., Desmeules, S., Gillespie, B., Depner, T., Klassen, P., Port, F.: Mortality risk for patients receiving hemodiafiltration versus hemodialysis: European results from the DOPPS. Kidney Int. **69**, 2087–2093 (2006)
8. Maduell, F., Moreso, F., Pons, M., Ramos, R., Mora-Macia, J., Carreras, J., Soler, J., Torres, F., Campistol, J., Martinez-Castellao, A.: High efficiency postdilutional online hemodiafiltration reduces all-cause mortality in hemodialysis patients. J. Am. Soc. Nephrol. **24**, 487–497 (2013)
9. Klinkmann, H., Falkenhagen, D., Stefoni, S., Bonomini, V.: Biocompatibility, the need for a systems approach. Contrib. Nephrol. **70**, 213–226 (1989)
10. Kiil, F.: Development of a parallel-flow artificial kidney in plastics. Acta Chir. Scand. Suppl. **253**(Suppl), 142–150 (1960)
11. Stewart, R., Cerny, J., Lipps, B., Holmes, G.: Hemodialysis with the capillary kidney. Univ. Mich. Med. Cent. J. **34**, 80–83 (1968)
12. Kuelz, M., Nederlof, B., Schneider, H.: In vitro and in vivo evaluation of a new dialyzer. Nephrol. Dial. Transplant. **17**, 1475–1479 (2002)
13. Gong, H., Zhang, X., Cheng, B., Sun, Y., Li, C., Li, T., Zheng, L., Huang, K.: Bisphenol A accelerates toxic amyloid formation of human islet amyloid polypeptide: a possible link between Bisphenol A exposure and type 2 diabetes. PLoS ONE **8**, 54198 (2013)
14. Kanno, Y., Okada, H., Kobayashi, T., Takenaka, T., Suzuki, H.: Effects of endocrine disrupting substance on estrogen receptor gene transcription in dialysis patients. Ther. Apher. Dial. **11**, 262–265 (2007)
15. Buteau, H., Velasco, G., Cristofari, M., Balaguer, P., Perrot-Applanat, M.: Xenoestrogens modulate vascular endothelial growth factor secretion in breast cancer cells through an estrogen receptor-dependent mechanism. J. Endocrinol. **196**, 399–412 (2008)
16. Krieter, D., Canaud, B., Lemke, H.D., Rodriguez, A., Morgenroth, A., von Appen, K., Dargoun, G.P., Wanner, C.: Bisphenol A in chronic kidney disease. Artif. Organs **37**, 283–290 (2012)

17. Tee, R., Cullinan, P., Welch, J., Burge, P.S., Newman-Taylor, A.: Specific IgE to isocyanates: a useful diagnostic role in occupational asthma. J. Allergy Clin. Immunol. **101**, 709–715 (1998)
18. Röckel, A., Klinke, B., Hertel, J., Baur, X., Thiel, C., Abdelhamid, S., Fiegel, P., Walb, D.: Allergy to dialysis materials. Nephrol. Dial. Transplant. **4**, 646–652 (1989)
19. Skarping, G., Dalene, M., Littorin, M.: 4,4′-Methylenedianiline in hydrolysed serum and urine from a worker exposed to thermal degradation products of methylene diphenyl di-isocyanate elastomers. Int. Arch. Occup. Environ. Health **67**, 73–77 (1995)
20. Bowry, S., Gatti, E., Vienken, J.: Contribution of polysulfone membranes to the success of convective therapies. Contrib. Nephrol. **173**, 110–118 (2011)
21. Fresenius Medical Care (2014) ESRD Patients, a global perspective Company Brochure
22. Streicher, E., Schneider, H.: Polysulphone membrane mimicking human glomerular basement membrane. Lancet **322**, 1136 (1983)
23. Kerr, P., Huang, L.: Membranes for hemodialysis. Nephrology **15**, 381–385 (2010)
24. Matsuda, T.: Biological responses at non-physiological interfaces and molecular design of biocompatible surfaces. Nephrol. Dial. Transplant. **4**(Suppl. 3), 60–66 (1988)
25. Schindler, R.: Inflammation and dialysate quality. Hemodial. Int. **10**, S56–S59 (2006)
26. Lonnemann, G.: Chronic inflammation in hemodialysis: the role of contaminated dialysate. Blood Purif. **18**, 214–223 (2000)
27. Hayama, M., Miyasaka, T., Mochizuki, S., Asahara, H., Tsujioka, K., Kohori, F., Sakai, K., Jinbo, Y., Yoshida, M.: Visualisation of distribution of endotoxin trapped in an endotoxin-blocking filtration membrane. J. Membr. Sci. **210**, 45–53 (2002)
28. Nakatani, T., Tsuchida, K., Sugimura, K., Yoshimura, R., Takemoto, Y.: Investigation of endotoxin adsorption with polyether polymer alloy dialysis membranes. Int. J. Mol. Med. **11**, 195–197 (2003)
29. Henrie, M., Ford, C., Andersen, M., Stroup, E., Diaz-Buxo, J., Madsen, B., Britt, D., Ho, C.: In vitro assessment of dialysis membrane as an endotoxin transfer barrier: geometry, morphology and permeability. Artif. Organs **32**, 701–710 (2008)
30. Weber, V., Linsberger, I., Rossmanith, E., Weber, C., Falkenhagen, D.: Pyrogen transfer across high- and low-flux hemodialysis membranes. Artif. Organs **28**, 210–217 (2004)
31. Thomas, M., Moriyama, K., Ledebo, I.: AN69: Evolution of the world's first high permeability membrane. Contrib. Nephrol. **173**, 119–129 (2011)
32. Valette, P., Thomas, M., Déjardin, P.: Adsorption of low molecular weight proteins to hemodialysis membranes: experimental results and simulations. Biomaterials **20**, 1621–1634 (1999)
33. Moachon, N., Boullanger, C., Fraud, S., Vial, E., Thomas, M., Quash, G.: Influence of the charge of low molecular weight proteins on their efficacy of filtration and/or adsorption on dialysis membranes with different intrinsic properties. Biomaterials **23**, 651–658 (2002)
34. Pascual, M., Schifferli, J.A.: Adsorption of complement factor D by polyacrylonitrile membranes. Kidney Int. **43**, 903–911 (1993)
35. Mori, H., Hiraoka, K., Yorifuji, R., Iwasaki, T., Gomikawa, S., Inagaki, O., Inoue, S., Takamitsu, Y., Fujita, Y.: Adsorption of human recombinant erythropoietin on dialysis membranes in vitro. Artif. Organs **18**, 725–728 (1994)
36. Cheung, A.K., Hohnholt, M., Leypoldt, J.K., DeSpain, M.: Hemodialysis membrane biocompatibility: the case of erythropoietin. Blood Purif. **9**, 153–163 (1991)
37. Opatrny Jr, K., Krouzecky, A., Wirth, J., Vit, L., Eiselt, J.: The effects of a polyacrylonitrile membrane and a membrane made of regenerated cellulose on the plasma concentrations of erythropoietin during hemodialysis. Artif. Organs **22**, 816–820 (1998)
38. Groth, T., Synowitz, J., Malsch, G., Richau, K., Albrecht, W., Lange, K.-P., Paul, D.: Contact activation of plasmatic coagulation on polymeric membranes measured by the activity of kallikrein heparinized plasma. J. Biomat. Sci. Polmer Edn. **8**, 797–807 (1997)
39. Rollason, G., Sefton, M.: Measurement of the rate of thrombin production in human plasma in contact with different materials. J. Biomed. Mat. Res. **26**, 675–693 (1992)
40. Vogler, E., Siedlecki, C.: Contact activation of blood-plasma coagulation. Biomaterials **30**, 1857–1869 (2009)

41. Sperling, C., Fischer, M., Maitz, M., Werner, C.: Blood coagulation on biomaterials requires the combination of distinct activation processes. Biomaterials **30**, 4447–4456 (2009)
42. Verresen, L., Waer, M., Vanrenterghem, Y., Michielsen, P.: Angiotensin-converting-enzyme-inhibitors and anaphylactic reactions to high-flux membrane dialysis. Lancet **336**, 1360–1362 (1990)
43. Tielemans, C., Madhoun, P., Lenaers, M., Schandene, L., Goldman, M., Vanherweghem, J.L.: Anaphylactoid reactions during hemodialysis on AN69 membranes in patients receiving ACE inhibitors. Kidney Int. **38**, 982–984 (1990)
44. Parnes, E.L., Shapiro, W.B.: Anaphylactoid reactions in hemodialysis patients treated with the AN69 dialyzer. Kidney Int. **40**, 1148–1152 (1991)
45. Brunet, P., Jaber, K., Berland, Y., Baz, M.: Anaphylactoid reactions during hemodialysis and hemofiltration: role of associating AN69 membrane and angiotensin I converting enzyme inhibitors. Am. J. Kidney Dis. **9**, 444–447 (1992)
46. Krieter, D., Grude, M., Lemke, H.D., Fink, E., Bönner, G., Schölkens, B., Schulz, E., Müller, G.A.: Anaphylactoid reactions during hemodialysis in sheep are ACE inhibitor dose-dependent and mediated by bradykinin. Kidney Int. **53**, 1026–1035 (1998)
47. Brophy, P., Mottes, T., Kudelka, T., McBryde, K., Gradner, J., Maxvold, N., Bunchman, T.: AN-69 membrane reactions are pH-dependent and preventable. Am. J. Kidney Dis. **38**, 173–178 (2001)
48. Renaux, J., Thomas, M., Crost, T., Loughraieb, N., Vantard, G.: Activation of the kalikrein-kinin system in hemodialysis: role of membrane electronegativity, blood dilution and pH. Kidney Int. **55**, 1097–1103 (1999)
49. Shiba, M., Tadokoro, K., Sawanobori, M., Nakajima, K., Suzuki, K., Juji, T.: Activation of the contact system by filtration of platelet concentrates with a negatively charged white cell-removal filter and measurement of venous blood bradykinin level in patients who received filtered platelets. Transfusion **37**, 457–462 (1997)
50. Krieter, D.H., Steinke, J., Kerkhoff, M., Fink, E., Lemke, H.D., Zingler, C., Müller, G.A., Schuff-Werner, P.: Contact activation in low-density lipoprotein apheresis systems. Artif. Organs **29**, 47–52 (2005)
51. Adam, A., Montpas, N., Keire, D., Désormeaux, A., Brown, N.J., Marceau, F., Westenberger, B.: Bradykinin forming capacity of oversulfated chondroitin sulfate contaminated heparin in vitro. Biomaterials **31**, 5741–5748 (2010)
52. Désormeaux, Al, Moreau, M.E., Lepage, Y., Chanard, J., Adam, A.: The effect of electronegativity and angiotensin-converting enzyme inhibition on the kinin-forming capacity of polyacrylonitrile dialysis membranes. Biomaterials **29**, 1139–1146 (2008)
53. Gretz, N., Bowry, S., Vienken, J., Odenwälder, W., Strauch, M.: Simple approach to heparin-free dialysis. Nephrol. Dial. Transplant. **8**, 990 (1993)
54. Lavaud, S., Paris, B., Maheut, H., Randoux, C., Renaux, J.L., Rieu, P., Chanard, J.: Assessment of the heparin-binding AN69 ST hemodialysis membrane: II. Clinical studies without heparin administration. ASAIO J. **51**, 348–351 (2005)
55. Kessler, M., Gangemi, C., Gutierrez Martones, A., Lacombe, J., Krier-Coudert, M., Galland, R., Kielstein, J., Moureau, F., Loughraieb, N.: Heparin-grafted dialysis membrane allows minimal systemic anticoagulation in regular hemodialysis patients: a prospective proof-of-concept study. Hemodial. Int. **17**, 282–293 (2013)
56. Sugaya, H., Sakai, Y.: Polymethylmethacrylate: from polymer to dialyzer. Contrib. Nephrol. **125**, 1–8 (1998)
57. Fabbrini, P., Sirtori, S., Casiraghi, E., Pieruzzi, F., Genovesi, S., Corti, D., Brivio, R., Gregorini, G., Como, G., Carati, M., Vignano, M., Stella, A.: Polymethylmethacrylate membrane and serum free light chain removal: enhancing adsorption properties. Blood Purif. **35**(Suppl 2), 52–58 (2013)
58. Locatelli, F., Andrulli, S., Pecchini, F., Pedrini, L., Agliata, S., Lucchi, L., Farina, M., La Milia, V., Grassi, C., Borghi, M.: Effect of high-flux dialysis on the anemia of haemodialysis patients. Nephrol. Dial. Transplant. **15**, 1399–1409 (2000)
59. Goeksel, T., Xie, W., Ritzerfeld, M., Heidenreich, S., Mann, H.: Prurigo nodularis and dialyzer membrane. Blood Purif. **35**(Suppl 2), 26–27 (2013)

60. Narita, I., Aichi, B., Omori, K., Sato, F., Ajiro, J., Saga, D., Kondo, D., Skatsume, M., Maruyama, S., Kazama, J., Akazawa, K., Gejyo, F.: The effect of polymethylmethacrylate dialysis membranes on uremic pruritus. Kidney Int. **69**, 1626–1632 (2006)
61. Schwarzbeck, A., Wittenmeier, K.-W., Hällfritzsch, U., Frank, J.: Anaphylactoid reactions ACE inhibitors and extracorporeal hemotherapy. Nephron **65**, 499–500 (1993)
62. Nakano, A.: Ethylene vinyl alcohol co-polymer as a high-performance membrane. An EVOH membrane with excellent biocompatibility. Contrib. Nephrol. **173**, 164–171 (2011)
63. Sirolli, V., Ballone, E., Di Stante, S., Amoroso, I., Bonomini, M.: Cell activation and cellular-cellular interactions during hemodialysis. Int. J. Artif. Organs **25**, 529–537 (2002)
64. Ito, S., Suzuki, C., Tsuji, S.: Platelet activation through interaction with hemodialysis membranes induces neutrophils to produce reactive oxygen species. J. Biomed. Mater. Res. **77A**, 294–303 (2006)
65. Ivanovich, P., Chenoweth, D., Schmidt, R., Klinkmann, H., Boxer, L., Jacob, H., Hammerschmidt, D.: Symptoms and activation of granulocytes and complement with two dialysis membranes. Kidney Int. **24**, 758–763 (1983)
66. Urbani, A., Louisell, S., Sirolli, V., Bucci, S., Amoroso, L., Pavone, B., Pieroni, L., Sacchetta, P., Bonomini, M.: Proteomic analysis of protein adsorption capacity of different haemodialysis membranes. Mol. BioSyst. **8**, 1029–1039 (2012)
67. Averbukh, Z., Modai, D., Sandbank, J., Berman, S., Cohn, M., Galperin, E., Cohen, N., Dishi, V., Weissgarten, J.: Red eye syndrome: clinical and experimental experience in a new aspect of diffusive eosinophilic infiltration? Artif. Organs **25**, 437–440 (2001)
68. Sunohara, T., Masuda, T.: Cellulose triacetate as a high-performance membrane. Contrib. Nephrol. **173**, 156–163 (2011)
69. Ronco, C., Tetta, C.: Extracorporeal blood purification: more than diffusion and convection. Does this help? Curr. Opin. Care **13**, 662–667 (2007)
70. Ronco, C.: Sorbents; from bench to bedside. Can we combine membrane separation processes and adsorbent based solute removal? Int. J. Artif. Organs **29**, 819–822 (2006)
71. Bouman, C., van Olden, R., Stoutenbeek, C.: Cytokine filtration and adsorption during pre- and postdilution hemofiltration in four different membranes. Blood Purif. **16**, 261–268 (1998)
72. Vanholder, R., de Smet, R., Glorieux, G., Argilés, A., Baurmeister, U., Brunet, P., Clark, W., Cohen, G., de Deyn, P., Deppisch, R., Descamps-Latscha, B., Henle, T., Jörres, A., Lemke, H.D., Massy, Z., Passlick-Deetjen, J., Rodriguez, M., Stegmayr, B., Stenvinkel, P., Tetta, C., Wanner, C., Zidek, W.: Review on uremic toxins: Classification, concentration, and interindividual variability. Kidney Int. **63**, 1934–1963 (2003)
73. Klammt, S., Wojak, H., Mitzner, A., Koball, S., Rychly, J., Reisinger, E., Mitzner, S.: Albumin-binding capacity (ABiC) is reduced in patients with chronic kidney disease along with an accumulation of protein-bound uraemic toxins. Nephrol. Dial. Transplant. **27**, 2372–2383 (2012)
74. Varshney, A., Rehan, M., Subbarao, N., Rabbani, G., Khan, R.: Elimination of endogenous toxin, creatinine from blood plasma depends on albumin conformation: site specific uremic toxicity & impaired drug binding. PLoS ONE **6**, 17230 (2011)
75. Henne, W., Pohle, R., Lawitzki, F.: Dialysis membrane for hemodialysis. German Patent 2705734 C3 (1978)
76. Tijink, M., Kooman, J., Wester, M., Sun, J., Saiful, S., Joles, J., Borneman, Z., Wessling, M., Stamatialis, D.: Mixed matrix membranes: a new asset for blood purification therapies. Blood Purif. **37**, 1–3 (2014)
77. Weissinger, E., Kaiser, T., Meert, N., deSmet, R., Walden, M., Mischak, H., Vanholder, R.: Proteomics: a novel tool to unravel the patho-physiology of uraemia. Nephrol. Dial. Transplant. **19**, 3068–3077 (2004)
78. Maduell, F., Arias-Guillen, M., Fontseré, N., Ojeda, R., Rico, N., Vera, M., Elena, M., Bedini, J., Wienecke, P., Campistol, J.: Elimination of large uremic toxins by a dialyzer specifically designed for high-volume convective therapies. Blood Purif. **37**, 125–130 (2014)
79. Lamy, T., Henri, P., Lobbedez, T., Comby, E., Ryckelynck, J., Ficheux, M.: Comparison between on-line high-efficiency hemodiafiltration and conventional high-flux hemodialysis for polycloncal free light chain removal. Blood Purif. **37**, 93–98 (2014)

Chapter 14
Polymers in Wound Repair

Antonio Francesko, Margarida M. Fernandes, Guillem Rocasalbas, Sandrine Gautier and Tzanko Tzanov

Abstract Efficient dermal wound care implies providing a healing environment at the site of injury. Current repair techniques, including polymeric dressings, are able to accelerate only the healing of epidermal and partial thickness acute wounds based on maintaining the area moist. However, these are not efficient in treatment of full-thickness and chronic wounds, which lack in inborn regenerative elements and are highly prone to infections. For this reason the research interest is nowadays shifted towards functional biomaterials to tackle severe skin deteriorations by providing a beneficiary for healing pro-active and pathogen-free environment. Recent advances in molecular biology and materials science together with better understanding of wound pathophysiology allowed for designing of new wound care approaches that rely on biochemical stimuli to promote wound closure. Biopolymers that couple intrinsic antimicrobial and wound repair properties with hydrophilicity appear as suitable dressing platforms. These can be further upgraded using various bio-entities (therapeutic molecules, cells) with the ability to address specific targets in the biochemical environment of wounds in order to stimulate the healing process. This chapter summarises the abundant experimental and clinical data on polymers in advanced wound dressings, scaffolds for dermal regeneration and platforms for drug delivery.

Keywords Polymers · Biopolymers · Active agents · Wound healing · Advanced dressings

---

A. Francesko · M.M. Fernandes · T. Tzanov (✉)
Grup de Biotecnologia Molecular i Industrial, Edifici Gaia, Department of Chemical Engineering, Universitat Politècnica de Catalunya, Rambla Sant Nebridi, 22, 08222 Terrassa, Spain
e-mail: tzanko.tzanov@upc.edu

G. Rocasalbas · S. Gautier
KitoZyme S.A., Parc Industriel Des Hauts-Sarts, Zone 2, Rue Haute Claire 4, 4040 Herstal, Belgium

F. Puoci (ed.), *Advanced Polymers in Medicine*, DOI 10.1007/978-3-319-12478-0_14

Abbreviations

bFGF	Basic fibroblast growth factor
BSA	Bovine serum albumin
ECM	Extracellular matrix
GAGs	Glycosaminoglycans
GM-CSF	Granulocyte macrophage colony stimulating factor
HA	Hyaluronic acid
HClO	Hypochlorous acid
MMPs	Matrix metalloproteinases
MPO	Myeloperoxidase
NPWT	Negative pressure wound therapy
PDGF-BB	Platelet-derived growth factor BB
PRP	Platelet rich plasma
PHMB	Polyhexamethylene biguanide
ROS	Reactive oxygen species
SF	Silk fibroin
VEGF	Vascular endothelial growth factor

Wounds: Formation and Repair

Skin Integrity and Its Function

Skin, the largest organ in the human body composed of epidermis, dermis and hypodermis, has several important functions, including regulation of water, electrolyte balance and thermoregulation. The outer epidermis forms a protective barrier to keep the water in the body and prevent pathogens from entering in addition to helping the skin to regulate body temperature. This layer is a stratified scaly epithelium composed of proliferating basal and differentiated suprabasal keratinocytes. The stratum corneum is the outermost part of epidermis with specific barrier properties. It consists of non-viable cells and is very firm but pliable and wrinkled. The underlying dermis is composed of a very dense fibre network—extracellular matrix (ECM), dominating the mechanical behaviour of the total skin, and therefore providing structural support to the organ. This gel-like matrix, secreted locally by the cells that it surrounds, is composed of a variety of polysaccharides and proteins: collagen fibrils, microfibrils, and elastic fibres, embedded in proteoglycans. An intricate network of these macromolecules, assembled in close association with the surface of the cell that produced them, provides the unique structure of the ECM, exhibiting high tensile strength combined with the substantial elasticity and compressibility. The deepest skin layer, the hypodermis or subcutaneous adipose tissue, is composed of loose fatty connective tissue. All skin layers contain blood vessels, lymph vessels, nerve endings, sweat glands and hair follicles.

Acute Wounds and Healing Process

According to the Wound Healing Society (www.woundheal.org), a wound is the result of disruption of normal anatomic structure and function of a tissue. A dermal wound is defined as a break in the integrity of the skin, raised due to external or internal noxious stimulus, which leads to an inadequate performance of the skin functions. It is therefore vital to restore the skin integrity and consequently functions as soon as possible. A completely healed wound implies that the affected part of the skin has returned to its normal anatomical structure and function, and similar appearance within a reasonable period of time [1]. The primary causes of acute wounds include mechanical injuries due to external factors such as abrasion and tear, after a frictional contact between the skin and hard surfaces, including penetrating wounds caused by knives and firearm shots, surgical incisions, etc. Burns and chemical injuries arise from radiation, electricity, corrosive chemicals and thermal sources, among others. Another classification of wounds is based on the number of skin layers and area of skin affected. Based on this it is possible to distinguish between an epidermal (superficial) wound and an injury involving both the epidermis and dermis that in addition affects the blood vessels and is referred to as a partial thickness wound. Full thickness skin wounds occur when the underlying subcutaneous fat or deeper tissues are damaged in addition to the epidermis and dermal layers. Epidermal and partial thickness wounds can regenerate due to the self-healing capacity of the body for re-epithelisation. Conversely, in the full-thickness wounds regenerative elements that reside in dermis are completely destroyed and the epithelisation is possible only on the wound edges.

Normal wound healing involves a complex series of orchestrated events leading to the repair of injured tissues. These dynamic events occur as a sequential cascade of processes requiring the coordinated completion of a variety of cellular activities correlating with the appearance of different cell types in the wound during various stages of the healing process [2]. Acute wounds heal in a very orderly and efficient manner characterised by four overlapping phases: haemostasis, inflammation, cell migration/proliferation, and maturation (remodelling) phase. After injury the bleeding flush out bacteria and antigens from the injury site, also causing aggregation of the platelets now accumulated at the site that form a haemostatic plug and prevent an excessive loss of blood. In addition, platelets release growth factors and adhesive proteins to activate cells in the surrounding area. During the inflammatory phase neutrophils arrive at the site of the injury, liberating phagocytes and a variety of enzymes and reactive oxygen species (ROS), crucial for wound cleaning and the prevention of infections [3]. Phagocytes engulf dead cells (necrotic tissue) previously liquefied by a simultaneous enzymatic (protease) action to a yellowish slough with bad odour. The inflammatory phase occurs almost simultaneously with haemostasis and lasts for about 3 days in normal healing process. However, if the action of the inflammatory factors is prolonged or they are found in counts higher than normal, the process is harmful for healthy cells—the common situation found in chronic wounds [4]. The migration phase involves the movement of keratinocytes and fibroblasts to the injured area to replace damaged and lost tissue. These cells regenerate from the margins, rapidly growing over the wound to cause epithelial thickening. Accompanied proliferative phase is characterised by the ingrowth of capillaries and lymphatic vessels into the wound and collagen synthesis by fibroblasts giving the skin strength and form. The newly formed granulation tissue and ECM consist mainly of glycosaminoglycans (GAGs), proteoglycans and collagen. During the angiogenesis (formation of new blood vessels) the fibroblasts transform into myofibroblasts that bring the margins of the wound together in order to reduce its size. The final phase of wound healing is the transformation of granulation tissue into a scar, characterised by a decreased inflammation. Myofibroblasts further undergo apoptosis and a new collagenous matrix replaces the provisional one [4]. The described cascade occurs in normal wound healing, with a reestablishment of the equilibrium between scar formation and scar remodelling, the longest part of the healing (up to two years) marking the end of the wound healing process.

Chronic Wounds and Impaired Healing

In contrast to acute wounds, abnormal response to an injury leads to formation of non-healing (chronic) wounds. Chronic wounds can affect many anatomical regions as a result of different underlying pathologies and accordingly are classified as venous leg ulcers, arterial ulcers, neuropathic ulcers, pressure ulcers (decubitus), vasculitis, etc. Except for serious burns that also cannot heal, all the conditions leading to chronic ulceration are more prevalent in the individuals with low mobility and elderly population. In addition, the increased occurrence and longevity of these ulcers are further compounded by the detrimental effects ageing has on the skin.

A chronic wound arises after disruption of the acute wound healing process at one or more of its phases, impairing the reestablishment of anatomical and functional integrity of the affected tissue in a physiologically appropriate length of time. Various factors can cause the failure of the normal healing process and trigger chronic inflammatory responses: foreign bodies introduced deep into the wound at the time of injury, inadequate management of already infected wounds, poor nutritional status of a patient, aged skin with reduced ability to fight infections, underlying diseases such as diabetes and anaemia that compromise the circulation resulting in poor delivery of blood cells and oxygen to the wound, etc. The disruption of the acute healing process is usually expressed in its inflammatory phase. The caused prolonged inflammation leads to an excessive matrix deposition and loss of tissue function [5].

Despite the different underlying aetiology, most chronic wounds show a similar behaviour and progress. This is because these ulcers share the specific biological markers which significantly differentiate from the environment of acute wounds. In acute wounds there is a balance between production and degradation of molecules (e.g. collagen); in chronic wounds this balance is disturbed in favour of degradation. Chronic ulcer fluids contain elevated level of neutrophils and neutrophil-derived enzymes compared with acute wound fluids due to their continuous influx during the prolonged inflammation [5]. Neutrophils undergo apoptosis at the site of injury and release oxidative enzyme myeloperoxidase (MPO). Under physiological conditions MPO catalyses the generation of hypochlorous acid (HClO), the most powerful ROS in human body, creating oxidative stress and impairing the healing process. The cytotoxicity of this reaction allows the killing of bacteria in the first line of defence. However, the HClO reacts with most biological molecules, including natural protease inhibitors. In healing wounds the production and activity of proteolytic enzymes, such as matrix metalloproteinases (MMPs) and serine proteases (e.g. elastase), are tightly regulated by counteraction of their natural inhibitors [6]. During granulation tissue formation levels of MMPs have been shown to be decreased compared to levels found in chronic wounds. In normal levels, these proteases play a role in cellular migration. In chronic wounds the generation of HClO induces disturbed ratio proteases/inhibitors [7], so that most of the enzymes are uninhibited [8]. In increased levels these proteases have detrimental effect on wound healing by uncontrolled digestion of the ECM and the growth factors [6].

Wound Management

Effective wound management depends on understanding a number of different factors such as the underlying mechanism of wound formation, the type of wound, the healing process and general condition of a patient in terms of health (e.g. diabetes, aged patient). First, in order to inspect a wound correctly for the proper treatment choice, it is indispensable to remove the necrotic tissue and foreign material from the areas around the wound. The removal of the dead tissue is known as wound debridement and could be carried out using several methods. Surgical removal with scalpel and/or scissors is the most effective and precise, however, can only be undertaken by highly skilled and trained practitioners. Wound irrigation, on the other hand, implies rehydration of necrotic tissue using e.g. hydrogel dressings and further its autolytic digestion by the enzymes accumulated in the wound site [9]. Here the outcome depends on many individual factors in the treated patient, and thus, little control over the process is granted. The more efficient alternative is the enzymatic removal of the necrotic tissue after liquefying using bacterial or animal derived collagenases. Despite being more controllable than the autolytic digestion, the biggest disadvantage of all enzymatic methods still remains much longer duration compared to the surgical debridement. Besides to assure establishing of the proper diagnosis of the wound, another objective of debridement is to provide a favourable environment at the surface of the wound in which healing could take place in combination with proper treatment strategy [10].

Depending on the wound type, the cause and its position on the body, nowadays the management involves one or the combination of the several available treatment options: topical application of antibiotics and/or antiseptics, multiple dressing changes per day and, recently, costly treatments involving the application of local mechanical stresses or energy to a wound—negative pressure wound therapy (NPWT) and mist ultrasound therapy.

Epicutaneous application of antimicrobial agents is, thus far, the most effective way to treat wound infections. However, such therapy is directed only to the ulcers with severe microorganism contamination. Moreover, the biggest concern is the overdoses due to the accumulation of immunoreactive compounds at the wound site [11].

NPWT consists of the controlled application of sub-atmospheric pressure to the local wound environment, using a sealed wound dressing connected to a vacuum pump. Studies suggested that NPWT assists in wound healing by providing a moist environment, stimulating circulation to the wound bed, decreasing bacterial colonisation and increasing the rate of granulation tissue formation [12]. However, the negative side of NPWT is a cost of the treatment and lack of an overall plan of care for the patients suffering different kind of ulcers. Although a consistent evidence of the benefit of NPWT in the treatment of diabetes-associated chronic leg ulcers together with safety of the treatment was demonstrated [13], its effectiveness compared to conventional/advances dressing treatments is still disputable [14, 15]. Moreover, the evaluation on "mixed wounds" was of poor quality and therefore requires better quality research to be conducted.

Another novel technology using non-contact, kilohertz-range ultrasound therapy is gaining popularity, especially in chronic wound management. Cells at the site of injury absorb the energy from the ultrasound wave and initiate signalling pathways with direct implications for the healing process. The therapy uses a low frequency, low intensity ultrasound to provide enough energy to stimulate healthy cells, but insufficient to damage them. The vibration of micron-sized bubbles, formed during sonication [16], within inter- and intracellular fluids causes changes in the cellular membrane potentials and cellular activities within the tissues. Ultrasound therapy has been shown to increase the healing rate in recalcitrant diabetic foot ulcers and other lower extremity wounds [17] however, it is rather cost-ineffective compared to standard wound care.

Compared to the above described physical methods for wound management the usage of modern polymer-based dressing materials is cheaper and more effective. Both synthetic polymers and biopolymers, e.g. chitosan, are easily processed into desired shape and design, and stabilised using different techniques for extended shelf-life [18]. Many of these macromolecules display beneficial features for the treatment of wounds, however, the variability in wound pathophysiology makes difficult to develop a dressing material that meets all the criteria for optimum healing. Much research is currently being undertaken to design wound dressings that can stimulate the healing taking into account all (or at least majority) of the factors impairing healing.

Polymer Dressings in Wound Treatment

Factors Influencing Dressing Choice

Many sophisticated dressings are nowadays available to the wound care practitioner, these made of a wide range of polymeric materials. Polymers may be used alone or in combinations thereof, being processed in different dressing designs such as films, foams, fibrous materials, beads, hydrogels, hydrocolloids or even pharmaceutical sprays comprising nano/micro-particulate systems. Depending on their composition and design, the polymeric dressings and formulations may be used to absorb exudate, provide and maintain a beneficial for wound healing moist environment, combat odour or infection, relieve pain, or promote debridement at the wound surface. Some dressings simply absorb exudate or wound fluid and may therefore be suitable for application to a variety of different wound types. Others have a more specific function and as such have a limited application being only suitable for the treatment of particular types of wounds or applied during one phase of the healing process. Due to the variations between pathophysiology of different wounds it is difficult to develop a dressing that meets all the criteria for optimum healing. Wound healing is a dynamic process and the performance requirements of a dressing can change as the wound progresses towards healing. For this reason, in most clinical cases a combination of individual component dressings that feature different functional properties is necessary in order to achieve effective wound healing in a reasonable time.

Nowadays, the design of a dressing is dominated by the hydrocolloids, useful for clean, granulating, epidermal wounds with low to medium exudate, but inefficient on infected and exuding wounds. Currently, polyurethane foams are promoted as an alternative to hydrocolloids or even used with them in combination carriers, without significant improvement in the healing rate of difficult to treat chronic ulcers. Nevertheless, the design of a dressing depends on the type of the wound, its thickness, position on the body, exudate volume, the stage of the healing process (early, late) and age of the affected individual. The modern dressings are most frequently found in the design of thin films/coatings, (hydro)gels and foam sheets (i.e. sponges) [10].

Thin transparent film dressings have low absorption capacity, thus are not useful for wounds with significant exudates. Films are mostly used for the later stage healing, when the wound exudates are minimised, or to simply cover the damaged area and protect the wound from external factors. Available in thickness ranging from μm to mm, these dressings are prepared by different methods (usually casting followed by evaporation) using one or more polymers. Sometimes films are used as top layers to keep other dressings in place, e.g. over ointment or hydrogel dressing. If applied alone, transparent films allow for on-site inspection of the healing progress without removal of the dressing. Thus, in advanced treatment strategies films/coatings bearing active functions could be an ideal solution for the combined wound treatment and monitoring of the wound status.

Hydrogels are highly absorbent water-insoluble networks of polymer chains with high degree of flexibility similar to that of the natural tissue. The hydrogels are normally classified according to the nature of network formation as physical and chemical hydrogels. The physical hydrogels are obtained by reversible electrostatic interactions (e.g. polyelectrolyte complexes) or through secondary interactions (e.g. hydrogen bonds), whereas the chemical hydrogels are covalently cross-linked. Hydrogels are useful for exudative wounds because of their high absorptive capacity, in addition to maintaining the moisture at the wound site and permitting the oxygen penetration. In addition, they provide excellent pain relief by reducing potential irritation and cooling the wound. Nevertheless, during application hydrogels should be covered by an outer layer of tape, netting or roll bandage. They were found particularly useful for the treatment of deep partial thickness wounds.

Hydrophilic foam dressings are permeable to oxygen and water vapour. They usually have a hydrophobic backing and some have an adhesive surface to make the application easier. Sponges are more easily saturated with wound exudates than hydrogels, hence their changing frequency is considerably higher, especially during early wound healing characterised with large amounts of exudates. Foam dressings are ideally suited for dry and semi-dry superficial and partial thickness wounds, in addition to chronic ulcers since they provide padding that can relieve pressure over bony prominences. From a technological point of view, the manufacturing of a foam dressing is commercially attractive consisting of an easy process of freeze-drying of a moulded suspension of the dressing components.

Synthetic Polymers as Dressing Materials

Besides the classification on their function and design, wound dressings can be categorised according to the type of material employed for their manufacturing: synthetic or naturally occurring polymers [19]. Synthetic polymers are mainly used as platforms for actuation and delivery of active agents, but also provide an optimal microenvironment for cell proliferation, migration and differentiation when used in biosynthetic skin grafts. Synthetic polymers used for permanent coverage (skin equivalents) should be fully biocompatible and with good mechanical properties. Biodegradability of synthetic polymers is the desired property when localised delivery of active compounds from temporary dressings/templates is required. Besides functionalisation with both organic and inorganic active agents, synthetic polymers are often used in a combination with biopolymers and further processed in different dressing designs [20]. Synthetic polymers show a superior mechanical strength compared to natural macromolecules, thus by their cross-linking or blending the mechanical properties of the latter are improved, whereas a bioactive component is added to the inert synthetic platform. Features of some of the most used synthetic polymers in wound healing are summarised below.

Polyurethanes are copolymers with repetitive urethane groups in their structures. This class of synthetic polymers have gained acceptance in the biomedical field due to their exceptional strength and biocompatibility. The physical properties of polyurethanes vary from brittle to very elastic. The biomedically acceptable polyurethanes are non-toxic and have elastomeric properties accompanied by good toughness, tear resistance and abrasion resistance. Such materia+ls favour reepithelialisation during wound healing [21]. Polyurethane foams are designed to absorb large amounts of exudates and maintain a moist wound environment and as such are not used on low exudating ulcers as this would cause dryness of the wound site. Examples of polyurethane foams on the market are Smith&Nephew's Allevyn® and Mölnlycke's Lyofoam®.

Due to its low toxicity, low allergic properties and high biocompatibility with body tissues and blood, **silicon** is extensively used for preparation of biomedical materials [22]. Being also resistant to biodegradation, silicone is used in the preparation of permanent implant elastomers for soft tissue repair and in combination with biopolymers as support materials for wound treatment and diagnosis [23, 24]. Silicones aid to the wound treatment modalities as an occlusive contact medium, being generally accepted as the only materials able to manage hypertrophic (burn related) scarring without significant side effects [25]. In addition, silicon-based dressings on the market, e.g. Safetac®, are generally regarded as easily changeable and painless upon replacement.

Teflon, a polymer synthesised by polymerisation of tetrafluoroethylene at high temperature and pressure, is an inert non-carcinogenic material. It is easily processed into desired shapes and facile to apply to the injured area [26]. Teflon is frequently used in a combination with another polymeric dressing to lower the adherence of the latter at the wound site, aiding to painless bandage removal.

Biopolymers as Dressing Materials

Modern industries necessarily exploit renewable resources, promoting environmentally friendly and beneficial technologies. Constant improvement in quality of products and competitive technologies for their generation is a must in order to keep competitive market positions. Biopolymers, due to their intrinsically beneficial properties for a broad spectrum of applications, are gaining importance as raw materials in many industrial sectors. They comply with the requirements for the medical/pharmaceutical materials, being biodegradable, biocompatible and in most cases not causing immune response in organism, in addition to integration with a particular cell type/tissue upon application.

The biomaterials used in skin repair should display intrinsic biocompatibility and biodegradability at the ideal rate corresponding to the rate of new tissue formation [27]. Besides these biomaterials, their degradation products should also not be toxic, immunogenic and carcinogenic. Polysaccharides and proteins, being natural components of all living structures and displaying the above properties, are up to date the most suitable candidates for fabrication of wound dressing materials.

Chitin and its deacetylated derivative **chitosan** are suitable bioplatforms that can be further improved by targeted functionalisation for skin repair. For example, the unique biological properties of chitosan characterised with human cell biocompatibility, human serum biodegradability, non-toxicity, antibacterial and haemostatic properties justify the use of this biopolymer in skin repair processes. The haemostatic activity of chitosan is exploited in early treatment of wounds [28], especially in large injuries subjected to heavy bleeding [29]. Many haemostatic products on the market consist thus, fully or partially, of chitosan. Moreover, chitosan aids to a rapid closure of full-thickness wounds due to its supportive effect to the fast growing of new blood vessels (angiogenesis) in the injured tissue [30]. Chitin and chitosan can be prepared in a variety of forms targeting particular application, i.e. healing of a certain wound type or on different position on the body. Films, hydrogels, fibres, powders and micro-/nanoparticles, entirely or partially composed of chitosan, have been demonstrated and continue to be evaluated for their benefits in wound healing [18].

Glycosaminoglycans are important components of connective tissues where their chains are covalently linked to a protein to form proteoglycans. As highly hydrophilic structures GAGs possess especially high affinity for physiological fluids to promote swelling [31]. **Chondroitin sulphate** is an important structural component of cartilage and materials made from this GAG are biocompatible and non-immunogenic. Chondroitin sulphate acts as surrogate extracellular matrix, serving as a repository for cytokines and growth factors, important bioentities for the healing process [32], and providing structural frameworks for fibroblasts during the epithelial regeneration. **Hyaluronic acid** (HA) is an intracellular component of connective tissues such as the synovial fluid of joints and an important part of ECM. The most important property of HA is its effect on angiogenesis: whereas high molecular weight HA inhibits angiogenesis, HA oligosaccharide units are proangiogenic [33, 34]. HA readily interacts with proteins, growth factors and tissue components with a vital importance in acceleration of dermal tissue repair [35]. Regarding the HA-based biomaterials, cross-linked hydrogel films have been produced for the use as polymeric drug delivery platforms with improved exploitation characteristics [36]. Furthermore, the biological properties of HA have been also combined with other biomaterials for the production of tissue engineering scaffolds or membranes [37, 38].

Alginic acid, a natural polysaccharide derived from brown algae, is well-known absorbent which dressings regardless of design easily conform to the shape of a wound and adapt to a wound bed. In addition, alginic acid and its salts are haemostatic agents; hence their application in the treatment of large injuries and burns. They are applied in the form of a gel and sponges produced from calcium alginate. An example of a calcium alginate on the market is Suprasorb A from Lohmann&Rauscher, a dressing that creates a clean wound environment for heavily exuding wounds due to its high absorbency. This dressing absorbs large exudate volumes and rapidly forms a gel through the exchange of calcium ions from the wound dressing with the sodium ions in the wound exudate. The gel binds to the exudate, trapping bacteria and tissue debris. When the dressing is changed, the exudate, bacteria and tissue debris are removed with the alginate fibres. Some studies also indicated that calcium alginate increases cellular activity properties during the healing process of diabetic foot ulcers [39].

Among proteins, **collagen** and derived hydrolysates (i.e. **gelatines**) showed vast potential for efficient wound treatment as dressings and drug delivery systems. Collagen is a major constituent of connective tissue and a principal structural protein of many organs. In living beings collagen is produced by fibroblasts and stimulates the wound healing cellular and molecular cascade, development of new tissue and wound debridement. Materials made from collagen thus provide both structural and biological support for the various cells involved in dermal tissue regeneration, and as cell scaffolds are expected to replace native collagen-based ECM [40]. Collagen-based pharmaceutical formulations related to skin conditions include suspensions for dermal and wound topical injection, collagen suture and catguts, sponges for coating of affected joints in full-thickness ulcers, and wound dressing materials in various designs such as sponges, resorbable membranes, films, hydrogels, nano- and micro-fibre scaffolds for cell support [41]. Furthermore, both collagen and gelatine matrices can be medicated, thus serving as reservoirs for drug delivery. Their use for delivery of different antibiotics has been discussed extensively [42]. These biopolymers are also frequently conjugated with other biomaterials and even with animal skin substitutes. For example, Promogran®—a blend of collagen and regenerated cellulose, is the only clinically proved advanced dressing that promotes chronic wound healing. Promogran® inhibits MMPs by: (i) sequestering these cationic enzymes in the negatively charged regenerated cellulose dressing component, and (ii) deviating the enzymes from the ECM hydrolysis using the collagen component as a decoy MMP substrate [43, 44].

Other proteins are recently being evaluated for the treatment of many types of wounds. **Fibrin**, **keratin**, **silk fibroin** (SF), **bovine serum albumin** (BSA), and combinations thereof and with other biomaterials, interact with the wound environment to promote/accelerate healing rates. These biomaterials are processed in many ways to achieve natural-based wound dressings, templates for delivery of bioactive agents and scaffolds to support cellular growth. Fibrin-like haemostatic materials are useful for cleaning and treatment of full-thickness skin lesions [45], keratin-based matrices showed potential as chronic wound dressings because of their interaction with the proteolytic wound environment to facilitate the healing process [46], SF-containing films and sponges are being extensively investigated in animal models for both superficial and full-thickness skin defects healing [47–49], whereas electrospun nanofibres made entirely from a globular BSA are intended for suturing and acceleration of wound closure wound [50].

Although beneficiary for healing of many types of wounds, biopolymers are efficient in the tissue repair processes only to a certain extent, being limited in interaction at molecular level with wound pathogens. These natural macromolecules attracted much attention as dressing materials due to their biodegradability, where material degradation and the new tissue formation should be parallel processes, normally the case in the treatment of acute wounds. The situation with chronic wounds is more complicated due to very low stability of these materials in contact with the fluids containing elevated levels of hydrolytic enzymes: e.g. lysozyme cleaves chitosan-based materials [51], whereas collagen is a natural substrate of several MMPs. Moreover, the use of biopolymers in wound management has not yet been clearly translated into a platform for widespread clinical use, as the existing studies only offer evidences for beneficial properties of the biopolymers as dressing platforms and not as active agents.

Role of Polymers in Advanced Wound Treatment

Over recent years, many new polymeric dressings, but few new dressing types appeared on the market. The healing concept of most dressings relies on maintaining of a moisture environment, without any active agent involved. Regardless of the polymer component and the bandage design, a major focus of advanced

Scheme 14.1 The concept of advanced wound healing products

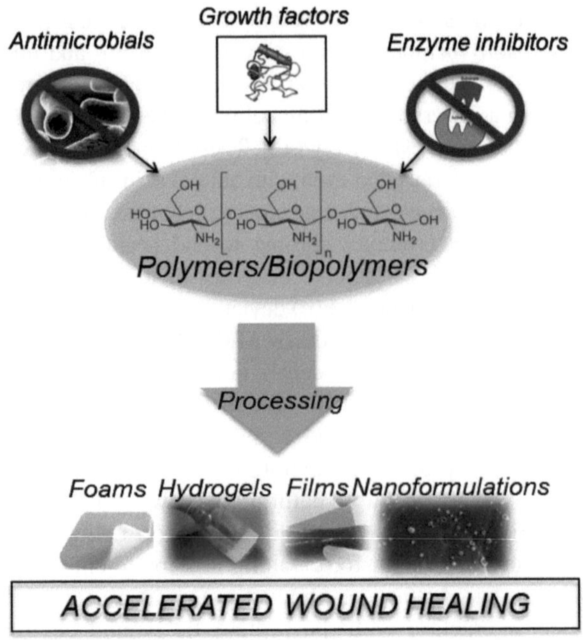

wound care in recent years has been the development of new dressings able to accelerate wound healing by erasing the chronicity factors, combining as many as possible functional properties in one [10]. Managing chronic or non-healing ulcers especially requires a systematic multi-professional approach and a willingness to consider also the patient's perspective to promote the most favourable conditions for healing. Despite all polymer-based materials promote wound repair to a certain extent, these materials exploit only the intrinsic properties of the matrix itself without any active agents to interact with the chronicity factors at the molecular level. The multifactorial nature of virtually all non-healing wounds requires biochemical stimuli to halter the events governing the ECM breakdown and impaired healing. Such effect can be expected only in case of controlled application of bioactive molecules, e.g. antimicrobials, enzyme inhibitors and growth factors.

From the point of view of a researcher, new bioactive wound dressings and formulations have been an area of tremendous growth following our understanding on the details of the wound repair. An orderly, predictable sequence of wound regeneration is driven by numerous cellular mediators, i.e. growth factors. The advanced wound products thus aim to accelerate repair by promoting/augmenting the activities of these mediators in non-healing conditions (Scheme 14.1). Although in many cases the role of polymers in such products is merely to provide a structural support, they are also crucial to maintain moisture environment, critical in the wound bed to promote growth factors, cytokines and migration of cells [52].

Accelerating Wound Healing with Active Agents—New Therapeutic Trends to be Combined with Polymers

Growth Factors and Cytokines

Growth factors are naturally occurring substances, secreted proteins and steroid hormones, capable of modulating cellular processes during tissue regeneration. They stimulate migration, infiltration, proliferation, and differentiation of mainly fibroblasts and keratinocytes by a complex signalling network. Accordingly, the capacity for wound repair can be augmented through the well-guided treatment involving these factors [53, 54]. The most promising growth factors that require clinical testing are vascular endothelial growth factor (VEGF) and basic fibroblast growth factor (bFGF). The most known platelet-derived growth factor BB (PDGF-BB) is the only one successfully completed randomized double-blind clinical trials in conjunction with standard wound care [55], which led to FDA approval for treatment of diabetic ulcers in a gel form under the trade name Regranex®. Nevertheless, new trends are moving towards mimicking the natural ways of healing in order to bring to the injury site a set of biological supplements to accelerate the functional recovery of the tissue, instead of relying on single-agent therapies. For example, activated autologous platelet rich plasma (PRP), known as plasma rich in growth factors (PRGF-Endoret®), an autologous blood platelet concentrate product recently classified as a medication in Spain, which, when activated, releases a set of growth factors that stimulate the regenerative phase of wound healing [56].

Cytokines are small proteins that modulate the immune response to stimulate tissue remodelling. Cell signaling culminates in an inflammatory phase of healing, which large part is regulated by both pro-inflammatory and anti-inflammatory cytokines. Interleukin-1, which in vitro stimulates most of the human cells, was tested in pressure ulcer patients with inconclusive results [57]. Similarly, granulocyte macrophage colony stimulating factor (GM-CSF) has been also showed promising for wound treatment in vitro, mainly due to the stimulation of VEGF production [58]. Other studies have given encouraging results in clinical trials on patients with venous stasis ulcers [59] and diabetic-foot ulcers [60]. However, cytokines should not be considered individually, because in vivo they function in complex networks and cascades, frequently exhibiting antagonism (the effects of one cytokine may be inhibited by another cytokine). The overall outcome of a biological response during inflammation thus reflects the balance between pro-inflammatory and anti-inflammatory cytokines [61]. This makes a combined cytokine therapy, with optimal stimulatory factors for wound repair, an attractive intervention for chronic diseases in general [62]. Nevertheless, both in vitro and in vivo studies on optimal synergistic combinations, duration and additional adjuvant therapies are required to precede clinical trials in order to assess the full potential of cytokines as biologic wound supplements.

Antimicrobials and Antiseptics

As infections still remain a feared complication in wounds, the purpose of applying antimicrobial agents is mainly to prevent or combat microbial colonisation. Sustained delivery of antimicrobials, e.g. antibiotics and silver, to wound sites from polymeric dressings is a preferred option than topical administration that often results in toxic reactions due to overdoses. Regardless of the administration approach, these antimicrobials effectively reduce microbial bioburden in infected wounds. However, silver toxicity to mammalian systems is still not fully investigated [63], whereas the excessive use of both antibiotics and silver led to the emergence of bacterial resistance [64, 65]. Further widespread use of antibiotics/silver is not desirable because it can only further contribute to the risk of developing microbial resistance, ultimately weakening our ability to counteract infections.

Current alternatives to antibiotics are antiseptics, with different mechanisms of inhibition of bacterial colonisation and growth. Although not as efficient as antibiotics, antiseptics are less toxic, active against broader spectrum of microorganisms, whereas resistance to antiseptics occurs less frequently [66]. For example, polyhexamethylene biguanide (PHMB) is an antiseptic with very low risk to induce bacterial resistance. An example of PHMB in conjunction with polymers is Suprasorb X + PHMB dressing of Lohmann&Rauscher, a calcium alginate with physically entrapped antiseptic, released into the wound upon application due to swelling.

Enzyme Inhibitory Agents

Abnormal redox state during the prolonged inflammation in non-healing ulcers calls for the use of redox drugs. MMPs are a group of metalloenzymes, where the catalytic Zn^{2+} in the active centre is coordinated by a redox-sensitive cysteine residue. Displacement, e.g. upon oxidation, of the cysteine ligand leads to the activation of the enzyme [67]—a mechanism termed "cysteine switch". The MMP activation/inhibition could be redox-regulated by e.g. thiol compounds affecting the sulfhydryl/disulphide state of the switch [68]. A non-specific regulation of MMPs activity could be achieved by zinc chelation. Since thiols combine metal chelating and redox functions [69], thiolated polymers are expected to control the activities of these enzymes via a combination of these two mechanisms. On the other hand, MPO is an oxidative enzyme able to produce HClO, overwhelming the natural shield of protease inhibitors, enabling their accumulation in the chronic wound site [70]. The prevention of MPO-derived HClO accumulation can be envisaged at two levels by: (i) using competitive amounts of substrates to avoid the enzyme chlorination activity and HClO production, and (ii) application of HClO scavengers. As thiols inhibit HClO production [71], the use of thiol-bearing compounds would be an integrated approach for attenuation of both oxidative and proteolytic enzyme activities.

Similar effects on both enzymes are expected using polyphenolic antioxidants. Plant polyphenolic extracts of varying structures from simple molecules to highly polymerised compounds are well-known for their antioxidant capacity and scavenging activity over free radical and non-radical reactive species [72], metal-chelating capability [73] and inhibitory activity over radical-generating enzymes [74]. Plant polyphenols also possess anti-inflammatory [75], antimicrobial [76] and wound healing promoting properties [77]. Some polyphenolic extracts are widely used in the therapy of skin conditions, skin damages such as burns, and as protective component in cosmetic formulations [78, 79]. Various polyphenolic extracts are reported as efficient inhibitors of both MPO [80] and MMPs [81].

Although majority of active agents are effective in preclinical models of dermal repair, most fail to demonstrate the healing improvements when applied topically or systemically in clinical settings. Their limited clinical success is attributed to short half-lives and lack of robust and approved delivery systems. Proper assembling of active agents with biocompatible delivery templates would ensure their stability during the application. For example, if the biopolymeric materials with intrinsic antimicrobial properties are upgraded with bioactive compounds to provide the biochemical stimuli in difficult to treat wounds, an integrated strategy for their efficient management could be achieved. Moreover, controllable enzymatic inhibition could be expected by tuning the degree of biopolymer functionalisation (e.g. biopolymer thiolation, dosed biopolymer impregnation with polyphenols). This would be a step forward towards the regulation of the optimal enzyme/inhibitors ratio necessary for healing. Additionally, if sustained delivery to targeted tissue compartments is achieved, prolonged effects may be expected with improved tissue repair outcomes. Currently, many novel systems based on synthetic and natural polymers are being developed and investigated as active agent delivery systems.

Next Generation Wound Dressings and Formulations Combining Polymers and Active Agents

Advances in biomaterials engineering and assembling/conjugation with biological agents allowed for application of novel wound healing therapies. Properly engineered hybrid biomaterials allow for accelerated recovery of damaged tissue by interfering with the wound healing process at the molecular level. Typically, two approaches for assembling active agents with biomaterials in wound repair are distinguished: (i) permanent immobilisation of the active agent onto polymeric matrix, and (ii) physical encapsulation of the active agent in the polymeric delivery system (matrix or template). The former approach involves chemical or enzymatic binding between the components where the active agent acts from the platform without being released to the wound. The advantage of this approach is the minimisation of the side effects due to the accumulation of immunoreactive compounds at the wound site, i.e. overdoses. The second approach is achieved by simple loading (impregnation) or encapsulation for programmed release of active agent [18]. If the delivery of an active in a consistent and sustained fashion over long periods of time is assured, the possibility of adverse effects and frequency of the dressing change also decrease.

Polymeric scaffolds that provide slow release of growth factors and cytokines have demonstrated the ability to attract cells through local signalling processes and stimulate the regenerative processes [82, 83]. Additionally, if these bioentities are integrated with biomaterials with beneficial for wound repair properties, enhanced wound healing properties to target more significant clinical utility are expected [84]. Among various biopolymers, gelatine, alginate, collagen and hyaluronic acid have been thus designed into gel matrices, porous sponges and microparticulate systems and used to deliver growth factors while maintaining their activity [85–89]. In one of the first studies of this type, a bilayer dressing comprising gelatine sponge and elastomeric synthetic polyurethane membrane used as the external layer was loaded with bFGF encapsulated in microparticles to achieve prolonged release [90]. The application of this hybrid wound dressing provided an optimum healing milieu for the proliferating cells and regenerating tissues in pig's skin defect models. Actually, most of the growth factors and cytokines are proteins that easily interact with other biopolymers, which makes the choice of an appropriate (bio)material critical to achieve enhanced and sustained release, and thus its action at the wound site. In one unicentre randomised control trial the autologous PRP was evaluated in the combination with a protease modulating Promogran®. The results in 51 patients with diabetic foot ulcers (17 of whom received the combined therapy) showed that this combination reduced the ulcer area more than that when compared with the dressing or PRP alone, suggesting a synergistic interaction between these components [91]. Nevertheless, prior to the widespread clinical use, the integrated growth factors/active dressing therapies need to be optimised and further validated for management of different types of difficult to treat wounds, by assessing their potential in larger, multicentre clinical trials.

Both synthetic and natural polymers have been also investigated and continue to be evaluated as platforms for immobilisation or delivery of active agents. There are numerous examples of polymers that have been mixed with antimicrobial/antiseptic substances to develop antimicrobial dressings and enhance healing of many wound types: fibrous hydrocolloids, poyurethane foam films and silicone gels were combined with silver [92, 93]; antibiotics were impregnated onto various polymer matrices for their delivery in wounds such as gentamycin from collagen sponges [94], ofloxacin from silicone gel sheets [95, 96], and minocycline from chitosan [97] and chitosan-polyurethane film dressings [98]; whereas PHMB-incorporated alginate antiseptic dressing is already marketed under the trade name of Suprasorb X + PHMB [99–101]. Another concept to manage difficult to treat wounds, e.g. chronic ulcers, is to control the activities of oxidative and proteolytic enzymes in wound bed by bringing down their elevated levels into the ranges found in acute wounds to allow healing to progress. However, this task must be taken with precaution, as the total inhibition of these enzymes is not desirable because of their role in the reconstruction of the ECM and wound progression towards closure. In one attempt, an active dressing specifically targeted towards reducing local levels of collagenases in non-healing wounds was developed using two biopolymers, bovine collagen and oxidised regenerated cellulose [44]. When placed in the wound bed, the collagen component acts as a decoy substrate for the proteases, whereas the oxidised cellulose dislodges metal ions from the active centre of these enzymes. Although this composite is still a state-of-the-art dressing on the market meant specifically for chronic wound treatment, it addresses only attenuation of the activities of some proteases at the wound site. The concept is currently being complemented by addressing other common factors influencing non-healing nature of chronic wounds of various aetiologies. For example, in our previous works, collagen, gelatine, chitosan, hyaluronic acid, chondroitin sulphate were used individually or as composite platforms, further upgraded with different plant polyphenols and thiol compounds targeting attenuation of both proteolytic collagenases and oxidative MPO, in addition to inhibiting bacterial growth. The produced biopolymeric platforms were either impregnated or permanently modified with active agents using chemical or enzymatic methods. For example, collagen was cross-linked with naturally occurring genipin to improve its biostability in physiological fluids prior to be impregnated with polyphenolic extracts from *Hamamelis virginiana* [102]. These extracts were previously found to be efficient scavengers of radical and non-radical reactive species, act as MPO substrates to prevent the accumulation of ROS and irreversibly inhibit collagenase [103]. The loading of plant polyphenols on sponge-like collagen dressings has been achieved on the bases of their ability to interact with proteins and polysaccharides [104, 105]. These interactions determine the release patterns from the biopolymer platforms and the activity of the advanced dressing [106]. Accordingly, in the case of polymer composites, capacity of the attenuation and especially duration of the inhibition effect are tuneable by the biopolymer composition and selection of the polyphenolic compound, being lower for polysaccharide than for protein platforms for which the effect is maintained up to 5 days [107]. In another study, a multifunctional bioactive chitosan/gelatine hydrogel additionally stabilised with plant polyphenols was achieved using laccase-assisted gelation [108]. Whereas gelatine facilitated coupling reactions and gelation, chitosan was used as an antimicrobial dressing platform. The phenolic compounds were covalently bonded on the hydrogels and exerted both: (i) structural function stabilising the dressing, and (ii) bio-activity inhibiting deleterious wound enzymes to stimulate the wound healing process. Permanent immobilisation of active agents reduces risk from overdoses and adverse immune effects at the wound site. The modification of polymeric surfaces in such way is a key aspect in biotechnology nowadays, including development of substrates for regenerative medicine. By alteration of the surface functionality controlled biochemical interactions with body fluids can be achieved. Thiolated chitosan, a biodegradable conjugate obtained by different chemical coupling approaches, combines a series of interesting functions such as mucoadhesive [109], permeation-enhancing [110], in situ gelling and enzyme inhibition properties [111, 112]. This conjugate was further processed into functional nanoscale films/coatings built using a layer-by-layer approach for alternate deposition of oppositely charged polyelectrolytes [113]. Glycosaminoglycans, namely HA with different Mw and chondroitin sulphate, were used as counterions to cationic thiolated conjugates. The biopolymer thiolation degree was identified as a key factor to achieve control of the thickness/size of the multilayered films. In addition, tuneable inhibition/adsorption of the deleterious enzymes coupled to fibroblast attachment/proliferation was observed by ruling the biopolymer modification degree.

Polymer-Based Healing Solutions in the Market

Nowadays, more than 3,000 types of dressings overwhelm the wound management market. The characteristics of the various types of dressings depend on the intrinsic properties of the polymers employed for their preparation. The resulting products may be used individually or in combination to absorb exudate, combat odour and infection, relieve pain, promote autolytic debridement (wound cleansing) and/or provide and maintain a moist environment at the wound surface. An ideal marketable wound dressing should: (i) allow debridement, (ii), provide and maintain a moist wound environment, (iii) allow absorption, removal of blood and excess of wound exudate, (iv) permit gaseous exchange (water vapour and air), (v) prevent infection, (vi) provide thermal insulation, (vii) possess low adherence to allow non-painful dressing change, (viii) protect the wound from trauma, (ix) be cost effective, and (x) be biocompatible.

Taking into consideration the above properties, wide range of polymer-based materials are available to match particular wound requirements. Unfortunately, no single dressing can accomplish all these goals. Thus, the election of the appropriate dressing to a specific wound type is a difficult task and depends on factors related to the product itself, patient's health status, wound type and location, and economic parameters, as summarised in Table 14.1.

Nowadays wound dressings frequently comprise the combination of polymeric layers with different functions that provide to the dressing particular characteristics. Table 14.2 presents an overview of various types of most frequent polymer-based wound dressings available in the market.

Table 14.1 Factors influencing the election of a wound dressing

Product-related	Patient-related	Wound-related		Economic-related	
Conformability	Wound aetiology	Wound type	Superficial	Cost	Unit cost
Fluid handling	State of continence		Full thickness		Treatment cost
Sensitisation potential	Fragile or easily damaged skin		Cavity		Cost of alternative materials
Odour elimination	Known sensitivity to medicated dressings	Wound description	Necrotic	Availability	On prescription
Non-toxicity			Sloughy		In stores or pharmacy departments
Antibacterial activity			Granulating		Inclusion in local formularies
Haemostatic properties			Epithelialising		
Permeability to tissue fluid and microorganisms			Full thickness		
Ease of use		Wound characteristics	Dry		
Pain related factors			Moist		
			Heavily exuding		
			Malodorous		
			Excessively painful		
			Infected		
			Location/size		

Table 14.2 Polymer-based wound dressings currently available in the market

	Properties	Commercial name	Manufacturer	Polymer
Films	Thin polyurethane semi-permeable transparent sheet bounded to acrylamide or with acrylic adhesive layer	Mepore	Mölnlycke	Viscose (cellu-lose) xanthate
	Elastic, conforms to wound shape	Skintact	Robinson	
	Pain relief			
	Prevents scab formation	Cutifilm	Smith and Nephew	Polyurethane
	Allows continuous inspection	EpiView	Convatec	
	Autolytic debridement			
	Minimal capacity to balance moisture and fluid accumulation	Mefilm	Mölnlycke	Polyurethane
		Opsite Flexigrid	Smith and Nephew	Polyurethane
	Indicted for partial thickness wounds	Allevyn	Smith and Nephew	Polyurethane
		Flexipore	Activheal	Polyurethane
		Bioclusive	Systagenix	Polyurethane
		Release	Johnson & Johnson	Ethylene-methyl acrylate
		Cutinova Hydro	Smith & Nephew	Polyurethane
		Primapore	Smith and Nephew	
		Melolin	Smith and Nephew	
		OpSite Plus	Smith and Nephew	Polyurethane
		OpSite flexiflixs	Smith and Nephew	Polyurethane
		C-View	Aspen Medical	Polyurethane
		Blisterfilm	Coviden	
		Polyskin II	Coviden	
		Tegaderm	3 M	Polyurethane

(continued)

Table 14.2 (continued)

	Properties	Commercial name	Manufacturer	Polymer
Hydrogels	Cross-linked hydrophilic polymers with 90–95% water content. Hydrogel wound dressing sheets are three-dimensional networks of cross-linked hydrophilic polymers that are insoluble in water and interact with aqueous solutions by swelling	Carrasyn Hydrogel	Carrington	Acemannan
		Tagaderm Hydrogel	3 M	Guar gum
	Highly conformable and permeable Absorb large amounts of drainage	GranuGel	Convatec	
	Non-adhesive against the wound for easy removal	Intrsite Gel	Smith & Nephew	Carboxymethyl cellulose
	Indicated for partial- and full-thickness wounds, wounds with necrosis, minor burns and radiation tissue damage	Flexigel	Smith & Nephew	
		Curasol	Health Point	
		Aquaflo	Kendall	Polyoxyethylene glycol
		AquaForm	Robert Bailey	Propylene glycol
		Plurilon Gel	Coloplast	Carboxymethyl cellulose
		Sterigel	Seton	Hemicellulose
		Regranex Gel	Healthpoint Biotherapeutics	Carboxymethyl cellulose
		Bionect	Dara BioScience	Hyaluronic acid

(continued)

Table 14.2 (continued)

	Properties	Commercial name	Manufacturer	Polymer
Hydrocolloids	Hydrocolloid wound dressings are wafers, powders or pastes composed of gelatine, pectin or carboxymethyl cellulose. Absorption capability depends on thickness and composition. Wafers are self-adhering and available with or without an adhesive border and in a wide variety of shapes and sizes	Tegaderm Hydrocolloid	3 M HealthCare	Polyurethane
		Comfeel Plus contiur Dressing	Coloplast	Carboxymethyl cellulose and calcium alginate
	Useful on areas that require contouring, such as heels and sacral ulcers Powders and pastes require a secondary dressing	Comfeel Plus Ulcer Dressing	Coloplast	Carboxymethyl cellulose, hydroxyethyl cellulose and calcium alginate
	Indicated for partial- and full-thickness wounds with or without necrotic tissue	Comfeel	Coloplast	Carboxymethyl cellulose and calcium alginate
		Replicare	Smith & Nephew	
		Nu Derm	Syntagenix	
		Hydrocoll Basic	Hartmann	
		Aquacel	ConvaTec	Carboxymethyl cellulose
		DuoDerm Extra Thin	ConvaTec	Polyuretane
		Granuflex R.	ConvaTec	Polyuretane
		Combiderm	ConvaTec	

(continued)

Table 14.2 (continued)

	Properties	Commercial name	Manufacturer	Polymer
Alginate dressings	Alginate wound dressings are non-woven, non-adhesive pads and ribbons composed of natural polysaccharide fibres or xerogel derived from seaweed. On contact with exudate these dressings form a moist gel through a process of ion exchange	Ultec Pro	Kendall	Alginic acid
		Tegagel	Systagenix	Alginic acid
		Algisite M	Smith & Nephew	Alginic acid
		Algosteril	Beirsdorf	Alginic acid
	Soft and conformable, easy to pack, tuck or apply over irregular-shaped wounds	Comfeel SeaSorb	Coloplast	Alginic acid
		Nu-Gel	Johnson & Johnson	Alginic acid
		Comfeel Plus	Coloplast	Alginic acid
	Generally require a secondary dressing	Kaltostat	ConvaTec	Alginic acid
	Indicated for wounds with moderate to heavy exudate, such as pressure ulcers, infected wounds, diabetic ulcers and venous stasis ulcers	Sorbsan	Maersk	Alginic acid
		Tegagel	3 M Health Care	Alginic acid
		Melgisorb	Mölnlycke	Alginic acid
		Carraginate	Carrington	Alginic acid
		Curasorb	Kendall	Alginic acid
		Sorbalgon	Hartman USA, Inc.	Alginic acid
Foams	Foam dressings are sheets and other shapes of foamed polymer solutions (most commonly polyurethane) with small, open cells capable of holding fluids. They may be impregnated or layered in combination with other materials	Avance Foam Dressing Kits	Medela	Polyurethane
		ComfortFoam	DermaRite Industries	Silicone and polyurethane
	Absorption capability depends on thickness and composition	Flexan	Mylan Bertek Pharmaceuticals	Polyurethane
	The area in contact with the wound surface is non-adhesive for easy removal. Available with an adhesive border and/or a transparent film coating that acts as a bacterial barrier	Lyofoam	Mölnlycke	Polyurethane
		ComfortFoam	DermaRite Industries	Silicone and polyurethane
	Indicated for partial- and full-thickness wounds	Optifoam	Medline Industries	Polyurethane

(continued)

Table 14.2 (continued)

	Properties	Commercial name	Manufacturer	Polymer
Collagen	Collagen wound dressings are available in the form of gels, pads, particles, pastes, powders, sheets or solutions derived from bovine, porcine or avian sources	BIOPAD	Angelini Pharma, Inc	Type I Collagen
		Stimulen Collagen Powder	Southwest Technologies	Modified collagen
	Some interact with wound exudate to form a gel	BGC Matrix	Mölnlycke	Collagen and β-glucan
	Usually require a secondary dressing	BIOSTEP* Collagen Matrix	Smith & Nephew	Collagen
	Indicated for partial- and full-thickness pressure ulcers, venous ulcers, donor sites, surgical wounds, vascular ulcers, diabetic ulcers, second-degree burns, abrasions and traumatic wounds	CellerateRX® Gel	Wound Care Innovations	65 % type I collagen
		CellerateRX® Powder	Wound Care Innovations	95 % type I collagen
		Endoform Dermal Template	Hollister Wound Care	90 % collagen and 10 % ECM
Silicone	Silicone Sheet or gels, some bound to polyamide net or designed as a wound contact layer with secondary dressings	CICA-CARE	Smith & Nephew	Silicone
		Mepiform	Mölnlycke	Silicone
	Reduce scar tissue	NovaGel	Mölnlycke	Silicone
	Atraumatic removal from the wound and surrounding skin	Mepitel	Mölnlycke	Silicone
		Metipac	Mölnlycke	Silicone
	Fluid impermeable	Metiplex	Mölnlycke	
	Prevent maceration			
	Long wearing times			
	Transparent			
	Indicated for second degree burns; chronic leg ulcers and paediatric patients			

Conclusions

Polymers in the form of dressings and pharmaceutical formulations are already an integral part of modern wound care. Synthetic polymers have good mechanical properties, near-limitless supply, and are easy to process into suitable designs for wound repair, including appropriate pore size and scaffold geometry. However, these advantages are countered by their minimal intrinsic bioactive properties. Biopolymer dressings, on the other hand, interact with dermal tissue and cells to accelerate the acute healing process, but they have little effects on healing of complex wounds. In line with this, advanced wound repair is currently directed towards stimulation of physiological repair at molecular level. Combining synthetic and/or biopolymer dressing with the therapeutic potential of bioactive molecules has emerged as an exciting field of research for enhanced wound repair. The rationale for the development of these next generation composites lies in their superior efficacy in preclinical models relative to the application of their components alone. Many approaches for assembling polymers with therapeutically relevant compounds are established technologies with few of these already commercialised based on the available clinical evidences. Nevertheless, the large amount of research being conducted is likely to result in additional approvals, and more advanced polymer-based dressings will certainly attain market in the next few years, considering their current preclinical/clinical evaluation.

Future Perspectives

Polymer dressings are an important segment of the medical and pharmaceutical wound management market worldwide. Both low- and high-tech products ranging from traditional inert synthetic bandages to bioactive solutions for which preparation emergent technologies are employed find the place on this dynamic market. Despite the wide variety of products available, complex non-healing wounds are still a challenge to manage and accordingly attract a great deal of attention among the research community. Their treatment represents a huge health burden and drain on healthcare resources due to the intensive medical intervention required. Furthermore, as elderly individuals become the fastest-growing segment of the population, the complex wounds occurrence will have an even more pronounced economic impact in the future. Therefore, new solutions such as advanced dressings to facilitate chronic wound healing are needed.

The advanced wound care market is constantly growing and includes an array of competing technologies and solutions that can be classified according to the materials from which they are produced. Polymer-based hydrocolloids, hydrogels, thin films and foam sheets are its largest sector. They also include few bioactive dressings and skin substitutes on the market that combine polymers with various therapeutics, antimicrobials, enzyme inhibitors and/or biological supplements acting on specific molecular targets in wound environment. In near future it is expected that polymers will be exploited more efficiently since they can be easily modified via chemical or biochemical techniques. Permanent functionalisation of polymer matrices with bioactive agents will allow their acting from the polymer matrix, without being release to the wound and thus avoiding risk of overdoses and associated adverse effects.

One of the main reasons of the high cost of managing complex wounds, besides the cost of the materials, is the time of hospitalisation. The decision-making in their treatment is therefore crucial and is required to be at the same time fast and accurate. Currently, the clinicians often visually inspect the wound to evaluate the infection status or rely on time-consuming and costly biopsy analyses requiring special equipment. Among the most recent advances in this area are remote monitoring devices evaluating wound-related parameters such as margin, volume, depth and area or off-site diagnostic kits relying on different detection markers, but often requiring painful wound fluid collection [114]. In order to increase the patient's comfort and at the same time provide reliable diagnosis, the wound care market should soon move from intuitive choices to proactive strategies for simultaneous healing and monitoring of the wound status. New point-of-care devices will be developed under the EU project InFact - Functional materials for fast diagnosis of wound infection (grant agreement n° FP7-609198), in order to implement a solution for fast infection diagnosis into an active wound dressing and thus complement the healing of wounds colonised with microorganisms. Such simple tool integrated into a next generation wound dressings will enable clinicians to assess the wound status rapidly avoiding painful wound fluid collection. The role of polymers in such devices will be equally important as in the nowadays modern dressings. Besides providing the structural support, various polymers will be employed to assemble the test components of a novel diagnostic tool, e.g. sample path (cellulose), conjugate pad (usually a polyester), assay matrix (nitro-cellulose membrane), absorbent pad (cellulose fibre sheets) and adhesive backing (polystyrene, vinyl or polyester) are employed in lateral flow devices.

References

1. Lazarus, G.S., et al.: Definitions and guidelines for assessment of wounds and evaluation of healing. Wound Repair Regener. **2**(3), 165–170 (1994)
2. Stadelmann, W.K., Digenis, A.G., Tobin, G.R.: Physiology and healing dynamics of chronic cutaneous wounds. Am. J. Surg. **176**(2, Supplement 1): 26S–38S (1998)
3. Weiss, S.J.: Tissue destruction by neutrophils. N. Engl. J. Med. **320**(6), 365–376 (1989)
4. Martin, P., Leibovich, S.J.: Inflammatory cells during wound repair: the good, the bad and the ugly. Trends Cell Biol. **15**(11), 599–607 (2005)
5. Diegelmann, R.F.: Excessive neutrophils characterize chronic pressure ulcers. Wound Repair Regener. **11**(6), 490–495 (2003)
6. Trengove, N.J., et al.: Analysis of the acute and chronic wound environments: the role of proteases and their inhibitors. Wound Repair Regener. **7**(6), 442–452 (1999)
7. Wang, Y., et al.: Myeloperoxidase inactivates timp-1 by oxidizing its n-terminal cysteine residue. J. Biol. Chem. **282**(44), 31826–31834 (2007)

8. Saarialho-Kere, U.K.: Patterns of matrix metalloproteinase and TIMP expression in chronic ulcers. Arch. Dermatol. Res. **290**(1), S47–S54 (1998)
9. Falabella, A.F.: Debridement and wound bed preparation. Dermatol. Ther. **19**(6), 317–325 (2006)
10. Boateng, J.S., et al.: Wound healing dressings and drug delivery systems: a review. J. Pharm. Sci. **97**(8), 2892–2923 (2008)
11. Atiyeh, B.S., et al.: Effect of silver on burn wound infection control and healing: review of the literature. Burns **33**(2), 139–148 (2007)
12. Gupta, S., et al.: Guidelines for managing pressure ulcers with negative pressure wound therapy. Adv. Skin Wound Care **17**, 1–16 (2004)
13. Xie, X., McGregor, M., Dendukuri, N.: The clinical effectiveness of negative pressure wound therapy: a systematic review. J. wound care **19**(11), 490–495 (2010)
14. Noble-Bell, G., Forbes, A.: A systematic review of the effectiveness of negative pressure wound therapy in the management of diabetes foot ulcers. Int. Wound J. **5**(2), 233–242 (2008)
15. Ubbink Dirk, T., et al.: Topical negative pressure for treating chronic wounds. Cochrane Database Syst. Rev. **16** (2008). doi: CD001898
16. Suslick, K.S., Grinstaff, M.W.: Protein microencapsulation of nonaqueous liquids. J. Am. Chem. Soc. **112**(21), 7807–7809 (1990)
17. Ennis, W.J., et al.: Evaluation of clinical effectiveness of mist ultrasound therapy for the healing of chronic wounds. Adv. Skin Wound Care: J. Prev. Healing **19**(8), 437–446 (2006)
18. Francesko, A., Tzanov, T.: Chitin, chitosan and derivatives for wound healing and tissue engineering. In: Nyanhongo, G.S., Steiner, W., Gübitz, G. (eds.) Biofunctionalization of Polymers and their Applications, pp. 1–27. Springer, Berlin (2011)
19. Queen, D., et al.: A dressing history. Int. Wound J. **1**(1), 59–77 (2004)
20. Mogoşanu, G.D., Grumezescu, A.M.: Natural and synthetic polymers for wounds and burns dressing. Int. J. Pharm. **463**(2), 127–136 (2014)
21. Wright, K.A., et al.: Alternative delivery of keratinocytes using a polyurethane membrane and the implications for its use in the treatment of full-thickness burn injury. Burns **24**(1), 7–17 (1998)
22. Jansson, E., Tengvall, P.: In vitro preparation and ellipsometric characterization of thin blood plasma clot films on silicon. Biomaterials **22**(13), 1803–1808 (2001)
23. Losi, P., et al.: Luminal surface microgeometry affects platelet adhesion in small-diameter synthetic grafts. Biomaterials **25**(18), 4447–4455 (2004)
24. Whelan, J.: Smart bandages diagnose wound infection. Drug Discov. Today **7**(1), 9–10 (2002)
25. Van den Kerckhove, E., et al.: Silicones in the rehabilitation of burns: a review and overview. Burns **27**(3), 205–214 (2001)
26. Raphael, K.G., et al.: Self-reported systemic, immune-mediated disorders in patients with and without proplast-teflon implants of the temporomandibular joint. J. Oral Maxillofac. Surg. **57**(4), 364–370 (1999)
27. Kim, I.-Y., et al.: Chitosan and its derivatives for tissue engineering applications. Biotechnol. Adv. **26**(1), 1–21 (2008)
28. Ueno, H., et al.: Accelerating effects of chitosan for healing at early phase of experimental open wound in dogs. Biomaterials **20**(15), 1407–1414 (1999)
29. Wedmore, I., et al.: A special report on the chitosan-based hemostatic dressing: experience in current combat operations. J. Trauma Acute Care Surg. **60**(3), 655–658 (2006)
30. Pietramaggiori, G., et al.: Effects of poly-N-acetyl glucosamine (pGlcNAc) patch on wound healing in db/db mouse. J. Trauma Acute Care Surg. **64**(3), 803–808 (2008)
31. Dhanasingh, A., et al.: Tailored hyaluronic acid hydrogels through hydrophilic prepolymer cross-linkers. Soft Matter **6**(3), 618–629 (2010)
32. Gilbert, M.E., et al.: Chondroitin sulfate hydrogel and wound healing in rabbit maxillary sinus mucosa. Laryngoscope **114**(8), 1406–1409 (2004)
33. West, D., et al.: Angiogenesis induced by degradation products of hyaluronic acid. Science **228**(4705), 1324–1326 (1985)
34. Perng, C.-K., et al.: In vivo angiogenesis effect of porous collagen scaffold with hyaluronic acid oligosaccharides. J. Surg. Res. **168**(1), 9–15 (2011)

35. Park, S.-N., et al.: Biological characterization of EDC-crosslinked collagen–hyaluronic acid matrix in dermal tissue restoration. Biomaterials **24**(9), 1631–1641 (2003)
36. Luo, Y., Kirker, K.R., Prestwich, G.D.: Cross-linked hyaluronic acid hydrogel films: new biomaterials for drug delivery. J. Controlled Release **69**(1), 169–184 (2000)
37. Lin, Y.-C., et al.: Synthesis and characterization of collagen/hyaluronan/chitosan composite sponges for potential biomedical applications. Acta Biomater. **5**(7), 2591–2600 (2009)
38. Chang, C.-H., et al.: Gelatin–chondroitin–hyaluronan tri-copolymer scaffold for cartilage tissue engineering. Biomaterials **24**(26), 4853–4858 (2003)
39. Dumville, J., et al., *Alginate dressings for healing diabetic foot ulcers.* Cochrane Database Syst. Rev. **15**(2) (2012)
40. Cen, L., et al.: Collagen tissue engineering: development of novel biomaterials and applications. Pediatr. Res. **63**(5), 492–496 (2008)
41. Parenteau-Bareil, R., Gauvin, R., Berthod, F.: Collagen-based biomaterials for tissue engineering applications. Materials **3**(3), 1863–1887 (2010)
42. Ruszczak, Z., Friess, W.: Collagen as a carrier for on-site delivery of antibacterial drugs. Adv. Drug Deliv. Rev. **55**(12), 1679–1698 (2003)
43. Cullen, B., et al.: Mechanism of action of PROMOGRAN, a protease modulating matrix, for the treatment of diabetic foot ulcers. Wound Repair Regener. **10**(1), 16–25 (2002)
44. Cullen, B., et al.: The role of oxidised regenerated cellulose/collagen in chronic wound repair and its potential mechanism of action. Int. J. Biochem. Cell Biol. **34**(12), 1544–1556 (2002)
45. Rothwell, S., et al.: Wound healing and the immune response in swine treated with a hemostatic bandage composed of salmon thrombin and fibrinogen. J. Mater. Sci. Mater. Med. **20**(10), 2155–2166 (2009)
46. Vasconcelos, A., Cavaco-Paulo, A.: Wound dressings for a proteolytic-rich environment. Appl. Microbiol. Biotechnol. **90**(2), 445–460 (2011)
47. de Moraes, M.A., Beppu, M.M.: Biocomposite membranes of sodium alginate and silk fibroin fibers for biomedical applications. J. Appl. Polym. Sci. **130**(5), 3451–3457 (2013)
48. Liu, T.-L., et al.: Cytocompatibility of regenerated silk fibroin film: a medical biomaterial applicable to wound healing. J. Zhejiang Univ. Sci. B **11**(1), 10–16 (2010)
49. Zhu, X., et al.: Activation of T lymphocytes on local trauma after implantation of regenerated porous silk fibroin film. J. Clim. Rehabil. Tissue Eng. Res. **15**, 7061–7065 (2011)
50. Dror, Y., et al.: Nanofibers made of globular proteins. Biomacromolecules **9**(10), 2749–2754 (2008)
51. Jin, R., et al.: Injectable chitosan-based hydrogels for cartilage tissue engineering. Biomaterials **30**(13), 2544–2551 (2009)
52. Sibbald, R.G., Woo, K.Y., Queen, D.: Wound bed preparation and oxygen balance—a new component? Int. Wound J. **4**, 9–17 (2007)
53. Werner, S., Grose, R.: Regulation of wound healing by growth factors and cytokines. Physiol. Rev. **83**(3), 835–870 (2003)
54. Barrientos, S., et al.: Perspective article: growth factors and cytokines in wound healing. Wound Repair Regener. **16**(5), 585–601 (2008)
55. Steed, D.L., Study Group, t.D.U.*: Clinical evaluation of recombinant human platelet—derived growth factor for the treatment of lower extremity diabetic ulcers. J. Vasc. Surg. **21**(1), 71–81 (1995)
56. Anitua, E., et al.: Platelet-rich plasma: preparation and formulation. Operative Tech. Orthop. **22**(1), 25–32 (2012)
57. Vande Berg, J., Robson, M., Mikhail, R.: Extension of the life span of pressure ulcer fibroblasts with recombinant human interleukin-1 beta. Am. J. Pathol. **146**(5), 1273–1282 (1995)
58. Cianfarani, F., et al.: Granulocyte/macrophage colony-stimulating factor treatment of human chronic ulcers promotes angiogenesis associated with de novo vascular endothelial growth factor transcription in the ulcer bed. Br. J. Dermatol. **154**(1), 34–41 (2006)
59. Da Costa, R.M., et al.: Randomized, double-blind, placebo-controlled, dose- ranging study of granulocyte-macrophage colony stimulating factor in patients with chronic venous leg ulcers. Wound Repair Regener. **7**(1), 17–25 (1999)

60. Cruciani, M., et al.: Are granulocyte colony-stimulating factors beneficial in treating diabetic foot infections?: a meta-analysis. Diabetes Care **28**(2), 454–460 (2005)
61. Kavanaugh, A.: Combination cytokine therapy: the next generation of rheumatoid arthritis therapy? Arthritis Care Res. **47**(1), 87–92 (2002)
62. Pellegrini, M., Mak, T., Ohashi, P.: Fighting cancers from within: augmenting tumor immunity with cytokine therapy. Trends Pharmacol. Sci. **31**(8), 356–363 (2010)
63. Lansdown, A.B.G.: Silver 2: toxicity in mammals and how its products aid wound repair. J. Wound Care **11**(5), 173–177 (2002)
64. Howell-Jones, R.S., et al.: A review of the microbiology, antibiotic usage and resistance in chronic skin wounds. J. Antimicrob. Chemother. **55**(2), 143–149 (2005)
65. Landsdown, A., Williams, A.: Bacterial resistance to silver in wound care and medical devices. J Wound Care **16**(1), 15–19 (2007)
66. Gilbert, P.: Avoiding the resistance pitfall in infection control. Does the use of antiseptic products contribute to the spread of antibiotic resistance? Ostomy Wound Manage **52**(10 A Suppl): 1S–3S (2006)
67. Giles, N.M., et al.: Metal and redox modulation of cysteine protein function. Chem. Biol. **10**(8), 677–693 (2003)
68. Gu, Z., et al.: S-nitrosylation of matrix metalloproteinases: signaling pathway to neuronal cell death. Science **297**(5584), 1186–1190 (2002)
69. Andreassen, O.A., et al.: N-acetyl-L-cysteine improves survival and preserves motor performance in an animal model of familial amyotrophic lateral sclerosis. NeuroReport **11**(11), 2491–2493 (2000)
70. Fu, X., et al.: Hypochlorous acid oxygenates the cysteine switch domain of pro-matrilysin (MMP-7). J. Biol. Chem. **276**(44), 41279–41287 (2001)
71. Van Antwerpen, P., et al.: Thiol-containing molecules interact with the myeloperoxidase/H2O2/chloride system to inhibit LDL oxidation. Biochem. Biophys. Res. Commun. **337**(1), 82–88 (2005)
72. Rice-Evans, C.A., Miller, N.J., Paganga, G.: Structure-antioxidant activity relationships of flavonoids and phenolic acids. Free Radic. Biol. Med. **20**(7), 933–956 (1996)
73. Mira, L., et al.: Interactions of flavonoids with iron and copper ions: a mechanism for their antioxidant activity. Free Radic. Res. **36**(11), 1199–1208 (2002)
74. Pauff, J.M., Hille, R.: Inhibition studies of bovine xanthine oxidase by luteolin, silibinin, quercetin, and curcumin. J. Nat. Prod. **72**(4), 725–731 (2009)
75. Ding, Z., et al.: Anti-inflammatory effects of scopoletin and underlying mechanisms. Pharm. Biol. **46**(12), 854–860 (2008)
76. Geyid, A., et al.: Screening of some medicinal plants of Ethiopia for their anti-microbial properties and chemical profiles. J. Ethnopharmacol. **97**(3), 421–427 (2005)
77. Kim, H., et al.: Enhanced wound healing by an epigallocatechin gallate-incorporated collagen sponge in diabetic mice. Wound Repair Regener. **16**(5), 714–720 (2008)
78. Masaki, H., Atsumi, T., Sakurai, H.: Protective activity of hamamelitannin on cell damage of murine skin fibroblasts induced by UVB irradiation. J. Dermatol. Sci. **10**(1), 25–34 (1995)
79. Deters, A., et al.: High molecular compounds (polysaccharides and proanthocyanidins) from Hamamelis virginiana bark: influence on human skin keratinocyte proliferation and differentiation and influence on irritated skin. Phytochemistry **58**(6), 949–958 (2001)
80. Kato, Y., et al.: Inhibition of myeloperoxidase-catalyzed tyrosylation by phenolic antioxidants in vitro. Biosci. Biotechnol. Biochem. **67**(5), 1136–1139 (2003)
81. Madhan, B., et al.: Role of green tea polyphenols in the inhibition of collagenolytic activity by collagenase. Int. J. Biol. Macromol. **41**(1), 16–22 (2007)
82. Chen, R., Mooney, D.: Polymeric growth factor delivery strategies for tissue engineering. Pharm. Res. **20**(8), 1103–1112 (2003)
83. Lee, K., Silva, E.A., Mooney, D.J.: Growth factor delivery-based tissue engineering: general approaches and a review of recent developments. J. R. Soc. Interface **8**(55), 153–170 (2011)
84. Koria, P.: Delivery of growth factors for tissue regeneration and wound healing. BioDrugs **26**(3), 163–175 (2012)

85. Ulubayram, K., et al.: EGF containing gelatin-based wound dressings. Biomaterials **22**(11), 1345–1356 (2001)
86. Kolambkar, Y.M., et al.: An alginate-based hybrid system for growth factor delivery in the functional repair of large bone defects. Biomaterials **32**(1), 65–74 (2011)
87. Değim, Z.: Use of microparticulate systems to accelerate skin wound healing. J. Drug Target. **16**(6), 437–448 (2008)
88. Takemoto, S., et al.: Preparation of collagen/gelatin sponge scaffold for sustained release of bFGF. Tissue Eng. Part A **14**(10), 1629–1638 (2008)
89. Matsumoto, Y., Kuroyanagi, Y.: Development of a wound dressing composed of hyaluronic acid sponge containing arginine and epidermal growth factor. J. Biomater. Sci. Polym. Ed. **21**(6), 126–715 (2010)
90. Huang, S., et al.: Wound dressings containing bFGF-impregnated microspheres. J. Microencapsul. **23**(3), 277–290 (2006)
91. Kakagia, D.D., et al.: Synergistic action of protease-modulating matrix and autologous growth factors in healing of diabetic foot ulcers. A prospective randomized trial. J. Diabetes Complications **21**(6), 387–391 (2007)
92. Leaper, D.J.: Silver dressings: their role in wound management. Int. Wound J. **3**(4), 282–294 (2006)
93. Leaper, D.: Silver dressings: their role in wound management. Int Wound J. **3**(4), 282–294 (2006)
94. Fong, J., Wood, F.: Nanocrystalline silver dressings in wound management: a review. Int. J. Nanomed. **1**(4), 441–449 (2006)
95. Rutten, H., Nijhuis, P.: Prevention of wound infection in elective colorectal surgery by local application of a gentamicin-containing collagen sponge. Eur. J. Surg. Suppl. **578**, 31–35 (1997)
96. Sawada, Y., et al.: Treatment of dermal depth burn wounds with an antimicrobial agent-releasing silicone gel sheet. Burns **16**(5), 347–352 (1990)
97. Sawada, Y., et al.: An evaluation of a new lactic acid polymer drug delivery system: a preliminary report. Br. J. Plast. Surg. **47**(3), 158–161 (1994)
98. Galandiuk, S., et al.: Absorbable, delayed-release antibiotic beads reduce surgical wound infection. Am. Surg. **63**(9), 831–835 (1997)
99. Aoyagi, S., Onishi, H., Machida, Y.: Novel chitosan wound dressing loaded with minocycline for the treatment of severe burn wounds. Int. J. Pharm. **330**(1–2), 138–145 (2007)
100. Kingsley, A., et al.: Suprasorb X + PHMB: antimicrobial and HydroBalance action in a new wound dressing. Wounds UK **5**(1), 72–77 (2009)
101. Glover, D., Wicks, G.: Suprasorb X + PHMB: the clinical evidence. J. wound care. ACTIVA healthcare Supplement, 15–21 (2009)
102. Elzinga, G., et al.: Clinical evaluation of a PHMB-impregnated biocellulose dressing on paediatric lacerations. J Wound Care **20**(6), 280–284 (2011)
103. Antonio, F., et al.: Cross-linked collagen sponges loaded with plant polyphenols with inhibitory activity towards chronic wound enzymes. Biotechnol. J. **6**(10), 1208–1218 (2011)
104. Díaz-GonzáLez, M., et al.: Inhibition of deleterious chronic wound enzymes with plant polyphenols. Biocatal. Biotransform. **30**(1), 102–110 (2012)
105. Haslam, E.: natural polyphenols (vegetable tannins) as drugs: possible modes of action. J. Nat. Prod. **59**(2), 205–215 (1996)
106. Madhan, B., et al.: Stabilization of collagen using plant polyphenol: role of catechin. Int. J. Biol. Macromol. **37**(1–2), 47–53 (2005)
107. Tang, H.R., Covington, A.D., Hancock, R.A.: Structure–activity relationships in the hydrophobic interactions of polyphenols with cellulose and collagen. Biopolymers **70**(3), 403–413 (2003)
108. Francesko, A., et al.: Functional biopolymer-based matrices for modulation of chronic wound enzyme activities. Acta Biomater. **9**(2), 5216–5225 (2013)
109. Rocasalbas, G., et al.: Laccase-assisted formation of bioactive chitosan/gelatin hydrogel stabilized with plant polyphenols. Carbohydr. Polym. **92**(2), 989–996 (2013)

110. Roldo, M., et al.: Mucoadhesive thiolated chitosans as platforms for oral controlled drug delivery: synthesis and in vitro evaluation. Eur. J. Pharm. Biopharm. **57**(1), 115–121 (2004)
111. Föger, F., Schmitz, T., Bernkop-Schnürch, A.: In vivo evaluation of an oral delivery system for P-gp substrates based on thiolated chitosan. Biomaterials **27**(23), 4250–4255 (2006)
112. Kast, C.E., et al.: Chitosan-thioglycolic acid conjugate: a new scaffold material for tissue engineering? Int. J. Pharm. **256**(1–2), 183–189 (2003)
113. Kast, C.E., Bernkop-Schnürch, A.: Thiolated polymers—thiomers: development and in vitro evaluation of chitosan–thioglycolic acid conjugates. Biomaterials **22**(17), 2345–2352 (2001)
114. Francesko, A., et al.: GAGs-thiolated chitosan assemblies for chronic wounds treatment: control of enzyme activity and cell attachment. J. Mater. Chem. **22**(37), 19438–19446 (2012)

Chapter 15
Polymers in Cardiology

Katrin Sternberg, Raila Busch and Svea Petersen

Abstract Polymers have found widespread applications in cardiology, in particular in coronary vascular intervention as stent platforms, coating matrices for drug-eluting stents (DES) and drug-coated balloons (DCB) and for transcatheter valve therapy. Besides permanent polymers, biodegradable polymers came in focus of current research and development for medical applications, as they degrade once their function is fulfilled, which might efficiently reduce observed hypersensitivity reactions. After reviewing polymers used for cardiovascular applications, the book chapter deals with possible surface modification reactions of the polymers including the provision with a local drug delivery function and/or biofunctionalization in order to selectively control cell-implant interactions. These functionalizations can be furthermore designed to enhance bio- and hemo-compatibility, which is of special interest for cardiovascular implants and devices. A general discussion of bio- and hemo-compatibility of polymers for cardiovascular applications and corresponding evaluation methods is additionally given. With our own published data, we finally highlight exemplary polymer applications in cardiology as polymer-based biodegradable stent platforms, biodegradable polymeric coatings for DES and hydrogel-based coatings for DCB. Moreover, developed biofunctionalization strategies of polymers are discussed with regard to their application in cardiology.

K. Sternberg (✉)
Aesculap AG, Research and Development, Am Aesculap-Platz, 78532 Tuttlingen, Germany
e-mail: katrin.sternberg@aesculap.de

R. Busch
Ernst-Moritz-Arndt University of Greifswald, Clinic for Internal Medicine B,
Ferdinand-Sauerbruch-Straße, 17475 Greifswald, Germany

S. Petersen
University of Rostock, Institute for Biomedical Engineering,
Friedrich-Barnewitz-Street 4, 18119 Rostock, Germany

F. Puoci (ed.), *Advanced Polymers in Medicine*, DOI 10.1007/978-3-319-12478-0_15

Keywords Polymers · Cardiology · Implant · Drug-eluting stent · Drug-coated balloon · Transcatheteraortic valve therapy · Local drug delivery · Biofunctionalization · Biocompatibility · Hemocompatibility

Abbreviations

AFM	Atomic force microscopy
ASTM	American Society for Testing and Materials
BMS	Bare metal stent
BTHC	n-butyryl tri-n-hexyl citrate
BVS	Bioresorbable vascular scaffold
DCB	Drug-coated balloon
DDES	Dual drug-eluting stent
DES	Drug-eluting stent
EC	Endothelial cells
ECM	Extra cellular matrix
EPC	Endothelial progenitor cells
ePTFE	Expanded poly(tetrafluoroethylene)
FACS	Flow cytometry
HA	Hyaluronic acid
HBOEC	Human blood outgrowth endothelial cells
IgG	Immunoglobulin G
LDD	Local drug delivery
LDPE	Low-density poly(ethylene)
P(3HB)	Poly(3-hydroxybutyrate)
P(4HB)	Poly(4-hydroxybutyrate)
PA	Polyamides
PAA	Poly(acrylic acid)
PAAm	Poly(acrylamide)
PAH	Poly(anhydride)
PBMA	Poly(n-butyl methacrylate)
PC	Phosphorylcholine polymer
PCL	Poly(ε-caprolactone)
PCU	Polycarbonate urea urethane
PDLLA	Poly(D,L-lactide)
PE	Poly(ethylene)
PET	Poly(ethylene terephthalate)
PEVA	Poly(ethylene-co-vinyl acetate)
PGA	Poly(glycolide)
PHA	Polyhydroxyalkanoates
PHB	Poly(hydroxybutyrate)
PLGA	Poly(lactide-co-glycolide)
PLA	Polylactide
PLLA	Poly(L-lactide)

PMMA	Poly(methyl methacrylate)
PNIPAAm	Poly(N-isopropyl acrylamide)
POE	Poly(ortho esters)
POSS	Polyhedral oligomeric silsesquioxane
PP	Poly(propylene)
PPFC	Parallel plate flow chamber
PS	Poly(styrene)
PTD-PC	Polytyrosine-derived polycarbonate
PTFE	Poly(tetrafluoroethylene)
PTX	Paclitaxel
PUR	Poly(etherurethanes)
PVDF-HFP	Poly(vinylidene fluoride)-hexafluoropropylene
PVP	Poly(vinylpyrrolidone)
SA/AA	Salicylic acid/adipic acid
SIBS	Poly(styrene-b-isobutylene-b-styrene)
SIR	Sirolimus
SMC	Smooth muscle cell
TA	Transapical
TAVI	Transcatheter aortic valve implantation
TF	Transfemoral
VEGF	Vascular endothelial growth factor

Introduction

Besides metals, ceramics and composites polymers are a main type of biomaterials, which are intended to interface with biological systems with the purpose to evaluate, treat, augment or replace any tissue, organ or function of the body [1, 2]. Fast it becomes clear that polymers are most useful for medical treatments associated with soft tissues, whereas metals and ceramics are better suitable for the treatment of harder tissues such as bone [3].

Today, polymer-based biomaterials take a key function in modern medicine. Amongst others they are applied in different medical devices, such as cardiovascular implants, intraocular lenses, suture materials, cochlea implants, soft tissue implants, as well as drug delivery systems. In this context, multifunctional materials which include functionalities, such as degradation capability, drug release capability, sensitivity against external stimuli or biomimetic functionality are of great interest for the medical device development. It can be assumed that multifunctional polymers will make an important contribution to therapeutic and diagnostic treatments in regenerative medicine, minimally invasive medicine and nanomedicine in the future [4, 5]. This required special polymeric biomaterials, which fulfill the specific demands of these application fields by their functionality and biocompatibility. In this context, an important advantage of polymers is that they can be designed with a great variance of polymeric architectures and thus chemical and physical properties by use of a broad spectrum of chemical synthesis strategies. Therefore, polymers offer a great potential for the adaptation of biomaterials to the interaction possibilities of the human organism. However, it is desired that the polymeric materials do not interact non-specifically with biological components, such as proteins or cells in order to allow specific interactions by integration of defined signal molecules into the polymeric network or onto the polymer surface by means of different biofunctionalization methods [6].

A great challenge is that only very few polymers can be used so far, which were specifically developed for manufacturing of medical devices. Instead of that, polymers are used, which are well-established in technical application areas. They were selected for the intended medical application by means of different in vitro and in vivo tests [5]. Nevertheless, correlating problems in biocompatibility to material properties is still insufficient, which makes the deduction of strategies for the polymer development. Thus, the future tasks for the development of multifunctional polymer materials intended for medical applications are not only to decide which functionality and property should have the highest priority in these combinations but also to improve and develop test methods for their adequate evaluation [5]. Therefore, the present chapter is not only focused on the review of polymers used in coronary vascular interventions as stent platforms, coating matrices for drug-eluting stents and drug-coated balloons, and for transcatheter valve therapy but also on the description of methods for their surface modification and the evaluation of their bio- and hemo-compatibility.

State of the Art

Due to the entering of drug-eluting stents (DES) in the European market in 2002, polymers were used with increasing demand regarding their potential as implant material for coronary applications. DES are vascular stents which allow the delivery of drugs in a controlled manner to arterial wall. The controlled local drug release should reduce or prevent in-stent restenosis as a result of thrombosis, inflammation as well as increased migration and proliferation of smooth muscle cells. The most DES consists of three components: (1) the stent platform, (2) the pharmacologically active substance (drug), and (3) the drug carrier, usually a polymeric matrix, which controls the drug release. Despite their high efficacy regarding the inhibition of in-stent restenosis, the first generation of DES based on biostable (non-biodegradable) polymeric drug carriers, such as poly(ethylene-co-vinyl acetate) (PEVA), poly(n-butyl methacrylate) (PBMA) and poly(styrene-b-isobutylene-b-styrene) block copolymer (SIBS), and potential cytotoxic drugs, such as sirolimus (SIR) and paclitaxel (PTX), came under scrutiny when incidences of death or myocardial infarction were reported after DES implantation [7]. In particular, late thrombosis and delayed healing were identified as potential risks associated with DES [8–10]. Furthermore, cases of hypersensitivity were observed in connection with DES implantations [11, 12]. In this context, it was stated that beside the stent platform and the drug the polymeric drug carrier is a target for the biocompatibility improvement of such implants. Therefore, DES coatings on the basis of biodegradable polymers were developed. The advantages of these DES are that (1) they offer the antirestenotic benefit of a standard DES, (2) they offer the safety benefit of an uncoated bare metal stent (BMS) [13], and (3) the coating polymers degrade once their function is fulfilled, which might efficiently reduce observed hypersensitivity reactions. To eliminate the presence of a permanent implant completely degradable coronary stents (scaffolds) on the basis of polymers, such as polylactides (PLA), or drug-coated balloons (DCB) were developed. A major benefit of temporary scaffolds over permanent BMS and DES platforms is that they fulfill both requirements, the prevention of recoil immediately after scaffold implantation as well as the restoration of vasomotion and long-term positive remodeling of the stented vessel [14]. From this it follows that polymers intended as scaffold materials degrade in a moderate period of 6–9 months to 2 years and the degradation products are biocompatible and do not induce undesired inflammation reactions [15]. On the other hand, due to the fact that PTX-coated balloons using low-molecular excipients showed a clear inferiority regarding their deliverability in comparison to uncoated balloon catheters [16], it can be supposed that also hydrophilic polymers, such as poly(vinylpyrrolidone) (PVP) or hyaluronic acid (HA), with high swelling and lubricious properties will be of great interest in the future also in this field [17, 18]. Another cardiovascular intervention, where polymeric implant materials could be used with increasing scope, is the transcatheter aortic valve implantation or replacement (TAVI or TAVR) usually performed in an interdisciplinary team of cardiologists and heart surgeons. Within the clinically established TAVI procedure the replacement of the aortic valve can be carried out less invasively using a catheter where the self-expanding or balloon-expandable valve prosthesis consisting of a metal stent structure and a tri-leaflet valve fashioned out of porcine or bovine pericardium is mounted. As recommended TAVI are established for the treatment of high-risk, multimorbid patients with severe aortic stenoses which are no candidates for the open-heart surgical replacement. Since it is known that biological valves based on xenogenic pericardium tend to calcify and have a decreased durability in comparison to mechanical valves [19] also valve materials based on synthetic polymers, such as polycarbonate urea urethanes and polyesters, are under consideration [20–23]. These examples demonstrate impressively that polymers became more important also for cardiological applications.

Well-Established Polymers for Cardiovascular Applications

Polymers used for such medical devices can be broadly classified regarding their origin into synthetic and natural polymers as well as regarding their stability into biostable and biodegradable polymers.

Synthetic and Natural Polymers

Due to the ease of polymer syntheses, the controlled adjustment of polymer properties, the high reproducibility and the rapid availability synthetic polymers, such as poly(ethylene) (PE), poly(methyl methacrylate) (PMMA), polyurethanes (PUR), poly(glycolide) (PGA) and PLA, have historically been the material of choice for implants and other medical devices. Polymer syntheses can be realized via different reaction mechanisms which vary in complexity due to functional groups present in the reacting compounds. Thus, the exemplarily named PE can be manufactured by chain-growth polymerization of its unsaturated monomer ethylene that is able to break and then link with another ethylene molecule to form a repeating chain via a free radical mechanism mostly divided into the stages chain initiation, chain propagation, and chain termination. The attractiveness of synthetic polymers, such as low-density poly(ethylene) (LDPE) for colonization of vascular smooth muscle cells can be affected by grafting with biologically active substances, such as glycine and bovine serum albumin, determined by Parizek et al. [24]. In this study, an increased spreading and a higher concentration of focal adhesion proteins were observed for the modification with glycine whereas an enhanced cell growth was achieved with grafted bovine serum albumin [24]. Additionally, PMMA is routinely produced by chain-growth polymerization of methyl methacrylate using radical or anionic initiations. In conjunction with vascular applications recently the development of air-spun PLA nanofibers grafted with pendant oligo(ethylene oxide)-containing polymethacrylate as hydrophilic scaffold modification for vascular tissue engineering was described [25].

PUR, due to their excellent hemocompatibility well-established as scaffold materials for vascular grafts [26–29], can be synthesized by a stepwise addition reaction, therefore called step-growth polymerization, between isocyanate and alcohol bifunctional monomers. In addition to the mentioned polyaddition and as a further type of step-growth polymerizations polycondensation reactions are generally used for the synthesis of polyesters. During such polycondensation a diol reacts with a diacid under release of water as condensate. Aliphatic polyesters can be also obtained from cyclic diesters, such as glycolide for PGA and lactide for PLA, by ring-opening polymerization under very mild conditions using anionic, cationic or metal organic catalysts. The ring-opening polymerization is the most common synthesis method for such polyesters due to the fact that in contrast to the polycondensation reaction high molecular weight polymers can be achieved. A further demand for use of such synthetic polymers in biomedical applications is to tailor the materials properties by copolymerization with different monomers (e.g. statistical, alternating, periodic and block copolymers) or by variation of the polymer architecture (e.g. block, star, comb, brush and coil-cycle-coil macromolecules).

Regarding the medical use of the above named polyesters it can be stated that PGA is commonly used as suture material for different surgical applications [30]. Further examples are glycolide-containing, nanofibrous scaffolds blended with gelatin [31] or hollow fibers blended with poly(ε-caprolactone) (PCL) [32] for vascular tissue engineering, as well as glycolide-based local drug delivery systems [33–35]. In addition to these examples it can be pointed that PLA was intensely tested as temporary stent material in cardiology [36, 37], vessel surgery [38, 39] and urology [40–42].

Similar in chemical structure as the linear, synthetic polyesters PGA and PCL is the absorbable biopolymer poly(4-hydroxybutyrate) [P(4HB)]. PGA, P(4HB) and PCL differ merely structurally in the number of 1, 3 and 5 methylene groups in the polymer backbone [43]. However, PGA and PCL can be synthesized chemically, while P(4HB) belongs to the class of biopolyesters called polyhydroxyalkanoates (PHA) and is produced naturally by microorganisms. Since 2007, where the first medical device made from P(4HB) was launched as surgical suture material, additional P(4HB) products including devices for hernia repair, tendon and ligament repair, and plastic and reconstructive surgery are under consideration. Additionally, P(4HB)-based tissue engineering products are currently in development including vascular grafts and heart valves [43]. In addition to P(4HB) poly(3-hydroxybutyrate) [P(3HB)] is also a representative of PHA that was of interest as bio-derived and biodegradable thermoplastic implant material. However, P(3HB) could not become accepted for vascular applications due to the fact that it evoked extensive inflammatory responses and fibrocellular proliferation after implantation in porcine coronary arteries [44], P(3HB) was investigated recently regarding its potential for use in osteosynthesis implants [45]. Furthermore, it was demonstrated that electrospun P(3HB)-based meshes appear to be suitable in combination with endothelial-differentiated cells to improve vascularization in engineered bone tissues [46].

Biopolymers from natural origins generally degrade physiologically by hydrolysis, in most cases enzymatically catalyzed, and are very biocompatible as they and their degradation products are mostly well-known for the human organism. Certainly, they vary from source to source regarding their properties, their impurities and therefore the possibility of bacterial or viral contamination and antigenicity [3].

Collagen-based biomaterials can be divided in biomaterials retaining the native tissue structure, such as heart valves and vascular prostheses, and biomaterials prepared from purified collagen and reconstituted under different physical forms [47, 48]. An example for the first type are decellularized tissue matrices prepared by a combination of enzymatic and detergent treatments of collagen-rich tissues, such as xenogenic heart valves and blood vessels [49–52]. Examples for the second type are sponges used as hemostat and wound dressing, membranes for guided tissue regeneration, matrices for use in tissue engineering as well as coatings for prostheses and drug release systems [48, 53–59]. Furthermore, gelatin obtained from collagen by chemical hydrolysis was tested regarding its potential as coating matrix for polyester-based arterial prostheses as well as material for microencapsulating of drugs or preparing biodegradable hydrogels used as sealant for polyester vascular grafts or polymeric network for vascular tissue engineering [60–63].

Other examples of natural polypeptides in medical use are albumin and elastin. For example, crosslinked albumin gels were described as potential sealants for prosthetic vascular grafts [64]. In addition, albumin-based hydrogels were tested for enhancement of articular cartilage and intervertebral disc regeneration [65]. Interestingly, albumin was also investigated recently as dissolvable stent to provide intraluminal support during vascular anastomosis [66]. Moreover, cytocompatible, injectable elastin-based hydrogels with alterable gelation characteristics, favorable mechanical properties and structural stability for load bearing applications showed great potential for various biomedical applications [67]. Biomaterials derived from recombinant elastin-based block copolymers and processed in various forms including particles, films, gels and fiber networks were also studied for potential applications in medicine [68].

Beside polypeptides also polysaccharides and derivatives are used for vascular applications. Interesting fields for cellulose, starch, alginate, hyaluronic acid and chitosan are their utilization as matrices for drug delivery systems [69–73] as well as for alginate, hyaluronic acid and chitosan as scaffolds for vascular tissue engineering [74–76]. Heparin, the most biologically active member of the group of sulfated glycosaminoglycans, is used as antithrombotic and anticoagulant agent in the management of cardiovascular diseases in general as well as for the prevention of blood clotting on artificial vascular prostheses and heart valves. The improvement of the hemocompatibility of implant surfaces in direct contact with blood is still one of the most important areas in clinical and biomedical research [5, 48], and therefore many investigations were done to modify implant surfaces with heparin or heparin-like molecules [77–79].

Nevertheless, some of the listed examples demonstrate that the line between synthetic and natural polymers cannot be drawn clearly for all cases. Therefore, the category bio-inspired polymers was included that is promising for implant applications due to the possibility of generating materials that mimic the organism's own structural polymers in terms of structure and function [3]. Such polymers, mainly artificial or non-naturally occurring proteins like elastin-like proteins, can be synthesized by biosynthesis under controlled conditions so that they have from batch to batch reproducible and controllable properties. Furthermore, they have the advantage that they are not contaminated microbially [3]. Based on this knowledge Venkatraman et al. predicted that controlled synthesized, bio-inspired proteins could open up new possibilities for the development of vascular grafts as they form the bridge between synthetic materials such as poly(ethylene terephthalate) (PET) and expanded poly(tetrafluoroethylene) (ePTFE) on the one hand, as well as completely biological materials such as decellularized vascular tissues on the other hand [3].

Biostable and Biodegradable Polymers

Due to the fact that the application of an implant material can be permanently or temporary required biostable or biodegradable biomaterials are used. In case of polymers the term "biostable" is to view with the limitation that also biostable polymers, such as PE intended mainly for non-vascular applications such as acetabulum cups [80], but also vascular grafts [81], polyamides (PA) intended for suture materials [82] and polymeric meshes [83] as well as PET [84] and poly(etherurethanes) (PUR) [84, 85] intended primarily for vascular grafts, partially degrade in the long term by mechanical abrasion (e.g. observed for PE), hydrolysis (e.g. observed for PA and PET) or oxidation (e.g. observed for PUR) [86]. Furthermore, vascular grafts based on ePTFE have proven to be an adequate biostable conduit for bypass surgery [87, 88]. Another important group of biostable polymers are silicones which are well-established as implant material for intraocular lenses [89, 90], breast implants [91] and cochlear implants [92].

The above described examples demonstrate that a lot of implant applications should possess long-term stable performances in the organism. However, developments in tissue engineering, regenerative medicine and local drug delivery promoted the need of biomaterials with biodegradability. Typical representatives of biodegradable polymers are proteins and polysaccharides as natural polymers and aliphatic polyesters (polyhydroxycarboxylic acids), polyanhydrides and poly(ortho esters) as synthetic polymers. In order to be degradable, polymers must have chemical bonds cleavable under physiologic conditions. In this context, the integration of hydrolytically cleavable bonds is a conventional method to realize degradable polymeric materials synthetically. The hydrolytic degradation has the advantage that the degradation rate is at most independent from the position of implantation due to the fact that in all regions of the human organism water is present [86]. In contrast, the concentration of enzymes, which can catalyze the hydrolysis of bonds and therefore can cause an increase of cleavage velocity, is locally different. The list of factors that influence the degradation behavior of biodegradable polymers is long and ranges exemplarily from their chemical structure, their molecular weight and distribution, their crystallinity and the existence of ionic groups (polymer-dependent) over the sample geometry, the surface morphology and thus the surface-volume ratio, the sterilization and storage conditions (sample-dependent) to the kind of their implantation, the pH and enzymatic conditions, as well as the physisorption of proteins and as a result the fibrotic encapsulation which can possibly accelerate the degradation by autocatalytic action of degradation products (implantation-dependent) [86]. Two mechanisms are described for the biodegradation process: (1) the bulk degradation, where the degradation is favored in the polymer bulk material due to the fact that water can diffuse faster into the bulk than the polymer can degrade and (2) the surface erosion, where the diffusion velocity of water is slower than the degradation rate of the polymer. Therefore, during the homogeneous bulk degradation the molecular weight of the polymer is decreased continuously whereas during the heterogeneous surface erosion the molecular weight is only decreased in a thin surface layer and the molecular weight of the polymer bulk material is nearly influenced.

Polyhydroxycarboxylic acids, such as PGA, PLA, P(3HB), P(4HB) and PCL, degrade by bulk degradation which can be divided into the following three steps: The first step is characterized by water absorption, polymer swelling and ester bond cleavage, although no mass loss is observed. In the second step, the average molecular weight is significantly reduced and the polymer loses its mechanical strength. Due to the proceeding formation of carboxylic groups autocatalytic hydrolysis takes place. During the third step polymer fragmentation can be observed and thus mass loss of the test samples can be measured. The degradation of such implanted polymers are completed when the formed low-molecular fragments including the free hydroxycarboxylic acids are dissolved in the surrounding physiologic medium and then metabolized in the citric acid cycle (Krebs cycle) [86, 93].

As example for surface erodible polymers polyanhydrides can be named which degrade by surface erosion with linear mass loss due to the easily cleavable anhydride bonds. An additional increase of hydrophobicity could be achieved by integration of aliphatic diacids with long hydrocarbon chains (dimers of unsaturated fatty acids) or by aromatic monomer units [86]. Another interesting group of surface erodible polymers are poly(ortho esters) which were focused investigated regarding their potential as drug delivery systems [94–96].

Therefore, it can be stated that although various biodegradable polymers have been evaluated, hydrolytically degradable polyhydroxycarboxylic acids which can be supplied in sufficient amounts and in medical grade quality, are the polymers of choice for vascular applications so far.

Polymers for Cardiovascular Application

Polymers for Stent Platforms

The role of a fully biodegradable scaffold is to provide a temporary support of the blood vessel, so that the vessel will be free of a rigid metallic caging and can recover its physiological function after complete scaffold degradation [97]. Therefore, the absence of a permanent stent platform may reduce the requirements for a long-term dual antiplatelet therapy and facilitate the return of vessel vasomotion and late expansive (positive) remodeling. Several polymer-based biodegradable scaffolds with a broad range of degradation times were used in clinical studies, see Table 15.1 for an overview.

However, comprehensive clinical requirements in terms of stent deliverability and stent mechanics compared to BMS can not all be fulfilled easily with polymeric scaffolds. As first Tamai et al. [98] reported their clinical experiences with an absorbable coronary polymer scaffold made from PLLA, the Igaki-Tamai scaffold. The Igaki-Tamai scaffold had a self-expanding zigzag helical coil design, where the self-expansion of this scaffold was assisted by balloon-expansion. The obtained results of this first study in humans demonstrated a low restenosis rate and a re-intervention rate of 10.5 % at 6 months [98]. The first clinically investigated fully absorbable DES is the bioresorbable vascular scaffold (BVS) by Abbott Vascular (USA). The BVS is based on a balloon-expandable PLLA scaffold and a PDLLA coating containing everolimus [134]. The first BVS generation (BVS 1.0) was tested in different clinical studies and was found to be safe [97]. The second generation (BVS 1.1) was enhanced

Table 15.1 Overview of relevant polymer-based vascular scaffolds used in clinical studies according to [13, 97]

Scaffold	Manufacturer	Polymer	Coating	Drug	Resorption time (months)
Igaki-Tamai	Kyoto Medical	PLLA	None	None	24
BVS 1.0	Abbott Vascular	PLLA	PDLLA	Everolimus	24
BVS 1.1	Abbott Vascular	PLLA	PDLLA	Everolimus	24
DESolve	Elixir	PLLA	None	Myolimus	12–24
Amaranth	Amaranth	PLLA	None	None	3–6
ART18AZ	ART	PDLLA	None	None	3–6
REVA	REVA Medical	PTD-PC	None	None	24
ReZolve	REVA Medical	PTD-PC	None	Sirolimus	4–6
Ideal BioStent	Xenogenics	SA/AA polymer	Salicylate	Sirolimus	>12

PLLA poly(L-lactide), *PDLLA* (poly(D,L-lactide), *PTD-PC* polytyrosine-derived polycarbonate, *SA/AA* salicylic acid/adipic acid

regarding its radial strength, mechanical integrity and drug release kinetics with the purpose to establish a scaffold platform for the routine clinical practice and with the wish to be the fourth revolution in interventional cardiology [97]. Currently, scaffold developments of approximately 16 companies including many key and niche players such as the above mentioned and others are under consideration. Therefore, a lot of innovations can be awaited in this field in the future.

Polymers as Coating Matrices for Drug-Eluting Stents (DES)

As described in Chap. 2 DES consists typically of a stent platform, a drug and a polymeric drug carrier. For the optimization of the polymeric drug carrier and therefore for the effective prevention of delayed healing and hypersensitive foreign body reactions observed with first-generation DES advanced biocompatible permanent polymers, such as a biomimetic phosphorylcholine polymer (PC), the extremely biointert poly(vinylidene fluoride)-hexafluoropropylene (PVDF-HFP) or the BioLinx™ polymer customized regarding a optimized, sustained drug release profile, were used in second-generation DES coatings. Furthermore, biodegradable polymers, such as PLA and poly(lactide-co-glycolide) (PLGA), were studied to optimize DES coatings regarding their biocompatibility. Due to the fact that the polymeric coatings degrade over time and the DES transform into a BMS they are expected to cause lower stent thrombosis. Despite these refinements seen in the current polymer-based DES polymer-free DES have been investigated where the drug was embedded mostly into microporous or nanoporous metallic stent surfaces [15, 99]. This parallel development took place, because it is known that the degradation products of some biodegradable polymers are associated with tissue inflammation during the degradation process [44] and thus these coatings may also hold the risk to cause stent thrombosis [15]. Other disadvantages of polymer-based stent coatings could be that delaminations during the stent expansion (high plastic deformation) occur and their mechanical properties are impaired after sterilization due to the fact that the cleavage of chemical bonds leads to a post-crystallization and embrittlement of the polymer [99]. The main DES equipped with polymer coatings are summarized in Table 15.2. However, intense work on stent development has successfully led to DES the next generations of DES will further improve the endothelialization and enhance the arterial healing possibly using biocompatible, polymer-based abluminal or dual, side-selective coatings, as well as other innovative, polymer-free drug reservoirs.

Table 15.2 Overview of relevant DES equipped with polymer coatings according to [97, 99, 100]

DES	Manufacturer	Polymer coating	Coating thickness (μm)	Kind of polymer	Drug	Drug amount (μg/mm^2)
Cypher	Cordis	PEVA, PBMA	12.6	Biostable	Sirolimus	1.4
Taxus express	Boston Scientific	SIBS	16	Biostable	Paclitaxel	1.0
Endeavor	Medtronic	PC	4.1	Biostable	Zotarolimus	1.0
Endeavor resolute	Medtronic	BioLinx™ polymer	4.1	Biostable	Zotarolimus	1.0
Xience-V	Abbott Vascular	PBMA, PVDF-HFP	7.6	Biostable	Everolimus	1.0
Promus element	Boston Scientific	PBMA, PVDF-HFP	6	Biostable	Everolimus	1.0
BioMatrix	Biosensors	PLA	10	Biodegradable	Biolimus A9	1.56

PEVA poly(ethylene-co-vinyl acetate), *PBMA* poly(n-butyl methacrylate), *SIBS* poly(styrene-b-isobutylene-b-styrene) block copolymer, *PC* phosphorylcholine polymer, *PVDF-HFP* poly(vinylidene fluoride)-hexafluoropropylene, *BioLinx*™ hydrophobic C_{10}-polymer/hydrophilic C_{19}-polymer/poly(vinylpyrrolidone) (PVP), *PLA* polylactide

Table 15.3 Overview of relevant PTX-coated balloon catheters according to [109]

DCB	Manufacturer	Excipient	Drug	Drug amount (μg/mm^2)
SeQuent Please	B.Braun	Contrast medium (iopromide)	PTX	3.0
Dior II	Eurocor	Shellac	PTX	3.0
Pantera Lux	Biotronik	BTHC	PTX	3.0
Elutax	Aachen Resonance	3-Layer design	PTX	2.0
In.Pact Falcon	Medtronic Invatec	Urea	PTX	3.0

BTHC n-butyryl tri-n-hexyl citrate, *Elutax* first layer guarantees homogenous PTX coating and secure PTX attachment; second layer consists of micro crystals of pure PTX; third layer consists of hydrogel which enables better pushability and trackability

Polymers as Coating Matrices for Drug-Coated Balloons (DCB)

As alternative to DES DCB were developed since it was found that a single short exposure to PTX using non-ionic contrast media or balloon catheter coatings as carriers for local drug delivery provided similar protection from restenosis as the most efficacious DES [16, 101, 102]. Since these first preclinical observations more than 10 years ago different DCB concepts were proven (Table 15.3). Regarding their deliverability a clear inferiority of PTX-coated balloons using low-molecular excipients in comparison to uncoated balloon catheters was demonstrated [16]. Furthermore, it was stated that a PTX dose of 3 $\mu g/mm^2$ is effective and tolerable for the DCB utilization [16, 103–105].

While DES coatings are designed as a drug reservoir in order to allow a sustained drug release over a long time period, the development of DCB affords coatings which are robust enough to physically maintain the drug on the surface of the balloon during transit of the device through the vascular system and allow a rapid, uniform and efficient drug transfer to the vessel wall during a short balloon dilatation time. Coating additives of commercially available DCB, which all engage the drug PTX, are equipped in such a way to enhance the PTX transfer to the vessel wall [16, 106]. Some of them are well studied as e.g. the contrast agent iopromide [101], plasticizers such as n-butyryl tri-n-hexyl citrate (BTHC) [107] and urea [108] (Table 15.3). In addition, hydrophilic, polymer-based DCB coatings with high swelling and slippage properties could have a high potential and will be presented in more detail in section "DCB Equipped with Hydrogel-Based Coatings".

Polymers for Transcatheter Aortic Valve Therapy

Due to the demographic development and increasing elderly population a growing group of patients will decline from surgical valve replacement, because they are too ill or weak to withstand the stress of invasive surgical treatments. In consideration of avoiding the need of open heart surgery and its associated risks, TAVI represents an ideal answer. Mostly, valve prostheses consist of a cobalt chromium alloy (balloon-expandable) or nitinol (self-expanding) stent structure where a tri-leaflet valve composed of porcine or bovine pericardium is mounted (Table 15.4).

Although no perseverative anticoagulation is required biological valves based on xenogenic pericardium demonstrated a decreased durability due to the fact that they tend to calcify in comparison to mechanical valves [19]. Thus, functional synthetic valves were developed. Exemplarily noted is a novel nanocomposite material described by Rahmani et al. [20, 23] that composed of a polycarbonate urea urethane (PCU) as soft segment and a hard segment derived from polyhedral oligomeric silsesquioxane (POSS) nanoparticles through covalent bonding forming pendant chain functional groups. The POSS-PCU nanocomposite demonstrated superior mechanical properties compared to porcine and bovine pericardial tissues. Additionally, it possessed enhanced resistance to calcification and thrombosis with superior in vivo biostability [20]. Furthermore, textile, less fragile

Table 15.4 Exemplary overview of valve prostheses consisting of xenogenic pericardium

Prosthesis	Manufacturer	Stent	Valve
Sapien-XT	Edwards	Cobalt chromium alloy, balloon expandable	Bovine pericardium
CoreValve	Medtronic	Nitinol, self-expanding	Porcine pericardium
JenaValve	JenaValve	Nitinol, self-expanding	Porcine root valve (TA), porcine pericardium (TF)
Portico	St. Jude	Nitinol, self-expanding	Bovine pericardium (TA), porcine pericardium (TF)
Engager	Medtronic	Nitinol, self-expanding	Bovine pericardium
Lotus	Boston Scientific, Sadra Medical	Braided nitinol	Bovine pericardium

TA transapical, *TF* transfemoral

polyester-based leaflets were designed as alternative to xenogenic, biologic materials [21, 22]. Based on these examples can be stated that also synthetic, polymeric materials could be an alternative replacement for valve leaflets.

Surface Modification of Polymers Intended for Local Drug Delivery and Biofunctionalization

The Objective of Surface Modification for Polymers Used in Cardiology

Much effort is invested in the novel design and synthesis of polymers to be used as biomaterial for the fabrication of implants with appropriate mechanical properties, durability and functionality. In dependence of the application, requirements might differ considerably, ranging from high mechanical stress resistance especially interesting for endoprostheses to high transparency in ophthalmologic implants. Also in the confined field of cardiology, polymers with various properties are used in a wide range of applications. For instance, the pumping bladder in an artificial heart should withstand a millions of cycles without failure while a stent platform needs to allow for a high degree of deformation. These functions are generally governed by the bulk composition of the polymers. The biological response to the devices or the composing polymers is in contrast largely controlled by the surface chemistry and structure. The rationale for the surface modification of polymers is according to Ratner et al. [110] therefore straightforward: retaining the key physical properties of a biomaterial while modifying only the outermost surface to influence the biointeraction. Commonly observed interactions of any material with a biological system or system containing biomolecules cover adsorption or adhesion processes of proteins and bacteria or platelets as well as phagocytosis and fibrous encapsulation. Especially relevant polymer-blood, -cell and -tissue interactions in cardiology are in detail reviewed in Chap. 5. Effective surface modification of polymers should mediate these interactions with the purpose of improved tissue-interface related-biocompatibility without modifying the mechanical properties and functionality of the device. In principal there are two categories of surface modifications. The first involves the overcoating of an existing surface by coating, grafting or thin film deposition of a material having a different composition and properties than the bulk material. The second category involves the chemical altering of atoms, compounds or molecules in the existing surface. Both strategies are relevant for polymer surface modification in cardiology. While coating technologies are mainly applied for the provision of cardiovascular implants with a polymer-based drug-delivery function [section "Polymer-Based Local Drug Delivery (LDD) Systems"], chemical surface modification can be applied for both, drug delivery and stable functionalization with biomolecules (section "Biofunctionalization of Polymers"); all with the purpose of mediating the cell-implant interaction.

Polymer-Based Local Drug Delivery (LDD) Systems

Classification of Polymer-Based LDD Systems

In general, polymer-based drug delivery systems can be broadly classified into physically and chemically controlled systems. Diffusion-controlled drug release is an example of a physical mechanism that is based on the diffusion of a drug molecule through a certain coating or matrix, mostly of polymeric nature. Besides the benefit that the drug is fixed on the implant's surface and relatively protected against mechanical stress, the thickness and type of polymeric coating allow a wide range of control over the drug release characteristics [111, 112]. In a further iteration of this approach, diffusion-controlled LDD systems can be divided into matrix and membrane systems, where the drug is either directly incorporated within or surrounded by the polymeric coating. Amongst others, these polymer-based LDD systems can be obtained by dip-coating and spray-coating techniques where the intended polymer and drug are either handled in the same solution, which might be a mixture of two solvents if needed, or separately for matrix and membrane systems, respectively. Polymers applied are rather hydrophobic to retard water interpenetration and thereby guarantee sustained drug release. If degradation of the device is desired, hydrolyzable polymers as polyesters with slower degradation than drug diffusion rate can be used for these systems. Table 15.5 provides an overview of polymers used in controlled drug release. Chemically controlled LDD systems offer another strategy for drug release. In these systems, drug release is achieved by degradation or swelling of the drug carrier or by cleavage of chemically bound drugs or biomolecules. For degradation-controlled systems polyanhydrides and poly(ortho esters), possessing highly labile groups that ensure rapid hydrolysis of polymer chains encountering water molecules and retarded water permeation by designing the polymers with

Table 15.5 Summary of commonly applied polymers in drug delivery (DD) systems

Polymer	Application
Chitosan	Biodegradable matrix for swelling-controlled DD
Dextrane	Biodegradable matrix for stimulus-responsive DD
Hyaluronic acid (HA)	Biodegradable matrix for swelling-controlled DD
Poly(acrylic acid) (PAA)	Permanent matrix for pH-sensitive DD
Poly(acrylamide) (PAAm)	Permanent matrix for stimulus-responsive DD
Poly(anhydride) (PAH)	Biodegradable matrix for degradation-controlled DD
Poly(n-butyl methacrylate) (PBMA)	Permanent matrix for diffusion-controlled DD
Poly(ε-caprolactone) (PCL)	Biodegradable matrix for diffusion-controlled DD
Poly(ethylene-co-vinyl acetate) (PEVA)	Permanent matrix for diffusion-controlled DD
Poly(glycolide) (PGA)	Biodegradable matrix for diffusion-controlled DD
Poly(hydroxybutyrate) (PHB)	Biodegradable matrix for diffusion-controlled DD
Poly(lactide) (PLA)	Biodegradable matrix for diffusion-controlled DD
Poly(N-isopropyl acrylamide) (PNIPAAm)	Permanent matrix for temperature-sensitive DD
Poly(ortho esters) (POE)	Biodegradable matrix for degradation-controlled DD
Poly(styrene-b-isobutylene-b-styrene) (SIBS)	Permanent matrix for diffusion-controlled DD
Poly(vinylpyrrolidone) (PVP)	Permanent matrix for swelling-controlled DD

hydrophobic monomer units, are used [113]. In contrast for LDD-systems, controlled via swelling, more hydrophilic polymers as e.g. hyaluronic acid are required. However, both systems, diffusion- and chemically controlled, provide drug release independently of their need, possibly leading to ineffectiveness of the LDD system at time of interest. Having this in mind, it would be highly beneficial if the drug is delivered by a system that senses the signal caused by disease, judges the magnitude of the signal and then acts to release the right amount of drug in response [114]. Here, stimulus-responsive hydrophilic polymeric networks as poly(acrylic acid) or poly(N-isopropyl acrylamide) hydrogels with swelling properties dictated by changes in pH [115, 116] or temperature [117–119], respectively, came into discussion. The induction of hydrogel swelling by such physical and chemical stimuli allows control over release of incorporated or underlying drugs. However, the cited stimuli are rather non-specific. An alternative are specific chemo-responsive hydrogels, which are designed to contain internal non-covalent interactions based on pendant ligands and complementary receptors [120]. These crosslinks can be broken by soluble ligand or receptor competitors, which are specific for certain diseases and can diffuse into the gel displacing the internal affinity crosslinks. Subsequently, the degree of crosslinking decreases and drugs can be released. Besides glucose-responsive hydrogels with concanavalin A—glucose affinity crosslinks [121], antigen-responsive hydrogels, where antibody–antigen pairs, chemically grafted to the hydrogel network serve as reversible crosslinkers, are discussed in literature. Several model systems have been established [120, 122, 123], while the best studied is probably the one of Miyata et al. [124–127], which is based on immunoglobulin G (IgG) antigens and corresponding antibodies grafted onto a poly(acrylamide)-(PAAm-) hydrogel, forming affinity crosslinks cleavable in the presence of free antigen. In an own study, we provided a thorough in vitro characterization of PAAm-hydrogels regarding drug permeability with the purpose of exploring the applicability of such hydrogels for implant-associated LDD systems [128]. Within this study, we were furthermore able to demonstrate an antigen-triggered release of bovine serum albumin as model drug from a model implant-associated LDD system. The continuation of work will now focus on the real implementation of such stimulus-responsive hydrogels to implant surfaces and the use of natural biocompatible polymers, particularly those in the poly(saccharide) family (e.g. hyaluronic acid and chitosan).

Polymer-Based LDD in Cardiology

LDD entered the field of cardiology with the development of drug-eluting stents (DES) which revolutionized the treatment of coronary artery disease. Stents can generally be described as tubular scaffolds from a wire mesh or a slotted tube, which are either self-expanding or balloon-expandable. Typical biomaterials for stent manufacture are stainless steel and cobalt-chromium alloys for balloon-expandable stents, and nickel-titanium alloys (nitinol) for self-expanding stents [129]. DES are specialized vascular stents which allow the delivery of drugs in a controlled manner to arterial wall with the purpose to reduce or prevent in-stent restenosis as process of enhanced smooth muscle cell proliferation. As described the most DES consist of a polymeric matrix as drug carrier, which controls the drug release [130, 131]. Drug carriers used on the initial commercially available DES were permanent polymers as a blend of PEVA and PBMA in ratio of 50/50 % (w/w) (Cypher stent, Johnson & Johnson, USA) and the copolymer SIBS (Taxus stent, Boston Scientific, USA). These polymeric coating materials however raised the question about long-term biocompatibility. Therefore, the activities in DES development headed for more biocompatible and biodegradable materials as PLA [38, 132, 133] and copolymers, such as PLGA [134, 135], which are fully metabolized to carbon dioxide and water (Krebs cycle). These polyester-based drug reservoirs have the advantage that they degrade during or after the drug release so that they do not cause long-term foreign body reactions. In addition, degradable polymer blends of P(4HB) and PDLLA have been developed. Recently several design approaches to provide temporary absorbable stents, which may allow for restoration of vasomotion and long-term positive remodeling of the stented vessel [14], with an LDD-function are discussed. The first clinically available stent is equipped with a PDLLA-coating (BVS, Abbott, USA).

Biofunctionalization of Polymers

Techniques in Surface Activation

Due to the low abundance of available functional groups on the surface of most polymers, their surface activation is often a precursor to performing biofunctionalization in the sense of chemically attaching a bioactive compound. Techniques that modify surface properties by introducing random, non-specific groups or by coating the surface are less useful in bioconjugation to polymer surfaces. Used surface activation techniques should in contrast be tailored to introduce a specific functional group, which might be achieved amongst others by wet- and plasma-chemical processes, detailed in the following and in Table 15.6.

Wet-chemical surface activation. In wet-chemical surface modification, a material is treated with liquid reagents to generate reactive functional groups on the surface. In contrast to plasma and other energy source surface modification techniques, this method has a general higher penetration depth and therefore modification of three-dimensional scaffolds within pores is often feasible in a simple way [136]. For instance, oxygen-containing moieties were introduced to PE [137, 138] and PP by treatment with chromic acid and potassium permanganate in sulfuric acid [139, 140]. Carboxyl and hydroxyl groups were generated by base and acid hydrolysis of PMMA [141], and PCL [142] with concentrated sodium hydroxide and sulfuric acid. One has to note that hydrolysis time of polyesters needs to be thoroughly optimized in order to retain the properties of the bulk polymers. Subsequent conversion of the functional groups to isocyanate groups by treatment with 4,4′-methylenebis(phenyl isocyanate) allowed formation of terminal amino groups by addition of ammonia. In an own study, we have already applied this activation procedure for the immobilization of acetylsalicylic acid and vascular endothelial growth factor (VEGF) to PCL [142]. Generation of primary amines is also possible by wet-chemical treatment without the intermediate step of hydrolysis. For instance aminolysis with various diamines including hydrazine hydrate, 1,6-hexanediamine, ethylenediamine, and N-aminoethyl-1,3-propanediamine, as well as lithiated diamines [7, 19, 22–28] has been applied to introduce amines to PMMA [143, 144], PUR [145], PLLA [146, 147], and PLGA [148]. The simple these methods are, they are however non-specific and the degree of surface functionalization might therefore not be repeatable between polymers of different molecular weight, crystallinity, or tacticity. Moreover, hazardous chemical waste might be generated [149]. A clean alternative are ionized gas treatments, first of all plasma-chemical modifications, described in the following.

Plasma-chemical surface activation. In contrast to the above described wet-chemical methods plasma treatments can provide modification of the top nanometer of a polymer surface without using solvents or generating chemical waste and with less degradation and roughening of the material than many wet-chemical treatments [136]. The type of inserted functional groups can be varied by selection of the plasma gas (Ar, N_2, O_2, H_2O, CO_2, NH_3) and operating parameters (pressure, power, time, gas flow rate) [136]. For instance, surfaces of PCL [142, 150], PLLA [147], PA [18],

Table 15.6 Overview of polymers subjected to surface activation treatments

Surface treatment	Polymer	Generated function
Treatment with chromic acid	Poly(ethylene) (PE)	Oxygen-containing groups
	Poly(propylene) (PP)	
Acidic/basic hydrolysis	Poly(ε-caprolactone) (PCL)	Hydroxyl and carboxyl groups
	Poly(methyl methacrylate) (PMMA)	
Aminolysis	Poly(L-lactide) (PLLA)	Amine groups
	Poly(lactide-co-glycolide) (PLGA)	
	Poly(methyl methacrylate) (PMMA)	
	Poly(urethane) (PUR)	
Oxygen plasma	Polyamide (PA)	Oxygen-containing groups
	Poly(ε-caprolactone) (PCL)	
	Poly(ethylene) (PE)	
	Poly(ethylene terephthalate) (PET)	
	Poly(L-lactide) (PLLA)	
Carbon dioxide plasma	Poly(ethylene) (PE)	Carboxyl groups
	Poly(propylene (PP)	
	Poly(styrene) (PS)	
Ammonia plasma	Poly(ε-caprolactone) (PCL)	Amine groups
	Poly(L-lactide) (PLLA)	
	Poly(styrene) (PS)	
	Poly(tetrafluorethylene) (PTFE)	
Silanization	Polyamide (PA)	Amine-, epoxy-, vinyl-groups
	Poly(ε-caprolactone) (PCL)	
	Poly(ethylene terephthalate) (PET)	
	Poly(L-lactide) (PLLA)	
	Poly(methyl methacrylate) (PMMA)	
	Poly(tetrafluoroethylene) (PTFE)	

PE [137], and PET [151] were provided with oxygen containing functional groups by oxygen plasma exposition. Moreover, carbon dioxide plasma could be used to introduce carboxyl groups to PP [152], PS [153], and PE [152]. The generation of amine groups was in addition performed by ammonia plasma to PTFE [154] and PS [153]. In own studies we treated PCL [142] and PLLA [147] by ammonia plasma and qualified the generation of amine groups via fluorescent labelling. Results reveal less functional groups on these surfaces in comparison to chemically activated surfaces, which is in good agreement with the well-known low plasma penetration depth of only 10 nm. However, no correlation with the efficiency of subsequent immobilization of biomolecules could be observed [155]. Besides a standalone technique, plasma treatments are often used as a precursor to other surface modification techniques, as for example plasma activation followed by silanization, as in detail described in the following.

Surface activation via silanization. Although surface modification using silane monolayers is primarily applied on glass and silicone substrates as a means to couple an organic polymer, this is certain to be an emerging field in research for polymer surface modification [136]. Because the target surface functional group in glass or silicon silanization is a hydroxyl, silanization can be applied to polymer surfaces, which have been hydroxylated by for instance treatment with oxygen plasma. As organosilanes with various end functionalities including amine, epoxy and vinyl groups are available, silanization offers the potential of modifying polymer surfaces with a bunch of functional groups for different application. Moreover, self assembled monolayers, produced by silanization, provide a nearly crystalline and hence more defined surface functionalization than typical wet-chemical or ionized gas functionalization techniques [156]. In own studies we used organsilanes with epoxy and amine head groups for the chemical attachment of hyaluronic acid to PA [18] and VEGF [142] and antibodies [147] to polyester surfaces, respectively.

Techniques in Biomolecule Immobilization

Among the numerous reported methods for immobilizing biomolecules to surfaces physical adsorption via van der Waals or electrostatic interactions, physical entrapment within hydrogels, ligand–receptor pairing (as in biotin–avidin) and covalent attachment via cleavable or non-cleavable bonds are most commonly used (Fig. 15.1). In dependence of the applied immobilization protocol a short-term and long-term localization of the biomolecule on the implant surface can be achieved [110].

Thus, biofunctionalization can be either used to provide the implant with a drug delivery or a stable novel surface functionality. In an own study, we could show this wide range of modification possibilities by VEGF immobilization and delivery from PLLA surfaces [157]. Observed release profiles differed in dependence of the applied immobilization method. Fastest release was observed for VEGF entrapped in a PAA hydrogel, followed by physically adsorbed VEGF and covalently attached VEGF via hydrolyzable bonds with the slowest release rate. The release of physically adsorbed or entrapped VEGF is diffusion-controlled and starts immediately after insertion into the elution medium. Chemical attachment however affords the cleavage of covalent bonds prior to liberation of biomolecules. This was achieved in that case by the formation of ester bonds between the side chain hydroxyl groups of VEGF and N,N-disuccinimidyl carbonate-activated surface amino groups on the PLLA surface.

As detailed above most of biofunctionalization methods afford a previous surface activation, which might be combined with the grafting of an intermediary spacer between the surface and the biomolecule for multiplication of available functional groups on the surface. Here, multifunctional spacers

(a)
(b)
(c)
(d)
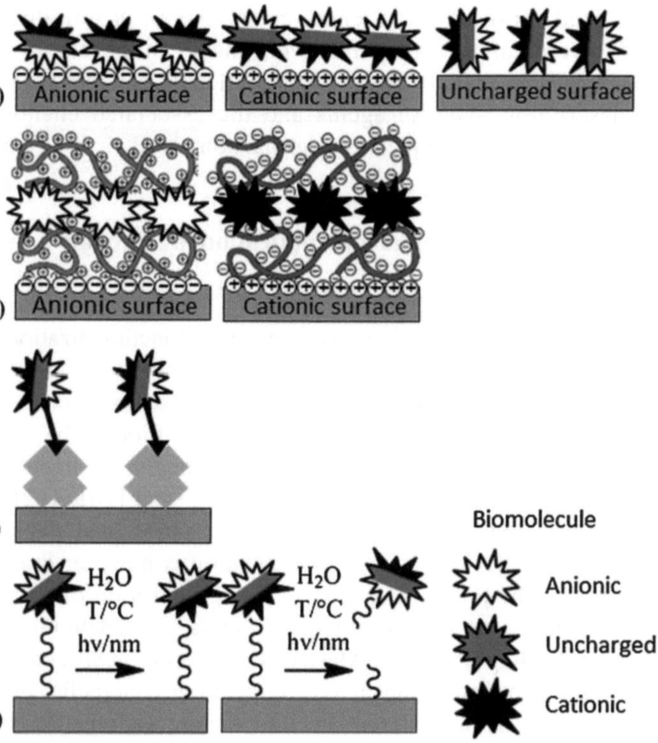

Fig. 15.1 Biomolecule immobilization strategies: **a** physical adsorption, **b** physical entrapment within hydrogel, **c** ligand–receptor pairing, and **d** covalent attachment

as poly(ethylenimine) or dendrimers with a wide range of terminal functional groups in defined quantity offer a way to increase this surface functionality [157, 158]. In addition, maintenance of biological activity is very important for hydrophobic polymer surfaces as these are often associated with non specific adsorption and denaturation. Besides the integration of hydrophilic PEG spacer [159], which effectively shield the compound from these issues, we investigated in an own study the inclusion of the peptide spacer $(GGAP)_4$ on PLLA surfaces. By this we reached efficient prevention of non-specific protein adsorption and enhanced bioactivity of subsequently covalently attached anti-CD34 antibodies [147].

A prerequisite for successful biomolecule immobilization is of course moreover that the specific functionality imparted to the inert surface must be compatible with the reactive sites on the compound to be covalently attached to that surface. While for adsorption processes the introduction of charged groups or simple modification of hydrophilic properties should be enough, covalent immobilization affords defined functional groups, including thiol, aldehyde, carboxylic acid, hydroxyl, and primary amine groups. These can be directly used for biomolecule attachment. However, most cases apply additional crosslinking agents, which can link the bioactive compound directly to the functionalized substrate (zero-length crosslinkers), or introduce themselves a spacer of several angstroms. Moreover, they can be stable or introduce hydrolyzable bonds in order to allow for biomolecule delivery from the surface. A detailed description of these agents and the associated chemistries can be found in Bioconjugate Techniques, by Hermanson [160].

Biofunctionalization of Polymers for Application in Coronary Vascular Intervention

In the field of cardiology, intensive research on biofunctionalization of polymers has been done since decades to develop novel surface designs for all types of endovascular implants in order to modulate their behavior in contact with blood and improve their bio-and hemocompatibility. Even prior to the development of DES this issue has been addressed by the establishment of stents, being coated with the anticoagulant heparin (e.g., Palmaz-Schatz stent [161, 162], Wiktor stent [163], and Jostent [164]), fibrin [165], cellulose [166], and phosphorylcholine (BiodivYsio stent [167]). Nowadays more attention is however drawn to the biofunctionalization of the polymer coating enabling activation of a cascade of biological processes that eventually regenerate or replace a functioning endothelium, referred to as prohealing approach. Materials promoting in situ endothelialization of vascular implants by capturing in vivo circulating endothelial progenitor cells (EPC) with the capacity to differentiate into mature endothelial cells (EC) and repopulate areas of vascular injury and endothelial disruption [168, 169]. The selection of the optimal target on the EPC surface in combination with an ideal capture molecule immobilized on the implant surface, which is decisive for the success of in situ endothelialization, is however still a challenge. A stainless steel-coated stent with a polysaccharide matrix covered by murine monoclonal anti-human antibodies directed towards the EPC surface marker CD34 is probably the most studied "EPC capture stent" nowadays. This Genous R-stent, developed by the company Orbus Medical Technologies in collaboration with Kutryk's group, has achieved CE approval and is commercially available since 2010. Although CD34 is not a specific marker of EPC, as only a small portion of the CD34-positive cells are actually EPC [170], first human clinical investigations of this technology demonstrated its safety and feasibility for the treatment of de novo coronary artery disease [171] and the long-term promotion of significant late regression of neointimal hyperplasia [172, 173]. Unfortunately, in spite of these initial promising clinical outcomes, following randomized clinical trials comparing the Genous R-stent with BMS (GENIUS STEMI) [174] and DES (TRIAS) [175–177] evidenced disappointing results with regard to late luminal loss. These results let to a general discussion of the Genous' clinical efficacy. As reaction to this discussion, novel surface modification strategies in order to increase availability of immobilized compounds and thereby biofunctionality of the modified surface and more selective capture molecules are searched. In this context, further antibodies than CD34 (e.g., anti-KDR) [178], against EPC selected aptamers [179], and materials mimicking the extra cellular matrix (ECM), are in focus of current research. From the plethora of insoluble and soluble macromolecules contained within ECM, the fibrillar protein collagen is probably the most commonly used coating on for example commercially available polyester vascular grafts [180]. Furthermore, besides the use of integer ECM components, various ECM peptide sequences as functional domains of proteins, glycoproteins, and proteoglycans have been isolated and grafted on biomaterials to control cell behavior, for example, REDV [181], PHSRN [182], RGD, and GRGDSP from fibronectin [183], laminin-derived recognition sequences, IKLLI, IKVAV [184] LRE, PDSGR, RGD, and YIGSR, and collagen type I derived sequence, DGEA [185]. However, these peptides, nicely reviewed by De Mel et al. [186], are not cell-selective as they bind to integrins, present on many cell types. To overcome this risk of low cell selectivity, Veleva et al. [187] used a combinatorial peptide library and phage display technique to isolate peptides, being more selective for human blood outgrowth endothelial cells (HBOEC). Indeed, selectivity of terpolymers, covalently coupled with these peptides, could be demonstrated for HBOEC in serum-free medium. The application of a coating combing both, an integer ECM component with functional peptide domains, might hence be very promising with regard to the creation of an optimal cell environment and thereby suppression of the foreign body reaction.

Biocompatibility of Polymers Used for Cardiovascular Applications

Interactions of Tissue- and Blood-Cells with the Polymer Surface Material

Diagnostic and therapeutical treatments implicate the contact between tissue, blood and the implanted material. In the cardiovascular field, a variety of biomaterial is implanted in heart and vessels, such as catheters, stents, heart valves and sondes for pacemakers and defibrillators. Using polymers for new technologies has been a revolutionary advance in the therapy of cardiovascular disease [47]. Nevertheless, there is increasing evidence that the polymer coating could be responsible for adverse effects (e.g. in-stent-restenosis, stent thrombosis, chronicle foreign body reactions). Therefore, a feasible biocompatible material should provide a complete re-endothelialisation of the surface, less thrombogenicity as well as anti-inflammatory properties in order to improve clinical outcomes.

Implantation of a polymer device into a vessel or tissue causes a complex inflammatory response inducing adhesive interactions between vascular cells (blood and tissue cells). During stenting, the endothelial layer is partially or completely destroyed. In animal experiments of vascular injury, denudation of endothelial cells results in platelet deposition followed by neointima formation [188–190]. In addition, complete coverage of endothelial cells is associated with attenuation or even stop of the growth of neointima from smooth muscle cells in the injured arterial segment [191, 192]. A poor endothelialisation promotes platelet aggregation, thrombus formation and stent-thrombosis. Therefore, the process of re-endothelialisation on the surface material requires sufficient biocompatible qualities of the underneath laying polymer surface. Recent studies have been demonstrated that proliferation, viability and function of endothelial cells, e.g. production of endothelial NO synthase, are dependent on the polymer surface [193, 194].

After stenting smooth muscle cells undergo complex phenotypic changes including migration and proliferation from the media towards the intima, and transition from a contractile to a synthetic phenotype [195]. Additionally, the release of cytokines and growth factors from white blood cells can induce increased smooth muscle cell growth and accumulation within the intima (neointima formation) leading to in-stent-restenosis.

Platelet adhesion and leukocyte rolling on injured endothelium are key events of this multistep process leading to platelet-leukocyte interaction, aggregation and activation of the coagulation cascade. Leukocyte rolling is mainly mediated by selectins (e.g. P-selectin) which interact with the leukocyte PSGL-1 receptor and by integrins (e.g. Mac-1) [196]. In terms of hemocompatibility, it is conceivable that slow rolling supports adhesion strengthening and spreading of polymorphnuclear cells and thus worsening hemocompatibility. Following monocyte adhesion and transmigration mediated by integrins, monocytes and monocyte-derived macrophages then secrete proinflammatory cytokines. These reactions can lead to chronic inflammatory responses. Chronic inflammation has been described as foreign body reaction where monocytes, macrophages and foreign body giant cells are present at the biomaterial interface for longer than 2 weeks [197]. Recent data from Busch et al. suggest differences in leukocyte activation and monocyte adhesion among various polymers (unpublished data). An explanation for this observation could be that biomaterials can modulate monocyte paracrine interactions to influence monocyte adhesion and viability [198]. Cohen et al. [199] demonstrated differences in monocyte activity on poly(ethylene glycol) hydrogels, poly(dimethyl siloxane), and tissue culture polystyrene in cultures with conditioned medium priming. Khandwekar et al. compared leukocyte adhesion on bare PCL surfaces and modulated PCL surfaces. They showed that leukocyte adhesion on bare PCL could even be more reduced when converting to a heparin-modified PCL [200].

Although red blood cells (erythrocytes) play only a minimal role in wound healing and blood-biomaterial interactions, the contact of red blood cells with the material can lead to hemolysis. Hemolysis is the breakage of the erythrocyte's membrane with the release of intracellular hemoglobin. Normally, red blood cells live for 110–120 days. After that, they naturally break down and are removed from the circulation by the spleen. Some diseases and medical devices cause red blood cells to break too soon requiring the bone marrow to accelerate the regeneration of red blood cells (erythropoesis). Medical devices for hemodialysis, heart-lung-bypass machines or mechanical heart valves induce more hemolysis than smaller implants like stents or catheters [201].

Testing Bio- and Hemo-compatibility of Polymers

Biocompatibility determines the interface reactions of blood and tissue cells with the surface of the biomaterial. In this context, the term "hemocompatibility" mainly refers to blood component reactions during contact with the biomaterial [202]. It is of great importance to test various polymer characteristics in detail before developing the elaborated design for in vivo application. Over the past years, a variety of methods have been established to determine hemo- and biocompatibility of polymer implants. In this chapter a summary of standardized and new methods is provided.

Complementary Perfusion Systems

Cell interactions with polymers are usually studied using cell culture techniques. In vitro evaluation of surface materials by directly seeding endothelial cells (ECs) and smooth muscle cells (SMCs) onto the biopolymers represents a common procedure to assess biocompatibility and cytotoxicity as well as cell morphology [203–205]. In this context, most in vitro studies analyzing the impact of material on tissue cells involve experiments under static conditions. However, in healthy vessels especially ECs are exposed to the blood stream. This pulsatile, laminar blood flow exerts shear stress on vascular endothelium, which induces anti-apoptotic signals and maintains an anti-inflammatory and non-thrombotic endothelial phenotype compared to ECs cultured under static conditions [206, 207]. Cell culture experiments represent a model in which one can study specific mechanisms involved in the biologic responses of blood and tissue cells to materials. During the last decades a variety of techniques has been developed to investigate vascular biology under hemodynamic conditions.

Parallel Plate Flow Chamber. The parallel plate flow chamber (PPFC) is a design most frequently used to study vascular cells under flow conditions. Here, cell culture media is circulated through the chamber at adjustable flow rates creating a defined laminar flow (Fig. 15.2).

A typical flow chamber consists of a polycarbonate corpus (bottom), a silicone gasket, which defines height and length of the flow channel (side walls) and a glass cover slip (top), which can be replaced by polymer foils. Under static cell culture conditions, the coverslip can be seeded with the cells of interest prior to the flow experiment. Additionally, these flow chambers are designed to allow fluorescence microscopic observation of a perfused cell layer. In this context PPFCs are suitable to measure the kinetics of cell attachment, detachment, and rolling on surfaces under flow conditions. Therefore, a range of studies refers to the adhesion of leukocytes and platelets on endothelial cells [208, 209]. Recently, Busch et al. [193] published a study which assessed a range of endothelial parameters in interaction with different stent materials using an in vitro perfusion system. However, these kind of experiments are limited by the rectangular geometry of the flow channel and do only allow for the investigation of cell monolayers over several hours.

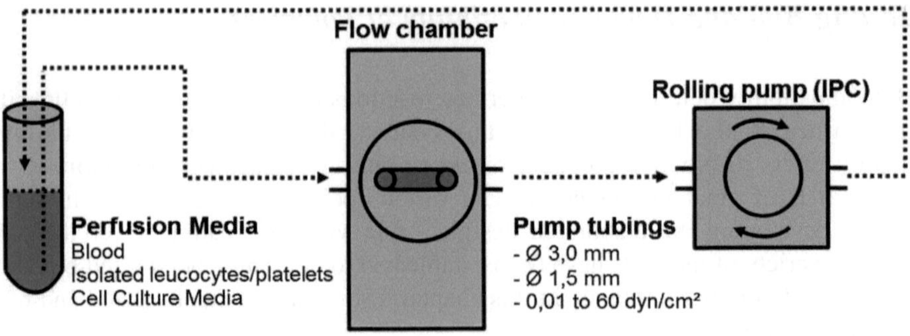

Fig. 15.2 Schematic diagram of an in vitro perfusion system for laminar shear stress conditions. Flow chamber contains the biomaterial with cultivated cells (e.g. HUVECs). Perfusion with full blood, isolated leukocytes, platelets or cell culture media. Rolling pump applies various volume rates. After perfusion, the perfused cells on the biomaterial (e.g. proliferation, vitality, PCR, Western blotting) and the supernatant (e.g. flow cytometry, ELISA) should be analyzed

Live Cell Imaging. To investigate the influence of the substrate regarding endothelial cell morphology in particular, it might be advisable to culture endothelial cells under flow conditions for several days. For that purpose, a specially designed *sticky-slide* (ibidi) can be utilized [210]. Different substrates can be mounted to the bottomless channel slide, which has been developed for microscopic applications. The slide can then be connected to the ibidi pump system and kept sterile for several days in a conventional incubator. Additionally, for example the cytoskeleton can be visualized and changes in morphology due to the substrate can be monitored by microscopic methods.

Tube Chamber System. To overcome the limitations of 2D cell culture models vessel-simulating bioreactors have been developed. Typically, a 3D bioreactor consists of a graft with an individual culture media reservoir to allow a transversal gas and media exchange between the perfused graft lumen and the outer chamber volume which simulates the interstitial tissue liquid. The porous graft (e.g. silicone, PTFE) is seeded with cells and the culture media is perfused through the construct. This procedure allows the in vitro cultivation of endothelial cells under fluid flow and results in a synthetic vessel [210, 211]. A special modification of a vessel-simulating flow-through cell has been developed by Neubert et al. and is particularly suitable for the evaluation of drug release and distribution from drug-eluting stents [212–214].

Cell Adhesion, Proliferation, and Cytotoxicity

To investigate cell material interactions, cultured cells are seeded on the polymer surfaces of interest and the extent of cell adhesion, proliferation, and viability is measured by standardized assays. Although in vitro experiments do not entirely reproduce the whole range of cellular responses to the implanted material, these methods provide a level of quantification which cannot be easily obtained in vivo.

Cell adhesion. For most applications the adhesion of cells is of fundamental interest being the initial event of cell attachment. A simple method to quantify adherent cells is to incubate cells over a surface for a period of time subsequently followed by the detachment of loosely adherent cells by gently washing the surface. Remaining cells can be labeled by fluorescent dyes and quantified using fluorescent measurements. Cell adhesion assays are also frequently used to assess monocyte or platelet adhesion on polymeric surfaces [215, 216]. In this context Hezi-Yamit et al. [217] did show that polymer hydrophilicity should be considered as a parameter to assess the biocompatibility of polymer surfaces. They showed that hydrophobic polymers such as PBMA or SIBS promote the adhesion of inflammatory activated monocytes while more hydrophilic polymers (e.g. PC (Phosphorylcholine) polymer) lead to less pro-inflammatory responses.

Cell proliferation. Endothelial growth is an essential factor after implantation. A continuous and healthy endothelial layer only prevents inflammatory and thrombotic events on the vessel wall. Besides, a healthy endothelium is crucial for regulating smooth muscle cell growth [218, 219]. Cell proliferation can be assessed by commercially available BrdU ELISA assay kits. On the basis of the study by Busch et al. [193] proliferation of ECs on hydrophobic permanent polymers (PEVA, PBMA) as well as biodegradable polymers [PLLA, P(4HB)] is reduced, whereas the polymeric blend PLLA/P(4HB) promotes EC growth. Data from this study do also show that SMC proliferation is influenced in the same way as EC growth and none of the polymers tested is able to enhance endothelial proliferation by simultaneously reducing smooth muscle cell growth.

Cytotoxicity. The determination of potential cytotoxicity is an important aspect of biomaterial testing standards such as ISO and ASTM (American Society for Testing and Materials), but does not provide a sufficient assertion regarding the biocompatibility of a biomaterial [220]. Cell viability is commonly determined with the MTT assay or the incorporation of resazurin. Both methods depend of the reduction of a non-fluorescent dye by enzymes of living cells. In a comprehensive study, the influence of several polymer films frequently used for coatings as well as newly developed polymers on endothelial and smooth muscle cell viability has been tested. Especially synthetic polymers such as PEVA and PBMA, but also biodegradable polyester P(4HB) show a significantly reduced cell viability, whereas PLLA and a polymeric blend PLLA/P(4HB) achieved better results than the control surface Thermanox™. Interestingly, under flow conditions only the polymeric blend PLLA/P(4HB) gained advantage over the control surface [193].

Endothelial Cell Function and Morphology

Developing of a polymer material as a medical implant also requires the investigation of the influence on endothelial cell function and gene expression [221, 222]. In healthy vessels the endothelial glycocalyx functions as a vasculoprotective layer on the luminal surface of ECs by sensing fluid flow and thereby, inducing endothelial NO synthase and NO release [223]. The study of Busch et al. [193]

underlines that common methods to assess cell adhesion, proliferation, and cytotoxicity under static conditions alone are not always sufficient to investigate the biocompatibility of polymer surfaces. For example P(3HB) shows an enhanced proliferation of ECs and SMCs as well as a reasonable cell viability under static conditions. However, under dynamic conditions cell viability is poor. Furthermore, the glycocalyx measured by fluorescence microscopy is augmented and clumpy indicating a disturbed endothelial function. However, ECs grown on PLLA based polymers show a high proliferation rate, excellent viability under static and dynamic conditions accompanied by a glycocalyx width within physiological range, which results in an enhanced gene expression of endothelial NO synthase under static and dynamic conditions.

The chemical and topographical properties of vascular implants are increasingly recognized as important cues having an impact on the response of vascular cells in vitro in terms of adhesion, proliferation, viability, migration, differentiation, and mechanotransduction signaling (e.g. endothelial NO synthase, PECAM-1) [224]. Cells attach to the polymer surface via focal adhesion point, connecting the cytoskeleton to the polymer surface. The formation of these interfaces can be affected indirectly by the topographical cues through orienting or organizing the cytoskeleton and polarizing cells with different functional behavior [225, 226]. Only recently atomic force microscopy (AFM) techniques have emerged to be suitable for probing micro- and nanomechanical properties of cell structures. This technique can be used to measure the elastic properties of cells adhered to different surfaces [227, 228].

Hemolysis Testing

Hemolytic activity is a requirement to be tested for any blood contacting medical devices. Many factors can induce hemolysis, such as shear forces, chemicals and the material/polymer itself [229]. The hemolytic activity of polymers has been investigated since decades. In 1975, Dillingham et al. [230] described in their article "Biological activation of polymers" hemolysis testing. Hemolysis is regarded as an especially significant screening test, which may not be measurable under in vivo conditions. There is however no clear consensus on the procedures of hemolysis testing due to insufficient comparative studies on the quality of the red blood cells used and the experimental conditions of testing. Henkelman et al. determined the effects of a number of incubation variables on the sensitivity and reproducibility of the hemolysis test using positively as well as negatively responding biomaterials and compared these results to those obtained according to the American Society for Testing and Materials (ASTM) standard [231]. According to ASTM F 756-00 [231] materials can be classified in three different categories according to their hemolytic index (hemolysis %). Materials with percentages of hemolysis over 5 % are considered hemolytic; while the ones with hemolytic index between 5 and 2 % are classified as slightly hemolytic. Finally, when the material presents a hemolysis percentage below 2 % it is considered as a non-hemolytic material.

Although a blood-compatible polymer should be non- or less-hemolytic, in practice several medical devices can cause hemolysis. Nevertheless, when hemolytic effects take place, it is important that the values of hemolysis are within acceptable limits and clinical benefits overcome the remaining risks.

A lot of studies performing hemolysis testing, like the work of Fischer et al. [232] refer to the method according to Parnham and Wetzig [233]: Whoole blood, collected in heparinized-tubes, from Wistar rats, is centrifugated, the pellet washed with PBS pH 7.4 and resuspended. The suspension of red blood cells is freshly to be prepared and used within 24 h. Polymers are added to the erythrocytes and incubated for 60 min at 37 °C. The release of hemoglobin is determinded by photometric analysis. Complete hemolysis is achieved using 0.2 % Triton X-100 yielding the 100 % control value.

Plasma Protein Adsorption

Proteins are a main constituent of blood plasma, e.g. with plasma concentrations ranging from 35 to 50 mg/ml for serum albumin and only 0–5 pg/ml for interleukin [234]. They are mediating for instance cell-cell interactions, coagulations cascade and inflammatory processes. Proteins can adsorb on the polymer, resulting in a surface protein layer with a thickness of 2–10 nm [235]. Adsorbed proteins are not bound indefinitely to the surface and the compositions may change over time. This phenomenon called Vroman effect occurs mainly on negatively charged hydrophilic surfaces [198]. Hydrophilicity has been described as a key determinant for the protein adsorption process. It has been known that hydrophobic surfaces (e.g. hydrophobic polymer) adsorb more proteins than hydrophilic surfaces (e.g. hydrophilic polymer). Surface hydrophilicity can be determined by static and dynamic water contact angle with water of more than 65° [236]. Protein and surface charge as well as conformational changes in protein structures have also been described as potential mechanisms for protein adsorption on polymers and may affect the biological activity of the protein. Several approaches for studying protein adsorption have been described. Hlady et al. [236] review various challenging methods like solution depletion techniques, optical (ellipsometry, variable angle reflectometry, surface plasmon resonance), spectroscopic, autoradiography and microscopic techniques.

Platelet Activation, Adhesion and Aggregation

Platelets adhere to polymeric surfaces through interaction with fibrinogen, von Willebrand factor, vitronectin and fibronectin [237]. The kinetics of platelet adhesion to artificial surfaces have been revealed to be very rapid and initiation of adhesion takes place in less than 5 s for hydrophobic surfaces and less than 30 s for hydrophilic surfaces. Platelet adhesion and aggregation, as a marker of prothrombotic potential of polymers, can be visualized by exposing human platelets to polymers [193]. In this study platelet adhesion and aggregation was visualized by SEM imaging and adjacent quantitative analysis. Besides that, platelet morphology on the polymer surface could be assessed. For instance, platelets adhered to PEVA, a biostable polymer, appeared conspicuous without any formation of pseudopodia whereas platelets on PLLA showed normal activated states. Furthermore, platelet activation can be evaluated by the release of soluble P-selectin, and collagen-induced platelet aggregation by the method of Born [238]. A further method to assess activation on polymers is the determination of platelet surface expression of cell adhesion molecules using flow cytometry (FACS). After dynamic perfusion of a physiologically concentrated leukocyte-platelet mixture over polymer surfaces, expression of CD 42b (GP Ib) which exhibits platelet activation can be determined by FACS analysis. GP Ib belongs to the GP Ib-IX-V complex which binds to the von Willebrand factor and facilitates initial platelet adhesion to endothelial cells on sites of vascular injury [196]. Expression of CD 62P (P-selectin), a cell adhesion molecule on the surface of activated platelets, can be used as marker for leukocyte-platelet aggregates, because activated platelets bind via P-selectin to the leukocyte receptor PSGL-1 [196].

Leukocyte Rolling and Adhesion

Injury induced during polymer implantation initiates an inflammatory response resulting in adhesion and extravasation of polymorphnuclear leukocytes to the implant site. Leukocyte rolling on the inner layer of the vessel wall is one of the first steps in this complex process. Therefore, it could be meaningful to measure leukocyte rolling velocity on polymer surfaces to estimate adherence of these blood cells to the material. In this regard, Goldmann and Lawrence introduced the definition of critical velocity implying the assumption that interaction between adhesion molecules takes place when a leukocyte moves with 70 % of the velocity of a freely moving leukocyte with the same distance from the vessel wall [239, 240]. In a recent study, leukocyte velocity on fibronectin coated bioabsorbable polymers was faster than on a Thermanox control surface (unpublished data) and only the minority of leukocytes roll on the flow channel when a shear stress of 1.5–5 dyne/cm^2 was applied. After hemodynamic perfusion, monocyte adhesion to the polymer surfaces can be determined using fluorescence microscopy of CD14+ stained cells. Despite leukocyte-platelet interactions are involved in tissue inflammation and thrombosis, especially after deposition of an implant/stent which leads to denudation of the vessel wall. There is only less research experience in evaluating leukocyte-platelet interactions with surface material. CD 11b/CD 18 (Mac-1) represents leukocyte activation as this receptor supports interactions with platelets and endothelial cells. Chang and Gorbet [241] showed that CD11b and leukocyte-platelet aggregates were upregulated upon contact with metal surfaces at pathological shear conditions. Another study investigated the effect of different synthetic polymers on CD11b/CD18 expression and the interactions between leukocytes and platelets [242].

Selected Own Examples

Polymer-Based Biodegradable Stent Platforms

Until today, several different degradable materials, both polymeric and metallic, with a broad range of mechanical properties and degradation times have been proposed for the application in absorbable stents. Among these developments are self-expanding fiber-based stents from PDLLA, PLLA and PLGA [243, 244] and balloon-expandable fiber-based stents from PLLA, polydioxanone, and poly(glycolide-co-ε-caprolactone) [245–247]. In own studies, we investigated the development of balloon-expandable slotted-tube stents based on different PLLA blend combinations. Extensive materials testing was performed regarding the thermo-mechanical and physico-chemical properties of different PLLA-based polymer blends. Results reveal that the addition of 22 % P(4HB) to PLLA allows the generation of a biodegradable polymeric stent with rapid expansion, low recoil, and high collapse pressure required for safe vascular stent application [248]. For instance, comparison of the tensile properties of the PLLA/P(4HB) blend with the cited PLLA tensile data [249] illustrates that the addition of 22 % P(4HB) to PLLA lowers the elastic modulus and the tensile strength by approx. 52 and 20 %, while elongation to break increases approximately 16-fold. Moreover, recorded DSC data indicate a marked reduction of crystallinity of the PLLA phase by approx. 49 % in the blended material compared to the referenced crystallinity data for pure PLLA [250]. Performed in vitro drug release studies reveal that the steady molecular weight decrease of the PLLA/P(4HB) blend material (60 % after 24 weeks) is more pronounced than with pure high molecular weight PLLA (28 % after 24 weeks) [249]. This accelerated degradation of the PLLA/P(4HB) blend material can be probably attributed in part to the lower molecular weight P(4HB) blend component, the lowered glass transition and the lower degree of crystallinity of the polymer blend, as compared to pure PLLA. Besides the mechanical properties biocompatibility of the stent platform was additionally improved by addition of the absorbable polyester P(4HB) as a blend partner. In an own recently published biocompatibility study of polymers including the two established biostable polymers used for drug-eluting stents PEVA and PBMA as well as the biodegradable polyester PLLA, P(3HB), P(4HB) and the above described blend of PLLA/P(4HB) in a ratio of 78/22 % (w/w), we could show, that only the polymeric blend of PLLA/P(4HB) achieved excellent endothelial markers of biocompatibility [193]. Moreover, data show that PLLA and P(4HB) tend to a more thrombotic response whereas the polymer blend is characterized by a lower thrombotic potential. Animal testing of this stent platform and a sirolimus-eluting version, which was subsequently developed, was performed in domestic pigs as an anastomotic support stent in the iliac artery. In this model the stent platform demonstrated patency and integrity over a follow-up time of 6 weeks under dual antiplatelet therapy with acetylsalicylic acid and clopidogrel with marked reduction of inflammation and neointimal growth for the DES [38, 251].

DES Equipped with Biodegradable Polymeric Coatings

Currently, a number of polymer coating materials, both biodegradable and non-degradable, as well as different drug classes, including anti-inflammatory compounds or immunomodulators, anti-proliferative agents, or drugs with effect on cell migration and extracellular matrix production, and drugs that promote vascular healing and re-endothelialization are under consideration [13]. In our own published studies, absorbable polymer stent coatings based on PLLA were developed. This research focused on the one hand on physicochemical characterization of the obtained coating with regard to morphology and the impact of processing parameters on polymer degradation [132] and on the other hand on the establishment of novel dual drug-eluting stents (DDES) with an abluminally focussed release of the potent anti-proliferative drug sirolimus and a luminally focussed release of atorvastatin with stabilizing effect on atherosclerotic deposits and stimulating impact on endothelial function [252]. During physicochemical characterization of established PLLA coatings, we observed that achieved structural integrity via a spray-coating process was maintained after crimping and full expansion of stent prototypes. Despite the fact that solution cast PLLA films exhibit high brittleness and low flexibility expansion of stents was obviously possible without evident coating cracking or delamination. In this study, we could furthermore confirm literature data [253, 254], by evidencing considerable loss of PLLAs molecular weight and increase in crystallinity upon irradiation sterilization. Thus coating mass of sterilized stents in an accelerated in vitro degradation study at 70 °C in phosphate buffer began to decrease earlier (after 14 days) as compared to the unsterile specimens (after 28 days). However, the rates of molecular weight reduction and mass loss of PLLA were found to be the same for unsterile and sterilized samples. The observed difference can be therefore dedicated to the initial difference in molecular weight, which already started to decrease with time for both specimen at the beginning of the degradation study. With these results, we could underline literature [255] that hydrolysis of PLLA proceeds in two steps. First a reduction of the polymer chain length by randomly distributed cleavage of ester bonds, without the formation of soluble components, takes place. In the second step of the degradation process actual mass loss and release of degradation products occurs.

The more recent study on DDES [253] presents in contrast an adapted spray-coating process for PLLA coatings allowing the formation of smooth form-fit polymer coatings at the abluminal and luminal side with 70 % respectively 90 % of the drug/polymer solution being deposited at the intended stent surface (Fig. 15.3). Although having a focus on in vitro drug release studies of the developed DDES, some important findings with regard to the PLLA coating were also made. In this context, we found that the total drug fraction released was more than doubled for sterilized DDES, tempered at 40 °C and even decupled for DDES tempered at 80 °C independently of sterilization in comparison to unsterile DDES, tempered at 40 °C. While no considerable differences are observed in molecular weight and the degree of crystallinity, which could be the reason of altered drug release

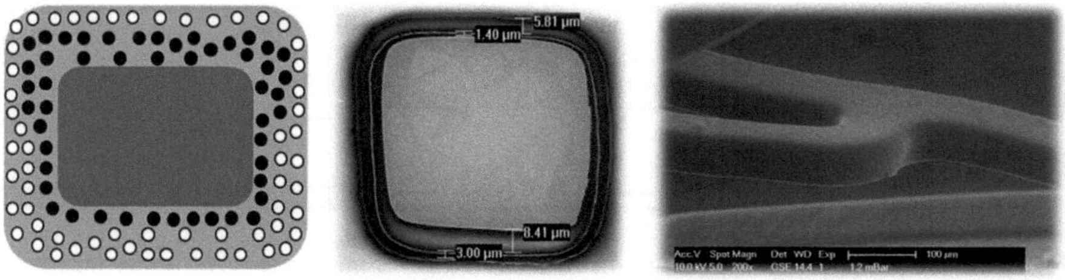

Fig. 15.3 Design of the dual drug-eluting stent. From *left* to *right* schematic representation of the dual drug-eluting stent, representative optical microscopy image of one representative strut cross section, representative electron micrograph

profiles, DSC-curves revealed the complete disappearance of the glass transition for sterilized and non-sterilized PLLA coatings, tempered at 80 °C. In accordance to literature, we possibly observe the densification of the amorphous phase and the increase of a so-called rigid amorphous fraction without change in the crystalline fraction [256, 257]. This might be associated with the formation of a non-linear drug distribution through the sample and partition towards the surface or within the mobile amorphous phase of the polymer due to exclusion from crystalline and rigid amorphous phases. As both mechanisms would lead to drug supersaturation in confined regions, drug release would be accelerated in comparison to samples, tempered at 40 °C with more homogeneous drug distribution. In summary, both studies highlight the importance of processing parameters for characteristics of the polymer coating and the resulting drug delivery properties.

DCB Equipped with Hydrogel-Based Coatings

Conventional DCB systems are often associated with considerable drug wash-off rates during transit of the device through the vascular system. For instance, Kelsch et al. [258] reported paclitaxel wash-off rates of up to 26–36 % for urea- or iopromide-based DCB, respectively, during an in vitro passage through a hemostatic valve and a guiding catheter. Having in mind that many of these interventional cardiovascular devices already incorporate a hydrophilic lubricious coating in order to ease movement through the vasculature [259, 260], we propose the use of the same hydrophilic coating as drug reservoir and transfer agent for DCB. When exposed to aqueous environments, these lubricious coatings may absorb a multiple of times its dry weight in water. One can hence presume that a previously embedded lipophilic drug as paclitaxel will be protected from elution until the coating is compressed leading to simultaneous release of water and drug. The envisaged mechanism is illustrated in Fig. 15.4.

In this regards, we investigated the use of the body-own and hence highly biocompatible biopolymer HA [18] and the pharmaceutically well-established synthetic polymer PVP [17] as drug reservoir and transfer agent for DCB. In both

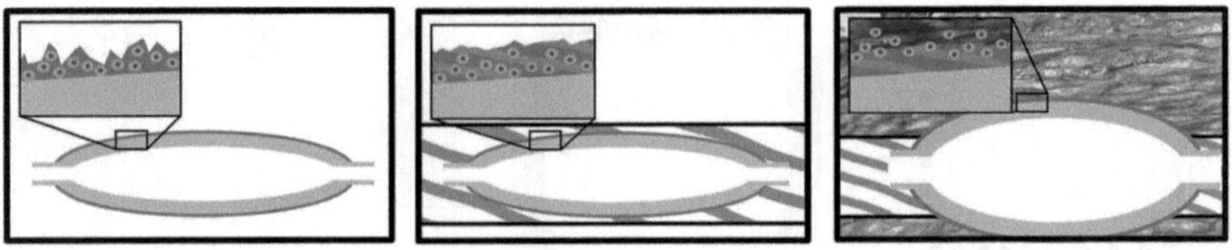

Fig. 15.4 Concept of hydrogel-based matrices for DCB. From *left* to *right* stable incorporation of drug within dry hydrogel on balloon surface, swelling of the hydrogel without loss of lipophilic drug upon balloon insertion to the vasculature, compression of the hydrogel and drug transfer to vessel wall upon balloon dilatation

cases we could show that crosslinking was essential for coating stability. While an inexpensive and biocompatible UV radiation process was applied for PVP, HA was crosslinked via different chemical crosslinking agents. Both methods afford drug incorporation after the crosslinking process due to possible photodecomposition during PVP crosslinking and involvement in polymerization during HA crosslinking, respectively. Moreover, crosslinking conditions have a considerable impact on drug delivery characteristics. For the PVP coating, we could show that short radiation times did not provide enough coating stability, associated with high wash off rates during DCB insertion and long radiation times lowered drug transfer efficiency upon balloon expansion. A 10 min radiation of PVP combined a minimized drug wash off rate of 34 % with an efficient drug transfer of 49 %, underlining the high potential of photochemically crosslinked PVP as coating matrix for DCB. Accordingly, the applied HA crosslinking procedure also influences transfer and release of paclitaxel. While crosslinking of HA with N-(3-dimethylaminopropyl)-N′-ethylcarbodiimide hydrochloride, yielding a rather low degree of crosslinking, provided coatings which allowed for an efficient paclitaxel transfer upon expansion in a vessel model, crosslinking with glutardialdehyde with a higher degree of crosslinking resulted in a slower drug release being more appropriate for implants with longer residence time in the body. Besides the application of hydrogels as matrix for DCB, their adjustability concerning the drug delivery characteristics can be considered as highly interesting for implant-associated LDD-systems in general.

Summary

The biological response to polymers as biomaterial is largely controlled by their surface chemistry and structure. Therefore, surface modification reactions, which should mediate the polymer-biological system interactions with the purpose of improved tissue-interface related-biocompatibility without modifying the mechanical properties and functionality of the device, are required. In principal, there are two categories which either involve the overcoating of an existing surface or the chemical altering of atoms, compounds or molecules in the existing surface. In this context and with regard to the application field of cardiology, we review coating technologies for the provision of cardiovascular implants with a polymer-based drug-delivery function and chemical surface modification for improved endothelialization. While we give an overview of the different control mechanisms and the applied polymers for polymer-based drug delivery systems, we provide information on surface activation and biofunctionalization techniques applied on the different polymers used in cardiology. The development of innovative polymer-based biodegradable implants and devices for cardiovascular applications moreover requires standardized as well as newly adapted methods for testing bio- and hemo-compatibility. In this context, we provide information on complementary in vitro perfusion systems, which should be used in order to provide physiological flow conditions. Besides the classical biocompatibility read-out parameter proliferation, cell function and vitality, tests for platelet adhesion, aggregation and leukocyte interactions become more and more important to account for clinical complications as thrombosis and chronical tissue reactions. Furthermore, the influence of polymer surface modifications should be addressed in future studies by for instance atomic force microscopy. After the presentation of theses test methods, we finally highlight own recent polymer-based developments for biodegradable coatings for DES with a dual drug delivery function, for stent platforms and for DCB matrices based on hydrogels.

References

1. Nair, L.S., Laurencin, C.T.: Biodegradable polymers as biomaterials. Prog. Polym. Sci. **32**, 762–798 (2007). doi:10.1016/j.progpolymsci.2007.05.017
2. Tian, H., Tang, Z., Zhuang, X., et al.: Biodegradable synthetic polymers: preparation, functionalization and biomedical application. Prog. Polym. Sci. **37**, 237–280 (2012). doi:10.1016/j.progpolymsci.2011.06.004
3. Venkatraman, S., Boey, F., Lao, L.L.: Implanted cardiovascular polymers: natural, synthetic and bio-inspired. Prog. Polym. Sci. **33**, 853–874 (2008). doi:10.1016/j.progpolymsci.2008.07.001
4. Lendlein, A., Hofmann, D., Scharnagl, N.: Abbaubare polymere in der medizin. Nachr. Aus. Chem. **59**, 117–120 (2011). doi:10.1515/NACHRCHEM.2011.59.2.117
5. Werner, C.: Nanomaterialien im Blut- und Gewebekontakt. Chem. Ing. Tech. **80**, 1661–1670 (2008). doi:10.1002/cite.200800109
6. Luxenhofer, R., Groll, J.: Makromolekulare Chemie 2010. Nachr. Aus. Chem. **59**, 324–334 (2011). doi:10.1515/NACHRCHEM.2011.59.3.324
7. Windecker, S., Meier, B.: Late coronary stent thrombosis. Circulation **116**, 1952–1965 (2007). doi:10.1161/CIRCULATIONAHA.106.683995
8. Farb, A., Burke, A.P., Kolodgie, F.D., Virmani, R.: Pathological mechanisms of fatal late coronary stent thrombosis in humans. Circulation **108**, 1701–1706 (2003). doi:10.1161/01.CIR.0000091115.05480.B0
9. Joner, M., Finn, A.V., Farb, A., et al.: Pathology of drug-eluting stents in humans: delayed healing and late thrombotic risk. J. Am. Coll. Cardiol. **48**, 193–202 (2006). doi:10.1016/j.jacc.2006.03.042
10. Lanzer, P., Sternberg, K., Schmitz, K.-P., et al.: Drug-eluting coronary stent very late thrombosis revisited. Herz **33**, 334–342 (2008). doi:10.1007/s00059-008-3080-x
11. Nebeker, J.R., Virmani, R., Bennett, C.L., et al.: Hypersensitivity cases associated with drug-eluting coronary stents: a review of available cases from the Research on Adverse Drug Events and Reports (RADAR) project. J. Am. Coll. Cardiol. **47**, 175–181 (2006). doi:10.1016/j.jacc.2005.07.071

12. Virmani, R., Kolodgie, F.D., Farb, A.: Drug-eluting stents: are they really safe? Am. Heart. Hosp. J **2**, 85–88 (2004). doi:10.1111/j.1541-9215.2004.03632.x
13. Garg, S., Serruys, P.W.: Coronary stents: looking forward. J. Am. Coll. Cardiol. **56**, S43–S78 (2010). doi:10.1016/j.jacc.2010.06.008
14. Grabow, N., Martin, D.P., Schmitz, K.-P., Sternberg, K.: Absorbable polymer stent technologies for vascular regeneration. J. Chem. Technol. Biotechnol. **85**, 744–751 (2010). doi:10.1002/jctb.2282
15. Sun, D., Zheng, Y., Yin, T., et al.: Coronary drug-eluting stents: from design optimization to newer strategies. J. Biomed. Mater. Res. A **102**, 1625–1640 (2014). doi:10.1002/jbm.a.34806
16. Berg, M.C., Kolodziej, H., Cremers, B., et al.: Drug-coated angioplasty balloon catheters: coating compositions and methods. Adv. Eng. Mater. **14**, B45–B50 (2012). doi:10.1002/adem.201180067
17. Petersen, S., Minrath, I., Kaule, S., et al.: Development and in vitro characterization of photochemically crosslinked polyvinylpyrrolidone coatings for drug-coated balloons. Coat. **3**, 253–267 (2013). doi:10.3390/coatings3040253
18. Petersen, S., Kaule, S., Teske, M., et al.: Development and in vitro characterization of hyaluronic acid-based coatings for implant-associated local drug delivery systems. J. Chem. (2013). doi:10.1155/2013/587875
19. Rippel, R.A., Ghanbari, H., Seifalian, A.M.: Tissue-engineered heart valve: future of cardiac surgery. World J. Surg. **36**, 1581–1591 (2012). doi:10.1007/s00268-012-1535-y
20. Rahmani, B., Burriesci, G., Mullen, M., Seifalian, A., Tzamtzis, S., Yap, J.: A new generation transcatheter heart valve with a novel nanocomposite material and fully retrievable design. J. Am. Coll. Cardiol. **60**(17), B34–B34 (2012). doi: 10.1016/j.jacc.2012.08.126
21. Heim, F., Durand, B., Chakfe, N.: Textile for heart valve prostheses: fabric long-term durability testing. J. Biomed. Mater. Res. B Appl. Biomater. **92**, 68–77 (2010). doi:10.1002/jbm.b.31490
22. Heim, F., Durand, B., Chafke, N.: Textile heart valve prosthesis: from fabric design criteria to early in-vivo performances. J. Heart Valve Dis. **22**, 361–367 (2013)
23. Rahmani, B., Tzamtzis, S., Ghanbari, H., et al.: Manufacturing and hydrodynamic assessment of a novel aortic valve made of a new nanocomposite polymer. J. Biomech. **45**, 1205–1211 (2012). doi:10.1016/j.jbiomech.2012.01.046
24. Parizek, M., Slepickova Kasalkova, N., Bacakova, L., et al.: Adhesion, growth, and maturation of vascular smooth muscle cells on low-density polyethylene grafted with bioactive substances. BioMed. Res. Int. **2013**, e371430 (2013). doi:10.1155/2013/371430
25. Ko, N.R., Sabbatier, G., Cunningham, A., et al.: Air-spun PLA nanofibers modified with reductively sheddable hydrophilic surfaces for vascular tissue engineering: synthesis and surface modification. Macromol. Rapid Commun. **35**, 447–453 (2014). doi:10.1002/marc.201300609
26. Theron, J.P., Knoetze, J.H., Sanderson, R.D., et al.: Modification, crosslinking and reactive electrospinning of a thermoplastic medical polyurethane for vascular graft applications. Acta Biomater. **6**, 2434–2447 (2010). doi:10.1016/j.actbio.2010.01.013
27. Hu, Z., Li, Z., Hu, L., et al.: The in vivo performance of small-caliber nanofibrous polyurethane vascular grafts. BMC Cardiovasc. Disord. **12**, 115 (2012). doi:10.1186/1471-2261-12-115
28. He, W., Hu, Z., Xu, A., et al.: The preparation and performance of a new polyurethane vascular prosthesis. Cell Biochem. Biophys. **66**, 855–866 (2013). doi:10.1007/s12013-013-9528-5
29. Han, J., Farah, S., Domb, A.J., Lelkes, P.I.: Electrospun rapamycin-eluting polyurethane fibers for vascular grafts. Pharm. Res. **30**, 1735–1748 (2013). doi:10.1007/s11095-013-1016-5
30. Pillai, C.K.S., Sharma, C.P.: Review paper: absorbable polymeric surgical sutures: chemistry, production, properties, biodegradability, and performance. J. Biomater. Appl. **25**, 291–366 (2010). doi:10.1177/0885328210384890

31. Hajiali, H., Shahgasempour, S., Naimi-Jamal, M.R., Peirovi, H.: Electrospun PGA/gelatin nanofibrous scaffolds and their potential application in vascular tissue engineering. Int. J. Nanomed. **6**, 2133–2141 (2011). doi:10.2147/IJN.S24312
32. Diban, N., Haimi, S., Bolhuis-Versteeg, L., et al.: Hollow fibers of poly(lactide-co-glycolide) and poly(ε-caprolactone) blends for vascular tissue engineering applications. Acta Biomater. **9**, 6450–6458 (2013). doi:10.1016/j.actbio.2013.01.005
33. Yi, F., Wu, H., Jia, G.-L.: Formulation and characterization of poly (D, L-lactide-co-glycolide) nanoparticle containing vascular endothelial growth factor for gene delivery. J. Clin. Pharm. Ther. **31**, 43–48 (2006). doi:10.1111/j.1365-2710.2006.00702.x
34. Yehia, S.A., Elshafeey, A.H., Elsayed, I.: A novel injectable in situ forming poly-DL-lactide and DL-lactide/glycolide implant containing lipospheres for controlled drug delivery. J. Liposome Res. **22**, 128–138 (2012). doi:10.3109/08982104.2011.631141
35. Amjadi, I., Rabiee, M., Hosseini, M.S., Mozafari, M.: Synthesis and characterization of doxorubicin-loaded poly(lactide-co-glycolide) nanoparticles as a sustained-release anticancer drug delivery system. Appl. Biochem. Biotechnol. **168**, 1434–1447 (2012). doi:10.1007/s12010-012-9868-4
36. Onuma, Y., Dudek, D., Thuesen, L., et al.: Five-year clinical and functional multislice computed tomography angiographic results after coronary implantation of the fully resorbable polymeric everolimus-eluting scaffold in patients with de novo coronary artery disease: the ABSORB cohort A trial. JACC Cardiovasc. Interv. **6**, 999–1009 (2013). doi:10.1016/j.jcin.2013.05.017
37. Bourantas, C.V., Papafaklis, M.I., Kotsia, A., et al.: Effect of the endothelial shear stress patterns on neointimal proliferation following drug-eluting bioresorbable vascular scaffold implantation: an optical coherence tomography study. JACC Cardiovasc. Interv. **7**, 315–324 (2014). doi:10.1016/j.jcin.2013.05.034
38. Bünger, C.M., Grabow, N., Kröger, C., et al.: Iliac anastomotic stenting with a sirolimus-eluting biodegradable poly-L-lactide stent: a preliminary study after 6 weeks. J. Endovasc. Ther. Off. J. Int. Soc. Endovasc. Spec. **13**, 630–639 (2006). doi:10.1583/06-1899R.1
39. Laaksovirta, S., Välimaa, T., Isotalo, T., et al.: Encrustation and strength retention properties of the self-expandable, biodegradable, self-reinforced L-lactide-glycolic acid co-polymer 80: 20 spiral urethral stent in vitro. J. Urol. **170**, 468–471 (2003). doi:10.1097/01.ju.0000076389.88489.af
40. Lumiaho, J., Heino, A., Kauppinen, T., et al.: Drainage and antireflux characteristics of a biodegradable self-reinforced, self-expanding X-ray-positive poly-L, D-lactide spiral partial ureteral stent: an experimental study. J. Endourol. Endourol. Soc. **21**, 1559–1564 (2007). doi:10.1089/end.2005.0085
41. Juuti, H., Kotsar, A., Mikkonen, J., et al.: The effect of pH on the degradation of biodegradable poly(L-lactide-co-glycolide) 80/20 urethral stent material in vitro. J. Endourol. Endourol. Soc. **26**, 701–705 (2012). doi:10.1089/end.2011.0199
42. Williams, S.F., Rizk, S., Martin, D.P.: Poly-4-hydroxybutyrate (P4HB): a new generation of resorbable medical devices for tissue repair and regeneration. Biomed. Tech. (Berl) **58**, 439–452 (2013). doi:10.1515/bmt-2013-0009
43. Van der Giessen, W.J., Lincoff, A.M., Schwartz, R.S., et al.: Marked inflammatory sequelae to implantation of biodegradable and nonbiodegradable polymers in porcine coronary arteries. Circulation **94**, 1690–1697 (1996)
44. Celarek, A., Kraus, T., Tschegg, E.K., et al.: PHB, crystalline and amorphous magnesium alloys: promising candidates for bioresorbable osteosynthesis implants? Mater. Sci. Eng. C Mater. Biol. Appl. **32**, 1503–1510 (2012). doi:10.1016/j.msec.2012.04.032
45. Zonari, A., Novikoff, S., Electo, N.R.P., et al.: Endothelial differentiation of human stem cells seeded onto electrospun polyhydroxybutyrate/polyhydroxybutyrate-co-hydroxyvalerate fiber mesh. PLoS ONE **7**, e35422 (2012). doi:10.1371/journal.pone.0035422
46. Garg, S., Serruys, P.W.: Coronary stents: current status. J. Am. Coll. Cardiol. **56**, S1–S42 (2010). doi:10.1016/j.jacc.2010.06.007

47. Freier, T., Sternberg, K., Behrend, D., Schmitz, K-P.: Health issues of biopolymers: polyhydroxybutyrate. In: Doi, Y., Steinbüchel, A. (eds.) Biopolymers, vol. 10, pp. 247–280. Wiley-VCH, Weinheim (2003)
48. Schmidt, C.E., Baier, J.M.: Acellular vascular tissues: natural biomaterials for tissue repair and tissue engineering. Biomaterials **21**, 2215–2231 (2000)
49. Hodde, J.: Naturally occurring scaffolds for soft tissue repair and regeneration. Tissue Eng. **8**, 295–308 (2002). doi:10.1089/107632702753725058
50. Heine, J., Schmiedl, A., Cebotari, S., et al.: Preclinical assessment of a tissue-engineered vasomotive human small-calibered vessel based on a decellularized xenogenic matrix: histological and functional characterization. Tissue Eng. Part A **17**, 1253–1261 (2011). doi:10.1089/ten.TEA.2010.0375
51. Tudorache, I., Cebotari, S., Sturz, G., et al.: Tissue engineering of heart valves: biomechanical and morphological properties of decellularized heart valves. J. Heart Valve Dis. **16**, 567–573 (2007). discussion 574
52. Tomizawa, Y.: Clinical benefits and risk analysis of topical hemostats: a review. J. Artif. Organs Off. J. Jpn. Soc. Artif. Organs **8**, 137–142 (2005). doi:10.1007/s10047-005-0296-x
53. Niiyama, H., Kuroyanagi, Y.: Development of novel wound dressing composed of hyaluronic acid and collagen sponge containing epidermal growth factor and vitamin C derivative. J. Artif. Organs Off. J. Jpn. Soc. Artif. Organs **17**, 81–87 (2014). doi:10.1007/s10047-013-0737-x
54. Wang, H.-L., Modarressi, M., Fu, J.-H.: Utilizing collagen membranes for guided tissue regeneration-based root coverage. Periodontol. 2000 **59**, 140–157 (2012). doi:10.1111/j.1600-0757.2011.00438.x
55. Langer, R., Vacanti, J.P.: Tissue engineering. Science **260**, 920–926 (1993)
56. Dumitriu, S., Popa V.I.: Polymeric Biomaterials. CRC Press, Boca Raton (2013)
57. Krenning, G., Moonen, J.-R.A.J., van Luyn, M.J.A., Harmsen, M.C.: Vascular smooth muscle cells for use in vascular tissue engineering obtained by endothelial-to-mesenchymal transdifferentiation (EnMT) on collagen matrices. Biomaterials **29**, 3703–3711 (2008). doi:10.1016/j.biomaterials.2008.05.034
58. Noishiki, Y., Ma, X.H., Yamane, Y., et al.: Succinylated collagen crosslinked by thermal treatment for coating vascular prostheses. Artif. Organs **22**, 672–680 (1998)
59. Marois, Y., Chakfé, N., Deng, X., et al.: Carbodiimide cross-linked gelatin: a new coating for porous polyester arterial prostheses. Biomaterials **16**, 1131–1139 (1995)
60. Li, D.X., Oh, Y.-K., Lim, S.-J., et al.: Novel gelatin microcapsule with bioavailability enhancement of ibuprofen using spray-drying technique. Int. J. Pharm. **355**, 277–284 (2008). doi:10.1016/j.ijpharm.2007.12.020
61. Manju, S., Muraleedharan, C.V., Rajeev, A., et al.: Evaluation of alginate dialdehyde cross-linked gelatin hydrogel as a biodegradable sealant for polyester vascular graft. J. Biomed. Mater. Res. B Appl. Biomater. **98**, 139–149 (2011). doi:10.1002/jbm.b.31843
62. Liu, Y., Chan-Park, M.B.: Hydrogel based on interpenetrating polymer networks of dextran and gelatin for vascular tissue engineering. Biomaterials **30**, 196–207 (2009). doi:10.1016/j.biomaterials.2008.09.041
63. Bos, G.W., Scharenborg, N.M., Poot, A.A., et al.: Proliferation of endothelial cells on surface-immobilized albumin-heparin conjugate loaded with basic fibroblast growth factor. J. Biomed. Mater. Res. **44**, 330–340 (1999). doi:10.1002/(SICI)1097- 4636(19990305)44:3<330:AID-JBM12>3.0.CO;2-O
64. Scholz, B., Kinzelmann, C., Benz, K., et al.: Suppression of adverse angiogenesis in an albumin-based hydrogel for articular cartilage and intervertebral disc regeneration. Eur. Cell Mater. **20**, 24–36 (2010). discussion 36–37
65. McCargar, R., Jenson, K., Dayton, A., et al.: Preparation of dissolvable albumin stents for vascular anastomosis with a 1.9 μm laser and in vitro mechanical strength assessments. Lasers Surg. Med. **44**, 330–338 (2012). doi:10.1002/lsm.22015
66. Fathi, A., Mithieux, S.M., Wei, H., et al.: Elastin based cell-laden injectable hydrogels with tunable gelation, mechanical and biodegradation properties. Biomaterials **35**, 5425–5435 (2014). doi:10.1016/j.biomaterials.2014.03.026

67. Kim, W., Chaikof, E.L.: Recombinant elastin-mimetic biomaterials: emerging applications in medicine. Adv. Drug Deliv. Rev. **62**, 1468–1478 (2010). doi:10.1016/j.addr.2010.04.007
68. Kolakovic, R., Peltonen, L., Laukkanen, A., et al.: Nanofibrillar cellulose films for controlled drug delivery. Eur. J. Pharm. Biopharm. Off. J. Arbeitsgemeinschaft Für Pharm Verfahrenstechnik EV **82**, 308–315 (2012). doi:10.1016/j.ejpb.2012.06.011
69. Santander-Ortega, M.J., Stauner, T., Loretz, B., et al.: Nanoparticles made from novel starch derivatives for transdermal drug delivery. J. Control. Release Off. J. Control Release Soc. **141**, 85–92 (2010). doi:10.1016/j.jconrel.2009.08.012
70. Gandhi, J.K., Opara, E.C., Brey, E.M.: Alginate-based strategies for therapeutic vascularization. Ther. Deliv. **4**, 327–341 (2013). doi:10.4155/tde.12.163
71. Dubuis, C., May, L., Alonso, F., et al.: Atorvastatin-loaded hydrogel affects the smooth muscle cells of human veins. J. Pharmacol. Exp. Ther. **347**, 574–581 (2013). doi:10.1124/jpet.113.208769
72. Fan, W., Yan, W., Xu, Z., Ni, H.: Erythrocytes load of low molecular weight chitosan nanoparticles as a potential vascular drug delivery system. Colloids. Surf. B Biointerfaces **95**, 258–265 (2012). doi:10.1016/j.colsurfb.2012.03.006
73. Bidarra, S.J., Barrias, C.C., Fonseca, K.B., et al.: Injectable in situ crosslinkable RGD-modified alginate matrix for endothelial cells delivery. Biomaterials **32**, 7897–7904 (2011). doi:10.1016/j.biomaterials.2011.07.013
74. Zhu, C., Fan, D., Wang, Y.: Human-like collagen/hyaluronic acid 3D scaffolds for vascular tissue engineering. Mater. Sci. Eng. C Mater. Biol. Appl. **34**, 393–401 (2014). doi:10.1016/j.msec.2013.09.044
75. Du, F., Wang, H., Zhao, W., et al.: Gradient nanofibrous chitosan/poly ε-caprolactone scaffolds as extracellular microenvironments for vascular tissue engineering. Biomaterials **33**, 762–770 (2012). doi:10.1016/j.biomaterials.2011.10.037
76. Shen, L., Wu, Y., Zhang, F., et al.: Assessment of an asymmetrical coating stent with sirolimus released from ablumial matrix in porcine model. Clin. Res. Cardiol. Off. J. Ger. Card. Soc. **101**, 917–927 (2012). doi:10.1007/s00392-012-0476-7
77. Ye, X., Wang, H., Zhou, J., et al.: The effect of heparin-VEGF multilayer on the biocompatibility of decellularized aortic valve with platelet and endothelial progenitor cells. PLoS ONE **8**, e54622 (2013). doi:10.1371/journal.pone.0054622
78. Bae, I.-H., Park, I.-K., Park, D.S., et al.: Thromboresistant and endothelialization effects of dopamine-mediated heparin coating on a stent material surface. J. Mater. Sci. Mater. Med. **23**, 1259–1269 (2012). doi:10.1007/s10856-012-4587-5
79. Mellon, S.J., Liddle, A.D., Pandit, H.: Hip replacement: landmark surgery in modern medical history. Maturitas **75**, 221–226 (2013). doi:10.1016/j.maturitas.2013.04.011
80. Galdbart, J.O., Branger, C., Andreassian, B., et al.: Elution of six antibiotics bonded to polyethylene vascular grafts sealed with three proteins. J. Surg. Res. **66**, 174–178 (1996). doi:10.1006/jsre.1996.0391
81. Tajirian, A.L., Goldberg, D.J.: A review of sutures and other skin closure materials. J. Cosmet. Laser Ther. Off. Publ. Eur. Soc. Laser Dermatol. **12**, 296–302 (2010). doi:10.3109/14764172.2010.538413
82. Ulrich, D., Edwards, S.L., Su, K., et al.: Human endometrial mesenchymal stem cells modulate the tissue response and mechanical behavior of polyamide mesh implants for pelvic organ prolapse repair. Tissue Eng. Part A **20**, 785–798 (2014). doi:10.1089/ten.TEA.2013.0170
83. Desai, M., Seifalian, A.M., Hamilton, G.: Role of prosthetic conduits in coronary artery bypass grafting. Eur. J. Cardio-Thorac. Surg. Off. J. Eur. Assoc. Cardio-Thorac Surg. **40**, 394–398 (2011). doi:10.1016/j.ejcts.2010.11.050
84. Farrar, D.J.: Development of a prosthetic coronary artery bypass graft. Heart Surg. Forum. **3**, 36–40 (2000)
85. Lendlein, A.: Polymere als implantatwerkstoffe. Chem. Unserer Zeit **33**, 279–295 (1999). doi:10.1002/ciuz.19990330505
86. Naoum, J.J., Arbid, E.J.: Bypass surgery in limb salvage: polytetrafluoroethylene prosthetic bypass. Methodist DeBakey Cardiovasc. J. **8**, 43–46 (2012)

87. Wise, S.G., Waterhouse, A., Kondyurin, A., et al.: Plasma-based biofunctionalization of vascular implants. Nanomed **7**, 1907–1916 (2012). doi:10.2217/nnm.12.161
88. Fujimoto, K., Honda, K., Wada, Y.R., et al.: Four-year experience with a silicone refractive multifocal intraocular lens. J. Cataract Refract. Surg. **36**, 1330–1335 (2010). doi:10.1016/j.jcrs.2010.02.021
89. Findl, O., Buehl, W., Bauer, P., Sycha, T.: Interventions for preventing posterior capsule opacification. Cochrane Database Syst. Rev. (2), CD003738 (2010). doi:10.1002/14651858.CD003738.pub3. Review. PMID: 20166069
90. Dieterich, M., Faridi, A.: Biological matrices and synthetic meshes used in implant-based breast reconstruction—a review of products available in Germany. Geburtshilfe Frauenheilkd **73**, 1100–1106 (2013). doi:10.1055/s-0033-1350930
91. Bohl, A., Rohm, H.W., Ceschi, P., et al.: Development of a specially tailored local drug delivery system for the prevention of fibrosis after insertion of cochlear implants into the inner ear. J. Mater. Sci. Mater. Med. **23**, 2151–2162 (2012). doi:10.1007/s10856-012-4698-z
92. Sisson, A.L., Schroeter, M., Lendlein, A.: Polyesters. In: Lendlein, A., Sisson, A. (eds.) Handbook Biodegradable Polymers, pp. 1–21. Wiley-VCH Verlag GmbH & Co. KGaA, Weinheim (2011)
93. Polak, M.B., Valamanesh, F., Felt, O., et al.: Controlled delivery of 5-chlorouracil using poly(ortho esters) in filtering surgery for glaucoma. Invest. Ophthalmol. Vis. Sci. **49**, 2993–3003 (2008). doi:10.1167/iovs.07-0919
94. Rothstein, S.N., Federspiel, W.J., Little, S.R.: A unified mathematical model for the prediction of controlled release from surface and bulk eroding polymer matrices. Biomaterials **30**, 1657–1664 (2009). doi:10.1016/j.biomaterials.2008.12.002
95. Palamoor, M., Jablonski, M.M.: Synthesis, characterization and in vitro studies of celecoxib-loaded poly(ortho ester) nanoparticles targeted for intraocular drug delivery. Colloids Surf. B Biointerfaces **112**, 474–482 (2013). doi:10.1016/j.colsurfb.2013.07.039
96. Iqbal, J., Gunn, J., Serruys, P.W.: Coronary stents: historical development, current status and future directions. Br. Med. Bull. **106**, 193–211 (2013). doi:10.1093/bmb/ldt009
97. Tamai, H., Igaki, K., Kyo, E., et al.: Initial and 6-month results of biodegradable poly-l-lactic acid coronary stents in humans. Circulation **102**, 399–404 (2000)
98. Patel, M.J., Patel, S.S., Patel, N.S., Patel, N.M.: Current status and future prospects of drug eluting stents for restenosis. Acta Pharm. Zagreb Croat **62**, 473–496 (2012). doi:10.2478/v10007-012-0036-8
99. Udipi, K., Chen, M., Cheng, P., et al.: Development of a novel biocompatible polymer system for extended drug release in a next-generation drug-eluting stent. J. Biomed. Mater. Res. A **85A**, 1064–1071 (2008). doi:10.1002/jbm.a.31664
100. Scheller, B., Speck, U., Romeike, B., et al.: Contrast media as carriers for local drug delivery successful inhibition of neointimal proliferation in the porcine coronary stent model. Eur. Heart J. **24**, 1462–1467 (2003). doi:10.1016/S0195-668X(03)00317-8
101. Speck, U., Scheller, B., Abramjuk, C., et al.: Neointima inhibition: comparison of effectiveness of non–stent-based local drug delivery and a drug-eluting stent in porcine coronary arteries1. Radiology **240**, 411–418 (2006). doi:10.1148/radiol.2402051248
102. Scheller, B., Hehrlein, C., Bocksch, W., et al.: Treatment of coronary in-stent restenosis with a paclitaxel-coated balloon catheter. N. Engl. J. Med. **355**, 2113–2124 (2006). doi:10.1056/NEJMoa061254
103. Tepe, G., Zeller, T., Albrecht, T., et al.: Local delivery of paclitaxel to inhibit restenosis during angioplasty of the leg. N. Engl. J. Med. **358**, 689–699 (2008). doi:10.1056/NEJMoa0706356
104. Werk, M., Langner, S., Reinkensmeier, B., et al.: Inhibition of restenosis in femoropopliteal arteries paclitaxel-coated versus uncoated balloon: femoral paclitaxel randomized pilot trial. Circulation **118**, 1358–1365 (2008). doi:10.1161/CIRCULATIONAHA.107.735985
105. Loh, J.P., Waksman, R.: Paclitaxel drug-coated balloons: a review of current status and emerging applications in native coronary artery de novo lesions. JACC Cardiovasc. Interv. **5**, 1001–1012 (2012). doi:10.1016/j.jcin.2012.08.005

106. Joner, M., Byrne, R.A., Lapointe, J.-M., et al.: Comparative assessment of drug-eluting balloons in an advanced porcine model of coronary restenosis. Thromb. Haemost. **105**, 864–872 (2011). doi:10.1160/TH10-11-0698
107. Cremers, B., Clever, Y., Schaffner, S., et al.: Treatment of coronary in-stent restenosis with a novel paclitaxel urea coated balloon. Minerva Cardioangiol. **58**, 583–588 (2010)
108. Arbeitsgruppe Interventionelle Kardiologie (AGIK) der Deutschen Gesellschaft für Kardiologie (DGK), Scheller, B., Levenson, B., et al.: Medikamente freisetzende Koronarstents und mit Medikamenten beschichtete Ballonkatheter: Positionspapier der DGK 2011. Kardiologe **5**, 411–435 (2011). doi:10.1007/s12181-011-0375-6
109. Ratner, B.D., Hoffman, A.S., Schoen, F.J., et al.: Biomaterials Science: An Introduction to Materials in Medicine, 1st edn. Academic Press, San Diego (1997)
110. Acharya, G., Park, K.: Mechanisms of controlled drug release from drug-eluting stents. Adv. Drug Deliv. Rev. **58**, 387–401 (2006). doi:10.1016/j.addr.2006.01.016
111. Sternberg, K., Petersen, S., Grabow, N., et al.: Implant-associated local drug delivery systems based on biodegradable polymers: customized designs for different medical applications. Biomed. Tech. (Berl) **58**, 417–427 (2013). doi:10.1515/bmt-2012-0049
112. Uhrich, K.E., Cannizzaro, S.M., Langer, R.S., Shakesheff, K.M.: Polymeric systems for controlled drug release. Chem. Rev. **99**, 3181–3198 (1999)
113. Qiu, Y., Park, K.: Environment-sensitive hydrogels for drug delivery. Adv. Drug Deliv. Rev. **53**, 321–339 (2001). doi:10.1016/S0169-409X(01)00203-4
114. Siegel, R.A., Firestone, B.A.: pH-dependent equilibrium swelling properties of hydrophobic polyelectrolyte copolymer gels. Macromolecules **21**, 3254–3259 (1988). doi:10.1021/ma00189a021
115. Tanaka, T.: Collapse of gels and the critical endpoint. Phys. Rev. Lett. **40**, 820–823 (1978). doi:10.1103/PhysRevLett.40.820
116. Hoffman, A.S.: Applications of thermally reversible polymers and hydrogels in therapeutics and diagnostics. J. Control. Release **6**, 297–305 (1987). doi:10.1016/0168-3659(87)90083-6
117. Bae, Y.H., Okano, T., Hsu, R., Kim, S.W.: Thermo-sensitive polymers as on-off switches for drug release. Makromol. Chem. Rapid Commun. **8**, 481–485 (1987). doi:10.1002/marc.1987.030081002
118. Aoki, T., Kawashima, M., Katono, H., et al.: Temperature-responsive interpenetrating polymer networks constructed with poly(acrylic acid) and poly(N, N-dimethylacrylamide). Macromolecules **27**, 947–952 (1994). doi:10.1021/ma00082a010
119. Zhang, R., Bowyer, A., Eisenthal, R., Hubble, J.: A smart membrane based on an antigen-responsive hydrogel. Biotechnol. Bioeng. **97**, 976–984 (2007). doi:10.1002/bit.21255
120. Tang, M., Zhang, R., Bowyer, A., et al.: A reversible hydrogel membrane for controlling the delivery of macromolecules. Biotechnol. Bioeng. **82**, 47–53 (2003). doi:10.1002/bit.10539
121. Lu, B., Xie, J., Lu, C., et al.: Oriented immobilization of Fab' fragments on silica surfaces. Anal. Chem. **67**, 83–87 (1995). doi:10.1021/ac00097a014
122. Lu, Z.R., Kopecková, P., Kopecek, J.: Polymerizable Fab' antibody fragments for targeting of anticancer drugs. Nat. Biotechnol. **17**, 1101–1104 (1999). doi:10.1038/15085
123. Miyata, T., Asami, N., Uragami, T.: A reversibly antigen-responsive hydrogel. Nature **399**, 766–769 (1999). doi:10.1038/21619
124. Miyata, T., Asami, N., Uragami, T.: Structural design of stimuli-responsive bioconjugated hydrogels that respond to a target antigen. J. Polym. Sci. Part B Polym. Phys. **47**, 2144–2157 (2009). doi:10.1002/polb.21812
125. Miyata, T., Asami, N., Okita, Y., Uragami, T.: Controlled permeation of model drugs through a bioconjugated membrane with antigen–antibody complexes as reversible crosslinks. Polym. J. **42**, 834–837 (2010). doi:10.1038/pj.2010.76
126. Miyata, T., Uragami, T., Nakamae, K.: Biomolecule-sensitive hydrogels. Adv. Drug Deliv. Rev. **54**, 79–98 (2002). doi:10.1016/S0169-409X(01)00241-1
127. Minrath, I., Arbeiter, D., Schmitz, K-P., et al.: In vitro characterization of polyacrylamide hydrogels for application as implant coating for stimulus-responsive local drug delivery. Polym. Adv. Technol. n/a–n/a (2014). doi:10.1002/pat.3294

128. Hanawa, T.: Materials for metallic stents. J. Artif. Organs Off. J. Jpn. Soc. Artif. Organs **12**, 73–79 (2009). doi:10.1007/s10047-008-0456-x
129. Kukreja, N., Onuma, Y., Daemen, J., Serruys, P.W.: The future of drug-eluting stents. Pharmacol. Res. Off J. Ital. Pharmacol. Soc. **57**, 171–180 (2008). doi:10.1016/j.phrs.2008.01.012
130. Grube, E., Gerckens, U., Müller, R., Büllesfeld, L.: Drug eluting stents: initial experiences. Z Für Kardiologie **91**(Suppl 3), 44–48 (2002)
131. Sternberg, K., Kramer, S., Nischan, C., et al.: In vitro study of drug-eluting stent coatings based on poly(l-lactide) incorporating cyclosporine A—drug release, polymer degradation and mechanical integrity. J. Mater. Sci. Mater. Med. **18**, 1423–1432 (2007). doi:10.1007/s10856-007-0148-8
132. Ge, J., Qian, J., Wang, X., et al.: Effectiveness and safety of the sirolimus-eluting stents coated with bioabsorbable polymer coating in human coronary arteries. Catheter Cardiovasc. Interv. Off J. Soc. Card. Angiogr. Interv. **69**, 198–202 (2007). doi:10.1002/ccd.20926
133. Serruys, P.W., Ong, A.T.L., Piek, J.J., et al.: A randomized comparison of a durable polymer Everolimus-eluting stent with a bare metal coronary stent: The SPIRIT first trial. EuroIntervention J. Eur. Collab. Work Group Interv. Cardiol. Eur. Soc. Cardiol. **1**, 58–65 (2005)
134. Pan, C.J., Tang, J.J., Weng, Y.J., et al.: Preparation and characterization of rapamycin-loaded PLGA coating stent. J. Mater. Sci. Mater. Med. **18**, 2193–2198 (2007). doi:10.1007/s10856-007-3075-9
135. Goddard, J.M., Hotchkiss, J.H.: Polymer surface modification for the attachment of bioactive compounds. Prog. Polym. Sci. **32**, 698–725 (2007). doi:10.1016/j.progpolymsci.2007.04.002
136. Kong, J.-S., Lee, D.-J., Kim, H.-D.: Surface modification of low-density polyethylene (LDPE) film and improvement of adhesion between evaporated copper metal film and LDPE. J. Appl. Polym. Sci. **82**, 1677–1690 (2001). doi:10.1002/app.2008
137. Bag, D.S., Kumar, V.P., Maiti, S.: Chemical modification of LDPE film. J. Appl. Polym. Sci. **71**, 1041–1048 (1999). doi:10.1002/(SICI)1097-4628(19990214)71:7<1041:AID-APP1>3.0.CO;2-R
138. Tao, G., Gong, A., Lu, J., et al.: Surface functionalized polypropylene: synthesis, characterization, and adhesion properties. Macromolecules **34**, 7672–7679 (2001). doi:10.1021/ma010941b
139. Sheng IS, E.: Effects of the chromic acid etching on propylene polymer surfaces. J. Adhes. Sci. Technol. **9**, 47–60 (1995). doi:10.1163/156856195X00284
140. Brown, L., Koerner, T., Horton, J.H., Oleschuk, R.D.: Fabrication and characterization of poly(methylmethacrylate) microfluidic devices bonded using surface modifications and solvents. Lab. Chip **6**, 66–73 (2006). doi:10.1039/b512179e
141. Wulf, K., Teske, M., Löbler, M., et al.: Surface functionalization of poly(ε-caprolactone) improves its biocompatibility as scaffold material for bioartificial vessel prostheses. J. Biomed. Mater. Res. B Appl. Biomater. **98B**, 89–100 (2011). doi:10.1002/jbm.b.31836
142. Fixe, F., Dufva, M., Telleman. P., Christensen, C.B.V.: Functionalization of poly(methyl methacrylate) (PMMA) as a substrate for DNA microarrays. Nucleic Acids Res. 32:e9 (2004). doi:10.1093/nar/gng157
143. Henry, A.C., Tutt, T.J., Galloway, M., et al.: Surface modification of poly(methyl methacrylate) used in the fabrication of microanalytical devices. Anal. Chem. **72**, 5331–5337 (2000). doi:10.1021/ac0006851
144. Zhu, Y., Gao, C., He, T., Shen, J.: Endothelium regeneration on luminal surface of polyurethane vascular scaffold modified with diamine and covalently grafted with gelatin. Biomaterials **25**, 423–430 (2004)
145. Zhu, Y., Gao, C., Liu, Y., Shen, J.: Endothelial cell functions in vitro cultured on poly(L-lactic acid) membranes modified with different methods. J. Biomed. Mater. Res. A **69**, 436–443 (2004). doi:10.1002/jbm.a.30007

146. Petersen, S., Strohbach, A., Busch, R., et al.: Site-selective immobilization of anti-CD34 antibodies to poly(L-lactide) for endovascular implant surfaces. J. Biomed. Mater. Res. B Appl. Biomater. **102**(2), 345–355 (2013)
147. Croll, T.I., O'Connor, A.J., Stevens, G.W., Cooper-White, J.J.: Controllable surface modification of poly(lactic-co-glycolic acid) (PLGA) by hydrolysis or aminolysis I: physical, chemical, and theoretical aspects. Biomacromolecules **5**, 463–473 (2004). doi:10.1021/bm0343040
148. Desai, S.M., Singh, R.P.: Surface modification of polyethylene. In: Albertsson, A.-C. (ed.) Long Term Properties of Polyolefins, pp. 231–294. Springer, Berlin (2004)
149. Oyane, A., Uchida, M., Yokoyama, Y., et al.: Simple surface modification of poly(epsilon-caprolactone) to induce its apatite-forming ability. J. Biomed. Mater. Res. A **75**, 138–145 (2005). doi:10.1002/jbm.a.30397
150. Kim, Y.J., Kang, I.K., Huh, M.W., Yoon, S.C.: Surface characterization and in vitro blood compatibility of poly(ethylene terephthalate) immobilized with insulin and/or heparin using plasma glow discharge. Biomaterials **21**, 121–130 (2000)
151. Aouinti, M., Bertrand, P., Poncin-Epaillard, F.: Characterization of polypropylene surface treated in a CO_2 plasma. Plasmas Polym. **8**, 225–236 (2003). doi:10.1023/A:1026392525543
152. Wang, M.-J., Chang, Y.-I., Poncin-Epaillard, F.: Acid and basic functionalities of nitrogen and carbon dioxide plasma-treated polystyrene. Surf. Interface Anal. **37**, 348–355 (2005). doi:10.1002/sia.2029
153. Crombez, M., Chevallier, P., Gaudreault, R.C., et al.: Improving arterial prosthesis neo-endothelialization: application of a proactive VEGF construct onto PTFE surfaces. Biomaterials **26**, 7402–7409 (2005). doi:10.1016/j.biomaterials.2005.05.051
154. Morent, R., De Geyter, N., Desmet, T., et al.: Plasma surface modification of biodegradable polymers: a review. Plasma Process. Polym. **8**, 171–190 (2011). doi:10.1002/ppap.201000153
155. Whitesides, G.M., Laibinis, P.E.: Wet chemical approaches to the characterization of organic surfaces: self-assembled monolayers, wetting, and the physical-organic chemistry of the solid-liquid interface. Langmuir **6**, 87–96 (1990). doi:10.1021/la00091a013
156. Petersen, S., Wulf, K., Schünemann, S., Teske, M., Schmitz, K.-P., Sternberg, K.: Biofunctionalization of polymer implant surfaces: from drug delivery to stable surface functionality. Biomed. Eng. Biomed. Tech. Biomed. Tech. (Berl) (2013). pii: /j/bmte.2013.58.issue-s1-C/bmt-2013-4052/bmt-2013-4052.xml. doi:10.1515/bmt-2013-4052
157. Bahulekar, R., Ayyangar, N.R., Ponrathnam, S.: Polyethyleneimine in immobilization of biocatalysts. Enzym. Microb. Technol. **13**, 858–868 (1991)
158. Dykes, G.M.: Dendrimers: a review of their appeal and applications. J. Chem. Technol. Biotechnol. **76**, 903–918 (2001). doi:10.1002/jctb.464
159. Holmberg, K., Tiberg, F., Malmsten, M., Brink, C.: Grafting with hydrophilic polymer chains to prepare protein-resistant surfaces. Colloids Surf. Physicochem. Eng. Asp. **123–124**, 297–306 (1997). doi:10.1016/S0927-7757(96)03810-1
160. Hermanson, G.T.: Bioconjugate Techniques. Academic Press, Waltham (2010)
161. Serruys, P.W., Emanuelsson, H., van der Giessen, W., et al.: Heparin-coated Palmaz-Schatz stents in human coronary arteries. Early outcome of the Benestent-II Pilot Study. Circulation **93**, 412–422 (1996)
162. Serruys, P.W., van Hout, B., Bonnier, H., et al.: Randomised comparison of implantation of heparin-coated stents with balloon angioplasty in selected patients with coronary artery disease (Benestent II). Lancet **352**, 673–681 (1998)
163. Vrolix, M.C.M., Legrand, V.M., Reiber, J.H.C., et al.: Heparin-coated Wiktor stents in human coronary arteries (MENTOR Trial). Am. J. Cardiol. **86**, 385–389 (2000)
164. Wöhrle, J., Al-Khayer, E., Grötzinger, U., et al.: Comparison of the heparin coated vs the uncoated Jostent–no influence on restenosis or clinical outcome. Eur. Heart J. **22**, 1808–1816 (2001). doi:10.1053/euhj.2001.2608
165. Holmes, D.R., Camrud, A.R., Jorgenson, M.A., et al.: Polymeric stenting in the porcine coronary artery model: differential outcome of exogenous fibrin sleeves versus polyurethane-coated stents. J. Am. Coll. Cardiol. **24**, 525–531 (1994)

166. Aggarwal, R.K., Ireland, D.C., Azrin, M.A., et al.: Antithrombotic potential of polymer-coated stents eluting platelet glycoprotein IIb/IIIa receptor antibody. Circulation **94**, 3311–3317 (1996)
167. Boland, J.L., Corbeij, H.A., Van Der Giessen, W., et al.: Multicenter evaluation of the phosphorylcholine-coated biodivYsio stent in short de novo coronary lesions: The SOPHOS study. Int. J. Cardiovasc. Interv. **3**, 215–225 (2000). doi:10.1080/14628840050515966
168. Asahara, T., Murohara, T., Sullivan, A., et al.: Isolation of putative progenitor endothelial cells for angiogenesis. Science **275**, 964–966 (1997). doi:10.1126/science.275.5302.964
169. Hristov, M., Erl, W., Weber, P.C.: Endothelial progenitor cells. Arterioscler. Thromb. Vasc. Biol. **23**, 1185–1189 (2003). doi:10.1161/01.ATV.0000073832.49290.B5
170. Peichev, M., Naiyer, A.J., Pereira, D., et al.: Expression of VEGFR-2 and AC133 by circulating human CD34+ cells identifies a population of functional endothelial precursors. Blood **95**, 952–958 (2000)
171. Aoki, J., Serruys, P.W., van Beusekom, H., et al.: Endothelial progenitor cell capture by stents coated with antibody against CD34: The HEALING-FIM (Healthy Endothelial Accelerated Lining Inhibits Neointimal Growth-First In Man) Registry. J. Am. Coll. Cardiol. **45**, 1574–1579 (2005). doi:10.1016/j.jacc.2005.01.048
172. Duckers, H.J., Silber, S., de Winter, R., et al.: Circulating endothelial progenitor cells predict angiographic and intravascular ultrasound outcome following percutaneous coronary interventions in the HEALING-II trial: evaluation of an endothelial progenitor cell capturing stent. EuroIntervention J. Eur. Collab. Work Group Interv. Cardiol. Eur. Soc. Cardiol. **3**, 67–75 (2007)
173. Duckers, H.J., Soullié, T., den Heijer, P., et al.: Accelerated vascular repair following percutaneous coronary intervention by capture of endothelial progenitor cells promotes regression of neointimal growth at long term follow-up: final results of the Healing II trial using an endothelial progenitor cell capturing stent (Genous R stent). EuroIntervention J. Eur. Collab. Work Group Interv. Cardiol. Eur. Soc. Cardiol. **3**, 350–358 (2007)
174. Bystroň, M., Cervinka, P., Spaček, R., et al.: Randomized comparison of endothelial progenitor cells capture stent versus cobalt-chromium stent for treatment of ST-elevation myocardial infarction. six-month clinical, angiographic, and IVUS follow-up. Catheter. Cardiovasc. Interv. Off. J. Soc. Card. Angiogr. Interv. **76**, 627–631 (2010). doi:10.1002/ccd.22612
175. Beijk, M.A.M., Klomp, M., Verouden, N.J.W., et al.: Genous™ endothelial progenitor cell capturing stent vs. the Taxus Liberté stent in patients with de novo coronary lesions with a high-risk of coronary restenosis: a randomized, single-centre, pilot study. Eur. Heart J. **31**(9), 1055–1064 (2009). doi:10.1093/eurheartj/ehp476
176. Beijk, M.A.M., Klomp, M., van Geloven, N., et al.: Two-year follow-up of the Genous™ endothelial progenitor cell capturing stent versus the Taxus Liberté stent in patients with de novo coronary artery lesions with a high-risk of restenosis: a randomized, single-center, pilot study. Catheter Cardiovasc. Interv. Off. J. Soc. Card. Angiogr. Interv. **78**, 189–195 (2011). doi:10.1002/ccd.23143
177. Klomp, M., Beijk, M.A., Varma, C., et al.: 1-year outcome of TRIAS HR (TRI-stent adjudication study-high risk of restenosis) a multicenter, randomized trial comparing genous endothelial progenitor cell capturing stents with drug-eluting stents. JACC Cardiovasc. Interv. **4**, 896–904 (2011). doi:10.1016/j.jcin.2011.05.011
178. Markway, B.D., McCarty, O.J.T., Marzec, U.M., et al.: Capture of flowing endothelial cells using surface-immobilized anti-kinase insert domain receptor antibody. Tissue Eng. Part C Methods **14**, 97–105 (2008). doi:10.1089/ten.tec.2007.0300
179. Hoffmann, J., Paul, A., Harwardt, M., et al.: Immobilized DNA aptamers used as potent attractors for porcine endothelial precursor cells. J. Biomed. Mater. Res. A **84**, 614–621 (2008). doi:10.1002/jbm.a.31309
180. Xue, L., Greisler, H.P.: Biomaterials in the development and future of vascular grafts. J. Vasc. Surg. **37**, 472–480 (2003). doi:10.1067/mva.2003.88
181. Hubbell, J.A., Massia, S.P., Desai, N.P., Drumheller, P.D.: Endothelial cell-selective materials for tissue engineering in the vascular graft via a new receptor. Biotechnol. Nat. Publ. Co. **9**, 568–572 (1991)

182. Ochsenhirt, S.E., Kokkoli, E., McCarthy, J.B., Tirrell, M.: Effect of RGD secondary structure and the synergy site PHSRN on cell adhesion, spreading and specific integrin engagement. Biomaterials **27**, 3863–3874 (2006). doi:10.1016/j.biomaterials.2005.12.012
183. Pierschbacher, M., Hayman, E.G., Ruoslahti, E.: Synthetic peptide with cell attachment activity of fibronectin. Proc. Natl. Acad. Sci. USA **80**, 1224–1227 (1983)
184. Tashiro, K., Sephel, G.C., Weeks, B., et al.: A synthetic peptide containing the IKVAV sequence from the A chain of laminin mediates cell attachment, migration, and neurite outgrowth. J. Biol. Chem. **264**, 16174–16182 (1989)
185. Weber, L.M., Hayda, K.N., Haskins, K., Anseth, K.S.: The effects of cell-matrix interactions on encapsulated beta-cell function within hydrogels functionalized with matrix-derived adhesive peptides. Biomaterials **28**, 3004–3011 (2007). doi:10.1016/j.biomaterials.2007.03.005
186. De Mel, A., Jell, G., Stevens, M.M., Seifalian, A.M.: Biofunctionalization of biomaterials for accelerated in situ endothelialization: a review. Biomacromolecules **9**, 2969–2979 (2008). doi:10.1021/bm800681k
187. Veleva, A.N., Heath, D.E., Cooper, S.L., Patterson, C.: Selective endothelial cell attachment to peptide-modified terpolymers. Biomaterials **29**, 3656–3661 (2008). doi:10.1016/j.biomaterials.2008.05.022
188. Schwartz, S.M., Haudenschild, C.C., Eddy, E.M.: Endothelial regneration. I. Quantitative analysis of initial stages of endothelial regeneration in rat aortic intima. Lab. Investig. J. Tech. Methods Pathol. **38**, 568–580 (1978)
189. Schwartz, S.M., Stemerman, M.B., Benditt, E.P.: The aortic intima. II. Repair of the aortic lining after mechanical denudation. Am. J. Pathol. **81**, 15–42 (1975)
190. Haudenschild, C.C., Schwartz, S.M.: Endothelial regeneration. II. Restitution of endothelial continuity. Lab. Investig. J. Tech. Methods Pathol. **41**, 407–418 (1979)
191. Tada, T., Reidy, M.A.: Endothelial regeneration. IX. Arterial injury followed by rapid endothelial repair induces smooth-muscle-cell proliferation but not intimal thickening. Am. J. Pathol. **129**, 429–433 (1987)
192. Doornekamp, F.N., Borst, C., Post, M.J.: The influence of lesion length on intimal hyperplasia after Fogarty balloon injury in the rabbit carotid artery: role of endothelium. J. Vasc. Res. **34**, 260–266 (1997)
193. Busch, R., Strohbach, A., Rethfeldt, S., et al.: New stent surface materials: the impact of polymer-dependent interactions of human endothelial cells, smooth muscle cells, and platelets. Acta Biomater. **10**, 688–700 (2014). doi:10.1016/j.actbio.2013.10.015
194. Busch AS, R.: Parameters of endothelial function are dependent on polymeric surface material. Biomed. Tech. (Berl) (2013). doi:10.1515/bmt-2013-4053
195. Chaabane, C., Otsuka, F., Virmani, R., Bochaton-Piallat, M.-L.: Biological responses in stented arteries. Cardiovasc. Res. **99**, 353–363 (2013). doi:10.1093/cvr/cvt115
196. Rinder, H.M., Bonan, J.L., Rinder, C.S., et al.: Dynamics of leukocyte-platelet adhesion in whole blood. Blood **78**, 1730–1737 (1991)
197. Anderson, J.M., Rodriguez, A., Chang, D.T.: Foreign body reaction to biomaterials. Semin. Immunol. **20**, 86–100 (2008). doi:10.1016/j.smim.2007.11.004
198. Tengvall, P., Lundström, I., Liedberg, B.: Protein adsorption studies on model organic surfaces: an ellipsometric and infrared spectroscopic approach. Biomaterials **19**, 407–422 (1998)
199. Cohen, H.C., Joyce, E.J., Kao, W.J.: Biomaterials selectively modulate interactions between human blood-derived polymorphonuclear leukocytes and monocytes. Am. J. Pathol. **182**, 2180–2190 (2013). doi:10.1016/j.ajpath.2013.02.022
200. Khandwekar, A.P., Patil, D.P., Shouche, Y., Doble, M.: Surface engineering of polycaprolactone by biomacromolecules and their blood compatibility. J. Biomater. Appl. **26**, 227–252 (2011). doi:10.1177/0885328210367442
201. Henkelman, S., Rakhorst, G., Blanton, J., van Oeveren, W.: Standardization of incubation conditions for hemolysis testing of biomaterials. Mater. Sci. Eng. C **29**, 1650–1654 (2009). doi:10.1016/j.msec.2009.01.002

202. Ratner, B.D.: Blood compatibility—a perspective. J. Biomater. Sci. Polym. Ed. **11**, 1107–1119 (2000)
203. Xu, H., Nguyen, K.T., Brilakis, E.S., et al.: Enhanced endothelialization of a new stent polymer through surface enhancement and incorporation of growth factor-delivering microparticles. J. Cardiovasc. Transl. Res. **5**, 519–527 (2012). doi:10.1007/s12265-012-9381-8
204. Mao, L., Shen, L., Niu, J., et al.: Nanophasic biodegradation enhances the durability and biocompatibility of magnesium alloys for the next-generation vascular stents. Nanoscale **5**, 9517–9522 (2013). doi:10.1039/c3nr02912c
205. Sgarioto, M., Adhikari, R., Gunatillake, P.A., et al.: Properties and in vitro evaluation of high modulus biodegradable polyurethanes for applications in cardiovascular stents. J. Biomed. Mater. Res. B Appl. Biomater. (2014). doi:10.1002/jbm.b.33137
206. Mukai, Y., Wang, C.-Y., Rikitake, Y., Liao, J.K.: Phosphatidylinositol 3-kinase/protein kinase Akt negatively regulates plasminogen activator inhibitor type 1 expression in vascular endothelial cells. Am. J. Physiol. Heart Circ. Physiol. **292**, H1937–H1942 (2007). doi:10.1152/ajpheart.00868.2006
207. Partridge, J., Carlsen, H., Enesa, K., et al.: Laminar shear stress acts as a switch to regulate divergent functions of NF-kappaB in endothelial cells. FASEB J. Off. Publ. Fed. Am. Soc. Exp. Biol. **21**, 3553–3561 (2007). doi:10.1096/fj.06-8059com
208. Ling, X., Ye, J.-F., Zheng, X.-X.: Dynamic investigation of leukocyte-endothelial cell adhesion interaction under fluid shear stress in vitro. Sheng Wu Hua Xue Yu Sheng Wu Wu Li Xue Bao Acta Biochim. Biophys. Sin. **35**, 567–572 (2003)
209. Taite, L.J., Rowland, M.L., Ruffino, K.A., et al.: Bioactive hydrogel substrates: probing leukocyte receptor-ligand interactions in parallel plate flow chamber studies. Ann. Biomed. Eng. **34**, 1705–1711 (2006). doi:10.1007/s10439-006-9173-x
210. Dunkern, T.R., Paulitschke, M., Meyer, R., et al.: A novel perfusion system for the endothelialisation of PTFE grafts under defined flow. Eur. J. Vasc. Endovasc. Surg. Off. J. Eur. Soc. Vasc. Surg. **18**, 105–110 (1999). doi:10.1053/ejvs.1999.0829
211. Rademacher, A., Paulitschke, M., Meyer, R., Hetzer, R.: Endothelialization of PTFE vascular grafts under flow induces significant cell changes. Int. J. Artif. Organs **24**, 235–242 (2001)
212. Neubert, A., Sternberg, K., Nagel, S., et al.: Development of a vessel-simulating flow-through cell method for the in vitro evaluation of release and distribution from drug-eluting stents. J. Control. Release Off. J. Control. Release Soc. **130**, 2–8 (2008). doi:10.1016/j.jconrel.2008.05.012
213. Seidlitz, A., Nagel, S., Semmling, B., et al.: Examination of drug release and distribution from drug-eluting stents with a vessel-simulating flow-through cell. Eur. J. Pharm. Biopharm. Off J Arbeitsgemeinschaft Für Pharm Verfahrenstechnik EV **78**, 36–48 (2011). doi:10.1016/j.ejpb.2010.12.021
214. Rudolph, A., Eickner, T., Seidlitz, A., et al.: Investigation of in vitro drug release behaviour of drug-eluting stents using a perfusion culture system. Biomed. Eng. Biomed. Tech. (2013)
215. Gerszten, R.E., Garcia-Zepeda, E.A., Lim, Y.C., et al.: MCP-1 and IL-8 trigger firm adhesion of monocytes to vascular endothelium under flow conditions. Nature **398**, 718–723 (1999). doi:10.1038/19546
216. Welt, F.G.P., Rogers, C.: Inflammation and restenosis in the stent era. Arterioscler. Thromb. Vasc. Biol. **22**, 1769–1776 (2002)
217. Hezi-Yamit, A., Sullivan, C., Wong, J., et al.: Impact of polymer hydrophilicity on biocompatibility: implication for DES polymer design. J. Biomed. Mater. Res. A **90**, 133–141 (2009). doi:10.1002/jbm.a.32057
218. Curcio, A., Torella, D., Indolfi, C.: Mechanisms of smooth muscle cell proliferation and endothelial regeneration after vascular injury and stenting: approach to therapy. Circ. J. Off. J. Jpn. Circ. Soc. **75**, 1287–1296 (2011)
219. Achneck, H.E., Sileshi, B., Parikh, A., et al.: Pathophysiology of bleeding and clotting in the cardiac surgery patient from vascular endothelium to circulatory assist device surface. Circulation **122**, 2068–2077 (2010). doi:10.1161/CIRCULATIONAHA.110.936773

220. Van Kooten, T.G., Klein, C.L., Köhler, H., et al.: From cytotoxicity to biocompatibility testing in vitro: cell adhesion molecule expression defines a new set of parameters. J. Mater. Sci. Mater. Med. **8**, 835–841 (1997)
221. Williams, D.F.: On the mechanisms of biocompatibility. Biomaterials **29**, 2941–2953 (2008). doi:10.1016/j.biomaterials.2008.04.023
222. O'Connor, R.S., Hao, X., Shen, K., et al.: Substrate rigidity regulates human T cell activation and proliferation. J. Immunol. Baltim. Md. 1950 **189**, 1330–1339 (2012). doi:10.4049/jimmunol.1102757
223. Gouverneur, M., Berg, B., Nieuwdorp, M., et al.: Vasculoprotective properties of the endothelial glycocalyx: effects of fluid shear stress. J. Intern. Med. **259**, 393–400 (2006). doi:10.1111/j.1365-2796.2006.01625.x
224. Kulangara, K., Leong, K.W.: Substrate topography shapes cell function. Soft Matter **5**, 4072–4076 (2009). doi:10.1039/B910132M
225. Lim, J.Y., Donahue, H.J.: Cell sensing and response to micro- and nanostructured surfaces produced by chemical and topographic patterning. Tissue Eng. **13**, 1879–1891 (2007). doi:10.1089/ten.2006.0154
226. Peterbauer, T., Yakunin, S., Siegel, J., et al.: Dynamics of spreading and alignment of cells cultured in vitro on a grooved polymer surface. J. Nanomater. **2011**, e413079 (2010). doi:10.1155/2011/413079
227. Takai, E., Costa, K.D., Shaheen, A., et al.: Osteoblast elastic modulus measured by atomic force microscopy is substrate dependent. Ann. Biomed. Eng. **33**, 963–971 (2005)
228. Simon, A., Cohen-Bouhacina, T., Porté, M.C., et al.: Characterization of dynamic cellular adhesion of osteoblasts using atomic force microscopy. Cytom. Part J. Int. Soc. Anal. Cytol. **54**, 36–47 (2003). doi:10.1002/cyto.a.10052
229. Kempe, D.S., Lang, P.A., Eisele, K., et al.: Stimulation of erythrocyte phosphatidylserine exposure by lead ions. Am. J. Physiol. Cell Physiol. **288**, C396–C402 (2005). doi:10.1152/ajpcell.00115.2004
230. Dillingham, E.O., Webb, N., Lawrence, W.H., Autian, J.: Biological evaluation of polymers. I. Poly(methyl methacylate). J. Biomed. Mater. Res. **9**, 569–596 (1975). doi:10.1002/jbm.820090605
231. F04 Committee: Practice for assessment of hemolytic properties of materials. ASTM International (2013)
232. Fischer, D., Li, Y., Ahlemeyer, B., et al.: In vitro cytotoxicity testing of polycations: influence of polymer structure on cell viability and hemolysis. Biomaterials **24**, 1121–1131 (2003). doi:10.1016/S0142-9612(02)00445-3
233. Parnham, M.J., Wetzig, H.: Toxicity screening of liposomes. Chem. Phys. Lipids **64**, 263–274 (1993)
234. Anderson, N.L., Anderson, N.G.: The human plasma proteome: history, character, and diagnostic prospects. Mol. Cell. Proteomics MCP **1**, 845–867 (2002)
235. Turbill, P., Beugeling, T., Poot, A.A.: Proteins involved in the Vroman effect during exposure of human blood plasma to glass and polyethylene. Biomaterials **17**, 1279–1287 (1996)
236. Hlady, V., Buijs, J., Jennissen, H.P.: Methods for studying protein adsorption. Methods Enzymol. **309**, 402–429 (1999)
237. Tsai, W.-B., Grunkemeier, J.M., McFarland, C.D., Horbett, T.A.: Platelet adhesion to polystyrene-based surfaces preadsorbed with plasmas selectively depleted in fibrinogen, fibronectin, vitronectin, or von Willebrand's factor. J. Biomed. Mater. Res. **60**, 348–359 (2002)
238. Born, G.V.R.: Aggregation of blood platelets by adenosine diphosphate and its reversal. Nature **194**, 927–929 (1962). doi:10.1038/194927b0
239. Goldman, A.J., Cox, R.G., Brenner, H.: Slow viscous motion of a sphere parallel to a plane wall—II Couette flow. Chem. Eng. Sci. **22**, 653–660 (1967). doi:10.1016/0009-2509(67)80048-4
240. Lawrence, M.B.: In vitro flow models of leukocyte adhesion. In: Ley, K. (ed) Physiology of Inflammation, pp. 204–221. Springer, New York (2001)

241. Chang, X., Gorbet, M.: The effect of shear on in vitro platelet and leukocyte material-induced activation. J. Biomater. Appl. **28**, 407–415 (2013). doi:10.1177/0885328212454689
242. Sirolli, V., Ballone, E., Amoroso, L., et al.: Leukocyte adhesion molecules and leukocyte-platelet interactions during hemodialysis: effects of different synthetic membranes. Int. J. Artif. Organs **22**, 536–542 (1999)
243. Uurto, I., Juuti, H., Parkkinen, J., et al.: Biodegradable self-expanding poly-L/D-lactic acid vascular stent: a pilot study in canine and porcine iliac arteries. J. Endovasc. Ther. Off. J. Int. Soc. Endovasc. Spec. **11**, 712–718 (2004). doi:10.1583/04-127MR.1
244. Venkatraman, S.S., Tan, L.P., Joso, J.F.D., et al.: Biodegradable stents with elastic memory. Biomaterials **27**, 1573–1578 (2006). doi:10.1016/j.biomaterials.2005.09.002
245. Venkatraman, S., Poh, T.L., Vinalia, T., et al.: Collapse pressures of biodegradable stents. Biomaterials **24**, 2105–2111 (2003)
246. Zilberman, M., Nelson, K.D., Eberhart, R.C.: Mechanical properties and in vitro degradation of bioresorbable fibers and expandable fiber-based stents. J. Biomed. Mater. Res. B Appl. Biomater. **74**, 792–799 (2005). doi:10.1002/jbm.b.30319
247. Welch, T.R., Eberhart, R.C., Chuong, C.-J.: The influence of thermal treatment on the mechanical characteristics of a PLLA coiled stent. J. Biomed. Mater. Res. B Appl. Biomater. **90**, 302–311 (2009). doi:10.1002/jbm.b.31286
248. Grabow, N., Bünger, C.M., Schultze, C., et al.: A biodegradable slotted tube stent based on poly(L-lactide) and poly(4-hydroxybutyrate) for rapid balloon-expansion. Ann. Biomed. Eng. **35**, 2031–2038 (2007). doi:10.1007/s10439-007-9376-9
249. Grabow, N., Bünger, C.M., Sternberg, K., et al.: Mechanical properties of a biodegradable balloon-expandable stent from poly(L-lactide) for peripheral vascular applications. J. Med. Devices **1**, 84–88 (2006). doi:10.1115/1.2355683
250. Grabow, N., Schlun, M., Sternberg, K., et al.: Mechanical properties of laser cut poly(L-lactide) micro-specimens: implications for stent design, manufacture, and sterilization. J. Biomech. Eng. **127**, 25–31 (2005)
251. Bünger, C.M., Grabow, N., Sternberg, K., et al.: Sirolimus-eluting biodegradable poly-L-lactide stent for peripheral vascular application: a preliminary study in porcine carotid arteries. J. Surg. Res. **139**, 77–82 (2007). doi:10.1016/j.jss.2006.07.035
252. Petersen, S., Hussner, J., Reske, T., et al.: In vitro study of dual drug-eluting stents with locally focused sirolimus and atorvastatin release. J. Mater. Sci. Mater. Med. **24**, 2589–2600 (2013). doi:10.1007/s10856-013-5001-7
253. Nugroho, P., Mitomo, H., Yoshii, F., Kume, T.: Degradation of poly(L-lactic acid) by γ-irradiation. Polym. Degrad. Stab. **72**, 337–343 (2001). doi:10.1016/S0141-3910(01)00030-1
254. Nuutinen, J.-P., Välimaa, T., Clerc, C., Törmälä, P.: Mechanical properties and in vitro degradation of bioresorbable knitted stents. J. Biomater. Sci. Polym. Ed. **13**, 1313–1323 (2002). doi:10.1163/15685620260449714
255. Pistner, H.: Osteosynthese mit bioresorbierbaren Materialien: Entwicklung einer Schraube vom Werkstoff bis zur klinischen Anwendung, Einhorn-Presse-Verlag (1999)
256. Sharon Xin, Lu, Cebe, P.: Effects of annealing on the disappearance and creation of constrained amorphous phase. Polymer **37**, 4857–4863 (1996). doi:10.1016/S0032-3861(96)00376-X
257. Delpouve, N., Saiter, A., Mano, J.F., Dargent, E.: Cooperative rearranging region size in semi-crystalline poly(L-lactic acid). Polymer **49**, 3130–3135 (2008). doi:10.1016/j.polymer.2008.04.045
258. Kelsch, B., Scheller, B., Biedermann, M., et al.: Dose response to Paclitaxel-coated balloon catheters in the porcine coronary overstretch and stent implantation model. Invest. Radiol. **46**, 255–263 (2011). doi:10.1097/RLI.0b013e31820577df
259. Kallmes, D.F., McGraw, J.K., Evans, A.J., et al.: Thrombogenicity of hydrophilic and nonhydrophilic microcatheters and guiding catheters. AJNR Am. J. Neuroradiol. **18**, 1243–1251 (1997)
260. Nagaoka, S., Akashi, R.: Low-friction hydrophilic surface for medical devices. Biomaterials **11**, 419–424 (1990)

Chapter 16
Recent Advances in Hemocompatible Polymers for Biomedical Applications

Elizabeth J. Brisbois, Hitesh Handa and Mark E. Meyerhoff

Abstract Blood-material interactions are critical to the success of implantable medical devices that are used in thousands of patients every day. Some common blood-contacting devices include catheters, stents, vascular grafts, heart valve prostheses, and extracorporeal circulation/membrane oxygenation systems. Among other complications, thrombosis and clot formation remains one of the major challenges in clinical application of these devices. The initial biological response of blood to a foreign surface is the rapid adsorption of plasma proteins, which is followed by platelet adhesion and activation, and ultimately thrombus formation. The key factors in clot formation are the chemical and physical nature of the surfaces and their interactions with the blood components, such as platelets and plasma proteins. Despite decades of research, an ideal non-thrombogenic surface is still yet to be identified and clinical use of these blood-contacting devices requires use of anticoagulation agents, increasing the risk of bleeding in patients. In this chapter, we will review some of the current and most promising strategies that have been used over the years to develop polymeric materials with improved hemocompatibility, including highly hydrophilic or hydrophobic surfaces, albumin coated surfaces, zwitterionic polymers, attached endothelial cells, patterned surfaces, immobilized heparin, and nitric oxide (NO) releasing/generating surfaces. We will also discuss some of the important techniques employed (using in vitro and in vivo models) to assess the hemocompatibility of any new material, including the measurement of platelet preservation, platelet and protein adhesion, the effect of flow rates on thrombosis, and the ultimate surface clot area.

Keywords Blood-surface interactions · Hemocompatibility · Heparin · Nitric oxide · Platelets · Polymers

E.J. Brisbois · H. Handa
Department of Surgery, University of Michigan, Ann Arbor, MI, USA

M.E. Meyerhoff (✉)
Department of Chemistry, University of Michigan, Ann Arbor, MI, USA
e-mail: mmeyerho@umich.edu

F. Puoci (ed.), *Advanced Polymers in Medicine*, DOI 10.1007/978-3-319-12478-0_16

Abbreviations

A-A	Arterio-arterlial
A-V	Arterio-venous
Alb	Albumin
Alg	Sodium alginate
APTT	Activated partial thromboplastin time
ATRP	Atom transfer radical polymerization
CysNO	*S*-nitrosocysteine
DACA	Diaminoalkyltrimethoxysilane
DBHD/N_2O_2	Diazeniumdiolated dibutylhexanediamine
DBHD	*N,N′*-dibutyl-1,6-hexanediamine
DMHD/N_2O_2	Diazeniumdiolated *N,N′*-dimethyl-1,6-hexanediamine
DMMSA	N,N-dimethyl-N-methacryloxyethyl-N-(3-sulfopropyl) ammonium
DMPAMS	N,N-dimethyl, N-(2-ethyl phosphate ethyl)-aminopropyltrimethy-oxysilane
DOS	Dioctyl sebacate
EC	Endothelial cells
ECC	Extracorporeal circulation
GPx	Glutathione peroxidase
GSH	Glutathione
GSNO	*S*-nitrosoglutathione
HEMA	2-hydroxyethyl methacrylate
IgG	Immunoglobulin
LPEI/N_2O_2	Diazeniumdiolated linear polyethylenimine
MDI	Methylene diphenyl isocyanate
NO	Nitric oxide
NOgen	NO-generating
NONOate	Diazeniumdiolate
NOrel	NO-releasing
P(PEGDMA)	Poly(poly(ethylene glycol) dimethacrylate)
PAAm	Polyacrylamides
PDMS	Poly(dimethylsiloxane)
PEG	Poly(ethylene glycol)
PEI	Polyethylenimine
PEGME	Poly(ethylene glycol) monomethyl ether
PEO	Poly(ethylene oxide)
PGA	Polyglycolic acid
PHEMA	Poly(hydroxyethyl methacrylate)
PLGA	Poly(lactic-*co*-glycolic acid)
PMEA	Poly(2-methoxyethyl acrylate)
PNVP	Poly(N-vinyl pyrrolidone)
PRP	Platelet-rich plasma
PS-CO_2	Carbon dioxide as plasma-treated polystyrene
PTFE	Polytetrafluoroethylene

PVA	Poly(vinyl alcohol)
PVC	Poly(vinyl chloride)
PVMMA	Poly(vinyl methyl ether-*co*-malic anhydride)
PVP	Poly(vinyl pyrrolidone)
RSNO	*S*-nitrosothiol
RSSR	Disulfide
SeCA	Selenocystamine
SeDPA	3,3′-diselenidedipropionic acid
SNAC	*S*-nitroso-*N*-acetyl-*L*-cysteine
SNAP	*S*-nitroso-*N*-acetylpenicillamine
SR	Silicone rubber
vWF	von Willebrand Factor

Introduction

Hemocompatibility of Common Blood-Contacting Devices

Blood-material interaction is critical to the success of implantable medical devices, including simple catheters, stents and grafts, insulation materials for electrical leads of pacemakers and defibrillators, and complex extracorporeal artificial organs, which are used in thousands of patients every day [1]. Polymers, including polyurethanes, silicone rubber (SR), and poly(vinyl chloride), are used extensively in the healthcare industry to fabricate such biomedical devices. Thrombosis is one of the primary problems associated with clinical application of blood-contacting materials, which can cause serious complications in patients and ultimately failure of the device's functionality [2]. Thrombus formation can lead to significant consequences such as complete obstruction of blood vessels in which stents are placed [3], occlusion of catheters [4] and small diameter vascular grafts [1], errant results from implantable chemical sensors [1], embolic complications with artificial hearts [5], and extensive blood damage and platelet consumption during extracorporeal membrane oxygenation [5]. Such complications can result in significantly increased medical costs, extended hospitalization, amputation, or increased morbidity. Despite a thorough understanding of the mechanisms of blood-surface interactions and decades of bioengineering research effort, the ideal non-thrombogenic prosthetic surface remains unidentified [5]. Over the last 50 years, much has been learned about foreign surface-induced thrombosis and the attempt to prevent it with systemic anticoagulation and surface modifications. In a clinical setting, many of these devices require the use of systemic anticoagulation (e.g., heparin) to avoid device failure [6]. The long-term use of anticoagulants can also have adverse effects, including hemorrhage and thrombocytopenia [7]. Despite these complications, heparin is still used as the standard anticoagulation therapy for patients on extracorporeal circulation (ECC), but the use of heparin does not prevent platelet activation and consumption.

Blood and the Coagulation Cascade

Biomaterial related thrombosis is a complex process, where the initial biological response when blood comes in contact with a foreign surface is protein adsorption, which is followed by platelet adhesion and activation, leading to thrombus formation (Fig. 16.1) [8]. Plasma proteins adsorb onto the surface of the implanted device (e.g., fibrinogen, fibronectin, von Willebrand factor (vWF), etc.) within seconds. These proteins further interact with receptors on the plasma membranes of platelets and facilitate platelet adhesion on the surface [9]. Upon contact with the foreign surface and platelet activation, a conformational change occurs, leading to the exposure of the glycoprotein GPIIb/IIIa receptor that binds platelets to fibrinogen [3]. Platelet activation also leads to conformation changes and the excretion of intracellular granulates containing agents (e.g., coagulation Factors V and VIII, adhesion molecules P-selectin and vWF, calcium ions, etc.) that further induce activation and aggregation of more platelets. This also activates the coagulation cascade, where a series of self-amplifying reactions triggered through surface contact (intrinsic pathway) or tissue factors (extrinsic pathway) ultimately converge at the final common pathway to form a thrombus (Fig. 16.2). Throughout the coagulation cascade, the normally inactive factors become enzymatically activated (e.g., Factor X becomes Factor Xa) by surface contact or cleavage by other activated enzymes. This sequence allows for rapid activation of other clotting factors and amplification of the entire coagulation cascade. When blood comes in contact with a foreign surface (biomedical device) protein adsorption will trigger the first step of the intrinsic pathway, with activation Factor XII to Factor XIIa. The presence of Factor XIIa will lead to the activation of Factor XI and eventually lead to the activation of Factor X and formation of thrombin (Factor II) in the common pathway [3]. Thrombin converts fibrinogen into fibrin and also activates Factor XIII, which cross-links and stabilizes fibrin into an insoluble gel that traps platelets and red blood cells in a thrombus on the surface within hours [9].

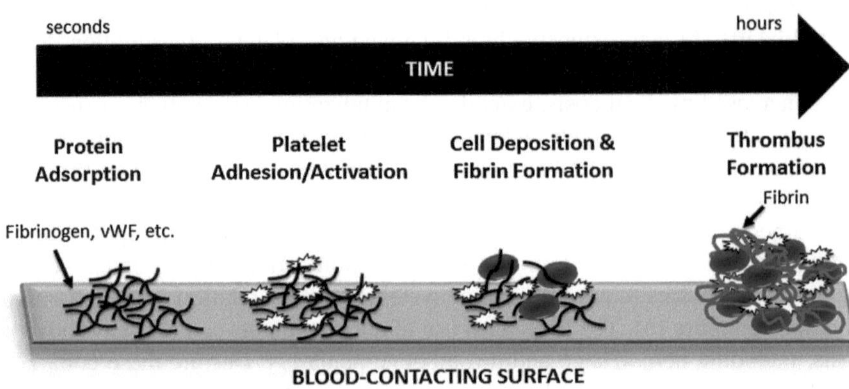

Fig. 16.1 Sequence of events leading to thrombus formation on blood-contacting surfaces (e.g., implanted medical devices)

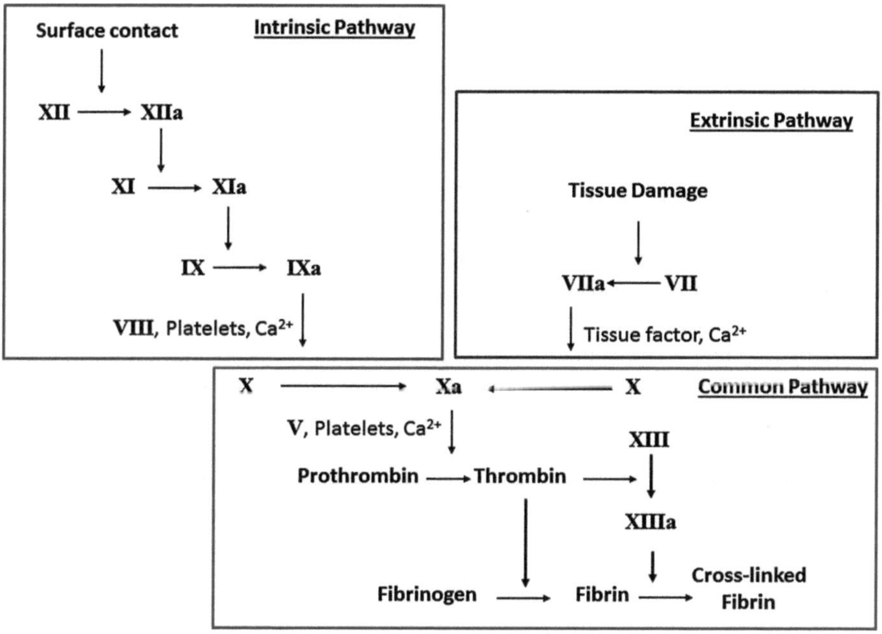

Fig. 16.2 Simplified schematic of the coagulation cascade, where clotting is initiated by either surface contact (intrinsic) or tissue factors (extrinsic) and ultimately converges at the common pathway to form thrombus

Improving Hemocompatibility of Biomedical Devices

In contrast to many polymers used in blood-contacting devices, the endothelial layer lining the human vasculature remains thrombus-free through several control mechanisms: a non-fouling phospholipid coating, membrane bound/released inhibitors of platelet and coagulation factors, as well as an efficient fibrinolytic system that removes fibrin deposits. Many of the major approaches for developing polymeric materials that are more hemocompatible are aimed at decreasing activation of key components of the coagulation cascade. Surface pacification is one approach, where the polymer surfaces aim to minimize protein adsorption (e.g., fibrinogen) and platelet adhesion/activation. Another approach is utilizing active polymer surfaces (e.g., immobilized heparin or nitric oxide (NO) release) that can interact with proteins, cells, and platelets to inhibit parts of the coagulation cascade. Research groups have worked to develop materials with suppressed blood-material interactions (e.g., polymeric materials which exhibit reduce protein and cell adhesion) and materials that mimic the non-thrombogenic endothelium. Polymers for blood-contacting devices are evaluated using various in vitro and in vivo testing methods, where protein and platelet adhesion are common markers to demonstrate the enhanced hemocompatibility properties of the material.

Overview of Current Technology/Strategies

Hydrophilic and Hydrophobic Materials

Protein adsorption on polymer surfaces is a well-recognized initiator of thrombus formation. Protein adsorption is dependent on a variety of material properties including surface charge, surface free energy, surface roughness, and a balance between hydrophobic and hydrophilic groups [10]. Ikada et al. [11] suggested that protein adhesion can be minimized when surface free energy is minimized, which occurs on strongly hydrophilic and strongly hydrophobic surfaces. One widely used approach has been to utilize hydrophilic surfaces in order to reduce protein adsorption and surface thrombogenicity. It has been concluded that hydrophilic polymers exert a steric repulsion effect towards blood proteins and cells [12, 13]. Hydrogels for blood contacting devices have been prepared using poly(vinyl alcohol) (PVA), polyacrylamides (PAAm), poly(N-vinyl pyrrolidone) (PNVP), poly(hydroxyethyl methacrylate) (PHEMA), poly(ethylene oxide) (PEO), poly(ethylene glycol) (PEG), poly(ethylene glycol) monomethyl ether (PEGME), and cellulose [14]. These hydrophilic materials strongly adsorb water, increasing its similarity to biological tissue and producing minimal interface tension with blood [15]. This strongly bound water also prevents cells and proteins from coming into contact with the polymer, reducing their adsorption to the surface [16].

Many hydrogels have poor mechanical properties, thus they have been grafted or coated onto other polymeric substrates and have improved hemocompatibility [15, 17–31]. Immobilization of PEG (–CH_2CH_2O–) is another popular means to make a polymer more protein and cell resistant [32]. Balakrishnan et al. demonstrated that PEGylated poly(viny chloride) had significantly less fibrinogen and platelet adsorption in comparison to a PVC control [21]. Li et al. reported that poly(poly(ethylene glycol) dimethacrylate) (P(PEGDMA)) grafted on silicone rubber reduced platelet adhesion by 90 % and also reduced plasma protein adsorption [26]. However, platelets still adsorbed on some PEG surfaces during in vivo experiments, despite the low protein adsorption observed during in vitro studies [33]. Plasma oxidation of polyethylene caused increased wettability with increased protein adsorption, but still reduced platelet adhesion [34]. Some hydrogels (e.g., cellulose) typically used as dialysis membranes/fibers are known to be thrombogenic, and therefore it can be concluded that low-protein adhesion does not necessarily result in hemocompatible surfaces [35]. Poly(2-methoxyethyl acrylate) (PMEA), which has been approved by the U.S. Food and Drug administration for medical use, not only exhibits lower protein adsorption and platelet adhesion than other hydrophilic surfaces, but it also reduces the amount of conformational changes that proteins undergo when adsorbed [16, 36]. This is of benefit since denaturation of adsorbed proteins can lead to platelet activation and subsequent thrombus formation, whereas, in contrast, when adsorbed proteins remain in their native confirmation, platelets cannot adhere (see discussion in Sect. "Albumin Coated Surfaces").

Strongly hydrophobic polymers are also known to have good hemocompatibility properties. Some hydrophobic polymers that are commonly used for medical applications include polyurethanes, silicones, polytetrafluoroethylene (PTFE), poly(vinyl chloride) (PVC), and polyethylene [37]. Very smooth silicone rubber and polyurethanes are known to have good thromboresistant properties [38, 39]. Hydrophobic polymers are conducive to non-specific protein adsorption (e.g., fibrinogen, albumin), and the adsorbed albumin appears to prevent subsequent protein adsorption [40]. It has been shown that increasing surface hydrophobicity also increases the amount of protein adsorbed, which, in turn, decreases the amount of conformational changes, potentially having a role in pacifying the surface [41]. For example, Elast-eon polymers (polyurethane and polydimethylsiloxane copolymers) are reported to have low surface energy and stronger binding to albumin (over fibrinogen) [42]. Alkyl chains have also been grafted on relatively hydrophilic polymers in order to increase the hydrophobicity of the surface [43–45]. Khorasani et al. [46] reported that both superhydrophobic and superhydrophilic surfaces were able to reduce platelet adhesion in comparison to controls. However, materials that are hydrophobic exhibit high protein adsorption and conformational changes of the adsorbed proteins [47, 48]. Polymeric materials with both hydrophilic and hydrophobic domains have also been reported to improve hemocompatibility (see Sect. "Patterned Modifications of Surfaces"). Ultimately, there is still no consensus as to which is better, hydrophilic or hydrophobic surfaces, for blood-contacting biomedical device applications [49].

Albumin Coated Surfaces

It is a widely accepted fact that protein adsorption is the first event that occurs upon foreign surface-blood contact. Human albumin (Alb) is the most abundant protein in the body with a concentration of 35–53 mg/mL in blood plasma. Due to its high concentration and low molecular weight, it is the first protein that adsorbs on the surface of implanted materials. Unlike fibrinogen, albumin is not known to have a peptide sequence that can facilitate binding of the platelet receptors and hence has been used as a coating to block non-specific platelet-surface interactions.

Since the early finding that Alb coated surfaces prevent adhesion of proteins and platelets [50], Alb has been extensively used as one of the strategies to develop hemocompatible surfaces. In one study, Alb was shown to significantly improve short-term thrombogenicity of Dacron arterial prostheses [51]. In another study, Guidoin et al. showed that Alb treatment does not affect the strength of polyester arterial prosthesis, but also found that within 1–2 weeks of implantation the Alb coating begins to disappear [52]. In a comparison of carbon dioxide gas plasma-treated polystyrene (PS-CO_2) coated Alb and PS-CO_2 treated Alb-heparin conjugate, albumin treated surfaces were found to be more effective in reducing platelet adhesion [53]. Albumin-heparin conjugate surface was also found to be suitable for endothelial cell seeding, which can further improve the hemocompatibility of the surfaces. Mohammad et al. demonstrated that combining Alb with Immunoglobulin G (IgG) results in a significant reduction in platelet adhesion in a 7 day in vitro study [54].

One of the limitations of Alb coating is that other proteins can displace Alb on the surface and reduce the long-term effectiveness of this approach. To prevent this displacement, covalent immobilization of Alb has been reported [55].

Another challenge with the Alb coating approach is that it adsorbs to hydrophobic surfaces more tightly than the hydrophilic surfaces, which necessitates increasing the hydrophobicity of the surface, a modification that is considered undesirable because platelets also adhere strongly to hydrophobic surfaces [56, 57]. Some other limitations of Alb coatings include conformational changes, physical degradation, and challenges with sterilization and shelf stability. In a recent study by the Latour group, it was shown that non-activated platelets can adhere to adsorbed Alb once a critical degree of adsorption-induced unfolding is reached [58, 59]. The platelet response shows a strong correlation with the degree of adsorption induced unfolding, very similar to the platelet adhesion response to adsorbed fibrinogen. These studies demonstrate the potential challenges with Alb coated surfaces, in that, while they may pacify the surface initially, the adsorbed Alb will show a time-dependent conformational change potentially leading to increased platelet adhesion/activation.

Patterned Modifications of Surfaces

Surfaces with patterns at the micro- and nanoscale level have also been investigated for their hemocompatibility properties. Copolymers containing both hydrophilic and hydrophobic domains (ABA-type block copolymers) have exhibited good antithrombotic properties [60–66], where the balance between the hydrophilicity and hydrobphobicity is important to enhance the biocompatibility [67]. Surfaces with hydrophilic/hydrophobic microdomains are reported to create an organized protein structure, albumin adsorbing on hydrophilic domains and fibrinogen adsorbing on hydrophobic domains, which suppresses platelet adhesion/activation [64, 68]. Okano et al. reported that copolymers composed of hydrophilic monomers, 2-hydroxyethyl methacrylate (HEMA) or poly(2-hydroxyethyl methacrylate) (PHEMA), and hydrophobic styrene had excellent thromboresistance properties, in terms of preventing platelet adhesion and deformation, during in vitro experiments [61, 62]. The PHEMA-styrene copolymer was coated on vascular grafts and had an occlusion time of 20 days (vs. 2 days for controls) when implanted in rabbits [61]. However, some of these ABA-type copolymers have the disadvantage that the hydrophilic segments have high surface free energy and bury themselves in the hydrophobic segments [69]. Oyane et al. [60] has reported a new block copolymer (PS-PME3MA) where the hydrophilic blocks remain at the surface when in contact with water. The PS-PME3MA polymer was found to be highly resistant to protein adsorption, cell adhesion, and platelet adhesion/activation.

Another type of surface modification that has been shown to exhibit improved hemocompatibility is attachment of hydrophilic polymer brushes, such as PEO [70, 71] or PEG [72–75]. These hydrophilic polymer brushes create an antifouling surface on the substrate due to steric repulsion. Long-chain polymer brushes have been attached to surfaces using physical adsorption or covalent binding techniques [76]. Polymer brushes that are more densely packed (high graft density) and have longer chain lengths further reduce protein adhesion and platelet adhesion/activation on the surface (Fig. 16.3) [77–79]. Stents coated with a chitosan-PEO coating were tested in

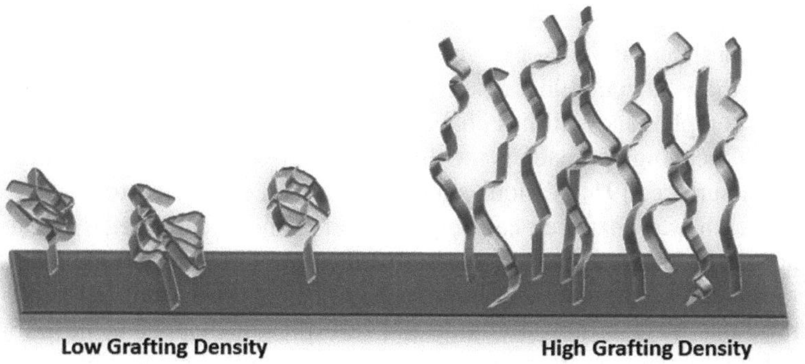

Fig. 16.3 Illustration showing relationship between polymer brush grafting density and chain length

an ex vivo porcine model, and had low platelet adhesion (similar to the endothelium) [80]. Dialysis membranes grafted with PEG brushes also had reduced platelet adhesion and improved hemocompatibility [72, 81, 82]. Tetraethylene glycol dimethyl ether grafted on polyethylene tubing was able to significantly reduce plasma protein (both fibrinogen and von Willebrand's factor) and platelet adsorption, in comparison to control tubing (PVC/Tygon, polyurethane, silicone, and polyethylene) [83]. Rodreguez-Emmenegger et al. recently reported an ultra-low fouling surface using poly[*N*-(2-hydroxypropyl) methacrylamide] (poly(HPMA)) brushes which was able to maintain the antifouling properties for up to two years of storage [84].

Attached Endothelial Cells

Another approach to making a surface more hemocompatible is to mimic the inner surface of blood vessels by attaching endothelial cells on the artificial surface, which provides an advantage in that the blood will come in contact with a surface that functions just like the endothelium. Endothelial cells (EC) line the inner walls of blood vessels and help in preventing thrombus formation by releasing anti-platelet agents such as nitric oxide (NO) and prostacyclin. Several research groups have used EC seeding on artificial surfaces for various biomedical applications including vascular grafts [85–87], stents [88], resorbable meshes [89], etc.

Williams and co-workers used a pressure sodding method to introduce EC cells into the luminal surface of PTFE grafts before implantation [86]. These grafts were tested for 12 weeks in carotid arteries of dogs. All of the control grafts clotted, whereas 86 % of the EC sodded grafts were found to be patent after the 12 week implantation period. To improve the hemocompatibility of vascular grafts, Taite et al. used NO releasing PU-PEG copolymer containing cell adhesive pentapeptide sequence to promote EC cell adhesion and migration [90]. In another study, Kutryk et al. [88] used xenotransplantation to seed endothelial cells on the surface of the stents to reduce blood contact with the stent surface.

Zünd and co-workers, seeded fibroblasts and ECs on polyglycolic acid (PGA) resorbable mesh as a precursor to vessels or cardiac valves [89].

Despite these encouraging results, EC proliferation and seeding on artificial surfaces is complex and still has challenges to overcome. One of the challenges of using the EC seeding approach is the difficulty in growing and maintaining the cells on artificial surfaces [91]. Various studies have been conducted to modify the surfaces in such a way that they can improve and promote endothelial cell adhesion. Kawamoto et al. showed that by plasma treatment of a PU surface, EC adhesion and proliferation can be dramatically improved [92]. In another study, Li and co-workers showed that increased proliferation and cell spreading can be achieved with arg-gly-asp (RGD) peptide grafted surfaces [93]. In yet another study, Yin et al. reported that mussel adhesive polypeptide mimic, containing dihydroxyphenylalanine and L-lysine (MAPDL) with PEG spacer, improved the cell attachment and growth and also reduced platelet adhesion in comparison to the controls [94]. Other challenges associated with the EC seeding approach include complex and expensive experimental procedures and long-term stability issues which still need to be addressed.

Zwitterionic Surfaces

Another effective approach to obtain a hemocompatible surface includes introducing a zwitterionic group, such as phosphobetaine, sulfobetaine or carboxylbetaine, to the substrate material (Fig. 16.4). These zwitterionic materials have been considered as biomimetic, antifouling, and hemocompatible materials because they contain phosphorylcholine-like groups which are present on the lipid bilayers of the cell membranes [95, 96]. Zwitterionic betaines have both anionic and cationic charged moieties in the same side chain which maintains an overall neutral charge. As discussed earlier, PEG and other hydrophilic materials, such as PEO and PHEMA, become hydrated via hydrogen bonding with water to prevent fouling. Zwitterionic materials can bind water molecules even more strongly (induced by electrostatic interactions) and hence can prevent significant change in protein conformation [97, 98].

There have been numerous publications showing the potential of zwitterion-based surfaces in resisting protein adsorption [95, 99], platelet adhesion [100–103],

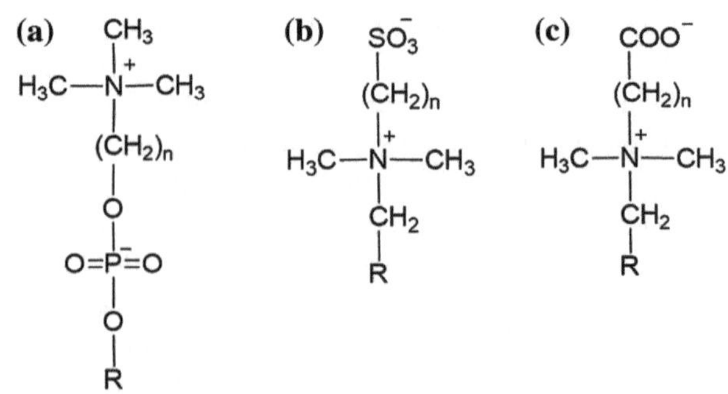

Fig. 16.4 Generic structures of phosphobetaines (**a**), sulfobetaines (**b**), and carboxylbetaines (**c**)

and consequently reduced thrombus formation compared to the control materials. Atom transfer radical polymerization (ATRP) is one of the commonly used methods to graft polymer surfaces with zwitterionic groups [97, 104–106]. Recently, various research teams have modified polymers using zwitterionic groups (carboxybetaine and sulfobetaine monomers) to mimic cell membrane surfaces [100, 102, 107, 108]. These surfaces have shown significantly lower fouling and platelet adhesion properties. In an another study, a zwitterionic silane coupling agent, N,N-dimethyl, N-(2-ethyl phosphate ethyl)-aminopropyltrimethyoxysilane (DMPAMS) was synthesized and studied for in vitro hemocompatibility [96]. Surfaces grafted with DMPAMS showed a steep drop in the water contact angle from 48° to 21.5°, indicating a more hydrophilic surface. At 200 mM surface concentration of DMPAMS, activated partial thromboplastin time (APTT) was prolonged from 28.8 s for the control to 37.8 s for the modified surface. Almost no platelet attachment was seen on the DMPAMS modified surface even after 3 h of blood contact. Lee et al. combined PEG with zwitterions for stent coating applications [109]. Significant reduction in protein adsorption and platelet adhesion was observed in addition to a substantial increase (compared to controls) in blood coagulation time for the zwitterionic-PEG grafted stents [109]. Polyurethane catheters grafted with a zwitterionic sulfobetain monomer (*N,N*-dimethyl-*N*-methacryloxyethyl-*N*-(3-sulfopropyl) ammonium, DMMSA) were also able to prevent platelet adhesion when soaked in platelet rich plasma (PRP) for 120 min [110]. Stents coated with phosphorylcholine, such as the commercial Bio*div Ysio* ™, have also been shown to exhibit enhanced hemocompatibility and increased endothelialization [111, 112].

Heparin Immobilization

Heparin (Fig. 16.5) is a highly sulfonated, anionic blood polysaccharide that binds to antithrombin III through ionic interactions, which inactivates thrombin and Factor Xa and thereby inhibits blood coagulation. Heparin has been clinically used since 1935 and is one of the most common anticoagulants employed during surgery and treatment of post-operative thrombosis and embolism [113]. However, systemic administration of anticoagulants, such as heparin, increases the risks of hemorrhage, thrombocytopenia, and thrombosis [7]. It is well known that some

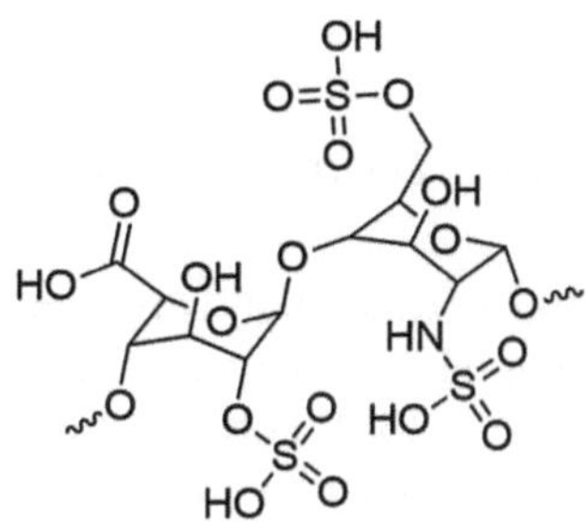

Fig. 16.5 Structure of a disaccharide sequence of heparin

heparinized and sulfonated materials have anticoagulant activity, resulting in prolongation of the blood clotting time [114]. Heparin immobilized on surfaces also suppresses platelet adhesion and protein adsorption [115]. Heparinization of surfaces is one of the most popular techniques to improve hemocompatibility and has been commercialized and used in the preparation of different medical devices (e.g., catheters, extracorporeal circuits, stents, grafts, etc.) [116, 117].

Heparin has been physically adsorbed, as well as ionically and covalently immobilized, on various polymer surfaces [117–122]. Ionic immobilization techniques require cationic residual groups in the polymer which interact with the ionic groups on heparin (e.g., COO^-, SO_4^{2-}, $NHSO_3^-$), while covalent binding of heparin utilizes the hydroxyl, carboxyl, or amino groups of heparin [120]. Heparin that is ionically bound to a surface will slowly be released due to ion-exchange with blood components, and this ultimately shortens the usage lifetime of the material [123]. The success of heparinized materials depends on the covalently bound heparin remaining in its native confirmation and its ability to complex with antithrombin III, which is most efficient when heparin is coupled by endpoint (vs. multipoint) attachment [124]. Michanetzis et al. [120] compared common heparin immobilization techniques, direct [125] and indirect [126] covalent binding, applied to the surfaces of commercially available polymers (silicone rubber, polyethylene, polypropylene, and poly(viny chloride)). While both techniques suffered from a low yield of immobilized heparin in comparison to the initial amount of heparin, the direct method produced a better heparinization yield (10.5 %) and both methods were able to improve the hemocompatibility in terms of reduced platelet activation and, therefore, an increased platelet retention rate. The anticoagulation properties of immobilized heparin have also been improved by using hydrophilic spacers (e.g., PEG), in comparison to heparin immobilized directly to the polymer. This reduces protein adsorption [127, 128]. Polyethylene tubing was modified with immobilized heparin via the method developed by Larm et al. [119] (commercialized as Carmeda ® BioActive Surface) and was able to maintain efficacy for up to 4 months when implanted in pigs [129]. The advantage of heparinized surfaces, in addition to the binding of antithrombin III, is the reduced/selective adhesion of certain plasma proteins, which alters the composition of the surface-adsorbed layer of proteins [130–133]. Heparin-coated devices, however, also suffer challenges, especially for long-term applications, due to heparin's short half-life and that surface-bound heparin only has ~1 % of the activity of free heparin [134]. Other immobilized direct thrombin inhibitors, such as hirudin, have demonstrated thromboresistant properties as well [116, 135].

Nitric Oxide (NO) Releasing/Generating Polymers

Nitric oxide (NO) is known to be a potent inhibitor of platelet activation and adhesion. Healthy endothelial cells exhibit an NO flux of $0.5-4.0 \times 10^{-10}$ mol cm^{-2} min^{-1} [136]. Polymeric materials with an NO flux that is equivalent to this level are expected to have similar anti-thrombotic properties. Nitric oxide is highly reactive under physiological conditions, thus a wide range of NO donor molecules, with functional groups that can store and release NO, have been studied for potential biomedical applications. Various reviews have been published that are devoted to a comprehensive discussion of different NO releasing/generating materials and their many potential biomedical applications [137–144]. The two major approaches to achieving localized NO release from polymeric surfaces are to (1) incorporate NO donor molecules or functional groups (e.g. diazeniumdiolates or *S*-nitrosothiols) into the polymer that will release the bound NO under physiological conditions (NO releasing polymers (NOrel)), or (2) incorporate catalysts into the polymers which can react with endogenous *S*-nitrosothiol (RSNO) species (present in blood) to locally generate NO (NO generating polymers (NOgen)) (Fig. 16.6). Nitric oxide has many other biological roles, including its antimicrobial action, which could potentially be utilized to also reduce the infection and biofilm formation that plagues many implantable biomedical devices. Thus, NO releasing/generating chemistries have the potential to create a dual-functioning material that is both antithrombotic and antimicrobial. Duration of the NO release can be tailored to fit the specific biomedical application of the device, and NO-generating materials can continuously generate NO in the presence of endogenous RSNO species (e.g., *S*-nitrosoglutathione (GSNO), *S*-nitrosocysteine (CysNO), etc.).

A wide variety of NO donor molecules have been investigated. The two most widely studied and used in combination with biomaterials are diazeniumdiolates and *S*-nitrosothiols. Diazeniumdiolates, also called NONOates, are relatively stable

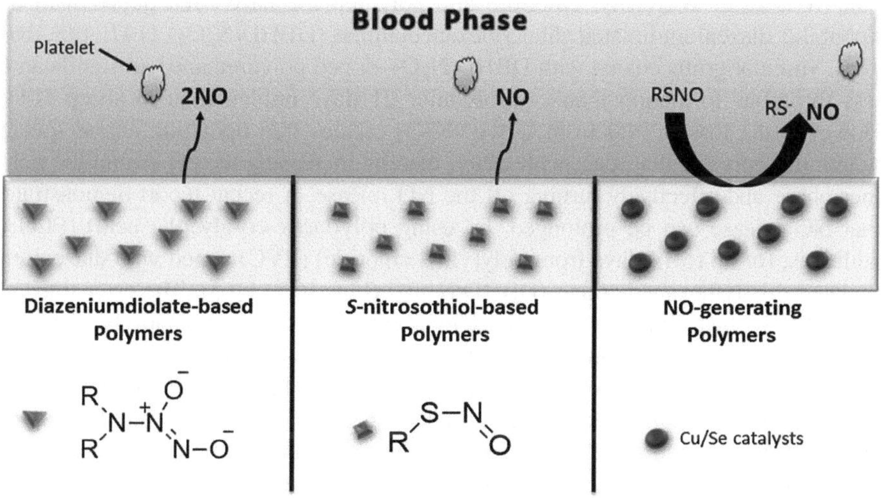

Fig. 16.6 Types of NO-releasing/generating polymers, where the NO that is released/generated can prevent activation of platelets that approach the polymer surface. Diazeniumdiolate-based materials undergo proton and thermal driven mechanisms to release NO. *S*-nitrosothiol (RSNO)-based polymers can release NO in the presence of heat, light, or metal ions (e.g., Cu^{+}). NO-generating materials consist of immobilized catalysts (e.g., Cu or Se compounds) that generate NO from endogenous RSNOs

species that undergo a proton or thermally driven mechanism to release two molecules of NO per diazeniumdiolate molecule. Diazeniumdiolates have been a popular NO donor that can easily be dispersed within polymers to facilitate localized NO release [145–149]. Mowery et al. [145] reported that water-soluble diamine-based diazeniumdiolates (e.g., DMHD/N_2O_2, diazeniumdiolated linear polyethylenimine (LPEI/N_2O_2)) leached from polymer matrices. Significant leaching of the NO donor species can result in non-localized NO release where the therapeutic action of NO occurs downstream from the biomedical device. Another concern with diazeniumdiolated-based polymers is the formation and leaching of some potentially carcinogenic decomposition products (e.g., *N*-nitrosamines) that are not intended for release into the bloodstream [145, 150]. To overcome the leaching concerns, strategies to covalently bind diazeniumdiolated functional groups to polydimethylsiloxane (PDMS) [151], xerogels [152–154], medical-grade polyurethanes [137, 155, 156], silica nanoparticles [157, 158], dendrimers [159–161], and other nanomaterials [138] have also been reported. Zhang et al. [151] covalently linked diaminoalkyltrimethoxysilane (DACA) to polydimethylsiloxane and then loaded this materials with NO under high pressure to form the diazeniumdiolated coating, DACA/N_2O_2-SR, which released NO for up to 20 days. The DACA/N_2O_2–SR was coated on extracorporeal circuits (ECC) and was able to reduce platelet consumption and thrombus formation during the 4 h blood flow in a rabbit model.

Attempts have also been made to add polymer top coats and/or create more lipophilic diazeniumdiolated species to minimize leaching into the aqueous phase and therefore maintain the localized NO release at the blood-polymer interface [147, 150, 162, 163]. Poly(vinyl chloride) and polyurethane have been doped with the lipophilic diazeniumdiolated dibutylhexanediamine (DBHD/N_2O_2) [147, 148, 164, 165]. Vascular grafts coated with DBHD/N_2O_2–doped polyurethane had significantly less thrombus formation than controls after 21 days implantation in sheep [148]. However, the loss of NO from DBHD/N_2O_2 creates free lipophilic amine species within the polymer that react with water, thereby increasing the pH within the polymer phase and effectively turning off the NO release. A recent report demonstrated that NO release can be prolonged, by using poly(lactic-co-glycolic acid) (PLGA) additives, for up to 14 days from poly(vinyl chloride) (PVC) doped with diazeniumdiolated dibutylhexanediamine (DBHD/N_2O_2) (Fig. 16.7) [165]. The ester linkages of the PLGA hydrolyze in the presence of water, producing lactic and glycolic acids that can act as proton sources to control the NO release from DBHD/N_2O_2-doped polymers. PLGAs can have varying hydrolysis rates, which is primarily determined by the copolymer ratio, the end group chemistry (either a free carboxylic acid or ester end group), and molecular weight. Handa et al. also demonstrated the importance of the inherent hemocompatibility of the base polymer (in which the NO chemistry is incorporated) [166]. By incorporating the same DBHD/N_2O_2 and PLGA chemistry into the Elast-eon E2As polymer (a copolymer with a mixed soft segment of poly(dimethylsiloxane) and poly(hexamethylene oxide) with a methylene diphenyl isocyante (MDI) hard segment), which inherently is more hemocompatible than PVC, the platelet count after 4 h of ECC (97 ± 10 % of baseline) was significantly improved over the PVC/DOS-based coating (79 ± 11 % of baseline) [165, 166].

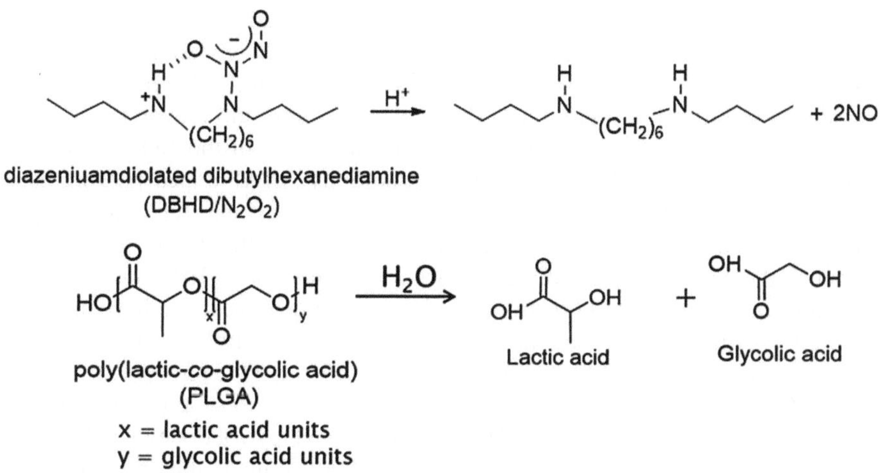

Fig. 16.7 Key reactions involved in NO release from diazeniumdiolated dibutylhexanediamine (DBHD/N_2O_2) in the presence of poly(lactic-*co*-glycolic acid) additive, that provides additional protons to drive the NO release reaction

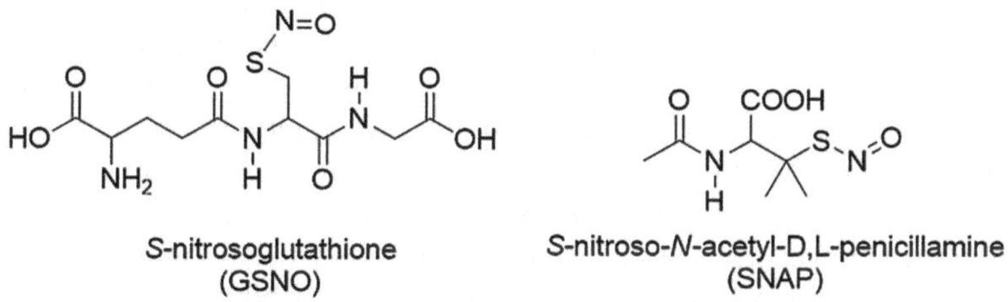

Fig. 16.8 Structures of example *S*-nitrosothiols species, *S*-nitrosoglutathione (GSNO) and *S*-nitroso-*N*-acetyl-D,L-penicillamine (SNAP)

Another widely studied class of NO donor molecules is *S*-nitrosothiol (RSNO) species (examples shown in Fig. 16.8). Physiological RSNOs, including *S*-nitrosoalbumin, *S*-nitrosocysteine (CysNO), and *S*-nitrosoglutathione (GSNO), are considered an endogenous reservoir of NO in vivo [167–169]. Other synthetic RSNOs, such as *S*-nitroso-*N*-acetylpenicillamine (SNAP) and *S*-nitroso-*N*-acetylcysteine (SNAC), have been shown to exhibit significant antimicrobial and antithrombotic effects [170–173]. It has also been demonstrated that RSNOs are both vasodilators and potent inhibitors of platelet aggregation [174–176]. RSNOs undergo thermal decomposition to release NO and produce a corresponding disulfide species (RSSR). The NO release from RSNOs can also be catalyzed by metal ions (e.g., Cu^+) [177] and by light, through irradiation at energies that correspond to the *S*-nitroso absorption bands at 340 and/or 590 nm [178–180]. Incorporation of RSNOs into polymers can extend the utility of these NO donors to be applicable in biomedical devices.

Low molecular weight RSNOs have been non-covalently dispersed within various polymer matrices [181–187]. Seabra et al. [182] prepared GSNO-doped poly(vinyl alcohol) and poly(vinyl pyrrolidone) blended films. This polymer matrix provided a stabilization effect on GSNO decomposition, in comparison to aqueous solutions of GSNO. However, due to leaching, 90 % of the NO was released during the first 24 h under physiological conditions. SNAP-doped polyurethanes (Tecoflex SG-80A and Tecophillic SP-60D-60) also exhibit rapid leaching of SNAP when soaked in buffer [186]. The rapid leaching of the RSNOs significantly shortened the duration of the NO release from these materials. Therefore, strategies to synthetically bind RSNO functionalities to the polymer backbone have also been explored. *S*-Nitrosothiol functionalities have been covalently bound to polymers such as xerogels [188, 189], polyurethanes [137, 190, 191], degradable polyesters [192–196], polyester/poly(methyl methacrylate) blends [197], poly(vinyl methyl ether-*co*-malic anhydride) (PVMMA) and poly(vinyl pyrrolidone) (PVP) [198], and poly(dimethylsiloxane) [199]. Dendrimers [200], fumed silica particles [180, 191], and silica nanoparticles [155, 156, 201] have also been synthetically modified with covalently bound RSNO functionalities and these materials can be doped into various polymer matrices to create coatings for biomedical devices.

Many of the RSNO-modified materials reported to date have not proven clinically useful due to their limited NO release lifetimes, low conversion to RSNO during synthesis, or lack of RSNO stability during storage. Recently, the RSNO-doping method has been revisited, utilizing more hydrophobic polymers. GSNO-doped Tygon, a proprietary plasticized poly(vinyl chloride) polymer, exhibited minimal leaching of GSNO during soaking under physiological conditions [187]. Incorporating SNAP into Elast-eon E2As created an NO-releasing polymer that is stable during storage (even at elevated temperatures), locally delivers NO under physiological conditions, significantly reduces the leaching of SNAP, and preserves platelets during a 4 h ECC study [186].

Due to the limited NO reservoir from NO donors that can be incorporated into polymers (either covalently bound or non-covalently dispersed), these NO releasing materials typically have a finite duration of NO release. Another approach to achieving localized NO delivery at a polymer/blood interface for a longer period of time is to use NO generating (NOgen) materials that utilize endogenous RSNOs and/or nitrite to locally generate NO at the blood-polymer interface. Various thiol-containing species (L-cysteine, 2-iminothiolane, and cysteine polypeptide) have been immobilized on polyethylene terephthalate and polyurethane, where the free thiol undergoes a transnitrosation reaction with circulating RSNOs (e.g., S-nitroso-albumin) [202, 203]. The resulting CysNO on the PET and PU surface decomposes to elevate the NO levels locally at the polymer/blood interface, which reduces platelet adhesion on the surface by more than 50 %. Other NOgen materials consist of catalysts (e.g., Cu (I/II) complexes or organoselenium species) that are immobilized within the polymer and are capable of locally generating NO from endogenous RSNOs and/or nitrite. Copper (II) sites within a polymer can be reduced to Cu(I) by endogenous reducing agents that are present in the blood (e.g., thiols, ascorbate). The Cu(I) sites then can reduce endogenous RSNOs in the blood (e.g., GSNO, CysNO, etc.) to NO and free thiolate anions in a catalytic manner [177]. Lipophilic copper complexes that were incorporated into polymers were able to reduce physiological levels of RSNOs and nitrite to locally generate NO [204–207]. Another reported NOgen polymer consists of copper nanoparticles (Cu^0) dispersed within a hydrophilic polymer (Tecophillic SP-60D-60), which was evaluated using a rabbit model for extracorporeal circulation (ECC) [208]. However, continuous infusion of SNAP was needed to supplement the endogenous RSNO levels in order to achieve good efficacy in reducing thrombus formation.

Organoselenium species have been studied as mimics of glutathione peroxidase (GPx), a selenoenzyme that protects cells from oxidative stress by reducing hydroperoxides using glutathione (GSH) [209], and investigated for their ability to generate NO from RSNOs [210]. Selenium catalysts are highly selective for reduction of RSNOs and exhibit no catalytic activity for nitrite or nitrate reduction [211]. Low molecular weight organoselenum species, selenocystamine (SeCA) and 3,3′-diselenidedipropionic acid (SeDPA), were immobilized on cellulose filter paper and polyethylenimine (PEI), demonstrating potential dialysis membrane applications [212]. In the presence of reducing agents at physiological pH, the diselenides can be converted into selenolates, which are the key intermediates that can reduce RSNOs into NO and thiolates [212]. Selenium species were also incorporated into layer-by-layer coatings containing alternating layers of sodium alginate (Alg) and selenium-modified PEI. Alg-PEI layer-by-layer films modified with SeDPA were able to generate physiological levels of NO from GSNO and also exhibited minimal leaching of catalytic sites after soaking in blood [211]. The Alg-PEI layer-by-layer coating was also modified to immobilize ebselen (2-phenyl-1,2-benzisoselenazol-3-(2H)-one), an aromatic selenium species with good GPx activity, and coated on catheters [213]. These selenium-based materials were able to generate physiological levels of NO from RSNOs; however, some reduction of NO flux was observed after soaking in blood, potentially from catalytic sites being blocked by adsorbed plasma proteins or low levels of catalyst species leaching into the solution. These NOgen polymers have an advantage in that they could potentially generate NO at the blood-polymer interface indefinitely, provided that the blood in contact with the polymer has adequate levels of RSNOs present at all times [214].

Methods to Assess Hemocompatibility

Extensive reviews on the various methods to evaluate the hemocompatibility of polymers and medical devices have been published (summarized in Table 16.1) [1, 215–223]. Clinical devices still suffer challenges due to thrombosis, even after standard testing as developed by the International Organization for Standardization (ISO 10993-4, "Selection of Tests for Interactions with Blood") [219, 224]. The ISO hemocompatibility testing requires evaluation of thrombosis, coagulation, hematology, platelet count and function, and immunology. Initial surface and physical-chemical characterization studies can provide useful information in order to correlate surface characteristics with hemocompatibility. Surface roughness, surface chemistry, surface charge distribution, and interfacial free energy are well known factors that

Table 16.1 Common surface characterization and blood compatibility tests used to evaluate the hemocompatibility of blood-contacting polymers

Surface Characterization	
Elemental and chemical composition	Porosity
	Roughness
Physical properties	Charge and charge density
	Elasticity
	Surface energy (wettability)

Blood Compatibility Testing	
In vitro Testing	Platelet adhesion (LDH assay)
Static (soaking in blood or plasma)	
Dynamic (agitators, centrifugation systems, flow chambers, Chandlerloops, closed loops)	Protein adsorption (fluorescent fibrinogen absorption assay)
	Circulating platelet, plasma fibrinogen, white blood cell counts
	Prothrombin time (PT), activated partial thromboplastin time (aPTT), and Thrombin clotting time (TCT)
In Vivo Models	
Coated or fabricated medical devices: Catheters Stents Vascular grafts Extracorporeal circuits Dialysis membranes Biomedical sensors	Platelet function via aggregation
	Flow cytometry (FACS) analysis of activation (e.g. P-selectin)
	Thrombus area on the device
	Embolism (e.g., visual, light scattering, Doppler ultrasound)
	Patency and occlusion time

can influence protein adsorption and cell-material surface interaction [225]. Many of the common hemocompatibility testing methods involve flowing blood through tubing (both in vitro and in vivo), and then conducting hemocompatibility evaluations of the blood exiting the test system. However, while they have potential to still be used as preliminary screening methods, in vitro static assays, such as fluorescent-based fibrinogen adsorption or platelet adhesion [164, 226], and dynamic systems (e.g. Chandler loops [227]) are limited due to the blood death over time. Various medical devices (e.g., catheters, stents, vascular grafts, dialysis membranes, etc.) have been fabricated or coated with polymers for evaluation in animal models in order to mimic clinical application. Arterio-venous (A-V) and areterio-arterial (A-A) shunt models have been used to test hemocompatibility, and they allow for evaluation of both local and systemic effects of the test polymer. For example, the rabbit model of thrombogenicity is a useful model of extracorporeal circulation, where the polymer is coated on the inner walls of Tygon tubing that form the ECC circuit [164, 208]. The ECC circuit is placed on the rabbit using an A-V shunt, and blood flows through the circuit for 4 h. This model allows a comprehensive evaluation of hemocompatibility (platelet preservation/consumption, plasma fibrinogen levels, and occlusion time) as well as the thrombus area in the ECC circuit after 4 h of blood flow.

Despite the encouraging results published for many of the polymer strategies discussed above, there are still some challenges with hemocompatibility testing and clinical application. For example, counting adhered platelets on the surface is a common method to evaluate hemocompatibility and has been used as a functional test for many of the polymers discussed above. This may be a good initial test; however, it does not provide the complete picture because platelets could be activated by the foreign surface and aggregate downstream from the device [223]. Similarly, during in vivo testing of a new material, any thrombus that forms on the surface may also be carried downstream. In addition, results from short-term in vitro testing cannot necessarily be used to predict long-term in vivo results [220]. Another challenge is the fact that research groups use a wide variety of testing methods and controls, so it remains unclear as to how significant the improvement is of these new materials over other materials (either published or clinically used) [220]. Defining standardized testing methods and appropriate controls/reference materials used by researchers (commercial, clinical, and academic) will help improve the advancement of novel materials to clinical application.

Conclusions

Over the last 50 years, much has been learned about blood-material interactions, and a variety of strategies have been reported to improve the hemocompatibility of blood-contacting medical devices. Materials reported to date primarily target different parts of the coagulation cascade (e.g., protein adsorption, platelet adhesion and activation, fibrin formation, etc.). Although many of the approaches described above are promising individually, combining two or more of these approaches may prove most beneficial. When these materials are effective, they may reduce or eliminate the need for administration of systemic anti-coagulation therapeutics (e.g. heparin) which is currently clinically utilized to reduce the risk of thrombus formation and other complications during use of blood-contacting devices. However, challenges still exist (e.g., shelf life and sterilization stability) and need to be addressed for some of the polymer approaches discussed here in order to achieve widespread clinical application. Standard testing methods should be utilized to test and compare the hemocompatibility of commercially available and new polymeric materials for biomedical applications.

References

1. Ratner, B.D.: The catastrophe revisited: blood compatibility in the 21st century. Biomaterials **28**(34), 5144–5147 (2007)
2. Colman, R.W.: Mechanisms of thrombus formation and dissolution. Cardiovasc. Pathol. **2**(3), 23–31 (1993)

3. Gorbet, M.B., Sefton, M.V.: Biomaterial-associated thrombosis: roles of coagulation factors, complement, platelets and leukocytes. Biomaterials **25**(26), 5681–5703 (2004)
4. Dwyer, A.: Surface-treated catheters—a review. In: Seminars in dialysis, pp 542–546. Wiley Online Library (2008)
5. Ratner, B.D.: Blood compatibility—a perspective. J. Biomater. Sci. Polym. Ed. **11**(11), 1107–1119 (2000)
6. Gaffney, A.M., Wildhirt, S.M., Griffin, M.J., Annich, G.M., Radomski, M.W.: Extracorporeal life support. BMJ 341 (2010)
7. Robinson, T.M., Kickler, T.S., Walker, L.K., Ness, P., Bell, W.: Effect of extracorporeal membrane oxygenation on platelets in newborns. Crit. Care Med. **21**(7), 1029–1034 (1993)
8. Horbett, T.A.: Principles underlying the role of adsorbed plasma proteins in blood interactions with foreign materials. Cardiovasc. Pathol. **2**(3), 137–148 (1993)
9. Schopka, S., Schmid, T., Schmid, C., Lehle, K.: Current strategies in cardiovascular biomaterial functionalization. Materials **3**(1), 638–655 (2010)
10. Brashm, J., Horbett, T.: Proteins at interfaces: physicochemical and biochemical studies. In: ACS Symposium Series, 1987, p 1. American Chemical Society, Washington, DC
11. Ikada, Y., Suzuki, M., Tamada, Y.: Polymer surfaces possessing minimal interaction with blood components. In: Polymers as biomaterials, pp 135–147. Springer, Heidelberg (1984)
12. Nagaoka, S., Mori, Y., Takiuchi, H., Yokota, K., Tanzawa, H., Nishiumi, S.: Interaction between blood components and hydrogels with poly (oxyethylene) chains. In: Polymers as biomaterials, pp 361–374. Springer, Heidelberg (1984)
13. Jeon, S., Lee, J., Andrade, J., De Gennes, P.: Protein—surface interactions in the presence of polyethylene oxide: I. Simplified Theo. J Colloid Interface Sci **142**(1), 149–158 (1991)
14. Peppas, N.A., Huang, Y., Torres-Lugo, M., Ward, J.H., Zhang, J.: Physicochemical, foundations and structural design of hydrogels in medicine and biology. Annu. Rev. Biomed. Eng. **2**, 9–29 (2000)
15. Okada, T., Ikada, Y.: Modification of silicone surface by graft polymerization of acrylamide with corona discharge. Makromol. Chem. **192**(8), 1705–1713 (1991)
16. Tanaka, M., Hayashi, T., Morita, S.: The roles of water molecules at the biointerface of medical polymers. Polym. J. **45**(7), 701–710 (2013)
17. Wang, H., Yu, T., Zhao, C., Du, Q.: Improvement of hydrophilicity and blood compatibility on polyethersulfone membrane by adding polyvinylpyrrolidone. Fibers Polym. **10**(1), 1–5 (2009)
18. Hanson, S.R., Harker, L.A., Ratner, B.D., Hoffman, A.: In vivo evaluation of artificial surfaces with a nonhuman primate model of arterial thrombosis. J. Lab. Clin. Med. **95**(2), 289–304 (1980)
19. Morra, M., Occhiello, E., Garbassi, F.: Surface modification of blood contacting polymers by poly (ethyleneoxide). Clin. Mater. **14**(3), 255–265 (1993)
20. Kwon, O.H., Nho, Y.C., Park, K.D., Kim, Y.H.: Graft copolymerization of polyethylene glycol methacrylate onto polyethylene film and its blood compatibility. J. Appl. Polym. Sci. **71**(4), 631–641 (1999)
21. Balakrishnan, B., Kumar, D., Yoshida, Y., Jayakrishnan, A.: Chemical modification of poly (vinyl chloride) resin using poly (ethylene glycol) to improve blood compatibility. Biomaterials **26**(17), 3495–3502 (2005)
22. Amiji, M.M.: Synthesis of anionic poly(ethylene glycol) derivative for chitosan surface modification in blood-contacting applications. Carbohydr. Polym. **32**(3–4), 193–199 (1997)
23. Wang, J., Pan, C.J., Huang, N., Sun, H., Yang, P., Leng, Y.X., Chen, J.Y., Wan, G.J., Chu, P.K.: Surface characterization and blood compatibility of poly(ethylene terephthalate) modified by plasma surface grafting. Surf. Coat. Technol. **196**(1–3), 307–311 (2005)
24. Okner, R., Domb, A.J., Mandler, D.: Electrochemically deposited poly(ethylene glycol)-based sol–gel thin films on stainless steel stents. New J. Chem. **33**(7), 1596–1604 (2009)
25. Nho, Y.C., Kwon, O.H.: Blood compatibility of AAc, HEMA, and PEGMA-grafted cellulose film. Radiat. Phys. Chem. **66**(4), 299–307 (2003)

26. Li, M., Neoh, K.G., Xu, L.Q., Wang, R., Kang, E.T., Lau, T., Olszyna, D.P., Chiong, E.: Surface modification of silicone for biomedical applications requiring long-term antibacterial, antifouling, and hemocompatible properties. Langmuir **28**(47), 16408–16422 (2012)
27. Jin, J., Jiang, W., Yin, J.H., Ji, X.L., Stagnaro, P.: Plasma proteins adsorption mechanism on polyethylene-grafted poly(ethylene glycol) surface by quartz crystal microbalance with dissipation. Langmuir **29**(22), 6624–6633 (2013)
28. Chung, C.W., Kim, H.W., Kim, Y.B., Rhee, Y.H.: Poly(ethylene glycol)-grafted poly(3-hydroxyundecenoate) networks for enhanced blood compatibility. Int. J. Biol. Macromol. **32**(1–2), 17–22 (2003)
29. Chiag, Y.C., Chang, Y., Chen, W.Y., Ruaan, R.C.: Biofouling resistance of ultrafiltration membranes controlled by surface self-assembled coating with PEGylated copolymers. Langmuir **28**(2), 1399–1407 (2012)
30. Bajpai, A.K.: Blood protein adsorption onto a polymeric biomaterial of polyethylene glycol and poly[(2-hydroxyethyl methacrylate)-co-acrylonitrile] and evaluation of in vitro blood compatibility. Polym. Int. **54**(2), 304–315 (2005)
31. Alibeik, S., Zhu, S., Brash, J.L.: Surface modification with PEG and hirudin for protein resistance and thrombin neutralization in blood contact. Colloids Surf. B **81**(2), 389–396 (2010)
32. Harris, J.M.: Poly (ethylene glycol) chemistry: biotechnical and biomedical applications. Springer, Heidelberg (1992)
33. Llanos, G.R., Sefton, M.V.: Immobilization of poly (ethylene glycol) onto a poly (vinyl alcohol) hydrogel: 2. Evaluation of thrombogenicity. J. Biomed. Mater. Res. **27**(11), 1383–1391 (1993)
34. Lee, J.H., Lee, H.B.: Platelet adhesion onto wettability gradient surfaces in the absence and presence of plasma proteins. J. Biomed. Mater. Res. **41**(2), 304–311 (1998)
35. Sefton, M., Gemmell, C., Gorbet, M. Nonthrombogenic treatments and strategies. Biomaterials Science: An Introduction to Materials in Medicine, pp. 456–470. Elsevier, New York (2004)
36. Tanaka, M., Motomura, T., Kawada, M., Anzai, T., Yuu, K., Shiroya, T., Shimura, K., Onishi, M., Akira, M.: Blood compatible aspects of poly(2-methoxyethylacrylate) (PMEA)—relationship between protein adsorption and platelet adhesion on PMEA surface. Biomaterials **21**(14), 1471–1481 (2000)
37. Nydegger, U., Rieben, R., Lämmle, B.: Biocompatibility in transfusion medicine. Transfus. Sci. **17**(4), 481–488 (1996)
38. Kolobow, T., Stool, E., Weathersby, P., Pierce, J., Hayano, F., Suaudeau, J.: Superior blood compatibility of silicone rubber free of silica filler in the membrane lung. ASAIO Trans. **20**, 269 (1974)
39. Szycher, M.: Biostability of polyurethane elastomers: a critical review. J. Biomater. Appl. **3**(2), 297–402 (1988)
40. Lassen, B., Malmsten, M.: Structure of protein layers during competitive adsorption. J. Colloid Interface Sci. **180**(2), 339–349 (1996)
41. Sivaraman, B., Fears, K.P., Latour, R.A.: Investigation of the effects of surface chemistry and solution concentration on the conformation of adsorbed proteins using an improved circular dichroism method. Langmuir **25**(5), 3050–3056 (2009)
42. Cozzens, D., Luk, A., Ojha, U., Ruths, M., Faust, R.: Surface characterization and protein interactions of segmented polyisobutylene-based thermoplastic polyurethanes. Langmuir **27**(23), 14160–14168 (2011)
43. Bahulekar, R., Tamura, N., Ito, S., Kodama, M.: Platelet adhesion and complement activation studies on poly (N-alkyl mono and disubstituted) acrylamide derivatives. Biomaterials **20**(4), 357–362 (1999)
44. Matsuda, T., Ito, S.: Surface coating of hydrophilic-hydrophobic block co-polymers on a poly (acrylonitrile) haemodialyser reduces platelet adhesion and its transmembrane stimulation. Biomaterials **15**(6), 417–422 (1994)

45. Hoffman, A.S., Cohn, D., Hanson, S.R., Harker, L.A., Horbett, T.A., Ratner, B.D., Reynolds, L.O.: Application of radiation-grafted hydrogels as blood-contacting biomaterials. Radiat. Phys. Chem. **22**(1), 267–283 (1983)
46. Khorasani, M., Mirzadeh, H.: In vitro blood compatibility of modified PDMS surfaces as superhydrophobic and superhydrophilic materials. J. Appl. Polym. Sci. **91**(3), 2042–2047 (2004)
47. Okubo, M., Hattori, H.: Competitive adsorption of fibrinogen and albumin onto polymer microspheres having hydrophilic/hydrophobic heterogeneous surface structures. Colloid Polym. Sci. **271**(12), 1157–1164 (1993)
48. Klose, T., Welzel, P.B., Werner, C.: Protein adsorption from flowing solutions on pure and maleic acid copolymer modified glass particles. Colloids Surf., B **51**(1), 1–9 (2006)
49. Sefton, M.V., Gemmell, C.H., Gorbet, M.B.: What really is blood compatibility? J. Biomater. Sci. Polym. Ed. **11**(11), 1165–1182 (2000)
50. Andrade, J., Hlady, V.: Protein adsorption and materials biocompatibility: a tutorial review and suggested hypotheses. In: Biopolymers/Non-Exclusion HPLC, pp 1–63. Springer, Heidelberg (1986)
51. Kottke-Marchant, K., Anderson, J.M., Umemura, Y., Marchant, R.E.: Effect of albumin coating on the in vitro blood compatibility of Dacron® arterial prostheses. Biomaterials **10**(3), 147–155 (1989)
52. Guidoin, R., Snyder, R., Martin, L., Botzko, K., Marois, M., Awad, J., King, M., Domurado, D., Bedros, M., Gosselin, C.: Albumin coating of a knitted polyester arterial prosthesis: an alternative to preclotting. Ann. Thorac. Surg. **37**(6), 457–465 (1984)
53. Bos, G.W., Scharenborg, N.M., Poot, A.A., Engbers, G.H., Beugeling, T., Van Aken, W.G., Feijen, J.: Blood compatibility of surfaces with immobilized albumin–heparin conjugate and effect of endothelial cell seeding on platelet adhesion. J. Biomed. Mater. Res. **47**(3), 279–291 (1999)
54. Mohammad, S., Olsen, D.: Immobilized albumin-immunoglobulin G for improved hemocompatibility of biopolymers. ASAIO J. **35**(3), 384–387 (1989)
55. Hoffman, A., Schmer, G., Harris, C., Kraft, W.: Covalent binding of biomolecules to radiation-grafted hydrogels on inert polymer surfaces. ASAIO J. **18**(1), 10–16 (1972)
56. Mikhalovska, L.I., Santin, M., Denyer, S.P., Lloyd, A.W., Teer, D.G., Field, S., Mikhalovsky, S.V.: Fibrinogen adsorption and platelet adhesion to metal and carbon coatings. Thromb. Haemost. **92**(11), 1032–1039 (2004)
57. Dion, I., Roques, X., Baquey, H., Baudet, E., Basse Cathalinat, B., More, N.: Hemocompatibility of diamond-like carbon coating. Bio-Med. Mater. Eng. **3**(1), 51–55 (1993)
58. Sivaraman, B., Latour, R.A.: The adherence of platelets to adsorbed albumin by receptor-mediated recognition of binding sites exposed by adsorption-induced unfolding. Biomaterials **31**(6), 1036–1044 (2010)
59. Sivaraman, B., Latour, R.A.: Delineating the roles of the GPIIb/IIIa and GP-Ib-IX-V platelet receptors in mediating platelet adhesion to adsorbed fibrinogen and albumin. Biomaterials **32**(23), 5365–5370 (2011)
60. Oyane, A., Ishizone, T., Uchida, M., Furukawa, K., Ushida, T., Yokoyama, H.: Spontaneous formation of blood-compatible surfaces on hydrophobic polymers: Surface enrichment of a block copolymer with a water-soluble block. Adv Mater **17**(19), 2329–2332 (2005)
61. Okano, T., Aoyagi, T., Kataoka, K., Abe, K., Sakurai, Y., Shimada, M., Shinohara, I.: Hydrophilic-hydrophobic microdomain surfaces having an ability to suppress platelet aggregation and their in vitro antithrombogenicity. J. Biomed. Mater. Res. **20**(7), 919–927 (1986)
62. Okano, T., Nishiyama, S., Shinohara, I., Akaike, T., Sakurai, Y., Kataoka, K., Tsuruta, T.: Effect of hydrophilic and hydrophobic microdomains on mode of interaction between block polymer and blood platelets. J. Biomed. Mater. Res. **15**(3), 393–402 (1981)
63. Sato, H., Nakajima, A., Hayashi, T., Chen, G.W., Noishiki, Y.: Microheterophase structure, permeability, and biocompatibility of A-B-A triblock copolymer membranes composed of poly (γ-ethyl L-glutamate) as the A component and polybutadiene as the B component. J. Biomed. Mater. Res. **19**(9), 1135–1155 (1985)

64. Nojiri, C., Okano, T., Jacobs, H.A., Park, K.D., Mohammad, S.F., Olsen, D.B., Kim, S.W.: Blood compatibility of PEO grafted polyurethane and HEMA/styrene block copolymer surfaces. J. Biomed. Mater. Res. **24**(9), 1151–1171 (1990)
65. Takahara, A., Tashita, J.-I., Kajiyama, T., Takayanagi, M., Macknight, W.J.: Microphase separated structure and blood compatibility of segmented poly (urethaneureas) with different diamines in the hard segment. Polymer **26**(7), 978–986 (1985)
66. Takahara, A., Tashita, J.-I., Kajiyama, T., Takayanagi, M., Macknight, W.J.: Microphase separated structure, surface composition and blood compatibility of segmented poly (urethaneureas) with various soft segment components. Polymer **26**(7), 987–996 (1985)
67. Sasaki, T., Ratner, B.D., Hoffman, A.S.: Radiation-induced co-graft polymerization of 2-hydroxyethyl methacrylate and ethyl methacrylate onto silicone rubber films. In: Abstracts of Papers of ACS. ACS, Washington, DC, Jan 1975
68. Okano, T., Uruno, M., Sugiyama, N., Shimada, M., Shinohara, I., Kataoka, K., Sakurai, Y.: Suppression of platelet activity on microdomain surfaces of 2-hydroxyethyl methacrylate-polyether block copolymers. J. Biomed. Mater. Res. **20**(7), 1035–1047 (1986)
69. Lewis, K.B., Ratner, B.D.: Observation of surface rearrangement of polymers using ESCA. J. Colloid Interface Sci. **159**(1), 77–85 (1993)
70. Chen, H., Zhang, Z., Chen, Y., Brook, M.A., Sheardown, H.: Protein repellant silicone surfaces by covalent immobilization of poly (ethylene oxide). Biomaterials **26**(15), 2391–2399 (2005)
71. Shen, M., Martinson, L., Wagner, M.S., Castner, D.G., Ratner, B.D., Horbett, T.A.: PEO-like plasma polymerized tetraglyme surface interactions with leukocytes and proteins: in vitro and in vivo studies. J. Biomater. Sci. Polym. Ed. **13**(4), 367–390 (2002)
72. Fushimi, F., Nakayama, M., Nishimura, K., Hiyoshi, T.: Platelet adhesion, contact phase coagulation activation, and C5a generation of polyethylene glycol acid-grafted high flux cellulosic membrane with varieties of grafting amounts. Artif. Organs **22**(10), 821–826 (1998)
73. Gorbet, M.B., Sefton, M.V.: Leukocyte activation and leukocyte procoagulant activities after blood contact with polystyrene and polyethylene glycol–immobilized polystyrene beads. J. Lab. Clin. Med. **137**(5), 345–355 (2001)
74. Hansson, K.M., Tosatti, S., Isaksson, J., Wetterö, J., Textor, M., Lindahl, T.L., Tengvall, P.: Whole blood coagulation on protein adsorption-resistant PEG and peptide functionalised PEG-coated titanium surfaces. Biomaterials **26**(8), 861–872 (2005)
75. Suggs, L.J., Shive, M.S., Garcia, C.A., Anderson, J.M., Mikos, A.G.: In vitro cytotoxicity and in vivo biocompatibility of poly (propylene fumarate-co-ethylene glycol) hydrogels. J. Biomed. Mater. Res. **46**(1), 22–32 (1999)
76. Gombotz, W.R., Guanghui, W., Horbett, T.A., Hoffman, A.S.: Protein adsorption to poly (ethylene oxide) surfaces. J. Biomed. Mater. Res. **25**(12), 1547–1562 (1991)
77. Norde, W., Gage, D.: Interaction of bovine serum albumin and human blood plasma with PEO-tethered surfaces: influence of PEO chain length, grafting density, and temperature. Langmuir **20**(10), 4162–4167 (2004)
78. Kizhakkedathu, J.N., Janzen, J., Le, Y., Kainthan, R.K., Brooks, D.E.: Poly (oligo (ethylene glycol) acrylamide) brushes by surface initiated polymerization: effect of macromonomer chain length on brush growth and protein adsorption from blood plasma. Langmuir **25**(6), 3794–3801 (2009)
79. Lai, B.F., Creagh, A.L., Janzen, J., Haynes, C.A., Brooks, D.E., Kizhakkedathu, J.N.: The induction of thrombus generation on nanostructured neutral polymer brush surfaces. Biomaterials **31**(26), 6710–6718 (2010)
80. Thierry, B., Merhi, Y., Silver, J., Tabrizian, M.: Biodegradable membrane-covered stent from chitosan-based polymers. J. Biomed. Mater. Res. A **75**(3), 556–566 (2005)
81. Wright, M.J., Woodrow, G., Umpleby, S., Hull, S., Brownjohn, A.M., Turney, J.H.: Low thrombogenicity of polyethylene glycol–grafted cellulose membranes does not influence heparin requirements in hemodialysis. Am. J. Kidney Dis. **34**(1), 36–42 (1999)
82. Sirolli, V., Di Stante, S., Stuard, S., Di Liberato, L., Amoroso, L., Cappelli, P., Bonomini, M.: Biocompatibility and functional performance of a polyethylene glycol acid-grafted cellulosic membrane for hemodialysis. Int. J. Artif. Organs **23**(6), 356–364 (2000)

83. Cao, L., Sukavaneshvar, S., Ratner, B.D., Horbett, T.A.: Glow discharge plasma treatment of polyethylene tubing with tetraglyme results in ultralow fibrinogen adsorption and greatly reduced platelet adhesion. J. Biomed. Mater. Res. A **79**(4), 788–803 (2006)
84. Rodriguez-Emmenegger, C., Brynda, E., Riedel, T., Houska, M., Šubr, V., Alles, A.B., Hasan, E., Gautrot, J.E., Huck, W.T.: Polymer brushes showing non-fouling in blood plasma challenge the currently accepted design of protein resistant surfaces. Macromol. Rapid Commun. **32**(13), 952–957 (2011)
85. Herring, M.B., Compton, R., Legrand, D.R., Gardner, A.L.: Endothelial cell seeding in the management of vascular thrombosis. Semin. Thromb. Hemost. **15**(2), 200–205 (1989)
86. Williams, S.K., Rose, D.G., Jarrell, B.E.: Microvascular endothelial cell sodding of ePTFE vascular grafts: improved patency and stability of the cellular lining. J. Biomed. Mater. Res. **28**(2), 203–212 (1994)
87. Zilla, P., Deutsch, M., Meinhart, J., Puschmann, R., Eberl, T., Minar, E., Dudczak, R., Lugmaier, H., Schmidt, P., Noszian, I.: Clinical in vitro endothelialization of femoropopliteal bypass grafts: an actuarial follow-up over three years. J. Vasc. Surg. **19**(3), 540–548 (1994)
88. Kutryk, M., van Dortmont, L., de Crom, R., van der Kamp, A., Verdouw, P., van der Giessen, W.: Seeding of intravascular stents by the xenotransplantation of genetically modified endothelial cells. Semin. Interv. Cardiol. **3**(3-4), 217–220 (1998)
89. Zünd, G., Hoerstrup, S.P., Schoeberlein, A., Lachat, M., Uhlschmid, G., Vogt, P.R., Turina, M.: Tissue engineering: a new approach in cardiovascular surgery; seeding of human fibroblasts followed by human endothelial cells on resorbable mesh. Eur. J. Cardiothorac. Surg. **13**(2), 160–164 (1998)
90. Taite, L.J., Yang, P., Jun, H.-W., West, J.L.: Nitric oxide-releasing polyurethane–PEG copolymer containing the YIGSR peptide promotes endothelialization with decreased platelet adhesion. J. Biomed. Mater. Res. B Appl. Biomater. **84**(1), 108–116 (2008)
91. L'heureux, N., Pâquet, S., Labbé, R., Germain, L., Auger, F.A.: A completely biological tissue-engineered human blood vessel. FASEB J **12**(1), 47–56 (1998)
92. Kawamoto, Y., Nakao, A., Ito, Y., Wada, N., Kaibara, M.: Endothelial cells on plasma-treated segmented-polyurethane: adhesion strength, antithrombogenicity and cultivation in tubes. J. Mater. Sci. Mater. Med. **8**(9), 551–557 (1997)
93. Li, J., Ding, M., Fu, Q., Tan, H., Xie, X., Zhong, Y.: A novel strategy to graft RGD peptide on biomaterials surfaces for endothelization of small-diamater vascular grafts and tissue engineering blood vessel. J. Mater. Sci. Mater. Med. **19**(7), 2595–2603 (2008)
94. Yin, M., Yuan, Y., Liu, C., Wang, J.: Development of mussel adhesive polypeptide mimics coating for in-situ inducing re-endothelialization of intravascular stent devices. Biomaterials **30**(14), 2764–2773 (2009)
95. Jiang, S., Cao, Z.: Ultralow-fouling, functionalizable, and hydrolyzable zwitterionic materials and their derivatives for biological applications. Adv. Mater. **22**(9), 920–932 (2010)
96. Wu, L., Guo, Z., Meng, S., Zhong, W., Du, Q., Chou, L.L.: Synthesis of a zwitterionic silane and its application in the surface modification of silicon-based material surfaces for improved hemocompatibility. ACS Appl. Mater. Interfaces **2**(10), 2781–2788 (2010)
97. Zhang, Z., Chen, S., Chang, Y., Jiang, S.: Surface grafted sulfobetaine polymers via atom transfer radical polymerization as superlow fouling coatings. J. Phys. Chem. B **110**(22), 10799–10804 (2006)
98. Ishihara, K., Nomura, H., Mihara, T., Kurita, K., Iwasaki, Y., Nakabayashi, N.: Why do phospholipid polymers reduce protein adsorption? J. Biomed. Mater. Res. **39**(2), 323–330 (1998)
99. Holmlin, R.E., Chen, X., Chapman, R.G., Takayama, S., Whitesides, G.M.: Zwitterionic SAMs that resist nonspecific adsorption of protein from aqueous buffer. Langmuir **17**(9), 2841–2850 (2001)
100. Jiang, Y., Rongbing, B., Ling, T., Jian, S., Sicong, L.: Blood compatibility of polyurethane surface grafted copolymerization with sulfobetaine monomer. Colloids Surf. B Biointerfaces **36**(1), 27–33 (2004)

101. Min, D.Y., Li, Z.Z., Shen, J., Lin, S.C.: Research and synthesis of organosilicon nonthrombogenic materials containing sulfobetaine group. Colloids Surf. B Biointerfaces **79**(2), 415–420 (2010)
102. Yuan, J., Lin, S., Shen, J.: Enhanced blood compatibility of polyurethane functionalized with sulfobetaine. Colloids Surf. B Biointerfaces **66**(1), 90–95 (2008)
103. West, S.L., Salvage, J.P., Lobb, E.J., Armes, S.P., Billingham, N.C., Lewis, A.L., Hanlon, G.W., Lloyd, A.W.: The biocompatibility of crosslinkable copolymer coatings containing sulfobetaines and phosphobetaines. Biomaterials **25**(7–8), 1195–1204 (2004)
104. Lobb, E.J., Ma, I., Billingham, N.C., Armes, S.P., Lewis, A.L.: Facile synthesis of well-defined, biocompatible phosphorylcholine-based methacrylate copolymers via atom transfer radical polymerization at 20 C. J. Am. Chem. Soc. **123**(32), 7913–7914 (2001)
105. Ma, H., Hyun, J., Stiller, P., Chilkoti, A.: "Non-fouling" oligo(ethylene glycol)- functionalized polymer brushes synthesized by surface-initiated atom transfer radical polymerization. Adv. Mater. **16**(4), 338–341 (2004)
106. Zhang, Z., Zhang, M., Chen, S., Horbett, T.A., Ratner, B.D., Jiang, S.: Blood compatibility of surfaces with superlow protein adsorption. Biomaterials **29**(32), 4285–4291 (2008)
107. Yuan, J., Zhang, J., Zhou, J., Yuan, Y., Shen, J., Lin, S.: Platelet adhesion onto segmented polyurethane surfaces modified by carboxybetaine. J. Biomater. Sci. Polym. Ed. **14**(12), 1339–1349 (2003)
108. Kitano, H., Tada, S., Mori, T., Takaha, K., Gemmei-Ide, M., Tanaka, M., Fukuda, M., Yokoyama, Y.: Correlation between the structure of water in the vicinity of carboxybetaine polymers and their blood-compatibility. Langmuir **21**(25), 11932–11940 (2005)
109. Lee, B., Shin, H.-S., Park, K., Han, D.: Surface grafting of blood compatible zwitterionic poly(ethylene glycol) on diamond-like carbon-coated stent. J. Mater. Sci. Mater. Med. **22**(3), 507–514 (2011)
110. Yuan, Y., Ai, F., Zang, X., Zhuang, W., Shen, J., Lin, S.: Polyurethane vascular catheter surface grafted with zwitterionic sulfobetaine monomer activated by ozone. Colloids Surf. B Biointerfaces **35**(1), 1–5 (2004)
111. Galli, M., Sommariva, L., Prati, F., Zerboni, S., Politi, A., Bonatti, R., Mameli, S., Butti, E., Pagano, A., Ferrari, G.: Acute and mid-term results of phosphorylcholine-coated stents in primary coronary stenting for acute myocardial infarction. Catheter Cardiovasc. Interv. **53**(2), 182–187 (2001)
112. Lewis, A., Tolhurst, L., Stratford, P.: Analysis of a phosphorylcholine-based polymer coating on a coronary stent pre-and post-implantation. Biomaterials **23**(7), 1697–1706 (2002)
113. Rabenstein, D.L.: Heparin and heparan sulfate: structure and function. Nat. Prod. Rep. **19**(3), 312–331 (2002)
114. Hylton, D.M., Shalaby, S.W., Latour, R.A.: Direct correlation between adsorption-induced changes in protein structure and platelet adhesion. J Biomed. Mater. Res. A **73A**(3), 349–358 (2005)
115. Ayres, N., Holt, D., Jones, C., Corum, L., Grainger, D.: Polymer brushes containing sulfonated sugar repeat units: synthesis, characterization, and in vitro testing of blood coagulation activation. J. Polym. Sci., Part A: Polym. Chem. **46**(23), 7713–7724 (2008)
116. Kidane, A.G., Salacinski, H., Tiwari, A., Bruckdorfer, K.R., Seifalian, A.M.: Anticoagulant and antiplatelet agents: their clinical and device application (s) together with usages to engineer surfaces. Biomacromolecules **5**(3), 798–813 (2004)
117. Sakiyama-Elbert, S.E.: Incorporation of heparin into biomaterials. Acta Biomater. **10**(4), 1581–1587 (2013)
118. Wan Kim, S., Jacobs, H.: Design of nonthrombogenic polymer surfaces for blood-contacting medical devices. Blood Purif. **14**(5), 357–372 (1996)
119. Larm, O., Larsson, R., Olsson, P.: A new non-thrombogenic surface prepared by selective covalent binding of heparin via a modified reducing terminal residue. Biomater. Med. Devices Artif. Organs **11**(2–3), 161–173 (1983)

120. Michanetzis, G., Katsala, N., Missirlis, Y.: Comparison of haemocompatibility improvement of four polymeric biomaterials by two heparinization techniques. Biomaterials **24**(4), 677–688 (2003)
121. Miyara, H., Harumiya, N., Mori, Y., Tanzawa, H.: A new antithrombogenic heparinized polymer. J. Biomed. Mater. Res. **11**(2), 251–265 (1977)
122. Goddard, J.M., Hotchkiss, J.H.: Polymer surface modification for the attachment of bioactive compounds. Prog. Polym. Sci. **32**(7), 698–725 (2007)
123. Engbers, G.H., Feijen, J.: Current techniques to improve the blood compatibility of biomaterial surfaces. Int. J. Artif. Organs **14**(4), 199–215 (1991)
124. Gölander, C., Arwin, H., Eriksson, J., Lundstrom, I., Larsson, R.: Heparin surface film formation through adsorption of colloidal particles studied by ellipsometry and scanning electron microscopy. Colloids Surf. **5**(1), 1–16 (1982)
125. Seifert, B., Romaniuk, P., Groth, T.: Bioresorbable, heparinized polymers for stent coating: in vitro studies on heparinization efficiency, maintenance of anticoagulant properties and improvement of stent haemocompatibility. J. Mater. Sci. Mater. Med. **7**(8), 465–469 (1996)
126. Bamford, C., Al-Lamee, K.: Studies in polymer surface modification and grafting for biomedical uses: 2. Application to arterial blood filters and oxygenators. Polymer **37**(22), 4885–4889 (1996)
127. Byun, Y., Jacobs, H.A., Kim, S.W.: Heparin surface immobilization through hydrophilic spacers: thrombin and antithrombin III binding kinetics. J. Biomater. Sci. Polym. Ed. **6**(1), 1–13 (1994)
128. Park, K.D., Okano, T., Nojiri, C., Kim, S.W.: Heparin immobilization onto segmented polyurethaneurea surfaces—effect of hydrophilic spacers. J. Biomed. Mater. Res. **22**(11), 977–992 (1988)
129. Arnander, C., Bagger-Sjoebaeck, D., Frebelius, S., Larsson, R., Swedenborg, J.: Long-term stability in vivo of a thromboresistant heparinized surface. Biomaterials **8**(6), 496–499 (1987)
130. Vroman, L.: The life of an artificial device in contact with blood: initial events and their effect on its final state. Bull. N. Y. Acad. Med. **64**(4), 352 (1988)
131. Wendel, H.P., Ziemer, G.: Coating-techniques to improve the hemocompatibility of artificial devices used for extracorporeal circulation. Eur. J. Cardiothorac. Surg. **16**(3), 342–350 (1999)
132. Keuren, J.F., Wielders, S.J., Willems, G.M., Morra, M., Lindhout, T.: Fibrinogen adsorption, platelet adhesion and thrombin generation at heparinized surfaces exposed to flowing blood. Thromb. Haemost. **87**(4), 742–747 (2002)
133. Weber, N., Wendel, H.P., Ziemer, G.: Hemocompatibility of heparin-coated surfaces and the role of selective plasma protein adsorption. Biomaterials **23**(2), 429–439 (2002)
134. Sperling, C., Houska, M., Brynda, E., Streller, U., Werner, C.: In vitro hemocompatibility of albumin–heparin multilayer coatings on polyethersulfone prepared by the layer-by-layer technique. J. Biomed. Mater. Res. A **76**(4), 681–689 (2006)
135. Werner, C., Maitz, M.F., Sperling, C.: Current strategies towards hemocompatible coatings. J. Mater. Chem. **17**(32), 3376–3384 (2007)
136. Vaughn, M.W.: Estimation of nitric oxide production and reaction rates in tissue by use of a mathematical model. Am. J. Physiol. Heart Circ. Physiol. **274**(6), H2163–H2176 (1998)
137. Frost, M.C., Reynolds, M.M., Meyerhoff, M.E.: Polymers incorporating nitric oxide releasing/generating substances for improved biocompatibility of blood-contacting medical devices. Biomaterials **26**(14), 1685–1693 (2005)
138. Seabra, A.B., Marcato, P.D., De Paula, L.B., Durán, N.: New strategy for controlled release of nitric oxide. J. Nano. Res. **20**, 61–67 (2012)
139. Riccio, D.A., Schoenfisch, M.H.: Nitric oxide release: Part I. Macromol. Scaffolds. Chem. Soc. Rev. **41**(10), 3731–3741 (2012)
140. Kim, J., Saravanakumar, G., Choi, H.W., Park, D., Kim, W.J.: A platform for nitric oxide delivery. J. Mater. Chem. B Mater. Biol. Med. **2**, 341–356 (2014)
141. Jen, M.C., Serrano, M.C., Van Lith, R., Ameer, G.A.: Polymer-based nitric oxide therapies: recent insights for biomedical applications. Adv. Funct. Mater. **22**(2), 239–260 (2012)

142. Halpenny, G.M., Mascharak, P.K.: Emerging antimicrobial applications of nitric oxide (NO) and NO-releasing materials. Anti-Infect. Agents Med. Chem. **9**(4), 187–197 (2010)
143. Eroy-Reveles, A.A., Mascharak, P.K.: Nitric oxide-donating materials and their potential in pharmacological applications for site-specific nitric oxide delivery. Future Med. Chem. **1**(8), 1497–1507 (2009)
144. Carpenter, A.W., Schoenfisch, M.H.: Nitric oxide release: Part II. Ther. Appl. Chem. Soc. Rev. **41**(10), 3742–3752 (2012)
145. Mowery, K.A., Schoenfisch, M.H., Saavedra, J.E., Keefer, L.K., Meyerhoff, M.E.: Preparation and characterization of hydrophobic polymeric films that are thromboresistant via nitric oxide release. Biomaterials **21**(1), 9–21 (2000)
146. Skrzypchak, A.M., Lafayette, N.G., Bartlett, R.H., Zhou, Z., Frost, M.C., Meyerhoff, M.E., Reynolds, M.M., Annich, G.M.: Effect of varying nitric oxide release to prevent platelet consumption and preserve platelet function in an in vivo model of extracorporeal circulation. Perfusion **22**(3), 193–200 (2007)
147. Batchelor, M.M., Reoma, S.L., Fleser, P.S., Nuthakki, V.K., Callahan, R.E., Shanley, C.J., Politis, J.K., Elmore, J., Merz, S.I., Meyerhoff, M.E.: More lipophilic dialkyldiamine-based diazeniumdiolates: synthesis, characterization, and application in preparing thromboresistant nitric oxide release polymeric coatings. J. Med. Chem. **46**(24), 5153–5161 (2003)
148. Fleser, P.S., Nuthakki, V.K., Malinzak, L.E., Callahan, R.E., Seymour, M.L., Reynolds, M.M., Merz, S.I., Meyerhoff, M.E., Bendick, P.J., Zelenock, G.B., Shanley, C.J.: Nitric oxide-releasing biopolymers inhibit thrombus formation in a sheep model of arteriovenous bridge grafts. J. Vasc. Surg. **40**(4), 803–811 (2004)
149. Smith, D.J., Chakravarthy, D., Pulfer, S., Simmons, M.L., Hrabie, J.A., Citro, M.L., Saavedra, J.E., Davies, K.M., Hutsell, T.C., Mooradian, D.L., Hanson, S.R., Keefer, L.K.: Nitric oxide-releasing polymers containing the [N(O)NO]- group. J. Med. Chem. **39**(5), 1148–1156 (1996)
150. Annich, G.M., Meinhardt, J.P., Mowery, K.A., Ashton, B.A., Merz, S.I., Hirschl, R.B., Meyerhoff, M.E., Bartlett, R.H.: Reduced platelet activation and thrombosis in extracorporeal circuits coated with nitric oxide release polymers. Crit. Care Med. **28**(4), 915–920 (2000)
151. Zhang, H., Annich, G.M., Miskulin, J., Osterholzer, K., Merz, S.I., Bartlett, R.H., Meyerhoff, M.E.: Nitric oxide releasing silicone rubbers with improved blood compatibility: preparation, characterization, and in vivo evaluation. Biomaterials **23**(6), 1485–1494 (2002)
152. Marxer, S.M., Rothrock, A.R., Nablo, B.J., Robbins, M.E., Schoenfisch, M.H.: Preparation of nitric oxide (NO)-releasing sol-gels for biomaterial applications. Chem. Mater. **15**(22), 4193–4199 (2003)
153. Nablo, B.J., Schoenfisch, M.H.: In vitro cytotoxicity of nitric oxide-releasing sol-gel derived materials. Biomaterials **26**(21), 4405–4415 (2005)
154. Hetrick, E.M., Schoenfisch, M.H.: Antibacterial nitric oxide-releasing xerogels: Cell viability and parallel plate flow cell adhesion studies. Biomaterials **28**(11), 1948–1956 (2007)
155. Koh, A., Carpenter, A.W., Slomberg, D.L., Schoenfisch, M.H.: Nitric oxide-releasing silica nanoparticle-doped polyurethane electrospun fibers. ACS Appl. Mater. Interfaces **5**(16), 7956–7964 (2013)
156. Koh, A., Riccio, D.A., Sun, B., Carpenter, A.W., Nichols, S.P., Schoenfisch, M.H.: Fabrication of nitric oxide-releasing polyurethane glucose sensor membranes. Biosens. Bioelectron. **28**(1), 17–24 (2011)
157. Shin, J.H., Metzger, S.K., Schoenfisch, M.H.: Synthesis of nitric oxide-releasing silica nanoparticles. J. Am. Chem. Soc. **129**(15), 4612–4619 (2007)
158. Shin, J.H., Schoenfisch, M.H.: Inorganic/organic hybrid silica nanoparticles as a nitric oxide delivery scaffold. Chem. Mater. **20**(1), 239–249 (2008)
159. Lu, Y., Sun, B., Li, C.H., Schoenfisch, M.H.: Structurally diverse nitric oxide-releasing poly(propylene imine) dendrimers. Chem. Mater. **23**(18), 4227–4233 (2011)
160. Stasko, N.A., Schoenfisch, M.H.: Dendrimers as a scaffold for nitric oxide release. J. Am. Chem. Soc. **128**(25), 8265–8271 (2006)

161. Sun, B., Slomberg, D.L., Chudasama, S.L., Lu, Y., Schoenfisch, M.H.: Nitric oxide-releasing dendrimers as antibacterial agents. Biomacromolecules **13**(10), 3343–3354 (2012)
162. Lantvit, S.M., Barrett, B.J., Reynolds, M.M.: Nitric oxide releasing material adsorbs more fibrinogen. J. Biomed. Mater. Res. A **101**(11), 3201–3210 (2013)
163. Wu, Y., Zhou, Z., Meyerhoff, M.E.: In vitro platelet adhesion on polymeric surfaces with varying fluxes of continuous nitric oxide release. J. Biomed. Mater. Res. A **81**(4), 956–963 (2007)
164. Major, T.C., Brant, D.O., Reynolds, M.M., Bartlett, R.H., Meyerhoff, M.E., Handa, H., Annich, G.M.: The attenuation of platelet and monocyte activation in a rabbit model of extracorporeal circulation by a nitric oxide releasing polymer. Biomaterials **31**(10), 2736–2745 (2010)
165. Handa, H., Brisbois, E.J., Major, T.C., Refahiyat, L., Amoako, K.A., Annich, G.M., Bartlett, R.H., Meyerhoff, M.E.: In vitro and in vivo study of sustained nitric oxide release coating using diazeniumdiolate-doped poly(vinyl chloride) matrix with poly(lactide-co-glycolide) additive. J. Mater. Chem. B Mater. Biol. Med. **1**(29), 3578–3587 (2013)
166. Handa, H., Major, T.C., Brisbois, E.J., Amoako, K.A., Meyerhoff, M.E., Bartlett, R.H.: Hemocompatibility comparison of biomedical grade polymers using rabbit thrombogenicity model for preparing nonthrombogenic nitric oxide releasing surfaces. J. Mater. Chem. B Mater. Biol. Med. **2**(8), 1059–1067 (2014)
167. Al-Sa'doni, H., Ferro, A.: S-nitrosothiols: a class of nitric oxide-donor drugs. Clin. Sci. **98**(5), 507–520 (2000)
168. Hogg, N.: Biological chemistry and clinical potential of S-nitrosothiols. Free Radical Biol. Med. **28**(10), 1478–1486 (2000)
169. Hogg, N., Singh, R.J., Kalyanaraman, B.: The role of glutathione in the transport and catabolism of nitric oxide. FEBS Lett. **382**(3), 223–228 (1996)
170. Langford, E.J., Brown, A.S., Wainwright, R.J., Debelder, A.J., Thomas, M.R., Smith, R.E.A., Radomski, M.W., Martin, J.F., Moncada, S.: Inhibition of platelet activity by S-nitrosoglutathione during coronary angioplasty. Lancet **344**(8935), 1458–1460 (1994)
171. Radomski, M.W., Rees, D.D., Dutra, A., Moncada, S.: S-nitroso-glutathione inhibits platelet activation in vitro and in vivo. Br. J. Pharmacol. **107**(3), 745–749 (1992)
172. Salas, E., Moro, M.A., Askew, S., Hodson, H.F., Butler, A.R., Radomski, M.W., Moncada, S.: Comparative pharmacology of analogues of S-nitroso-*N*-acetyl-DL-penicillamine on human platelets. Br. J. Pharmacol. **112**(4), 1071–1076 (1994)
173. De Souza, G.F.P., Yokoyama-Yasunaka, J.K.U., Seabra, A.B., Miguel, D.C., De Oliveira, M.G., Uliana, S.R.B.: Leishmanicidal activity of primary S-nitrosothiols against Leishmania major and Leishmania amazonensis: implications for the treatment of cutaneous leishmaniasis. Nitric Oxide **15**(3), 209–216 (2006)
174. Salas, E., Langford, E.J., Marrinan, M.T., Martin, J.F., Moncada, S., De Belder, A.J.: S-nitrosoglutathione inhibits platelet activation and deposition in coronary artery saphenous vein grafts in vitro and in vivo. Heart **80**(2), 146–150 (1998)
175. Albert, J., Daleskog, M., Wallen, N.H.: A comparison of the antiplatelet effect of S-nitrosoglutathione in whole blood and platelet-rich plasma. Thromb. Res. **102**(2), 161–165 (2001)
176. Ricardo, K.F.S., Shishido, S.M., De Oliveira, M.G., Krieger, M.H.: Characterization of the hypotensive effect of S-nitroso-N-acetylcysteine in normotensive and hypertensive conscious rats. Nitric Oxide-Biol. Ch **7**(1), 57–66 (2002)
177. Dicks, A.P., Swift, H.R., Williams, D.L.H., Butler, A.R., Al-Sa'doni, H.H., Cox, B.G.: Identification of Cu + as the effective reagent in nitric oxide formation from S-nitrosothiols (RSNO). J. Chem. Soc. Perkin Trans. **2**, 481–487 (1996)
178. Sexton, D.J., Muruganandam, A., Mckenney, D.J., Mutus, B.: Visible light photochemical release of nitric oxide from S-nitrosoglutathione: potential photochemotherapeutic applications. Photochem. Photobiol. **59**(4), 463–467 (1994)
179. Wood, P.D., Mutus, B., Redmond, R.W.: The mechanism of photochemical release of nitric oxide from S-nitrosoglutathione. Photochem. Photobiol. **64**(3), 518–524 (1996)

180. Frost, M.C., Meyerhoff, M.E.: Controlled photoinitiated release of nitric oxide from polymer films containing S-Nitroso-N-acetyl-dl-penicillamine derivatized fumed silica filler. J. Am. Chem. Soc. **126**(5), 1348–1349 (2004)
181. Shishido, S.L.M., Seabra, A.B., Loh, W., Ganzarolli De Oliveira, M.: Thermal and photochemical nitric oxide release from S-nitrosothiols incorporated in Pluronic F127 gel: potential uses for local and controlled nitric oxide release. Biomaterials **24**(20), 3543–3553 (2003)
182. Seabra, A.B., De Oliveira, M.G.: Poly(vinyl alcohol) and poly(vinyl pyrrolidone) blended films for local nitric oxide release. Biomaterials **25**(17), 3773–3782 (2004)
183. Seabra, A.B., De Souza, G.F.P., Da Rocha, L.L., Eberlin, M.N., De Oliveira, M.G.: S-nitrosoglutathione incorporated in poly(ethylene glycol) matrix: potential use for topical nitric oxide delivery. Nitric Oxide-Biol. Ch **11**(3), 263–272 (2004)
184. Seabra, A.B., Da Rocha, L.L., Eberlin, M.N., De Oliveira, M.G.: Solid films of blended poly(vinyl alcohol)/poly(vinyl pyrrolidone) for topical S-nitrosoglutathione and nitric oxide release. J. Pharm. Sci. **94**(5), 994–1003 (2005)
185. Simoes, M., De Oliveira, M.G.: Poly(vinyl alcohol) films for topical delivery of S-Nitrosoglutathione: effect of freezing-thawing on the diffusion properties. J. Biomed. Mater. Res. B Appl. Biomater. **93B**(2), 416–424 (2010)
186. Brisbois, E.J., Handa, H., Major, T.C., Bartlett, R.H., Meyerhoff, M.E.: Long-term nitric oxide release and elevated temperature stability with S-nitroso-N-acetylpenicillamine (SNAP)-doped Elast-eon E2As polymer. Biomaterials **34**(28), 6957–6966 (2013)
187. Joslin, J.M., Lantvit, S.M., Reynolds, M.M.: Nitric oxide releasing tygon materials: studies in donor leaching and localized nitric oxide release at a polymer-buffer interface. ACS Appl. Mater. Interfaces **5**(19), 9285–9294 (2013)
188. Riccio, D.A., Dobmeier, K.P., Hetrick, E.M., Privett, B.J., Paul, H.S., Schoenfisch, M.H.: Nitric oxide-releasing S-nitrosothiol-modified xerogels. Biomaterials **30**(27), 4494–4502 (2009)
189. Riccio, D.A., Coneski, P.N., Nichols, S.P., Broadnax, A.D., Schoenfisch, M.H.: Photoinitiated nitric oxide-releasing tertiary S-Nitrosothiol-modified xerogels. ACS Appl. Mater. Interfaces **4**(2), 796–804 (2012)
190. Coneski, P.N., Schoenfisch, M.H.: Synthesis of nitric oxide-releasing polyurethanes with S-nitrosothiol-containing hard and soft segments. Polym Chem. **2**(4), 906–913 (2011)
191. Frost, M.C., Meyerhoff, M.E.: Synthesis, characterization, and controlled nitric oxide release from S-nitrosothiol-derivatized fumed silica polymer filler particles. J. Biomed. Mater. Res. A **72A**(4), 409–419 (2005)
192. Coneski, P.N., Rao, K.S., Schoenfisch, M.H.: Degradable nitric oxide-releasing biomaterials via post-polymerization functionalization of cross-linked polyesters. Biomacromolecules **11**(11), 3208–3215 (2010)
193. Damodaran, V.B., Place, L.W., Kipper, M.J., Reynolds, M.M.: Enzymatically degradable nitric oxide releasing S-nitrosated dextran thiomers for biomedical applications. J. Mater. Chem. **22**, 23038–23048 (2012)
194. Damodaran, V.B., Reynolds, M.M.: Biodegradable S-nitrosothiol tethered multiblock polymer for nitric oxide delivery. J. Mater. Chem. **21**, 5870–5872 (2011)
195. Damodaran, V.B., Joslin, J.M., Wold, K.A., Lantvit, S.M., Reynolds, M.M.: S-Nitrosated biodegradable polymers for biomedical applications: synthesis, characterization and impact of thiol structure on the physicochemical properties. J. Mater. Chem. **22**, 5990–6001 (2012)
196. Seabra, A.B., Martins, D., Simoes, M., Da Silva, R., Brocchi, M., De Oliveira, M.G.: Antibacterial nitric oxide-releasing polyester for the coating of blood-contacting artificial materials. Artif. Organs **34**(7), E204–E214 (2010)
197. Seabra, A.B., Da Silva, R., De Souza, G.F.P., De Oliveira, M.G.: Antithrombogenic polynitrosated polyester/poly(methyl methacrylate) blend for the coating of blood-contacting surfaces. Artif. Organs **32**(4), 262–267 (2008)
198. Li, Y., Lee, P.I.: Controlled nitric oxide delivery platform based on S-nitrosothiol conjugated interpolymer complexes for diabetic wound healing. Mol. Pharm. **7**(1), 254–266 (2009)

199. Gierke, G.E., Nielsen, M., Frost, M.C.: S-Nitroso- N -acetyl-D-penicillamine covalently linked to polydimethylsiloxane (SNAP–PDMS) for use as a controlled photoinitiated nitric oxide release polymer. Sci. Technol. Adv. Mat. **12**(5), 055007 (2011)
200. Stasko, N.A., Fischer, T.H., Schoenfisch, M.H.: S-Nitrosothiol-modified dendrimers as nitric oxide delivery vehicles. Biomacromolecules **9**(3), 834–841 (2008)
201. Riccio, D.A., Nugent, J.L., Schoenfisch, M.H.: Stober synthesis of nitric oxide-releasing S-Nitrosothiol-modified silica particles. Chem. Mater. **23**(7), 1727–1735 (2011)
202. Duan, X., Lewis, R.S.: Improved haemocompatibility of cysteine-modified polymers via endogenous nitric oxide. Biomaterials **23**(4), 1197–1203 (2002)
203. Gappa-Fahlenkamp, H., Lewis, R.S.: Improved hemocompatibility of poly(ethylene terephthalate) modified with various thiol-containing groups. Biomaterials **26**(17), 3479–3485 (2005)
204. Oh, B.K., Meyerhoff, M.E.: Spontaneous Catalytic Generation of Nitric Oxide from S-Nitrosothiols at the Surface of Polymer Films Doped with Lipophilic Copper(II) Complex. J. Am. Chem. Soc. **125**(32), 9552–9553 (2003)
205. Oh, B.K., Meyerhoff, M.E.: Catalytic generation of nitric oxide from nitrite at the interface of polymeric films doped with lipophilic Cu (II)-complex: a potential route to the preparation of thromboresistant coatings. Biomaterials **25**(2), 283–293 (2004)
206. Hwang, S., Meyerhoff, M.E.: Polyurethane with tethered copper (II)–cyclen complex: preparation, characterization and catalytic generation of nitric oxide from S-nitrosothiols. Biomaterials **29**(16), 2443–2452 (2008)
207. Puiu, S.C., Zhou, Z., White, C.C., Neubauer, L.J., Zhang, Z., Lange, L.E., Mansfield, J.A., Meyerhoff, M.E., Reynolds, M.M.: Metal ion-mediated nitric oxide generation from polyurethanes via covalently linked copper(II)-cyclen moieties. J. Biomed. Mater. Res. Part B Appl. Biomater. **91B**(1), 203–212 (2009)
208. Major, T.C., Brant, D.O., Burney, C.P., Amoako, K.A., Annich, G.M., Meyerhoff, M.E., Handa, H., Bartlett, R.H.: The hemocompatibility of a nitric oxide generating polymer that catalyzes S-nitrosothiol decomposition in an extracorporeal circulation model. Biomaterials **32**(26), 5957–5969 (2011)
209. Mugesh, G., Singh, H.B.: Synthetic organoselenium compounds as antioxidants: glutathione peroxidase activity. Chem. Soc. Rev. **29**(5), 347–357 (2000)
210. Hou, Y., Guo, Z., Li, J., Wang, P.G.: Seleno compounds and glutathione peroxidase catalyzed decomposition of S-nitrosothiols. Biochem. Biophys. Res. Commun. **228**(1), 88–93 (1996)
211. Yang, J., Welby, J.L., Meyerhoff, M.E.: Generic nitric oxide (NO) generating surface by immobilizing organoselenium species via layer-by-layer assembly. Langmuir **24**(18), 10265–10272 (2008)
212. Cha, W., Meyerhoff, M.E.: Catalytic generation of nitric oxide from S-nitrosothiols using immobilized organoselenium species. Biomaterials **28**(1), 19–27 (2007)
213. Cai, W., Wu, J., Xi, C., Ashe Iii, A.J., Meyerhoff, M.E.: Carboxyl-ebselen-based layer-by-layer films as potential antithrombotic and antimicrobial coatings. Biomaterials **32**(31), 7774–7784 (2011)
214. Reynolds, M.M., Frost, M.C., Meyerhoff, M.E.: Nitric oxide-releasing hydrophobic polymers: preparation, characterization, and potential biomedical applications. Free Radical Biol. Med. **37**(7), 926–936 (2004)
215. Sefton, M.V., Gemmell, C.H., Gorbet, M.B.: What really is blood compatibility? J. Biomat. Sci-Polym. E **11**(11), 1165–1182 (2000)
216. Lemm, W., Unger, V., Bucherl, E.S.: Blood compatibility of polymers: in vitro and in vivo tests. Med. Biol. Eng. Comput. **18**(4), 521–526 (1980)
217. Kirkpatrick, C., Mittermayer, C.: Theoretical and practical aspects of testing potential biomaterials in vitro. J. Mater. Sci. Mater. Med. **1**(1), 9–13 (1990)
218. Sefton, M.V.: Perspective on hemocompatibility testing. J. Biomed. Mater. Res. **55**(4), 445–446 (2001)
219. Seyfert, U.T., Biehl, V., Schenk, J.: In vitro hemocompatibility testing of biomaterials according to the ISO 10993-4. Biomol. Eng. **19**(2), 91–96 (2002)

220. Braune, S., Grunze, M., Straub, A., Jung, F.: Are there sufficient standards for the in vitro hemocompatibility testing of biomaterials? Biointerphases **8**(1), 1–9 (2013)
221. Ratner, B.D.: Evaluation of the blood compatibility of synthetic polymers: consensus and significance. Contemporary Biomaterials: Material and Host Response, Clinical Applications, New Technology and Legal Aspects, pp. 193–204. Noyes Publications, Park Ridge (1984)
222. Hanson, S.R., Ratner, B.: Evaluation of blood-materials interactions. In: Biomaterials science: an introduction to materials in medicine, pp. 367–378. San Diego (2004)
223. Ratner, B.D., Horbett, T.A.: Chapter II.3.5—Evaluation of blood–materials interactions. In: Ratner BD, Hoffman AS, Schoen FJ, Lemons JE (eds) Biomaterials Science (Third Edition), pp. 617–634. Academic Press, Waltham (2013)
224. Sefton, M.V., Sawyer, A., Gorbet, M., Black, J.P., Cheng, E., Gemmell, C., Pottinger-Cooper, E.: Does surface chemistry affect thrombogenicity of surface modified polymers? J. Biomed. Mater. Res. **55**(4), 447–459 (2001)
225. Gristina, A.G.: Biomaterial-centered infection: microbial adhesion versus tissue integration. Science **237**, 1588–1595 (1987)
226. Tzoneva, R., Heuchel, M., Groth, T., Altankov, G., Albrecht, W., Paul, D.: Fibrinogen adsorption and platelet interactions on polymer membranes. J. Biomater. Sci. Polym. Ed. **13**(9), 1033–1050 (2002)
227. Haycox, C.L., Ratner, B.D.: In vitro platelet interactions in whole human blood exposed to biomaterial surfaces: Insights on blood compatibility. J. Biomed. Mater. Res. **27**(9), 1181–1193 (1993)

Chapter 17
Polymer Based Biosensors for Medical Applications

Solène Cherré and Noemi Rozlosnik

Abstract The objective of this chapter is to give an overview about the newest developments in biosensors made of polymers for medical applications. Biosensors are devices that can recognize and detect a target with high selectivity. They are widely used in many fields such as medical diagnostic, environmental monitoring and food safety. The detected element varies from a single molecule (such as glucose), a biopolymer (such as DNA or a protein) to a whole organism (such as bacteria). Due to their easy use and possible miniaturization, biosensors have a high potential to come out of the lab and be available for use by everybody. To fulfil these purposes, polymers represent very appropriate materials. Many nano- and microfabrication methods for polymers are available, allowing a fast and cheap production of devices. This chapter will present the general concept of a biosensor in a first part. The second part will focus on conducting polymers, used as electrode material in devices based on electrochemical detection. A third part will describe the molecularly imprinted technology, where the target is replicated in 3D negative form into the polymer.

List of Abbreviations

ATP	Adenosine triphosphate
COC	Cyclic olefin copolymer
CP	Conductive polymers or intrinsically conducting polymers
DNA	Deoxyribonucleic acid
EDC	1-Ethyl-3-(3-dimethylaminopropyl) carbodiimide hydrochloride
EGCG	Epigallocatechin-3-gallate

S. Cherré · N. Rozlosnik (✉)
Department for Micro-and Nanotechnology, Technical University of Denmark,
Kongens Lyngby, Denmark
e-mail: noemi.rozlosnik@nanotech.dtu.dk

F. Puoci (ed.), *Advanced Polymers in Medicine*, DOI 10.1007/978-3-319-12478-0_17

ELISA	Enzyme-linked immunosorbent assay
GOx	Glucose oxidase
IUPAC	International Union of Pure and Applied Chemistry
ITO	Indium tin oxide
LOD	Limit of detection
MIP	Molecularly imprinted polymer
NIP	Non imprinted polymer
NHS	N-Hydroxysuccinimide
NTA	Nitrilotriacetic acid
PANI	Polyaniline
PDMS	Polydimethylsiloxane
PEDOT	Poly(3,4-ethylenedioxythiophene)
PMMA	Poly(methyl methacrylate)
POC	Point of care
PPy	Polypyrrole
QD	Quantum dots
RNA	Ribonucleic acid
SELEX	Systematic evolution of ligands by exponential enrichment
ssDNA	Single stranded DNA
UV	Ultraviolet
v/v	Volume to volume

Introduction

Recently, Turner published a comprehensive review article about the history of biosensors [1]. The development of biosensors started 30 years ago when Clark and Lyons [2] described the first enzyme-electrode [3]. Biosensors rapidly emerged to high interest in research. Every year the number of papers published reporting about the development of a biosensor is growing. The start in the industry was however slower, but now the market is worth several billions of US dollars [3]. Biosensors find application in food safety, environment monitoring, defence, but the main field remains medical diagnostics with the great domination of the glucose biosensors.

Most biosensors are developed with the goal of being used outside laboratories, for home use, by the general practitioner or on field [Point of Care (POC) or field based sensors]. Therefore they have to be inexpensive and easy to use while giving highly accurate results.

In this chapter we will introduce the basics of biosensors and how plastic materials (polymers) can be used in these devices. The high variability and inexpensive nature of polymers makes them very attractive for application in this field. We will then present how conducting polymers can be integrated in biosensors as electrodes. The application of molecular imprinted polymers will also be described.

Biosensors

Definition of Biosensors

Biosensors are devices that have the main aim of detecting and possibly quantifying a so called analyte or target of interest in a highly specific and selective way. They are relatively small devices being easy to use in order to minimize the possible errors in manipulation. Ideally, the user should only have to add the sample into the device through an inlet to get a clear analytical result in a short time, preferably without the possibility of misinterpretation. The response from a biosensor could be for example a colour change, a numerical value or formation of a visible product. There is a wide range of analytes that can be detected in a biosensor: inorganic compound such as salts, small molecules for example glucose, large biomolecules such as DNA or proteins or even whole organisms such as bacteria. In the following parts, we will show examples of biosensors for various analytes.

The International Union of Pure and Applied Chemistry (IUPAC) gave the following definition for a biosensor in 1992:

> A device that uses specific biochemical reactions mediated by isolated enzymes, immunosystems, tissues, organelles or whole cells to detect chemical compounds usually by electrical, thermal or optical signals. [4]

From this definition, we can define the three main parts of a biosensor: (i) the analyte, (ii) the bioelement used for recognition of the analyte and (iii) the transducer, which detects the recognition event and further processes the signal. Figure 17.1 shows the working principle of a biosensor. The sensor on the left of Fig. 17.1 is exposed to an analyte for which the sensor is specific; therefore a binding or recognition event occurs, which generates a signal that the transducer detects. The sensor on the right of Fig. 17.1 is exposed to another analyte. Since the bioelement cannot recognize it, no detection signal will be processed.

Recognition Elements

In a biosensor, different types of bioelement can be used. In this section some of them will be described without the ambition of completeness. For more details on bioelements, the reader is referred to excellent reviews by Chambers et al. [5] and Bhalerao and Nistala [6]. Figure 17.2 shows some of the different types of bioelement. The main requirement for a good bioelement is that it is highly specific for the analyte with a high affinity. The affinity of the bioelement to the analyte is the limiting factor for the sensitivity of a biosensor [7].

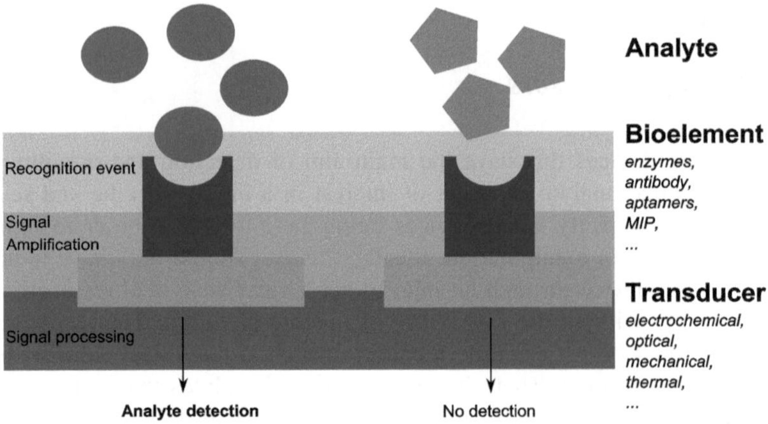

Fig. 17.1 Working principle of a biosensor. The analyte is specifically recognized by the bioelement. A biochemical reaction occurs upon the event of recognition leading to the generation of a signal, which can be amplified. Exposure of a biosensor to a non-specific analyte leads to no recognition signal

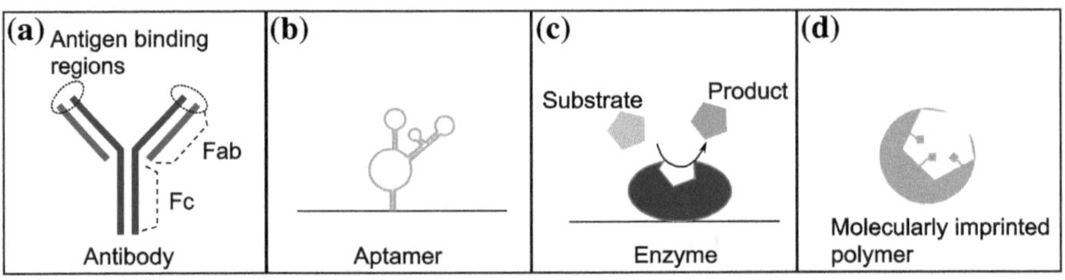

Fig. 17.2 Four different bioelements for a biosensor. **a** Antibodies are widely used in biosensors and other immunoassay due to the availability of antibodies against of wide range of targets. **b** Aptamers are oligonucleotides that specifically bind and recognize various targets. **c** Enzyme based biosensors have been extensively investigated. The high specificity of the enzyme for its target makes it very attractive for biosensor applications. **d** Molecular imprinted polymers (MIP) is a bioelement that is synthesized upon polymerisation of monomers around the target that can be separated leaving an imprint that can catch the target with a very high specificity

Enzymes

Widely used types of bioelement are **enzymes**. Enzymes are highly selective for their substrate (i.e. the analyte) and they catalyse the binding event. After binding of the substrate on the active sites, a chemical reaction occurs producing a measureable product, and releasing the enzyme for further reactions [8]. Often the enzyme-based biosensors are coupled with an electrochemical transducer. This is the case for example in case of enzyme-based glucose biosensors. The glucose oxidase (GOx) oxidizes glucose to gluconolactone, thereby using oxygen and producing H_2O_2 [9]. The consumption of oxygen can be measured by an oxygen electrode or the production of H_2O_2 can be measured amperometrically. The main disadvantage of enzymes is the cost and the time consuming purification that is required to have a concentration of enzymes high enough in the system.

Antibodies

The second—and probably most widely used—bioelements for analyte recognition in biosensor are **antibodies**. Antibodies are proteins produced by the immune system of many organisms. Their function is to recognize and neutralize pathogenic agents in a highly specific way. Due to their high specificity, each antibody molecule will recognize only one defined target. Antibodies are composed of two heavy chains and two light chains forming a "Y" having two antigen recognition sites (at the Fab regions) and a constant region (Fc region) as shown on Fig. 17.2.

Antibodies are produced by immunizing an animal (mouse, rabbit, horse, etc.) with the target. After some days, the serum of the animal will contain antibodies in high concentration against the injected target. The serum is collected and purified by affinity chromatography in order to obtain an antibody solution that is qualified as polyclonal, since it will contain several types of antibodies against one target (each type of antibody binding to a different binding site of the target.). Polyclonal antibodies solutions are relatively cheap to produce and find application amongst others in enzyme-linked immunosorbent assays (ELISA). However they might lack specificity for certain biosensors [6]. The specificity is improved by using monoclonal antibodies, which are mixtures of antibodies containing only one set of antibody against one particular binding site of the target. They are produced using the hybridoma technology where immortalized cancer cells are fused with antibody-producing B-cells in order to obtain a cell line producing one single set of antibody. With the progress of the recombinant technology, antibodies have also been developed having only the antigen-binding region (Fab fragment) and also antibodies carrying Fab and Fc fragments from different organisms. For biosensors, the Fc region is as well of great importance as it can be used for enhancement of the detection signal. Antibodies against the Fc region of a e.g. mouse antibody can be produced in a different organism (e.g. rabbit). Different markers (fluorescent molecules, biotin, gold particles, etc.) can then be conjugated to the Fc part of this second antibody that permits the detection of the binding event. This type of sandwich assay is widely used in ELISA and lateral flow assays like the pregnancy test.

Aptamers

Aptamers represent an attractive alternative to antibodies as bioelements. They are short ssDNA or RNA oligonucleotide sequences (20–40 bases) that fold into a 3D-structure that has a high selectivity and affinity for a defined target [10]. The 3D-structure is stabilized after binding to the target. Aptamers are smaller in size compared to antibodies and they can be synthesized chemically so that no batch-to-batch variation is introduced into the biosensor. Thank to this chemical synthesis, aptamers can easily be modified with alternative groups and conjugated to any kind of markers either at the 3′ or at the 5′ end of the sequence [11]. Aptamers are thermally stable as they can resist several cycles of denaturation/renaturation [11].

Aptamers can be developed against any type of target (metal ion, biomolecules, cells, etc.) [10]. The selection is usually run in a cycle called Systematic Evolution of Ligands by Exponential Enrichment (SELEX) [12]. A random pool of different aptamers is incubated with the target. The aptamers bound to the target are separated from the non-bound aptamers. After release of the target, the binding aptamers are driven through a new selection cycle. This process is repeated until the affinity of the aptamers to the target is high enough (dissociation constant in the nano- to picomolecular range). Recently, advancements in the SELEX technology have greatly reduced the time and costs required for the selection of an aptamer. This in vitro selection gives the possibility of selecting aptamers against non-immunogenic and toxic substances for which no antibodies can be developed [13].

Aptamer-based biosensors, also called aptasensor have gain a wide interest in the last years due to the advantages of aptamers compared to antibodies. Similar to antibodies, a variety of immobilization methods is available to bind aptamers to the sensor element. Aptasensors can be coupled to an electrochemical, optical or mass-sensitive transducer [13]. One of the successful examples for aptasensor was the detection of thrombin which was widely investigated [14]. Xiao et al. [15] have made an interesting development: a redox compound (methylene blue) was inserted into the thrombin aptamer. When the target bound to the aptamer, the induced conformation change inhibited the electron transfer from the methylene blue to the electrode. This change could be detected amperometrically.

Molecular Imprints

Going even more towards synthetic recognition bioelements, we would like to draw attention to **molecularly imprinted polymers (MIP)** that were first investigated by Mosbach and Wulff in the 1970s [16]. MIP will be described more in detailed in Sect. "Molecularly Imprinted Polymers (MIP): An Alternativeto Bioelement". Briefly, during the polymerization the monomers of the polymer are self-assembling around the target. After removing the target, an imprint of the target is remaining, which can be used as recognition element for the biosensor. MIP offer a greater chemical stability than biomolecules [17] and can be developed for most of the targets.

Other Recognition Elements

Further bioelements that are worth mentioning here are **whole cells** (eukaryotic cells or bacterial cells) such as the fibroblast cells which were used by Feng et al. [18] to develop a biosensor for the electrochemical measurement of the ATP concentration.

Another type of biosensor widely used is the DNA hybridization sensor. In this type of sensor, a **DNA probe** is immobilized on the transducer of the sensor. When the complementary strand hybridizes to the probe, a signal is generated that is then detected. As an example, the sensor developed by Nascimento et al. [19] detected bovine papillomavirus DNA electrochemically on a sensor functionalized with a specific probe of 27 bases.

Sensitivity and Selectivity of Biosensors

Sensitivity and selectivity are used to evaluate the biosensors. In the physical meaning, the **sensitivity** indicates how much the signal changes with a change of analyte concentration, while the **selectivity** shows how good the sensor can detect the analyte among the complex matrix of the sample (for example in blood, urine, saliva etc.). The **limit of detection (LOD)** is also often a measure of the quality of the sensor as it determines the lowest concentration of analyte that can still be detected by the sensor, i.e. gives a significant change in the sensor response. When the analyte is detected without any further labelling by a second probe, the literature refers to the sensors as label-free sensors [7]. Biosensors often are label-free sensors.

To increase the sensitivity and specificity of the biosensors in most cases the bioelement is immobilized on the active part of the biosensor. This process is called "functionalization". Without aiming to give a full list of methods the reader can find some of the most used processes for immobilization in the followings.

Functionalization

Several immobilization methods are available in order to functionalize the biosensor [6].

Absorption of the bioelement onto the surface of the biosensor is often used. This is a simple method since it only requires the incubation of the bioelement on the surface, but the amount of active bioelement on the surface is not well controlled [20]. Various types of non-covalent interactions can take place during the adsorption of the bioelement such as **attractive Van-der-Waals forces, electrostatic interactions, and hydrophobic interactions** [6, 21].

Covalent binding is often the most desirable methods of binding the bioelement as it is more controlled and reliable [6]. Covalent binding can be achieved using various linkers like 1-ethyl-3-(3-dimethylaminopropyl) carbodiimide hydrochloride (EDC) [22] or glutaraldehyde on materials containing OH-groups on the surface. Thiol group modified bioelements can bind to a gold surface. Silanes can be used to bind the bioelements on glass or on silicon.

The bioelement can also be **incorporated** into a porous material. In this case the analyte must be able to diffuse freely into the material in order to reach the bioelement. This offers a high surface-to-volume ratio but controlling the concentration of the bioelement is difficult. Enzymes are often entrapped in such a porous material.

Important is however that the immobilization does not affect the structure of the sites for analyte recognition as well as the function of the bioelement.

Transducer

Once the target is captured by the recognition element, the binding must generate a signal that can be detected by a transducer. The biosensing event can be only qualitative (analyte is there or not) or also quantitative (how much of the analyte is present in the tested sample). Several transduction methods are available, among others: optical, electrochemical or mechanical [23].

Optical Transducers

Optical methods require that a light or colour signal is produced by the recognition event. This could be for example light produced by an enzyme reaction. Fluorescence signalling is also often used in biosensors. Optical transduction can also be done in the form of a colorimetric assay, where the binding event results in a colour change of the recognition layer [24]. In lateral flow assays, nanoparticles are conjugated to the antibodies. During the recognition, the colour of the particles is changing, in most cases forming a coloured line on the sensor.

Electrochemical Transducers

Electrochemical transducers are also often integrated in biosensors. An extensive development has enabled the systems to become sensitive and highly specific for the substrates. The signal can easily be processed and analysed. The working principle of the electrochemical transducer is that the binding event can induce a change in the electrical properties of the system. Different types of devices are available [25]. If electroactive species are oxidized or reduced during the biochemical reaction, a current can be measured. This is an *amperometric detection*, which can be divided in two modes: amperometry when the potential is kept constant and voltammetry when the potential is varied [26]. Since the biomolecules are often not electroactive, a mediator can be added to the reaction chain, which will—in most cases—increase the sensitivity [26]. In *potentiometry*, the potential between working and reference electrode is measured when no current flows. By that, the ion activity of the sample can be measured, which is related to the concentration of analyte [27]. In the course of the biochemical reaction, the charges in the system are changed (for example: due to the production of electrons in an enzymatic reaction) [26, 28]. This change is then monitored. *Conductometric* sensors measure the change in the electrode resistance due to the binding event on the surface. Often AC voltage with small amplitude (10–20 mV) is used for measuring the impedance of an electrode system in *impedimetric* sensors. These sensors detect the changes of impedance upon changes on the electrode surface and/or in the solution [29]. Since the binding event is detected at the surface of the electrode, it has to occur in close proximity of this electrode; that is within the Debye length. The small size of aptamers meets this requirement and makes them a very attractive bioelement for electrochemical-based biosensors.

Other Transducers

Other transduction methods include **mass-sensitive methods** like the cantilever-based sensors [30]. Cantilevers are usually made of small silicon plate (length: 100 μm) with a low force constant. They are fixed at one end and can vibrate at the other end. Silicon can easily be functionalized with bioelements such as antibodies or aptamers. Upon binding of the analyte to the bioelement at the surface of the cantilever, the resonance frequency of the cantilever is changing, which can be detected with help of a laser beam shining the cantilever surface [31].

To summarize, biosensors are very versatile devices. There is a broad range of possible configurations regarding bioelements for analyte recognition, as well as for the signal transducer. In the next section we describe how the polymers are used for the development of biosensors.

Conductive Polymers in Biosensors

Polymers as Device Materials

Biosensors made of plastic materials emerged because of their favourable properties: cost effectiveness, suitability for mass replication based on injection moulding, excellent stability providing inexpensive, high-throughput, and large-scale devices with environmentally friendly disposability.

Several biocompatible polymers are known and used for device fabrication. The most commonly used materials are poly(methyl methacrylate) (PMMA), Cyclic olefin copolymer (COC) and polydimethylsiloxane (PDMS).

Recently several methods were developed for fast prototyping and mass production of micro- and nanostructures in polymers. Injection moulding is one of the techniques, which is commonly used with great success. Improvement in patterning, structuring [32] or bonding [33] of those materials is essential for the creation of low cost and portable biosensors. However, in this work, we do not focus on these fabrication methods, rather we describe some specific polymers which are commonly used in biosensor designs.

Polymers are mostly known for their insulating properties and their roles as dielectrics and resists [34]. However, a class of polymers can conduct electricity, and therefore they are called "**conductive polymers**" **(CP)**. The use of CPs as electrode materials is becoming more and more widespread for biological applications, especially in the field of biosensors [35], as they are cheaper and easier to produce than conventional metal electrodes.

Conductive Polymers as Electrode Materials

Polyaniline was the first CP polymer, which was described in the mid-19th century by Henry Letheby [36]. Since then numerous intrinsically CP have been developed, among others: polyacetylene, polythiophene, polypyrrole. CPs, also referred to as synthetic metals, have found applications in many fields. They are integrated for example in solar cells, rechargeable batteries and biomedical devices [37]. CPs are also very attractive for biosensors. In biosensors, CP can be used as excellent non-metallic electrodes. Numerous biosensors have been developed over the past 20 years with electrodes made of CP. The fabrication is fairly easy and flexible. This allows the biosensors to be single-use system; avoiding any risk of contamination and adaptation of the biosensors to new targets can be rapidly made. They are mostly biocompatible, can easily be synthesized and can be modified for immobilization of bioelements [38]. These conductive polymers are referred to as intrinsic conductive polymers in comparison to extrinsic conductive polymers that are a polymer matrix in which some metal particles have been entrapped [39].

Doping

The conducting process in polymers is rather complex. For the conducting process, the charge carriers have to be able to move in the material. This is achieved because the conjugated backbone of the polymer provides delocalized pi-orbitals that overlap continuously to allow free movement of the electrons [35, 40]. Besides delocalized electrons, the conductive polymers can have other charge carriers, which are often produced by doping with electron acceptors or donors [37]. The concept of polarons, bipolarons and solitons has been introduced to describe the charge defects introduced by the doping [41, 42]. Oxidation of the polymer creates holes (p-doping) while reduction adds electrons (n-doping) [34]. Different methods of doping can be applied [37]. For example, through *chemical doping* with iodine, the conductivity of polyacetylene could be increased over seven orders of magnitudes [37, 43, 44]. This discovery was rewarded the Nobel Prize in chemistry in 2000. *Electrochemical doping* can also be performed by the electropolymerization of the monomers. With this method, the ions come from the electrolyte solution [34]. The advantage of this method is that a polymer film is directly created on the electrode [45]. Photodoping introduces charge defects by irradiation of light [37].

In the following, three examples of conductive polymers will be discussed because these are the most commonly used in biosensors. Table 17.1 shows the chemical structures of polypyrrole, polyaniline and PEDOT, the three conductive polymers reviewed in this section.

Polyaniline

Polyaniline is a CP that has been known and used for a very long time. The synthesis of polyaniline, often abbreviated as **PANI**, is based on the oxidation of the monomer aniline. PANI has been reported to have a high conductivity (up to 103 S/m) [46, 47]. Thanks to its properties, it has found a wide range of sensing applications, inclusive in biosensors. The reader is referred to the excellent review of Dhand et al. [48]. Horseradish peroxidase (HRP) is an enzyme extensively incorporated in biosensors. It catalyzes the reduction of hydrogen peroxide (H_2O_2), a reactive oxygen species, which is produced by a wide range of

Table 17.1 Chemical structure of polypyrrole, PEDOT, polyaniline

Polypyrrole	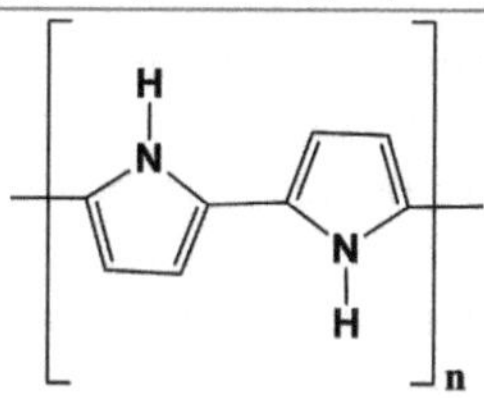
PEDOT	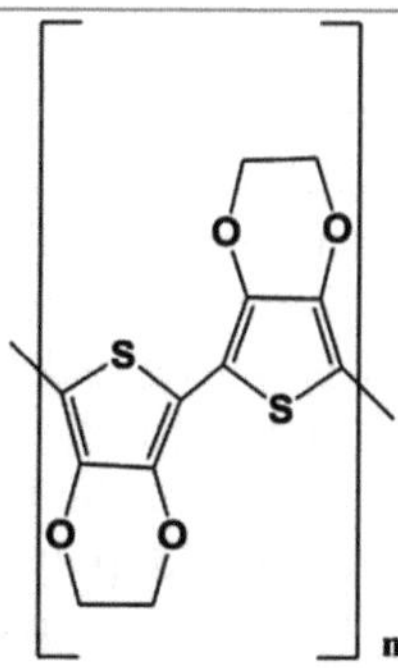
Polyaniline	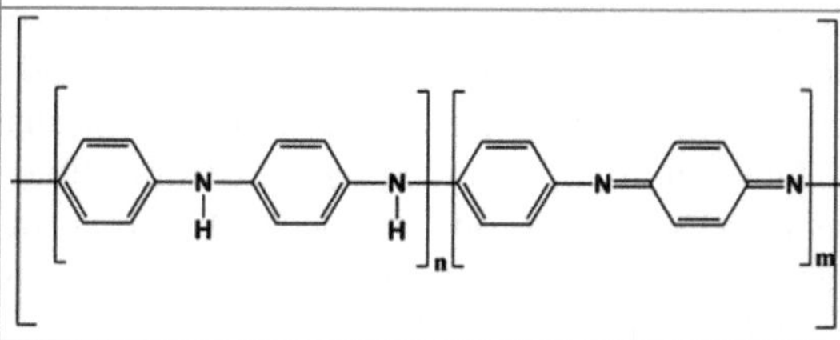

enzymatic reactions [49]. Detection of H_2O_2 is highly relevant in food and pharmaceutical industry. Chairam et al. [50] developed an enzyme based amperometric biosensor for the detection of H_2O_2. HRP was immobilized in the layer of conducting polymer poly(aniline-co-o-aminobenzoic acid) via electrostatic interactions. After mixing of the enzyme in the polymer, the mixture was simply cast onto a glassy carbon electrode. A layer of the biopolymer chitosan was then coated onto the HRP-p (Ani-co-o-Aba). This layer was used as a binder for the enzyme. This sensor showed a linear range from 10 to 1,000 μM with a detection limit of 1.8 μM. This novel and fast fabrication method showed excellent promising results for highly sensitive biosensors.

The biopolymer chitosan has also been used in combination with PANI films by Srivastava et al. [51]. They developed a modified PANI-gold electrode with immobilization of cholesterol oxidase on a chitosan matrix. First, nanocomposites of PANI and gold were prepared. After complete polymerisation, the nanocomposites were incorporated in chitosan. This mixture was then spin coated onto an indium tin oxide (ITO) glass. The success of the immobilization was assessed by cyclic voltammetry measurements that showed a lower current peak caused by the electrical hindrance of the immobilized enzyme. The biosensor was optimized for the detection of cholesterol. Cholesterol is oxidized by cholesterol oxidase which produces H_2O_2, that is oxidized producing electrons that are transferred to the electrodes via the redox mediator $Fe(CN)_6^{-3}$. The signal is a peak in current that increases with the cholesterol concentration. The biosensor was stable over the time and retained a 90 % cholesterol oxidase activity over two weeks.

Composites of gold and PANI on a glassy carbon electrode were also used by Xiang et al. [52] for the development of a glucose biosensor. They used a bienzymatic approach where glucose was oxidized thereby producing H_2O_2, which was reduced by cytochrome oxidase c, absorbed on the surface of the nanocomposites. This sensor enabled a direct electron transfer to the electrode material. The sensor has a detection limit of 0.01 mM.

A similar electrochemical based sensor was developed using nanocomposites of PANI, graphene and horse radish peroxidase on ITO glas [53]. This biosensor was able to measure very low concentration of anti-malaria drug in various pharmaceutical preparations and in different body fluids (urine, plasma and serum).

Similarly, nanocomposites of graphene and PANI were used by Ruecha et al. [54] to develop a paper based biosensor for the enzyme based detection of cholesterol and the electrochemical detection of the by-product H_2O_2 of the enzymatic reaction. Interestingly they incorporated polyvinylpyrrolidone in the modified electrode in order to improve the stabilization of the graphene concentration. Those biosensors based on composites of different materials often show a combination of the parameters of the materials and therefore offer a higher thermal stability, better conductivity and improved resistance to salts.

Tamer et al. [55] worked on the optimization of the fabrication of the composites PANI/gold nanorod for glucose detection. In this biosensor, the enzyme GOx was covalently bound to the electrode via the linker glutaraldehyde. This matrix offered a large surface to functionalize.

PANI has also been shown to be usable in combination with whole bacterial cells as bioelement. Anu Prathap et al. [56] developed a biosensor where recombinant *E. coli* bacteria were immobilized by adsorption into a PANI film. The bacteria had been previously transformed with the gene linA2, coding for an enzyme involved in the first step of the degradation of pesticide lindane. Using recombinant *E. coli* bacteria assured a higher robustness and better performances to the sensor compared to the wild type which has a slow degradation rate of lindane. The sensor was proved to be functional during two weeks if stored at 4 °C. It could detect lindane in the part per trillion concentrations. It was highly sensitive and selective since it could detect the three isomers of lindane but showed no response for two other common pesticides. The advantage of using a whole cell as bioelement is to overcome the lack of synthetic bioelement for certain targets and provide the sensor with a high specificity. The detection was based on the change of conductivity induced in the PANI film after production of HCl by the enzymatic reaction. Amperometric measurements were used to register the increase in current upon production of HCl.

PANI was also used in combination with carbon nanotubes to fabricate a sensor with cytochrome oxidase as bioelement [57]. This system could be used for different kinds of sensing events based on the enzymatic reduction of H_2O_2. The sensitivity of a biosensor based on a PANI film on a gold electrode was improved by using a composite of PANI with polypyrrole nanoparticles [58]. The sensor was used to detect glutamate in food products with an enzymatic reaction of the covalently bound glutamate oxidase.

Nanowires based biosensors offer a high sensitivity. Lee et al. [59] developed a biosensor based on a single PANI nanowire that was functionalized via the EDC and N-Hydroxysuccinimide (NHS) (EDC/NHS) chemistry with antibodies against immunoglobulin G (IgG) and Myo, two cardiac biomarkers. The nanowire was fabricated using the electrochemical growth method between two gold electrodes. The binding of either IgG or Myo was recorded by the increase of conductance of the wire. The PANI biosensor was highly selective and sensitive to its target with detection limits of 3 ng/mL for IgG and 1.4 ng/mL for Myo.

Polypyrrole

Polypyrrole (PPy) is a conducting polymer that has attracted high interest in the biosensor field. PPy forms a yellow film that that becomes darker upon polymerization. PPy is indeed biocompatible, enabling the CP for the application in the medical biosensor field and shows a high conductivity [42]. It is worth mentioning that PPy has recently found application in the drug delivery field [60]. The synthesis of PPy has been extensively studied and can be done chemically or by electropolymerization. The way that the synthesis is performed has a significant effect on the properties of the PPy film [42, 61]. High conductive polypyrrole can reach a conductivity of up to 200 S/cm. Doped PPy films are relatively stable in air. The degradation of polypyrrole films starts with the loss of dopants, followed by the degradation of the polymer backbone [62]. Polypyrrole films have been described as being planar chains along the direction of the film layer.

Xu et al. [63] recently presented a biosensor for thrombin sensing based on polypyrrole electrodes prepared by electropolymerization on platinum electrodes. They used pyrrole-nitrilotriacetic acid (pyrrole-NTA) monomers that were polymerized and complexed with Cu^{2+}. As bioelement, they immobilized a histidine labelled aptamer on the polypyrrole film through the histidine-NTA-Cu^{2+} interaction. The surface of this biosensor was shown to be non-adherent to proteins. The change of impedance was measured upon binding of the target to the aptamer. Thrombin was detected in the picomolar range (4.4×10^{-12} mol/L). Detection of the *E. coli* strain K12 was achieved by a DNA-based biosensor [64]. Short DNA sequences (25 base pairs) called hybridization probes were designed complementary to the sequence of the gene D-glucoronidase from *E. coli*. The DNA sequences were incorporated in the bulk of pyrrole that was electropolymerized onto a platinum electrode. The hybridization was measured by cyclic voltammetry with a clear difference between the amplitudes of the oxidation peaks resulting from the hybridization of a complementary sequence or from a non-complimentary sequence. The response of the biosensor could be obtained within 15–20 min which was much faster than any detection system involving culturing of the bacteria. Glucose biosensors have also been extensively investigated. They mainly use an enzyme-based system with GOx as bioelement and electrochemical detection. Olea et al. [65, 66] developed a new way to immobilize the enzyme GOx onto the biosensor surface. GOx was encapsulated in a multilamellar lipid vesicle before being incorporated into the polymer film. The comparison between free enzyme and encapsulated enzyme showed that the sensitivity was improved fivefold and that the stability of the biosensor was increased as well [67].

PEDOT

Poly(3,4-ethylenedioxythiophene) (PEDOT) is a conducting polymer developed as a derivative of polythiophene by Bayer AG in the late 1980s [68]. Even though developed later than other CP, it has rapidly gained a very high interest in the industry since it is very stable and can be processed in water. It has a high conductivity (400–1,000 S/cm [69]), while presenting a good light transmission. The synthesis is fast and can be done either by electropolymerization or chemical synthesis [70]. PEDOT is often doped with poly(styrene) sulfonate (PSS). Huang et al. [71] reported that doping PEDOT:PSS films with sorbitol and glycerol modified the morphology and thereby increased the conductivity. Iron tosylate is a smaller molecule, also used for doping PEDOT [72]. An important feature of PEDOT for biosensors and medical applications is that PEDOT is biocompatible and almost the only one which is stable in aqueous solution. PEDOT forms a light blue film in oxidized state that becomes dark blue in reduced state. PEDOT finds application in solar cells and in organic LED as well [73].

In the field of biosensors, PEDOT is mainly used to replace the metal microelectrodes.

The deposition of the CP thin film to the substrate is most commonly done by spin coating, dipping or spray coating [74] or by electropolymerization. The film can be patterned in several ways. The classical photolithography combined with dry etching requires cleanroom conditions. However micropatterns can be made outside of the cleanroom by soft lithography or by screen printing. Recently, Hansen et al. [75, 76] developed a novel patterning method of PEDOT through stamping of the film by an agarose stamp soaked in sodium hypochlorite. The stamp was patterned with the negative shape of the electrodes. The sodium hypochlorite over-oxidizes the PEDOT, which causes the loss of the conductivity, i.e. the CP is deactivated. The deactivated PEDOT can then easily be removed by rinsing the film with water.

The agarose patterning method was used to develop all-polymer biosensors based on different bioelements. Kiilerich-Pedersen et al. [77] established a biosensor that can detect viral infection within a few hours. This biosensor was based on an array of interdigitated electrodes made out of PEDOT doped with tosylate. Cells were cultivated on the surface of the sensor electrodes. After a few hours of incubation with viruses, the viral infection was registered by a decrease in impedance, even before any morphological change was seen in the cells. This is faster and requires less sample preparation compared to the traditional methods involving culture of the pathogens or detection of the pathogens genetic material by PCR.

The agarose stamping method was also used by Daprà et al. [78] for the fabrication of a biosensor for food safety. This biosensor was able to detect antibiotics (ampicillin and kanamycin) in the concentration range of respectively 100 pM and 1 μM and 10 nM to 1 nM, which are below the residual limits authorized in milk in the European Union. This sensor is highly flexible and the functionalization can be adapted to other pathogens. For example, Kiilerich-Pedersen et al. [79] used the sensor in order to detect influenza A viruses using aptamers as bioelements. The detection was carried out within only 15 min. This all-polymer biosensor has shown a great potential for POC devices in terms of easy production and usability, low cost and great flexibility. As shown by Rosati et al. [80], improvement of the design of the electrodes can improve the performances of this biosensor even further.

Residuals of phenolic compounds such as bisphenol A in water are of great concern for the health due to the highly toxic, carcinogenic and mutagenic nature of those compounds. Classical methods to detect phenol compounds are time-consuming and require a lot of preparation. Moczko et al. [81] developed a biosensor for fast amperometric detection of phenol compounds. A layer of PEDOT was screen printed on carbon electrodes. As bioelement the enzyme tyrosinase was entrapped in a screen printed biocompatible photopolymer as described by Andreescu et al. [82]. Tyrosinase was used to oxidize the phenol compounds thereby producing quinones that are electrochemically reduced. This biosensor allowed the rapid detection of phenolic compounds in water from the field. The use of PEDOT in this biosensor enabled an improved electrical conducting process with the electrodes showing a conductivity of $2{,}111 \pm 310$ S/cm.

PEDOT has also been used for glucose biosensors. Park et al. [83] created small containers where GOx was entrapped. The containers were closed by a layer of conductive PEDOT. Entrapping enzymes in microtubules was a new way to immobilize them and provided a higher conductivity.

Arter et al. [84] created an array of PEDOT nanowires. They incorporated the bacteriophage M13 into the PEDOT solution before polymerization. They tested the accessibility of the viruses by incubating the nanowires array with fluorescently labelled antibodies.

Molecularly Imprinted Polymers (MIP): An Alternative to Bioelement

Description and Synthesis of MIP

MIP have been developed by the pioneer groups of Günter Wulff [85] and Klaus Mosbach [86] in 1972 and in the 1980s. They have gained an increasingly large interest during the past years as it can be seen from the increase of publications related to this topic [87]. MIPs are synthetic polymer cavities with a shape, which is highly specific for a defined target by a high stereo-and regiospecificity [16]. MIPs are synthesized by mixing the target molecule or imprint with functional monomers. These pre-assembled complexes are mixed with cross-linking monomers that create a rigid polymer network. After polymerization, the imprint is removed leaving a cavity specific in shape and size for the imprint. The target molecule can then rebind to the MIP as shown in Fig. 17.3.

Two imprinting approaches can be distinguished: covalent and non-covalent [16]. In the covalent approach, the functional monomers covalently bind to the target. This offers a highly specific rebinding and more homogenous binding sites across the polymer network [17]. However, removal of the template is more complicated and the rebinding is slower [88]. In the non-covalent imprinting, the imprint and the functional monomers interact by electrostatic, ionic, or hydrophobic interaction or hydrogen bonding [16, 89]. Advantages of this non-covalent approach are the easy removal of the imprint from the MIPs by simply washing with appropriate solvents [90] and a faster rebinding of the target [85]. Moreover, the non-covalent interaction mimics better the interactions occurring in nature [17]. However, the risk of unspecific binding is higher [85].

The functional monomers have double functions. They undergo interactions with the target and have a point of interaction with the cross-linking polymer [86]. The choice of functional monomers depends on the affinity required between the functional monomers and the template. Commonly used functional monomers are acrylic and methacrylic polymers for interaction with amino groups, and vinylpyridine for interaction with carboxylic groups [86]. Commonly used cross linkers are ethyleneglycol dimethacrylate and dimethylbenzene [86]. Two other elements are also highly important for the preparation of the MIPs. First, the porogen, the

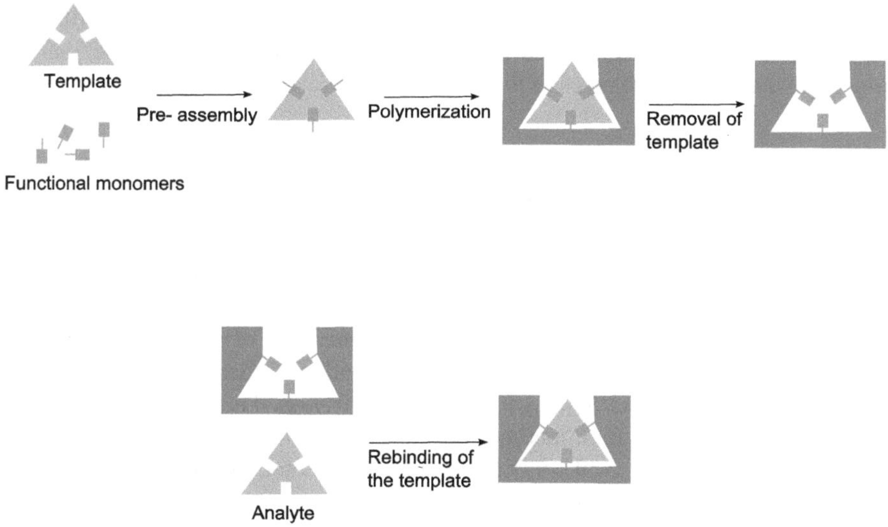

Fig. 17.3 The fabrication principle of molecularly imprinted polymers (MIP). The template and the functional monomers are pre-assembled through different kinds of interactions (covalent, hydrogen bonding, etc.). A polymer matrix is then polymerized around the pre-assembled complex. The template is removed. The analyte can then bind specifically to the MIP

solvent is responsible for the porosity in the material. Important is that the porogen does not interact with the functional monomers [86]. Typical porogens are DMF or DMSO [86]. Secondly, the polymerization initiator plays an important role. MIP are mostly synthesized by radical polymerization [17]. Polymerization can be initiated by irradiation with UV-light or by thermal induction [86]. The polymerization can be performed in situ by for example electropolymerization on the electrode of the biosensor. MIP can also be synthesized as a layer around silica beads.

MIPs have attracted a wide interest in sensing applications, but also in separation technology, as catalytically active polymers for mimics of enzymes [16] and in drug delivery [91]. In separation technology, MIP can be integrated in affinity chromatography columns. For biosensing applications, MIP can be used as alternative to the natural bioelements. They are more stable than antibodies [16] and suffer less from batch to batch variations. They can be made stable at extreme pH and temperatures [86]. Moreover, MIP can be developed against a wide range of targets, even against targets for which the development of antibodies is not easy [92], such as toxic targets or targets not inducing an immunogenic response. The development of MIPs against small targets is well established. However, developing MIPs against larger biomolecules such as DNA or proteins remains challenging [17]—among others—due to the entrapment of the target protein in the polymer matrix [93]. The MIP based sensor can be developed with different configurations [17]. Binding of the target to the MIP can induce a change in the sensor (e.g. electrical properties) that is then registered. The sensor can also be built based on competitive binding. In this configuration, the analyte has to compete for the MIP cavities with a fluorescently labelled reference analyte or has to displace already bound labelled reference analytes. A third possibility could be that the binding event induces changes in the polymer itself (e.g. optical changes) [17].

MIP and Electrochemical Biosensors

As previously described, electrochemical sensors are excellent biosensors. They are relatively inexpensive and less labour intensive than sensors based on other transducers. MIPs are excellent bioelements for this type of sensor. The advances of the technology have permitted the direct integration of these bioelements on the transducer surface for example by electropolymerization. This allows a very reproducible and rapid fabrication method for the sensors. The reader is also referred to the review of Malitesta et al. [94] about the new methods for electrosynthesis of MIPs and their integration on sensors.

Zeng et al. [95] fabricated MIPs in the conducting polymer PANI against the amino acid glycine, one of the major neurotransmitters. The MIPs were prepared by electrodeposition on carbon fiber electrodes. As control, they prepared so-called "Non Imprinted Polymers (NIP)" that were synthesized exactly like the MIPs but without the imprint L-glycine. The binding event was recorded by amperometric measurements. A significantly higher response was achieved with the MIPs compared to the NIPs, which made the authors conclude that specific L-glycine MIPs had been created during the synthesis.

Combining CP with MIPs is a very smart way to combine the biorecognition element within the transducer itself. Recently, Wen et al. [96] also developed a MIP based sensor using PANI. The so-called "molecularly imprinted electrochemical sensor (MIES)" was developed to detect creatinine, a widely used biomarker for—among others—muscular dystrophy. Creatinine and the functional monomer aniline were first preassembled around Fe_3O_4@PANI nanoparticles. The MIPs were deposited on a glassy carbon electrode using a magnetic field. A short electrodeposition step ordered the MIP on the surface. To remove the template, a negative potential was applied for 3 min. Binding was as well registered by amperometric measurements. The sensor showed a very high specificity for creatinine since no change in the signal was recorded when other compounds from blood plasma or urine were added. The long-term stability was tested over a month, after which the sensor had lost only 10 % of its response.

Similarly, Xue et al. [97] developed a dopamine MIES. The MIPs were directly synthesized around gold nanoparticles. They were electrodeposited on the surface of a gold electrode, interfaced with a layer of gold nanoparticles. The introduction of gold particles in MIP gave a higher conductivity of the sensor. The MIES was shown not to react to ascorbic acid and uric acid, two compounds that often interfere in dopamine samples. Khadro et al. [98] also described the development of a biosensor for creatinine as well as urea. The MIP were synthesized on a gold electrode. Electrochemical impedance spectroscopy (EIS) measurements were performed to detect the binding.

EIS was also used by Peeters et al. [99] to quantify the concentration of serotonin in blood plasma. MIP were prepared using a mixture of methacrylic acid and acrylamide as functional monomers. The polymerization with ethylene glycol dimethacrylate was conducted in a UV-oven during 12 h. MIP particles of 25 μm were synthesized with this method. The template molecules of serotonin were removed by extraction with solvents. The MIPs were placed on the electrode using an adhesive polymer. The flow cell for serotonin measurement had two channels in order to measure the response on the MIP (active channel) and on the NIP (reference channel) simultaneously. One main advantage of this sensor is that serotonin can be measured in blood plasma directly.

Duan et al. [100] developed an electrochemical sensor against the antioxidant substance epigallocatechin-3-gallate (EGCG) present in tea. They used poly(*o*-phenylenediamine) as functional monomer to create the MIP film by electropolymerization over the glassy carbon electrode. The imprint molecules were removed by washing the film with a combination of the methanol and acetic acid (90:10 v/v). Substances analogous to EGCG gave a significantly lower response than EGCG itself showing the high selectivity of the sensor. A response could be obtained with this sensor within 11 min, which makes the sensor highly appropriate for industrial use.

Yarman and Scheller [101] used an o-phenylenediamine-resorcinol mixture to create MIP against tamoxifen, a nonsteroidal anti-estrogen used in breast cancer therapy but considered as a doping substance. The MIP were electropolymerized on a glassy carbon electrode. Cyclic voltammetry and amperometric measurements were used to study the rebinding of tamoxifen. The authors showed the great selectivity of the sensor that gave a 2.3 times lower response to 4-hydroxy-tamoxifen, an intermediate of tamoxifen. However, this work suggested the incorporation of enzymes in order to decrease the interferences with other substances as well as decrease fouling of electrode surface.

MIP and Optical Biosensors

Quantum dots have excellent opto-electronic properties. Wang et al. [102] used them to develop a photoelectrochemical sensor. MIP were fabricated around the quantum dots CdTe QD using acrylamide as functional monomers and ethylene-glycol dimethacrylate as cross linker. Those MIPs@CdTe QD were dropped on the on paper screen-printed carbon working electrode where gold nanoparticles had been previously electrodeposited. The target was incubated on the sensor for one hour. After washing, the sensor was illuminated with UV light and the current intensity was registered in the presence of ascorbic acid solution. The gold nanoparticles allowed an improved electron transfer of the photocurrent. This photoelectrochemical sensor could measure the pesticide S-fenvalerate at the low concentration of 3.5×10^{-9} mol L^{-1}. This work showed a way to fabricate highly sensitive and reproducible sensors that has a great potential for application in the biomedical field as well. Surface plasmon resonance (SPR) is a technique by which changes happening on the surface (for example binding of an analyte) can be registered. MIPs are also well-appropriated elements for capture of the analyte for SPR measurements.

Cennamo et al. [103] developed a SPR based sensor with a MIP layer of about 150 nm. This sensor was able to specifically recognize L-nicotine and not D-nicotine at a low concentration relevant for samples in the field. Other examples of MIP based SPR sensors are the sensor by Verma and Gupta [104] detecting the antibiotics tetracycline and their vitamin B3 sensor [105] for which the MIPs were prepared in hydrogel. Lotierzo et al. [106] developed an SPR based sensor for domoic acid, a neurotoxin. They compared their sensor with a sensor based on monoclonal antibodies and found that the MIP based sensor could be regenerated without losing its functionality and had a three times lower detection limit compared to the immunosensor.

Zhou et al. [107] improved an immunosensor by using MIP instead of the primary antibody for the detection of hemoglobin. The MIP were prepared around magnetic beads ($Fe_3O_4@SiO_2$) using 3-aminobenzeneboronic acid as functional and cross linking monomer. The polymerization was initiated with ammonium persulfate at room temperature. After 14 h of incubation, the template was removed by elution in 1 % sodium dodecyl sulfate (SDS). For analytical purposes, the magnetic MIPs were incubated with the hemoglobin sample. This step allowed for the enrichment of hemoglobin in very low concentrated samples. Then, a detection antibody conjugated with $Ru@SiO_2$ was added. Those immunocomplexes were captured by a magnet. The tag on the detection antibody allowed the electrochemiluminescence detection of hemoglobin. Using MIP instead of antibodies, the sensor was more stable and less expensive to produce than with primary antibodies.

The optimization of the fabrication of MIPs is required for each application. Rahiminezhad et al. [108] propose to use a chemometric approach to find the optimal parameters to prepare MIPs against diazinon. A central composite design was developed for this approach with five essential factors that were the different amount of template, solvent, initiator, the ratio between the functional monomers and the cross linker as well as the polymerization temperature. With this approach, they could optimize the synthesis of MIPs. Constantly new fabrication methods are developed as the one proposed by Dechtrirat et al. [109]. Further development in the synthesis of MIP is expected to increase the use of MIP in biosensors.

Through the examples presented above, MIPs appear to be very promising novel bioelements. They are more stable and more reproducible than natural antibodies. They can be used in combination with various transducers (electrochemical, optical, immunosensors, etc.). The synthesis can be set up so that the MIPs are directly synthesized on the transducer. A large diversity of functional monomers and cross-linking polymers as well as synthesis methods is available. An easy fabrication and characterization of the MIP could give them the potential to be widely used in an industrial fabrication of the sensors.

Outlook

In recent years, major advances have been achieved in the biosensor field. The configuration possibilities have been extended. More and more bioelements have been developed, increasing the affinity to the target and therefore the selectivity of the sensors. Progresses in the technology allowed that transducers became more and more sensitive and precise. The biosensor field has gained a lot from the multidisciplinary approach. Combined efforts in biology, chemistry and physics have been the key to incredible biosensors able to detect analytes in complex environments such as blood plasma or urine. If the detection is possible directly in body fluids, and no further sample preparation or purification is required, the analysis is much faster and errors can be minimized. Moreover, this would mean that the analysis could be made outside specialized laboratories, by the general practitioner or even the patient himself.

Future direction and development in the biosensor field will be towards **non-invasive monitoring** of patients and towards **implantable biosensors** [1], as well as sensors that could be integrated into smart textiles [110]. This would be more comfortable both for the patients but also for the clinicians. Those sensors would allow a more regular and precise monitoring of the patient, whose therapy could be adapted going towards a personalized medicine. But once again, this can only be achieved in an interdisciplinary work. Polymers are highly appropriated materials in this field. It can be concluded that biosensors based on polymers have a great potential in the biomedical field and decisive advances can be expected in the next years.

References

1. Turner, A.: Biosensors: then and now. Trends Biotechnol. **31**(3), 119–120 (2013)
2. Clark, L.C., Lyons, C.: Electrode systems for continuous monitoring in cardiovascular surgery. Ann. N. Y. Acad. Sci. **102**, 29–45 (1962)
3. Turner, A.P.F.: Biosensors: sense and sensibility. Chem. Soc. Rev. **42**(8), 3184–3196 (2013)
4. McNaught, A.D., Wilkinson, A.: IUPAC Compendium of Chemical Terminology, 2nd edn. Blackwell Scientific Publications, Oxford (1997)
5. Chambers, J.P., et al.: Biosensor recognition elements. Current Issues Mole. Biol. **10**(1–2), 1–12 (2008)
6. Bhalerao, K., Nistala, G.: Biomolecular Components of a Biosensor. Series on Biomedical Nanotechnology, pp. 1–20. Pan Stanford Publishing, Singapore (2012)
7. Daniels, J.S., Pourmand, N.: Label-free impedance biosensors: opportunities and challenges. Electroanalysis **19**(12), 1239–1257 (2007)
8. Sharma, A., Rogers, K.R.: Biosensors. Meas. Sci. Technol. **5**(5), 461–472 (1994)
9. Wang, J.: Electrochemical glucose biosensors. Chem. Rev. **108**(2), 814–825 (2008)
10. Song, K.-M., Lee, S., Ban, C.: Aptamers and their biological applications. Sensors **12**(1), 612–631 (2012)
11. Jayasena, S.D.: Aptamers: an emerging class of molecules that rival antibodies in diagnostics. Clin. Chem. **45**(9), 1628–1650 (1999)
12. Hamula, C., et al.: Selection and analytical applications of aptamers. TrAC Trends Anal. Chem. **25**(7), 681–691 (2006)

13. Song, S., et al.: Aptamer-based biosensors. TrAC Trends Anal. Chem. **27**(2), 108–117 (2008)
14. Bini, A., et al.: Analytical performances of aptamer-based sensing for thrombin detection. Anal. Chem. **79**(7), 3016–3019 (2007)
15. Xiao, Y., et al.: Label-free electronic detection of thrombin in blood serum by using an aptamer-based sensor. Angew. Chem. Int. Ed. Engl. **44**(34), 5456–5459 (2005)
16. Mosbach, K.: Molecular imprinting. Trends Biochem. Sci. **19**(1), 9–14 (1994)
17. Haupt, K., Mosbach, K.: Molecularly imprinted polymers and their use in biomimetic sensors. Chem. Rev. **100**(7), 2495–2504 (2000)
18. Feng, X., et al.: A living cell-based biosensor utilizing G-protein coupled receptors: principles and detection methods. Biosens. Bioelectron. **22**(12), 3230–3237 (2007)
19. Nascimento, G.A., et al.: Electrochemical DNA biosensor for bovine papillomavirus detection using polymeric film on screen-printed electrode. Biosens. Bioelectron. **38**(1), 61–66 (2012)
20. Hopkins, N.E.: Antibody engineering for biosensor applications. In: Zourob, M. (ed.) Recognition Receptors in Biosensors SE-12 pp. 451–529. Springer, New York (2010). doi:10.1007/978-1-4419-0919-0_12
21. Dugas, V., Elaissari, A., Chevalier, Y.: Surface sensitization techniques and recognition receptors immobilization on biosensors and microarrays. In: Zourob, M. (ed.) Recognition Receptors in Biosensors SE-2 pp. 47–134. Springer, New York (2010). doi:10.1007/978-1-4419-0919-0_2
22. Hermanson, G.T.: Zero-length crosslinkers. In: Hermanson, G.T. (ed.) Bioconjug. Tech. pp. 259–273. Academic Press, Boston (2013)
23. Spichiger-Keller, U.E.: Chemical and Biochemical Sensors. In Spichiger-Keller U.E. (ed.) Chemical Sensors and Biosensors for Medical and Biological Applications, pp. 33–81. Wiley-VCH Verlag GmbH, German (1998). doi:10.1002/9783527612284.ch2
24. Liu, G.-Y., et al.: Colorimetric detection of carbenicillin using cationic polythiophene derivatives. Chin. J. Polym. Sci. **31**(11), 1484–1490 (2013)
25. Pohanka, M., Skládal, P.: Electrochemical biosensors—principles and applications. J. Appl. Biomed. **6**(2), 57–64 (2008)
26. Grieshaber, D., et al.: Electrochemical biosensors—sensor principles and architectures. Sensors **8**(3), 1400–1458 (2008)
27. Bakker, E., Pretsch, E.: Potentiometric sensors for trace-level analysis. Trends Anal. Chem. TRAC **24**(3), 199–207 (2005)
28. Janata, J.: Principles of Chemical Sensors. Springer, USA (2009)
29. Lisdat, F., Schäfer, D.: The use of electrochemical impedance spectroscopy for biosensing. Anal. Bioanal. Chem. **391**(5), 1555–1567 (2008)
30. Datar, R., et al.: Cantilever sensors: nanomechanical tools for diagnostics. MRS Bull. **34**(06), 449–454 (2009)
31. Lang, H., Hegner, M., Gerber, C.: Cantilever array sensors. Mater. Today **8**(4), 30–36 (2005)
32. Hierlemann, A., et al.: Microfabrication techniques for chemical/biosensors. Proc. IEEE **91**(6), 839–863 (2003)
33. Tsao, C.-W., DeVoe, D.: Bonding of thermoplastic polymer microfluidics. Microfluid. Nanofluid. **6**(1), 1–16 (2009)
34. Wynne, K.J., Street, G.B.: Conducting polymers. A short review. Ind. Eng. Chem. Prod. Res. Dev. **21**(1), 23–28 (1982)
35. Gerard, M.: Application of conducting polymers to biosensors. Biosens. Bioelectron. **17**(5), 345–359 (2002)
36. Hush, N.S.: An overview of the first half-century of molecular electronics. Ann. N. Y. Acad. Sci. **1006**(1), 1–20 (2003)
37. Malhotra, B.D., Chaubey, A., Singh, S.P.: Prospects of conducting polymers in biosensors. Anal. Chim. Acta **578**(1), 59–74 (2006)
38. Ates, M.: A review study of (bio)sensor systems based on conducting polymers. Mater. Sci. Eng. C: Mater. Biol. Appl. **33**(4), 1853–1859 (2013)
39. Dzugan, T.: Electrical properties of PEDOT. Electron Technol 2009 ISSE 2009 32ND Int SPRING Semin Electron Technol, pp. 101–104 (2009). doi:10.1109/ISSE.2009.5207058

40. Dai, L.: Conducting Polymers. Engineering Materials and Processes, pp. 41–80. Springer, London (2004)
41. Kivelson, S., Heeger, A.J.: Theory of the soliton-lattice to polaron-lattice transition in conducting polymers. Synth. Met. **17**(1–3), 183–188 (1987)
42. Kivelson, S., Heeger, A.J.: Intrinsic conductivity of conducting polymers. Synth. Met. **22**(4), 371–384 (1988)
43. Shirakawa, H., et al.: Synthesis of electrically conducting organic polymers: halogen derivatives of polyacetylene, (CH). J. Chem. Soc. Chem. Commun. **16**, 578–580 (1977)
44. Chiang, C.K., et al.: Synthesis of highly conducting films of derivatives of polyacetylene, (CH)x. J. Am. Chem. Soc. **100**(3), 1013–1015 (1978)
45. Vernitskaya, T.V., Efimov, O.N.: Polypyrrole: a conducting polymer; its synthesis, properties and applications. Russ. Chem. Rev. **66**(5), 443–457 (1997)
46. Ćirić-Marjanović, G.: Recent advances in polyaniline research: Polymerization mechanisms, structural aspects, properties and applications. Synth. Met. **177**, 1–47 (2013)
47. Lee, K., et al.: Metallic transport in polyaniline. Nature **441**(7089), 65–68 (2006)
48. Dhand, C., et al.: Recent advances in polyaniline based biosensors. Biosens. Bioelectron. **26**(6), 2811–2821 (2011)
49. Giannoudi, L., Piletska, E.V., Piletsky, S.A.: Development of biosensors for the detection of hydrogen peroxide.In: Giardi, M.T., Piletska E.V. (eds.) Biotechnological Applications of Photosynthetic Proteins: Biochips, Biosensors and Biodevices, pp. 175–191. Springer, New York (2006)
50. Chairam, S., Buddhalee, P., Amatatongchai, M.: A novel hydrogen peroxide biosensor based on horseradish peroxidase immobilized on poly(aniline-co-o-aminobenzoic acid) modified glassy carbon electrode coated with chitosan film. Int. J. Electrochem. Sci. **8**(8), 10250–10264 (2013)
51. Srivastava, M., et al.: A chitosan-based polyaniline-Au nanocomposite biosensor for determination of cholesterol. Anal. Methods **6**(3), 817–824 (2014)
52. Xiang, C., et al.: Bienzymatic glucose biosensor based on direct electrochemistry of cytochrome c on gold nanoparticles/polyaniline nanospheres composite. Talanta **110**, 96–100 (2013)
53. Radhapyari, K., et al.: Graphene-polyaniline nanocomposite based biosensor for detection of antimalarial drug artesunate in pharmaceutical formulation and biological fluids. Talanta **111**, 47–53 (2013)
54. Ruecha, N., et al.: Novel paper-based cholesterol biosensor using graphene/polyvinylpyrrolidone/polyaniline nanocomposite. Biosens. Bioelectron. **52**, 13–19 (2014)
55. Tamer U., et al. Fabrication of biosensor based on polyaniline/gold nanorod composite. Int. J. Electrochem. (2011)
56. Anu Prathap, M.U., et al.: Polyaniline-based highly sensitive microbial biosensor for selective detection of lindane. Anal. Chem. **84**(15), 6672–6678 (2012)
57. Batra, B., et al.: Fabrication of a cytochrome c biosensor based on cytochrome oxidase/NiO-NPs/cMWCNT/PANI modified Au electrode. J. Biomed. Nanotechnol. **9**(3), 409–416 (2013)
58. Batra, B., Kumari, S., Pundir, C.S.: Construction of glutamate biosensor based on covalent immobilization of glutamate oxidase on polypyrrole nanoparticles/polyaniline modified gold electrode. Enzym. Microbial Technol. **57**, 69–77 (2014)
59. Lee, I., et al.: Highly sensitive single polyaniline nanowire biosensor for the detection of immunoglobulin G and myoglobin. Biosens. Bioelectron. **26**(7), 3297–3302 (2011)
60. Geetha, S., et al.: Biosensing and drug delivery by polypyrrole. Anal. Chim. Acta **568**(1–2), 119–125 (2006)
61. Kang, H.C., Geckeler, K.E.: Enhanced electrical conductivity of polypyrrole prepared by chemical oxidative polymerization: effect of the preparation technique and polymer additive. Polymer **41**(18), 6931–6934 (2000)
62. Mohammad, F., Calvert, P.D., Billingham, N.C.: Thermal stability of electrochemically prepared polythiophene and polypyrrole. Bull. Mater. Sci. **18**(3), 255–261 (1995)

63. Xu, H., et al.: Label-free impedimetric thrombin sensor based on poly (pyrrole–nitrilotri-acetic acid)–aptamer film. Biosens. Bioelectron. **41**, 90–95 (2013)
64. Rodriguez, M.I., Alocilja, E.C.: Embedded DNA-polypyrrole biosensor for rapid detection of Escherichia Coli. IEEE Sens. J. **5**(4), 733–736 (2005)
65. Olea, D., Moreau, P., Faure, C.: Polypyrrole-glucose oxidase biosensor. Effect of enzyme encapsulation in multilamellar vesicles on film growth and morphology. J. Electroanal. Chem. **605**(2), 125–135 (2007)
66. Olea, D., Moreau, P., Faure, C.: Polypyrroleâ€ glucose oxidase biosensor. Effect of enzyme encapsulation in multilamellar vesicles on film growth and morphology. J. Electroanal. Chem. **605**(2), 125–135 (2007)
67. Olea, D., Viratelle, O., Faure, C.: Polypyrrole-glucose oxidase biosensor. Effect of enzyme encapsulation in multilamellar vesicles on analytical properties. Biosens. Bioelectron. **23**(6), 788–94 (2008)
68. Elschner, A., et al.: The Discovery and Development of Conducting Polymers, pp. 1–20. CRC Press, Boca Raton (2010)
69. Rozlosnik, N.: New directions in medical biosensors employing poly (3,4-ethylenedioxy thiophene) derivative-based electrodes. Anal. Bioanal. Chem. **395**(3), 637–645 (2009)
70. Corradi, R., Armes, S.P., Sciences, M.: Chemical synthesis of poly(3,4-ethylenedioxythiophene). Synth. Met. **84**(1), 453–454 (1997)
71. Huang, J., et al.: Investigation of the effects of doping and post-deposition treatments on the conductivity, morphology, and work function of poly(3,4-ethylenedioxythiophene)/ poly(styrene sulfonate) films. Adv. Funct. Mater. **15**(2), 290–296 (2005)
72. Elschner, A., et al.: The in situ polymerization of EDOT to PEDOT. PEDOT, pp. 91–111. CRC Press, Boca Raton (2010)
73. Reuter, K., Kirchmeyer, S., Elschner, A.: PEDOT–Properties and Technical Relevance, Handb. Thiophene-Based Mater. pp. 549–576. Wiley, Hoboken (2009)
74. Charlot, B., et al.: Micropatterning PEDOT:PSS layers. Microsyst. Technol. **19**(6), 895–903 (2012)
75. Hansen, T.S., et al.: Highly stretchable and conductive polymer material made from poly(3,4-ethylenedioxythiophene) and polyurethane elastomers. Adv. Funct. Mater. **17**(16), 3069–3073 (2007)
76. Hansen, T.S., et al.: Direct fast patterning of conductive polymers using agarose stamping. Adv. Mater. **19**(20), 3261–3265 (2007)
77. Kiilerich-Pedersen, K., et al.: Polymer based biosensor for rapid electrochemical detection of virus infection of human cells. Biosens. Bioelectron. **28**(1), 386–392 (2011)
78. Daprà, J., et al.: Comparative study on aptamers as recognition elements for antibiotics in a label-free all-polymer biosensor. Biosens. Bioelectron. **43**, 315–320 (2013)
79. Kiilerich-Pedersen, K., et al.: High sensitivity point-of-care device for direct virus diagnostics. Biosens. Bioelectron. **49**, 374–379 (2013)
80. Rosati, G., et al.: Performance improvement by layout designs of conductive polymer microelectrode based impedimetric biosensors. Electroanalysis **26**(6), 1400–1408 (2014)
81. Moczko, E., et al.: Biosensor employing screen-printed PEDOT:PSS for sensitive detection of phenolic compounds in water. J. Polym. Sci., Part A: Polym. Chem. **50**(11), 2286–2292 (2012)
82. Andreescu, S., Barthelmebs, L., Marty, J.-L.: Immobilization of acetylcholinesterase on screen-printed electrodes: comparative study between three immobilization methods and applications to the detection of organophosphorus insecticides. Anal. Chim. Acta **464**(2), 171–180 (2002)
83. Park, J., Kim, H.K., Son, Y.: Glucose biosensor constructed from capped conducting microtubules of PEDOT. Sens. Actuators B Chem. **133**(1), 244–250 (2008)
84. Arter, J.A., et al.: Virus-PEDOT nanowires for biosensing. Nano Lett. **10**(12), 4858–4862 (2010)
85. Wulff, G., Sarhan, A.: Über die Anwendung von enzymanalog gebauten Polymeren zur Racemattrennung. Angew. Chem. **84**(8), 364–364 (1972)
86. Arshady, R., Mosbach, K.: Synthesis of substrate-selective polymers by host-guest polymerization. Die Makromol. Chem. **182**(2), 687–692 (1981)
87. Dickert, F.: Molecular imprinting. Anal. Bioanal. Chem. **389**(2), 353–354 (2007)
88. Peng, Y., Britt D, Walsh M, Doyle T.: Macromolecule-Imprinted polymers. In: Irudayaraj, J. (ed.) Series on Biomedical Nanosensors, pp. 21–58. Pan Stanford Publishing, Singapore (2012)

89. Brüggemann, O.: Molecularly imprinted polymers: a new dimension in analytical bioseparation. In: Freitag, R. (ed.) Synthetic Polymers for Biotechnology and Medicine, pp. 134–161. Eurekah/Landes Bioscience, Georgetown (2003)
90. Puoci, F., et al.: Molecularly Imprinted Polymers (MIPs) in biomedical applications. Biopolymers **28**, 548–574 (2010)
91. Puoci, F., et al.: Molecularly imprinted polymers in drug delivery: state of art and future perspectives. Expert Opin. Drug Deliv. **8**(10), 1379–1393 (2011)
92. Yano, K.: Molecularly imprinted polymers for biosensor applications. TrAC Trends Anal. Chem. **18**(3), 199–204 (1999)
93. Spivak, D.A.: MIPS in biotechnology, perspective and reality. In: Piletsky, S.A., Turner, A. (eds.) Molecular Imprinting of Polymers, pp. 1–9. Eurekah/Landes Bioscience, Georgetown (2006)
94. Malitesta, C., et al.: MIP sensors–the electrochemical approach. Anal. Bioanal. Chem. **402**(5), 1827–1846 (2012)
95. Zeng, H., Wang, D., Yu, J.: A molecule-imprinted polyaniline membrane modified on carbon fiber for detection of glycine. Bio-Med. Mater. Eng. **24**(1), 1085–1091 (2014)
96. Wen, T., et al.: Novel electrochemical sensing platform based on magnetic field-induced self-assembly of Fe3O4@Polyaniline nanoparticles for clinical detection of creatinine. Biosens. Bioelectron. **56C**, 180–185 (2014)
97. Xue, C., et al.: Amperometric detection of dopamine in human serumby electrochemical sensor based on gold nanoparticles doped molecularly imprinted polymers. Biosens. Bioelectron. **49**, 199–203 (2013)
98. Khadro, B., et al.: Molecularly imprinted polymers (MIP) based electrochemical sensor for detection of urea and creatinine. Procedia Eng. **5**, 371–374 (2010)
99. Peeters M, Troost FJ, van Grinsven B, et al: MIP-based biomimetic sensor for the electronic detection of serotonin in human blood plasma. Sens. Actuators B Chem. **171–172**, 602–610 (2012). doi:10.1016/j.snb.2012.05.040
100. Duan, Y., et al.: Determination of epigallocatechin-3-gallate with a high-efficiency electrochemical sensor based on a molecularly imprinted poly(o -phenylenediamine) film. J. Appl. Polym. Sci. **129**(5), 2882–2890 (2013)
101. Yarman, A., Scheller, F.W.: The first electrochemical MIP sensor for tamoxifen. Sensors **14**(5), 7647–7654 (2014)
102. Wang, Y., et al.: A novel microfluidic origami photoelectrochemical sensor based on CdTe quantum dots modified molecularly imprinted polymer and its highly selective detection of S-fenvalerate. Electrochim. Acta **107**, 147–154 (2013)
103. Cennamo, N., et al.: High selectivity and sensitivity sensor based on MIP and SPR in tapered plastic optical fibers for the detection of l-nicotine. Sens. Actuators B: Chem. **191**, 529–536 (2014)
104. Verma, R., Gupta, B.D.: Optical fiber sensor for the detection of tetracycline using surface plasmon resonance and molecular imprinting. Analyst **138**(23), 7254–7263 (2013)
105. Verma, R., Gupta, B.D.: Fiber optic SPR sensor for the detection of 3-pyridinecarboxamide (vitamin B3) using molecularly imprinted hydrogel. Sens. Actuators B Chem. **177**, 279–285 (2013)
106. Lotierzo, M., et al.: Surface plasmon resonance sensor for domoic acid based on grafted imprinted polymer. Biosens. Bioelectron. **20**(2), 145–152 (2004)
107. Zhou, J., et al.: A single antibody sandwich electrochemiluminescence immunosensor based on protein magnetic molecularly imprinted polymers mimicking capture probes. Sens. Actuators B Chem **186**, 300–307 (2013)
108. Rahiminezhad, M., et al.: Application of response surface methodology to synthesize appropriate molecularly imprinted polymer for diazinon. Key Eng. Mater. **605**(605), 67–70 (2014)
109. Dechtrirat, D., et al.: Hybrid material for protein sensing based on electrosynthesized mip on a mannose terminated self-assembled monolayer. Adv. Funct. Mater. **24**(15), 2233–2239 (2014)
110. Affatato, L.: Smart textiles: a strategic perspective of textile industry. Adv. Sci. Technol. **80**, 1–6 (2013)

MIX
Papier aus verantwortungsvollen Quellen
Paper from responsible sources
FSC® C105338

If you have any concerns about our products,
you can contact us on
ProductSafety@springernature.com

In case Publisher is established outside the EU,
the EU authorized representative is:
Springer Nature Customer Service Center GmbH
Europaplatz 3, 69115 Heidelberg, Germany

Printed by Libri Plureos GmbH
in Hamburg, Germany